Moreton Morrell Site

WITHDRAWN

WITHDRAWN

KT-556-318

2

00079086

Introduction to Kinesiology

Studying Physical Activity

Shirl J. Hoffman, EdD

The University of North Carolina at Greensboro

Janet C. Harris, PhD

California State University, Los Angeles

Editors

WARWICKSHIRE COLLEGE
LIBRARY
ROYAL LEAMINGTON SPA & MORETON MORRELL
WARWICK NEW ROAD, LEAMINGTON SPA CV32 5JE
Tel: Leamington Spa 318070

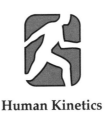

Human Kinetics

Library of Congress Cataloging-in-Publication Data

Introduction to kinesiology : studying physical activity / Shirl J. Hoffman, Janet C. Harris, editors.
      p. cm.
    Includes bibliographical references and index.
    ISBN 0-87322-676-3
     1. Kinesiology.   I. Hoffman, Shirl J., 1939-   II. Harris, Janet C.

    QP303 .I53 2000
    612.7'6--dc21

99-057432

ISBN: 0-87322-676-3 √

Copyright © 2000 by Human Kinetics Publishers, Inc.

All rights reserved. Except for use in a review, the reproduction or utilization of this work in any form or by any electronic, mechanical, or other means, now known or hereafter invented, including xerography, photocopying, and recording, and in any information storage and retrieval system, is forbidden without the written permission of the publisher.

Page 35: Children's Games (Kinderspiele), 1560 (panel) by Pieter the Elder Brueghel (c. 1515-69)
Kunsthistorisches Museum, Vienna, Austria/Bridgeman Art Library

Page 36: Children's Games (Kinderspiele): detail of bottom section showing various games, 1560 (oil on panel) by Pieter the Elder Brueghel (c. 1515-69)
Kunsthistorisches Museum, Vienna, Austria/Bridgeman Art Library
Ali Meyer / Bridgeman Art Library

Figures 1.4 and 1.5 reprinted, by permission, from National Strength and Conditioning Association, 2000, *Essentials of Strength and Conditioning*, 2d ed. (Champaign, IL: Human Kinetics). Figures 1.6 and 1.9, and photo on page 389 reprinted, by permission, from J.H. Wilmore and D.L. Costill, 1999, *Physiology of sport and exercise*, 2d ed. (Champaign, IL: Human Kinetics), 6, 64, 238. Photos of Gerald Kenyon, Franklin Henry, and Lawrence Rarick, reprinted, by permission, from J.D. Massengale and R.A. Swanson, Eds., 1997, *The history of exercise and sport science* (Champaign, IL: Human Kinetics). Photos on pages 438, 463, 469, 490, 492, 511, 517, 519, 536, 538, and 550 courtesy of the authors. Photo of Jeremy Howell © 1992 Triad Photography Group. Other credits appear with figure, table, or photo.

Developmental Editor: Christine M. Drews
Assistant Editor and Writing Consultant: John Wentworth
Assistant Editors: Melissa Feld and Sandra Merz Bott
Copyeditor: Patsy Fortney
Proofreaders: Pamela S. Johnson and Sarah Wiseman
Indexer: Patsy Fortney
Permission Manager: Heather Munson
Graphic Designer: Robert Reuther
Graphic Artist: Judy Henderson
Photo Editor: Clark Brooks
Cover Designer: Jack W. Davis
Photographer (cover): PhotoDisc Inc.
Art Manager: Craig Newsom
Illustrator: Matthew Hutton, except figures 1.4 and 1.5 by Mic Greenberg, figure 1.6 by Chuck Nivens, and figure 1.9 by Kristin Mount
Printer: United Graphics
Printed in the United States of America   10 9 8 7 6 5 4 3 2 1

WARWICKSHIRE COLLEGE
LIBRARY
Cl
612.76 HOF
Acc No:
00079086

Human Kinetics

Web site: http://www.humankinetics.com/

United States: Human Kinetics
P.O. Box 5076
Champaign, IL 61825-5076
1-800-747-4457
e-mail: humank@hkusa.com

Canada: Human Kinetics
475 Devonshire Road Unit 100
Windsor, ON N8Y 2L5
1-800-465-7301 (in Canada only)
e-mail: humank@hkcanada.com

Europe: Human Kinetics, P.O. Box IW14
Leeds LS16 6TR, United Kingdom
+44 (0)113-278 1708
e-mail: humank@hkeurope.com

Australia: Human Kinetics
57A Price Avenue
Lower Mitcham, South Australia 5062
(08) 82771555
e-mail: liahka@senet.com.au

New Zealand: Human Kinetics
P.O. Box 105-231, Auckland Central
09-523-3462
e-mail: humank@hknewz.com

To Claude Mourot Hoffman

Shirl J. Hoffman

To the many people who have inspired my lifelong learning

Janet C. Harris

Contents

Foreword

I want to tell you the story of the birth of *Introduction to Kinesiology*. Like most births, it came into being with considerable pain but also with great joy and satisfaction. I've helped bring nearly a thousand new books into existence at Human Kinetics, but this has been, unequivocally, the most challenging of them all.

The discipline of kinesiology—the science that studies physical activity—has evolved primarily from the profession of physical education over the last 50 years. The study of physical activity today is a thriving enterprise, and that study provides useful knowledge not only for physical education, but also for many new professions for which physical activity is central to the services provided. You'll discover the full story about the evolution of kinesiology and its related professions in this book.

I saw the need for this book more than 10 years ago. Most introductory books in our field were either introductions to physical education or the profession of teaching physical activity, or a mix of physical education and the sport and exercise sciences. When we began working on this book, a few books had been published that introduce people to the discipline of kinesiology or parts of the discipline, but no book had looked at the broad field of physical activity—the fundamental phenomenon of kinesiology. In this book, your editors and contributors introduce you to the experience (or "doing") of physical activity, the study of physical activity, and the practice of professions for which physical activity is core to the services provided.

This book is the first comprehensive "map" of the territory we call physical activity. It's not easy to map an emerging field. The boundaries of its various parts differ in clarity, with some parts well defined and others just beginning to emerge. There are differences of opinion about what parts should be included in the map and what these parts should be named. The major task of developing this book was to sort through these differences to obtain as much consensus as possible to describe the field clearly and accurately.

The book got an "icy" start back in February 1990, when I invited a team of respected scholars in the field to meet at Human Kinetics to develop a plan for this book. The group was greeted with an ice storm that knocked out the electrical power at our offices for five days. Fortunately, we had power at my home where we met for two days.

The team developed a good plan and contributors were asked to begin writing, but as outlines and drafts of the chapters were received, we began to realize the challenge before us. The chapters were not providing a clear map, and we were not using the same language to describe the map. We had not recognized the need to establish mapping tools, similar to longitude and latitude, to define the location of the various parts of the physical activity field. We went back to the drawing board to develop the tools—better definitions of the parts and a better plan for the whole of the parts.

The book began going through an evolution. Each time we sought to map the field, we discovered the inaccuracies of old maps, found new territories, and built new roads connecting the parts. The journey of discovery was often exhilarating, but at times painful because of the disagreement among the development team. Some of the initial team dropped out because they were unable to commit the time to the journey, or were not in agreement with the larger map. Others endured and contributed greatly to the journey.

My sincere thanks go to all who helped develop this book, not only the editors and contributors, but also many others who helped us see the field with greater clarity, even if we did not always agree. I especially want to recognize the editors, Shirl Hoffman and Janet Harris. At one time the book stalled and the path forward was not clear. Drs. Hoffman and Harris guided the book out of its conceptual fog by focusing its parts much more clearly. The editors have not only provided invaluable editorial guidance to the contributors, but they have also each written several chapters. Dr. Hoffman provides an especially unique description of the "doing" of physical activity in section 1.

This book would still be on a floppy disk if it were not for Chris Drews, the book's developmental editor. Chris not only helped the editors and contributors write the book, but she also successfully arbitrated many discussions to help reach consensus on critical content issues and made vital recommendations regarding the map itself. If I had the power, I would bestow on Chris an honorary doctorate for her contribution to this book.

We now have a comprehensive introductory text to the physical activity field. Of course, it's not the final word; it's only a start—but a good start. This book contains the content that every student who enters kinesiology or any physical activity profession should have. I hope that existing introductory courses will adopt this text, and also that the text will persuade curriculum developers to launch introductory kinesiology courses based on the content of this text.

I'm very proud to publish this book, not for the obvious business reasons as a publisher, but because I believe it will make an important contribution to kinesiology. Indeed, I believe it is the most important book Human Kinetics has published.

Rainer Martens
Publisher
December 1999

Preface to the Instructor

Writing an introductory text for any discipline is a daunting task, but it is especially so for kinesiology. Kinesiology is a young discipline undergoing rapid evolution, which, quite understandably, has raised issues about its nature, future, organization, purpose, name, and relationship to the professions. In one way or another, all of these issues converge in the writing of an introductory text. We have taken bold positions on some of these issues, such as the name for the discipline, the central phenomenon of study, and definitions of critical terms. Issues that seemed less critical to understanding the big picture of kinesiology purposely were kept in the background so as not to distract students from the primary theme of the text.

Even more problematic when writing an introductory text is the changing demographic landscape of students enrolling in departments of kinesiology. Gone are the days when physical education professors could confidently assume that all students entering as majors in their departments were planning to be physical education teachers and coaches. Now it is just as likely that students in the introductory course have their sights set on careers in sport management, athletic training, cardiac rehabilitation, fitness counseling and leadership, aquatic leadership, rehabilitative exercise, sport information, adapted physical education, or related professions. Some elect the kinesiology major as preparation for graduate study in physical therapy, chiropractic, podiatry, or medicine. Still others choose kinesiology as a course in liberal studies, without specific professional goals in mind. And of course, a substantial percentage of students come to the introductory course lacking any clear vision of what career they will pursue. The likelihood that this book would be used by students with a diverse range of needs and interests was foremost in our minds at every stage of the writing process.

In the search for the common ground on which all of these diverse students stand, we quickly came to the decision that Karl Newell (1990b) was correct: physical activity *is* the central phenomenon of study in kinesiology. It is a shared interest and curiosity about physical activity that unites students with these differing professional aspirations and makes kinesiology the logical discipline for them to study. For this reason we have given a great deal of attention to the phenomenon of physical activity. Students who lack insight into its pervasiveness and indispensability, or who doubt its worth in their personal or social lives, will not easily be convinced that a discipline of kinesiology is even needed. Although students may come to an introductory class in kinesiology with a wealth of knowledge and experience about physical activity, it is no guarantee that they will appreciate its variety, complexity, and elegance. Like art educators who must reorient students grown accustomed to viewing their world with category-hardened habits of seeing before they are to view it from a fresh and novel perspective, so the teacher of this introductory course must assist students in viewing physical activity in new and exciting ways if they are to appreciate fully the importance of the discipline of kinesiology.

The overarching purpose of this text, then, is to help students appreciate the importance of physical activity, to help them discern its relationship to the discipline of kinesiology, and to introduce them to the physical activity professions. The perspective on physical activity is broad, ranging far beyond exercise, sport, or health-related physical activity. By embracing an intentionally expansive view of physical activity and kinesiology, however, we have in no way diminished the emphasis currently given to sport and exercise in kinesiology. These have been and will continue to be the dominant forms of physical activity studied in the discipline. At the same time, the book will have missed its mark if it fails to expand students' conceptions of physical activity or fails to develop an appreciation for the potential contributions kinesiology can make to fields far removed from sport and exercise.

Plan of the Text

The text is organized around a model of kinesiology as a discipline that draws knowledge from three sources: participating in and observing physical activity, studying and conducting research, and delivering professional services. By defining the discipline as an integration of knowledge associated with experience, formal study, and professional practice, we hope to sensitize students to the critical importance of all three of these dimensions of the discipline.

Chapter 1 provides an overview of the book, offers key definitions, and presents the model around which the text is organized. Section 1 (chapters 2 through 4) focuses on experiencing physical activity, casting a wide lens on the many ways our physical activity experiences contribute to our understanding of kinesiology. Chapter 2 introduces students to "The Spheres of Physical Activity Experience," our way of helping students appreciate the indispensability of physical activity, not only in sport and exercise, but also in work, rehabilitation, daily living, and other spheres of existence. Chapter 3 directs attention to the importance of physical activity experiences, concentrating on the physical effects of experience. The intent here is to help students appreciate the beneficial effects and limitations of physical activity experiences while also portraying kinesiologists and physical activity professionals as "experience specialists" whose skill lies in designing and manipulating physical activity experiences to bring about predetermined ends.

The editors were aware of how easily discussions of the benefits of physical activity experiences can—often quite unintentionally—lead students to appreciate only the physical aspects of physical activity. Chapter 4 takes a more holistic approach by exploring the subjective aspects of physical activity. It invites students to consider the deep emotional and spiritual meanings, as well as the many different kinds of knowledge, to be gleaned from physical activity.

Section 2 (chapters 5 through 12) introduces students to the academic subdisciplines of kinesiology. They are portrayed as elements in three spheres of scholarly study of physical activity: the sociocultural, behavioral, and biophysical spheres. The schematics are intended to help students enrolled in subdisciplinary courses such as motor learning, exercise physiology, and sport history to understand how the subdisciplines fit within the larger picture of kinesiology and to appreciate the knowledge boundaries constructed around these areas of study.

The authors of the chapters in section 2, eminent scholars in their own subdisciplines, provide a general overview of each area of study with an eye toward helping students understand the particular contribution it makes to the discipline of kinesiology. Each chapter covers the major historical events in the development of the subdiscipline, the research methods used in the subdiscipline, what professionals such as biomechanists, exercise physiologists, and others do in the course of their professional work, and how students' present knowledge can form a foundation for more advanced study. Each chapter presents practical, real-world applications from the subdiscipline in order to help students understand why the subdiscipline is important and how it may relate to a variety of professional endeavors.

Section 3 (chapters 13 through 17) is designed to help students begin thinking about professions in which physical activity plays a central role. Throughout this section, authors have kept in mind that many students entering kinesiology departments may have tentative professional goals at best. To this end, chapter 13 takes a general approach to the physical activity professions, introducing students to what it means to be a professional and what will be required of them if they are to become a professional. Students are led through a series of steps intended to assist them in determining whether they are suited by interest, talent, and motivation to a career in kinesiology.

Chapters 14 through 17 include a wealth of information about clusters of careers drawn from the spheres of professional practice. Each chapter focuses on a collection of professional opportunities within a sphere, including health and fitness, therapeutic exercise, teaching and coaching, and sport management. The authors of each chapter explain the need for professions in that sphere and offer a brief historical background. In addition, each chapter includes an analysis of work settings in the sphere, "up-close views" of specific professions, an overview of educational qualifications needed to practice in the sphere, resources, case studies and profiles of working professionals, and a section devoted to "inside advice" for those planning careers in that cluster of professions. We believe this section will help students make intelligent career choices earlier, and help them match their career aspirations with their overall strengths.

We included interaction exercises throughout the text in order to involve students more actively in their learning. These exercises are intended to encourage students to engage more deeply with the content, putting themselves into the pictures they are reading about. Rather than simply reading about the discipline, we hope that students will envision themselves as professionals and begin to take steps toward their career goals.

Acknowledgments

Such a far-ranging text is much too ambitious a project for one or two people to take on, which is why we recruited some of the very best scholars and professionals to accompany us on this challenging adventure. Each brought to the project a unique educational background and professional experiences, yet all shared our commitment to producing a text that would effectively orient undergraduate students to the exciting world of physical activity and the discipline of kinesiology. We believe their contributions have added a richness and comprehensiveness that would not have been possible from a single author.

It is important to recognize, however, that although this book features the work of many authors, it is not an anthology or a collection of only marginally related chapters. Rather, it is in every sense of the word a textbook organized around a central theme; structured to accomplish the intended purposes; and integrated as to terminology, concepts, objectives, and even graphics. Ensuring this level of consistency proved to be an amazingly complex task, not only for the editors but also for the editorial staff at Human Kinetics.

Ultimately, the task of pulling together the diverse contributions, putting them in context, designing a structure for the text, defining and describing the discipline, tackling thorny issues, ironing out apparent inconsistencies, and interpreting the material in the text fell to the editors. Any errors that have been made, whether of omission or commission, should be attributed to us, not to others who have so generously given of their time and effort to this project.

Attempting to single out individuals who have contributed to the completion of the book runs the risk of inadvertent omissions. Our sincere appreciation has been earned by the contributing authors who persevered through a long and often arduous process, met unreasonable deadlines, and revised manuscripts more times than they might have thought necessary. This text is as much theirs as it is ours. Several of our colleagues began the journey but for one reason or another weren't able to finish. We hope they are satisfied with the finished product. Obvious debts of gratitude are owed to those who have served as our mentors and to the thousands of students who attended our classes over the past several decades. The overarching model for this book was the product of many hours of discussion and spirited debate between the editors when we were colleagues on the faculty at University of North Carolina at Greensboro. The camaraderie, support, and stimulation from our colleagues there helped form our ideas about the discipline that figure prominently in this text.

At home the quiet support and encouragement Claude Mourot Hoffman willingly gave to her husband was appreciated more than she knows. Among family, Larry and Mary Ann Harris weathered changes with less support at times than their daughter would have preferred.

Finally, we owe an enormous debt of gratitude to Chris Drews, developmental editor at Human Kinetics, for her skillful work in bringing this manuscript to completion. Both of us came to a new understanding of the importance of having a hardworking, cordial, patient, tactful, and talented developmental editor. The project may well have not been completed without Chris's untiring efforts.

Shirl J. Hoffman
Janet C. Harris

Preface to the Student

Most students enter college having decided on a major before they know a great deal about it. Many have not asked themselves the fundamental questions, such as, Why is the major important? What types of careers do people in the major enter after graduating? What subjects do students in the major study, and how is the course of study organized? Not knowing the answers to these questions at the beginning of their undergraduate experience makes it very difficult to put their course work in perspective and worse, can leave them questioning the value of many of the courses they are required to take. If you have decided to major or are considering a major in kinesiology, you may not know much about the field of study and may have only vague ideas concerning the career opportunities available to you.

This is why this textbook was written. It is intended to help you understand what the discipline of kinesiology is, why it is important, what kinesiology majors study, what types of knowledge they acquire over the course of four years, and what types of careers are available to kinesiology students. It also is intended to help you reach an early decision, not only about whether you want to major in kinesiology, but also about what type of career most interests you. You may see no pressing need to decide on a career at this early stage of your college experience, but, as you will see in this book, there are advantages to identifying early the career path you want to follow.

Kinesiology may be a term you have never heard before. In fact, you may be enrolled in a major called "exercise and sport science" or "physical education and exercise science" or some other name. This is one of the confusing things about this major; the discipline is known by many titles. Actually, this isn't all that uncommon for a young and evolving area of study such as kinesiology; it simply hasn't been around long enough for everybody to agree on a single term! Over the past decade, however, more and more scholars and college and university departments have decided to use the term *kinesiology*. For this reason it has been selected as the title of this text.

Because kinesiology integrates knowledge from a variety of sources and draws on theories, concepts, and principles from many other disciplines, it's not easy to describe or explain it to students. This text presents the discipline in a new and, we believe, exciting way. We were concerned that you understand not only the enormous breadth of the discipline, but also how the many parts of the discipline fit together. In the pages that follow, you will learn that physical activity is the centerpiece of the discipline. This may be the most important point in the book. It means that whether you plan to be a sports administrator, athletic trainer, physical education teacher, or physical or occupational therapist, you have an interest in and curiosity about physical activity.

Just as the discipline of psychology is the study of human behavior and the discipline of biology is the study of life forms, the discipline of kinesiology is the study of physical activity. But don't interpret *study* to mean only reading books, writing papers, and taking exams. Kinesiology integrates knowledge from three different, yet related, sources: your experiences performing and observing physical activity, the formal study of physical activity, and professional practice centered in physical activity. This is a new approach to understanding the interrelationships of the parts of the discipline.

Section 1 of the text will spark your thinking about physical activity, why it is important, and how it intersects our lives at a variety of different junctures we call *spheres of physical activity experience*. If you think that sport and exercise are what kinesiologists study, you are correct; but you are not correct if you think these are the only forms of physical activity that kinesiologists study. Here you will come to appreciate the fact that kinesiology also makes contributions to our understanding and improvement of physical activity performances in venues far beyond the athletic field or exercise gym. In this section human experience in physical activity is presented as a unique source of knowledge. You will also come to appreciate the fact that humans are endowed with a unique ability to plan and engage in physical activity experiences in order to improve the quality of their lives. After reading this section, you should have come to view kinesiologists as physical activity experts who, through planned physical activity experiences, help people realize their individual goals. This section also will help you appreciate the fact that physical activity touches us at many different levels, the physical for sure, but also at the cognitive, emotional, and spiritual levels.

Whereas section 1 invites you to reflect on the knowledge gained through the experiences of participating in and watching physical activity, section 2 presents a broad, "once over lightly" coverage of the knowledge to be derived from the scholarly study of physical activity. The chapter titles in this section are an outline of the core body of academic (theoretical) knowledge that all kinesiology students should master before they graduate. To help you better organize this vast body of knowledge in your mind, we have grouped it into larger categories called *spheres of scholarly study*. The chapters are authored by nationally recognized scholars who are particularly skilled at introducing you to their areas of specialized study. Keep in mind that each chapter is intended only to introduce you to the area of study, not to provide you with all of the scholarly knowledge you will need to master in that area before you graduate.

Section 3 introduces you to the world of professional practice. Students enrolled in kinesiology departments often have widely disparate career goals, from becoming an athletic trainer or physical educator to becoming a corporate fitness leader, cardiac rehabilitation specialist, or many others. Each of these is a form of professional practice. In this section we have grouped the many possible careers into *spheres of professional practice* according to similarities in the types of work and general educational requirements. The chapters are authored by outstanding scholars in various areas of professional practice. They are eminently qualified to describe the different types of work done by physical activity professionals as well as offer details concerning what you can do to develop yourself into an outstanding professional.

As you read through the text, don't skip over the objectives listed at the beginning of each chapter; they are your map for the pages that follow. Also, a number of "interactive items" intended to engage your thinking about points in the text are sprinkled throughout the chapters. Don't miss the unique opportunity they offer for learning. Also, make sure to focus on each key point and to think back over what you have read. The study questions at the end of each chapter will direct you to what the authors believe are some of the most important points they have covered. Good luck in your reading, and good luck in your career in kinesiology!

1

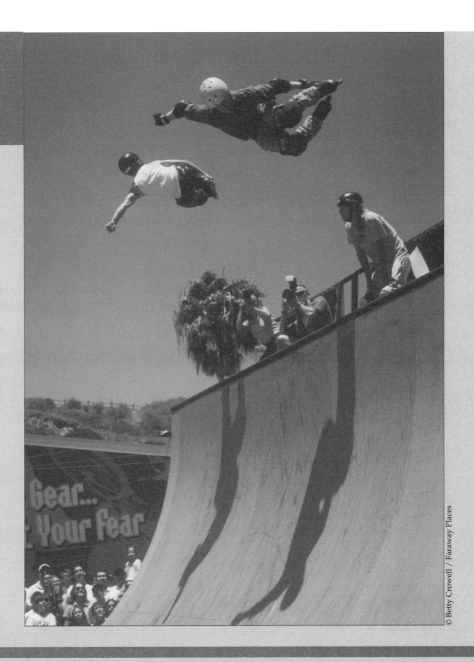

© Betty Crowell / Faraway Places

Discovering the Field of Physical Activity

Shirl J. Hoffman and Janet C. Harris

In this chapter . . .

Have you been physically active today? Of course you have. At the very least, you managed to get out of bed, walk to the bathroom, get dressed, eat breakfast, and perhaps make your way to class, all of which require hundreds of different movements. These movements are remarkable, not only for their complexity, but also for their variety. Physical activity is so interwoven into your life that it's probably far easier to count the number of ways in which you weren't physically active than the ways in which you were.

A moment's reflection will convince you that our lives are an endless universe of physical activity. We walk, reach, run, lift, leap, throw, grasp, wave, push, pull, and perform thousands of other movements as part of living a normal human existence. Physical activity is essential in our work. It is essential to our daily tasks around the house. It is an important means of expressing ourselves through gesture, art, and dance. Our health depends on performing regular forms of vigorous physical activity, and we rely on various forms of recreational physical activity for fun and enjoyment.

But more than this, physical activity is part of our nature. It is an important means by which we explore and discover our world, and it helps define us as human beings. A significant part of our lifetimes is spent learning to master a broad range of physical activities, from the earliest skills of reaching, grasping, and walking to enormously complex skills such as hitting a baseball, performing a somersault, or playing the piano. Most of us master a broad range of physical activities at a moderate level of competence. Others manage to achieve spectacular physical feats such as bench pressing 310 kilograms (683 lb), running 201 kilometers (125 miles) in 24 hours, diving to 124 meters (407 ft), or climbing Mt. Everest at over 8,840 meters (29,002 ft).

This chapter is intended to arouse your curiosity about physical activity and cause you to appreciate its complexity, its universality, and its importance to human life. It will help you understand how the discipline of kinesiology is organized to study physical activity. Because you've been physically active during your whole life, you have the advantage of bringing to your reading of this book a wealth of experiences and knowledge about physical activity. At the same time, you probably haven't thought about physical activity or experienced it quite like you will be asked to do here. In fact, at times it may be necessary for you to set aside past experiences and assumptions so that you can examine physical activity from a fresh and exciting point of view.

The authors wish to acknowledge Rainer Martens' contributions to the conceptualization of this chapter.

CHAPTER OBJECTIVES

In this chapter we will:

- Help you appreciate the pervasiveness and diversity of physical activity in human life
- Introduce you to ways of defining and thinking about physical activity
- Introduce you to the discipline of kinesiology and its relationship to physical activity
- Familiarize you with the types of knowledge about physical activity acquired through experience, scholarly study, and professional practice
- Introduce you to the notion of a profession and physical activity career possibilities

As you can see, we have a lot to accomplish in this chapter, so if you're feeling a bit drowsy, you might want to take a brisk walk, run a few miles, or play a favorite sport with friends before you go any further. When you come back, you will be rejuvenated and ready to learn about the fascinating subject of physical activity.

Overview

Thanks to scientific investigation, people are now more aware than ever of the importance of physical activity to our cognitive, emotional, and physical well-being. One indication of this is the rise in popularity of college and university curriculums devoted to the study of physical activity. This interest in studying physical activity has been fueled in part by an explosion of career opportunities for college-trained professionals who have an in-depth knowledge of the scientific and humanistic bases of physical activity, along with training in professional practice. Career possibilities now extend well beyond the traditional professions of teaching physical education and coaching. Physical therapy, cardiac rehabilitation, sport management, athletic training, and fitness leadership and management are just a few of the careers that are likely to require formal academic preparation in kinesiology.

Coupled with this growing recognition of the importance of physical activity is the realization that something as vital to human life as physical activity deserves to be studied as seriously and systematically as other respected disciplines in higher education such as biology, psychology, and sociology. Disciplines are organized bodies of knowledge that are considered worthy of study. Kinesiology is now acknowledged by scholars as the discipline that studies physical activity. This book calls special attention to the unique way kinesiology is learned. You may have noticed in the college courses you've taken that not all disciplines are learned in the same way. For example, art is learned through reading and writing and artistic exploration through projects in the studio. History, literature, and philosophy are learned largely through intensive reading, writing, memorization, thinking, and discussion. Reading, writing, memorization, thinking, and discussion are also important when learning chemistry and biology, but these disciplines also involve active participation in laboratory exercises. Kinesiology is learned partly in the same way as these other disciplines, and partly in a different way.

Like most other disciplines, part of kinesiology is learned through planned and systematic scholarly study. This involves much reading, writing, memorization, thinking, and discussion. As we have noted, scholarly study is used in such disciplines as history, literature, and psychology. It is also used to master subjects in the kinesiology curriculum such as sport history, motor development and learning, exercise physiology, biomechanics, and sport psychology. Where does the knowledge contained in such subjects come from? Mostly from the work of scholars who have added to the knowledge base through systematic research and scholarship. The knowledge we have of sport history or philosophy of sport, for example, is derived through the scholarly efforts of kinesiologists who are sport historians and sport philosophers. The knowledge we have of biomechanics of physical activity is derived from kinesiologists who conduct research in biomechanics laboratories at universities. All knowledge about physical activity produced through research by kinesiologists is part of the discipline of kinesiology. Much of this knowledge is included in college and university kinesiology curriculums. In addition, knowledge about physical activity produced by scholars in other disciplines (e.g., psychology, physiology, history) becomes incorporated into the discipline of kinesiology if it is used in further research by kinesiologists, or if it is included in college and university kinesiology curriculums.

But kinesiology is learned in other ways as well. Kinesiology students also gain knowledge about physical activity, their own selves, and the world around them through performing and watching physical activity. In this text performing and watching physical activity constitute "experiencing" physical activity. Thus, experiencing physical activity is another source of knowledge about physical activity; it is actually a second way of learning kinesiology. When knowledge derived from experiencing physical activity is included in college or university kinesiology curriculums it becomes part of the body of knowledge of kinesiology.

A third way of learning in kinesiology is through professional practice, although here the focus is not so much on knowledge about physical activity as it is on how physical activity can be used to bring about predetermined ends. This is what physical activity professionals such as physical education teachers or cardiac rehabilitation specialists do: they systematically manipulate the physical activity experiences of others to achieve certain predetermined ends. Where does this knowledge come from? Some of this knowledge used to guide professionals is derived from actually engaging in professional practice, although, as we shall see, knowledge gained from experiencing physical activity and the scholarly study of physical activity are very important in professional practice as well. Another way of explaining this is that exercise therapists, teachers and coaches, athletic trainers, and other physical activity professionals develop a rich knowledge base of professional practice as they perform their daily tasks. If this knowledge is grounded in careful, systematic observations of the effects of their manipulations of physical activity on others such as students, patients, and clients, it often becomes incorporated into kinesiology curriculums offered by colleges and universities and is taught to students. As such it also is part of the discipline of kinesiology.

You will notice that we have carefully defined kinesiology as knowledge derived from experiencing physical activity, scholarly study of physical activity, and professional practice centered in physical activity, *but only when that knowledge is embedded in a college or university curriculum in kinesiology and/or used by kinesiologists in their physical activity research.* The reason for this is to clarify precisely what is part of the discipline and what is not. Physical activity is a pervasive phenomenon that reaches far beyond the university curriculum. It is performed, studied, and is the center of professional practice in many venues outside the college or university setting. It may be important and valuable in its own right, but it does not constitute the "doing" of kinesiology any more than a businessperson who uses elementary psychological principles to motivate her sales force is "doing" psychology. The discipline of psychology remains tied to the college and university curriculum, and to the research of psychologists. Similarly, the principles of kinesiology may be used in many ways outside the discipline but kinesiology per se remains a function of curriculums and research in colleges and universities.

There is another reason to limit our conception of kinesiology to that knowledge contained in college or university curriculums and/or used in research. It tends to be more highly organized and more scientifically verifiable than physical activity knowledge that is not. To illustrate, we tend to have much more confidence in the suggestions of a university faculty member in kinesiology who specializes in fencing than those of a lawyer who fences as a hobby. We have more confidence in the scientific validity of statements concerning an exercise program offered by a kinesiologist than those offered by a television exercise guru who lacks formal training in kinesiology. And, we are more likely to trust a kinesiologist specializing in pedagogy to recommend how we should organize a large group of young children for instruction in gymnastics than a volunteer coach who has no formal training in kinesiology.

Many people experience physical activity (e.g., walk through a supermarket collecting groceries, play pickup basketball), study physical activity (e.g., read popular trade books on fitness or sports), or engage in a form of "professional" practice (e.g., volunteer youth league coach) outside the confines of the university curriculum, but these do not necessarily constitute "doing" kinesiology.

Later in this chapter you will learn how all three components of knowledge about physical

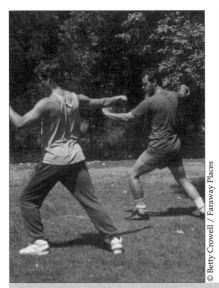
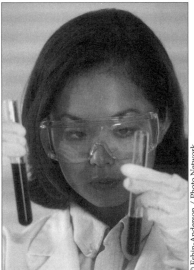
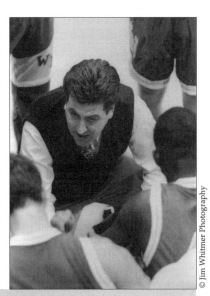

The discipline of kinesiology includes experiencing, studying, and practicing a profession in physical activity. Knowledge gained from any of these three sources that is included in a university curriculum is part of the discipline of kinesiology.

activity fit together to make up the discipline of kinesiology. The most complete knowledge of kinesiology is gained from engaging in all three components—experience, scholarly study, and professional practice—although knowledge from each component is valuable in its own right. These three components are depicted in figure 1.1. This figure will be repeated throughout the book to remind you of the component of physical activity that is currently being discussed in the text.

🗝️ Experiencing physical activity, scholarly study of physical activity, and professional practice centered in physical activity are the three sources of physical activity knowledge that make up the discipline of kinesiology.

What Is Physical Activity?

We have already said that kinesiology is the discipline that deals with physical activity. Just as human behavior is the focal point of the discipline of psychology and life forms are the focal point of biology, so physical activity is the focal point of the discipline of kinesiology. But what is physical activity? At first you might think this is a silly question. Everybody knows what it is, so

why waste time defining it? But definitions can be very important, especially in scientific and professional fields where terms may be defined somewhat differently than they are in everyday language. These definitions, called **technical definitions**, ensure that people working within a science or profession share a common understanding. Thus, before we go much further, let's be sure that we all have the same understanding of what physical activity is. We must be careful in formulating our technical definition, since it will specify the types of human activities that form the centerpiece of kinesiology.

In everyday life, throwing a javelin, driving a car, walking, performing a cartwheel, swimming, digging a ditch, hammering a nail, and typing at a keyboard all would be described as examples of physical activity, as would the "kick" you exhibit when the doctor taps your patellar tendon to test your reflexes, the blinking of your eye, the peristaltic action of your small intestine brought on by muscular contractions, the contraction of your diaphragm when you sneeze, and the action of your throat muscles when you swallow. But are all of these muscular actions of concern to kinesiologists? Not really. Although all are examples of human movement, they're really too diverse in form and purpose for any single discipline to study. Indeed, if all forms of human movement were to be the focus of kinesiology,

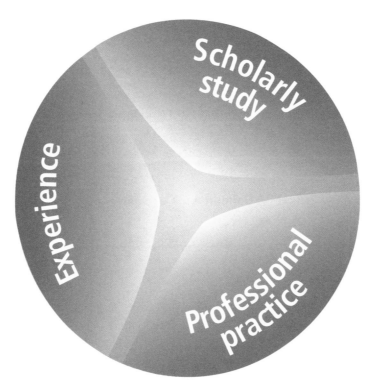

Figure 1.1 Sources of knowledge in kinesiology.

This would be a good time to wrestle with some fundamental questions about physical activity. Perhaps the most fundamental question of all is, What exactly *is* physical activity? Before you continue reading this chapter, think carefully about the following questions. Take time to compare your answers with those of your classmates.

1. What are your favorite physical activities? Name at least three.
2. Why do you believe that all of the activities you have listed are *physical* activities?
3. What characteristics do they all share that cause you to consider them to be *physical* activities?
4. Do you have hobbies that are *not* physical activities? Why do you believe they are not?

After you have thought about or discussed these questions, write your own definition of physical activity. Keep this handy to compare with the definition we will propose in the next few pages.

then kinesiologists would study everything humans do, since any time we do anything, we move!

For this reason, kinesiologists use a much different definition of physical activity than people use in everyday language. The discipline requires a definition that isn't too *inclusive* (e.g., all human movement) or too *exclusive* (e.g., only human movement related to sports) (see figure 1.2).

Consider, for example, how physical activity is defined in the surgeon general's report: "bodily movement that is produced by the contraction of skeletal muscle *and that substantially increases energy expenditure*" [italics added] (U.S. Department of Health and Human Services, 1996, p. 21). This definition limits physical activity to voluntary or purposeful behaviors (contraction of the skeletal muscles as opposed to involuntary muscles). This

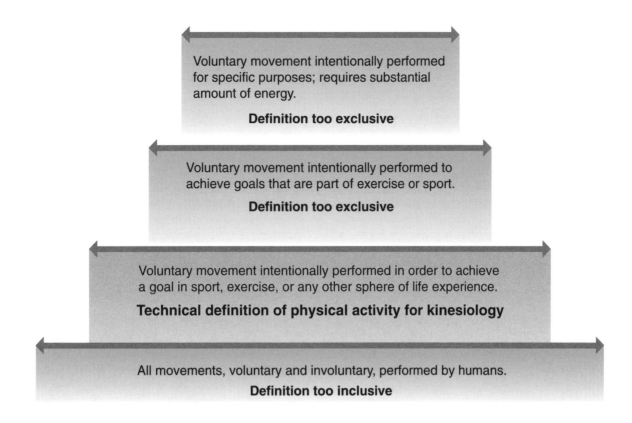

Voluntary movement intentionally performed for specific purposes; requires substantial amount of energy.
Definition too exclusive

Voluntary movement intentionally performed to achieve goals that are part of exercise or sport.
Definition too exclusive

Voluntary movement intentionally performed in order to achieve a goal in sport, exercise, or any other sphere of life experience.
Technical definition of physical activity for kinesiology

All movements, voluntary and involuntary, performed by humans.
Definition too inclusive

Figure 1.2   Only movement that is voluntary and performed for a specific purpose meets the technical definition of physical activity.

seems like a sensible thing to do since most of the time kinesiologists are interested in the ways in which people carry out intentional or planned actions, not simplistic physiological responses.

But if you read the definition carefully, you will see that the surgeon general's approach narrows the definition much further. Only voluntary movement that "substantially increases energy expenditure" meets this technical definition of physical activity. However, although many types of physical activity that interest kinesiologists do require substantial amounts of energy, many others do not. For example, scholars and professionals in the physical activity field are interested in such tasks as bowling, passing a football, shooting a basketball, handwriting, gardening, swimming, or taking a leisurely walk, activities that don't always substantially increase energy expenditure. The surgeon general's technical definition, then, seems too restrictive because it eliminates many types of physical activity that interest kinesiology scholars and professionals.

What about limiting our technical definition to include only those physical activities that are

directly related to exercise and sport? Some would point out that since kinesiology has its historical roots in exercise and sport (a point emphasized in chapter 6), and since most students entering the field have their sights set on a career in exercise and/or sport, this definition might seem to make a great deal of sense.

But even though these two categories of physical activity receive the most attention in contemporary kinesiology—and they certainly take center stage in this text—it doesn't seem wise to ignore the fact that the study of kinesiology also includes the study of other, more wide-ranging forms of physical activity. Examples include basic postural mechanisms, the physiology and body mechanics of work, the development of reaching and grasping behaviors in infants, and the daily life support activities of the elderly. Physical activity professionals teach children how to perform fundamental movement patterns such as hopping, running, skipping, or expressive physical activities such as dance, while those working in rehabilitation programs teach patients to recover lost capacities to walk, sit, rise from a chair, or drive a car. As the range of occupations open to graduates of kinesiology departments continues to expand, clearly a technical definition of physical activity that reaches beyond exercise and sport is in order.

The definition of physical activity used in this text takes its cue from Professor Karl Newell (1990a) who defined physical activity as *intentional, voluntary movement directed toward achieving an identifiable goal*. Notice three things about this definition: First, it does not stipulate that the activity must require substantial amounts of energy. Large-muscle activities typically require the highest levels of energy, but the definition doesn't limit physical activity only to these. Swimming, lifting barbells, running marathons, and rollerblading are physical activities, but so are typing, handwriting, sewing, and surgery.

Second, whether or not the activity takes place in a sport or exercise setting is irrelevant, according to this definition. Surely, shooting a basketball is a form of physical activity, but so is tossing a piece of paper into the wastebasket. Pole vaulting is a physical activity, and so is jumping over a fence. Swinging a baseball bat is a physical activity, but so is swinging a sledgehammer.

Third, according to this definition, simply moving your body doesn't constitute physical activity. Movement includes any change in the position of your body parts relative to each other. Think about it. When you move you always alter the position of one or more of your body parts relative to some other body part. But movement by itself does not constitute physical activity. Only movement that is intentional and voluntary—purposefully directed toward an identifiable goal—meets our technical definition of physical activity. This excludes all involuntary reflexes and all physiological movements such as peristalsis, swallowing, or blinking an eye. It also excludes voluntary movements that are not performed with an intentional goal in mind. The repetitive movements of a compulsive-obsessive psychiatric patient, or thoughtlessly scratching your head

What Is and Is Not Physical Activity?

Read each question and circle Yes if it is physical activity and No if it is not physical activity.

Yes   No   1. You're running on a hot day and experience muscle spasms in your hamstrings. Spasms involve contraction of your hamstring muscles. Are the spasms an example of physical activity?

Yes   No   2. A mosquito keeps buzzing around your head, and you swat it.

Yes   No   3. A car backfires and the noise startles you, making you blink.

Yes   No   4. You're asleep and a friend raises and lowers your arm without your knowing it. Is your arm's movement physical activity?

Yes   No   5. In the previous example, was your friend performing physical activity?

Yes   No   6. A physical therapist helps a patient move her leg through a full range of motion. Is the patient engaged in physical activity?

Yes   No   7. Your coach tells you to do a series of conditioning exercises, and you do them even though you don't really want to.

Yes   No   8. You try to hit a golf ball off the tee but you miss.

Yes   No   9. Sitting still before you compete in a wrestling match, your heart pounds against your chest. Is the movement of your heart physical activity?

Yes   No   10. While listening to a boring lecture, you drum your fingers on the desk unknowingly.

Answers: 1. No; 2. Yes; 3. No; 4. No; 5. Yes; 6. Yes; 7. Yes; 8. Yes; 9. No; 10. No or pulling on your earlobe, are examples of human movement that fall outside the technical definition of physical activity.

🔑 Physical activity is movement that is intentional, voluntary, and directed toward achieving an identifiable goal. This excludes human movements that are involuntary such as reflexes, or those performed aimlessly and without a specific purpose.

What Is Kinesiology?

Kinesiology is a discipline or body of knowledge that focuses on physical activity. The discipline derives and incorporates knowledge from three different yet related sources:

- Experiencing physical activity (experiential knowledge)
- Studying the theoretical and conceptual bases of physical activity (theoretical knowledge)
- Professional practice centered in physical activity (professional practice knowledge)

We have already mentioned that this book emphasizes the unique way that kinesiology is studied. Typically, we associate the term *study* only with learning theoretical material through reading, writing, memorization, thinking, and discussion. However, experience with physical activity, theories and concepts about physical activity, and professional practice are all important sources of information for kinesiologists. For this reason, this text has been divided into three sections, each of which examines a distinct source of knowledge that is incorporated into the discipline of kinesiology.

Figure 1.3 depicts the three major dimensions of kinesiology. You will notice that each dimension corresponds to a different source of knowledge of physical activity (figure 1.1). The part of the figure marked A1 represents disciplinary knowledge acquired from our experiences with physical activity. Usually, this involves performing physical activity, but we can also acquire knowledge by observing others perform. This experiential knowledge, described in section 1 of this book, is often acquired through physical activity classes (e.g., classes in soccer, weight training, swimming) offered in kinesiology departments. Experiential knowledge that is included in a formal college or university kinesiology curriculum is part of the discipline of kinesiology. So far, experiential knowledge has not been divided into formal subdisciplines within the discipline of kinesiology.

It is possible, of course, to acquire experiential knowledge through physical activities you are involved in outside of a formal college or university curriculum; this kind of experiential knowledge is represented by part A2 of figure 1.3. This knowledge is on the fringes of the discipline. For example, you might take tennis lessons at a private club, play tennis on weekends with friends, take martial arts lessons at a commercial center, work out on your own at a campus fitness center, play intramural football in a recreational league, or train for firefighting through the fire department. You can often learn extremely valuable things from such experiences, but this knowledge is not a central part of the kinesiology discipline unless it is formally incorporated into college and university kinesiology classes. These aspects of experiencing physical activity are also discussed in section 1 of this text.

Part B1 of figure 1.3 represents disciplinary knowledge acquired from the scholarly study of theories and concepts about physical activity. This theoretical knowledge is divided into categories or subdisciplines. Taken together, the subdisciplines constitute the spheres of scholarly study examined in section 2 of this book. This disciplinary knowledge is taught in its most systematic and comprehensive form in college and university curriculums, usually in departments of kinesiology.

However, because physical activity is such a broad category of human behavior, other university departments sometimes engage in the scholarly study of physical activity as well, as represented by part B2 in figure 1.3. For example, departments of drama, dance, and music sometimes teach about the scholarly aspects of physical activity, as do departments of engineering and medicine. This knowledge, however, is on the fringes of kinesiology, and it is not covered in this book. Departments of kinesiology are the only academic units within colleges and universities that identify the unified study of physical

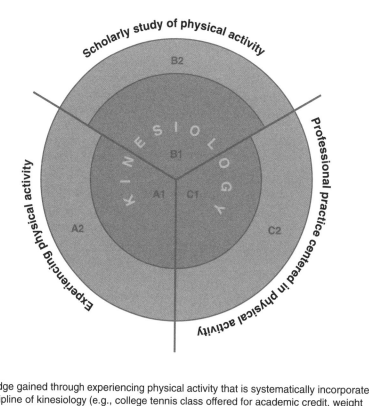

A1 Knowledge gained through experiencing physical activity that is systematically incorporated into the discipline of kinesiology (e.g., college tennis class offered for academic credit, weight training class offered for academic credit).

A2 Knowledge gained through experiencing physical activity that is *not* incorporated into the discipline of kinesiology (e.g., learning a dramatic stage movement, taking tennis lessons at a country club, playing Little League baseball, firefighting).

B1 Knowledge gained through scholarly study of physical activity that is systematically incorporated into the discipline of kinesiology (e.g., sport history, exercise physiology, motor development).

B2 Knowledge gained through scholarly study of physical activity that is *not* systematically incorporated into the discipline of kinesiology (e.g., research about playing a musical instrument, reading a popular book on fitness).

C1 Knowledge gained through professional practice centered in physical activity that is systematically incorporated into the discipline of kinesiology (e.g., knowledge gained in roles such as certified athletic trainer or elementary physical education teacher that is included in university kinesiology classes).

C2 Knowledge gained through professional practice centered in physical activity that is *not* systematically incorporated into the discipline of kinesiology (e.g., knowledge gained in roles such as certified athletic trainer or elementary physical education teacher that is *not* included in university kinesiology classes).

Figure 1.3 The discipline of kinesiology in colleges and universities.

activity *as their sole mission*. Also, you will have noticed many books and magazines on the shelves of your bookstore that deal with sports and fitness. Many of these are not based in science or systematic analysis and are not part of the discipline of kinesiology.

Part C1 of the model in figure 1.3 represents disciplinary knowledge acquired from profes-

sional practice centered in physical activity— professional practice such as managing a fitness center, teaching physical education, engaging in personal training, or working in cardiac rehabilitation. This **professional practice knowledge** becomes part of the discipline when it is discovered or tested in professional settings and is incorporated by faculty into college and university kinesiology classes, usually classes focused on preparing students for specific physical activity professions. Professional practice knowledge usually deals with appropriate ways of manipulating physical activity experiences. For example, fitness counseling, athletic training, physical education, and sport management rely on professional practice knowledge. This component of physical activity knowledge is described in more detail in section 3 of this book. So far, professional practice knowledge has not been divided into formal subdisciplines within the discipline of kinesiology.

Of course, not all knowledge acquired through professional practice is incorporated into the kinesiology curriculum. For example, a coach who is planning drills for her team may rely more on knowledge gained from people who coached her in the past than from the latest scientific information on skill learning. Sometimes such knowledge is effective; after all, a coach is not likely to use it unless she detects that it is effective for preparing her players. But often such knowledge is flawed from a scientific standpoint. The good results the coach observed may have less to do with her actions than with other factors she didn't take into account. This is one reason why some of the knowledge gained through professional practice is not incorporated into the discipline. Such knowledge is located on the perimeter of C2 in figure 1.3 to indicate this.

Professional practice knowledge is most valuable when combined with knowledge from the other dimensions of kinesiology (experience and scholarly study). Together, these can provide an important framework for conceiving of and using knowledge about professional practice. Sometimes, people who possess only a fraction of the disciplinary knowledge (represented in parts A1, B1, and C1) assume professional roles anyway. How is this possible? Because in some cases the demand for physical activity professionals is so great that institutions hire those who lack adequate qualifications. School districts, for example, sometimes hire coaches, and fitness centers sometimes hire personal trainers, who have little or no background in kinesiology. Obviously, it is possible to develop a modest level of competency in almost any profession without mastering the knowledge one should understand. Through trial and much error such a person may "muddle through." But this can be dangerous.

You may have known or heard about laypersons, for example, who managed to learn enough about the law to represent themselves in court. But the risk of such a person making a mistake is high. By the same token, an unqualified individual who assumes the role of a physical activity professional lacks the informed judgment of one who has studied kinesiology.

Let's quickly review our description of kinesiology. It is a discipline or body of knowledge that concentrates on physical activity—knowledge acquired through experience or performance of physical activity, scholarly study of theories and concepts about physical activity, and professional practice centered in physical activity. Because it is a formal discipline it typically is taught in a college or university by highly trained individuals known as kinesiologists, just as psychology is taught in universities by psychologists, and biology by biologists. Departments of kinesiology are staffed by faculty who, taken together, understand the broad knowledge base of the discipline. Their curriculums—organized sequences of classes—are structured in ways that offer maximal opportunities for integrating all three types of knowledge.

> The discipline of kinesiology consists of experiential knowledge, theoretical knowledge, and professional practice knowledge. Experiential knowledge derives from experiencing physical activity; theoretical knowledge derives from systematic research about physical activity; and professional practice knowledge derives from and contributes to the process of delivering physical activity services.

The Focus of Kinesiology

Because kinesiology is historically linked to physical education (see chapter 6), two specific forms of physical activity—exercise and sport—currently receive primary attention from kinesiologists. This is why exercise and sport are the focal points of this book. **Exercise** is a specific form of physical activity that we engage in for purposes of improving performance, health, and/or bodily appearance. Running or lifting weights to increase your fitness (improve your health) or to lose body fat (change the appearance of your body) is exercise, as is weight training by bodybuilders hoping to increase the size and definition of their muscles to achieve an ideal "look." Working out in order to increase strength or cardiovascular endurance is also exercise. Exercise performed for the express purpose of conditioning your body to improve your athletic performance, or your performance in other physical activities, is known as **training** (see chapter 3).

Sport is a form of physical activity in which skilled movement is performed in order to achieve a goal in a manner specified by established rules. The rules exist for the sole purpose of creating the game. Obviously, some people engage in exercise and sport simultaneously. For example, you might compete in racquetball with the hope of getting good enough to win your city's championship, but also in order to get

enough exercise to improve your body's functioning or appearance.

What are your favorite forms of exercise? What sports do you most enjoy? Are there physical activities you participate in that do not seem to fit our definitions of exercise and sport?

Preparing fitness leaders and consultants, teachers and coaches, cardiac and neuromuscular rehabilitation specialists, sport management specialists, athletic trainers, strength training specialists, and numerous other physical activity professionals is the primary mission of kinesiology. In some cases, a degree in kinesiology is appropriate for students interested in dance and other forms of expressive movement (e.g., dra-

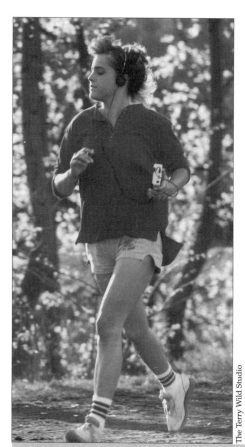

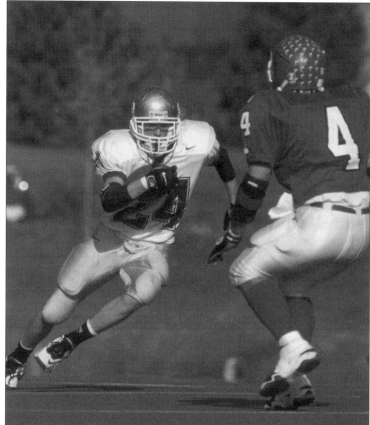

The Terry Wild Studio

© Human Kinetics

Exercise and sport are the primary focus of physical activity studied in kinesiology.

matic arts). And increasingly, students are pursuing undergraduate kinesiology degrees as liberal studies subjects, with no plans to enter a physical activity profession but with a great deal of interest in learning about physical activity in human life.

Many undergraduates pursue master's degrees in kinesiology after graduation in order to become more knowledgeable about their chosen physical activity profession. Sometimes students pursue undergraduate degrees in kinesiology as **preprofessional** preparation for graduate training in an allied health profession such as physical therapy, occupational therapy, or medicine. And a few students continue their studies with the goal of earning doctoral degrees in kinesiology in order to become college or university faculty members.

Professionals trained in kinesiology share a common interest in and curiosity about physical activity in its broadest dimensions. At the same time, they also tend to develop rather specialized orientations depending upon their professional role. For example, practitioners working in the area of cardiovascular fitness may be most interested in vigorous, sustained forms of physical activity involving the large muscles of the body. They are especially interested in how such experiences can alter the physiological functioning of the body. Physical education teachers may entertain a much more comprehensive perspective of physical activity. Their interests span cardiovascular fitness activities, sport skills, and (if they are elementary teachers) developmental activities in throwing, catching, running, and hopping. In addition, they may have a special interest in physical activity that develops social responsibility and other personal traits in children. Professionals working in athletic training or rehabilitation exercise are particularly interested in physical activity as a medium of rehabiliation. Sport marketers have a different orientation to physical activity altogether. Their interests center on making physical activity appealing to paying audiences by promoting and staging performances that are attractive to the largest number of people. Thus, in addition to developing an understanding and appreciation for physical activity, it will also be important for you to develop a deep understanding of physical activity in the context of whatever specialized professional practice you choose to enter.

Exercise and sport are the principal forms, but not the only forms, of physical activity studied by kinesiologists. Exercise includes any physical activity performed for the purpose of improving performance, health, and/or bodily appearance. Sport includes any physical activity that people perform in order to attain a goal in a manner dictated by rules that exist solely to create the game.

Why Kinesiology?

Scholars have debated at length the label that would best characterize an academic discipline focused broadly on physical activity. For many years, the label *physical education* was appropriate for the rather limited mission of kinesiology departments—preparing school physical education teachers and coaches. But the term hardly captures the essence of a discipline that now contains extensive knowledge about physical activity used in a wide range of professions. Many names have been proposed for the discipline. Your department might be called "exercise and sport science," "kinesiology," "human performance," "health and human performance," "human movement science," or "physical education," to list only a few examples of the many names in existence today.

While none of these names is "wrong," most scholars emphasize the need for a single term broad enough to describe the entire discipline. Although not all scholars believe that *kinesiology* is the best descriptor (Locke, 1990; Siedentop, 1990), we believe that it is, not only because the term has been adopted by a growing number of departments at prestigious universities, but also because it best characterizes a discipline that deals with many different forms of physical activity in many different professional settings. (We recognize that "kinesiology" is sometimes applied more narrowly to the subdiscipline called "biomechanics"; see chapter 11.)

Support for the label *kinesiology* has come from the American Academy of Physical Education, an honorary society of approximately 120 scholars. The nearly 70-year-old academy undertook a two-year study of the matter in 1990 and decided that the name of the organization should be changed to the American Academy of Kinesiology and Physical Education. So, regardless of the name of the department in which you are enrolled, you are encouraged to refer to the discipline as kinesiology.

The Holistic Nature of Kinesiology

When you complete this introductory study of kinesiology, we hope you will be convinced of the holistic nature of physical activity. **Holism** is a characteristic of humanity that underscores the interdependence and interrelatedness of mind, emotions, body, and spirit. Although it is quite common for people to think of kinesiology as a discipline that deals exclusively with body movement, in reality physical activity involves our minds, emotions, and souls every bit as much as our bodies. We find it convenient to speak of *physical* activity because the physical aspects are readily observable, but in reality it could also be defined as *cognitive* activity, *emotional* activity, and even *soul* activity. Thus, studying kinesiology will take you far beyond the study of the biological aspects of physical activity. It includes an analysis of the psychological antecedents and outcomes of sport and exercise; the sociological, philosophical, and historical foundations of physical activity; the dynamics of skill development, performance, and learning; and the human processes involved in the teaching and learning of physical activity.

Think about the last time you went for a run or a brisk walk. First, you may have stretched a bit to warm up your muscles and started slowly as your body continued to warm up. You probably realize that you didn't have to think that much about controlling the muscles involved (except when that dog chased you). Like most well-learned skills, your muscle contractions occurred almost automatically, as did the increase in your heart rate, the depth and frequency of your breathing, and the onset of perspiration. Of course, you were able to direct your attention to your running form when you wanted to, adjusting the length or frequency of your stride or altering your posture. You also could enjoy the scenery you passed, the calmness of a lake, the beauty of a mountain trail. And, if you're like most runners, you may have simply let your mind wander, solving problems, thinking of the day ahead of or behind you, or dreaming dreams.

In fact, most people find physical activities such as running or walking so easy that they rarely think about the marvelous human capacities that allow us to perform them. It's easy to forget how wonderfully complex the human body is. If you continue with your studies in kinesiology, you'll study anatomy and physiology along with advanced courses in exercise physiology, biomechanics, sport and exercise psychology, and motor behavior. These will help you understand and appreciate the many mechanisms and systems that enable our bodies to perform physical activity.

Also, through your studies in philosophy of physical activity you will come to appreciate the holistic nature of human beings and how impossible it is to separate our bodies from "ourselves." Although it is easier to talk about our bodies or body parts such as the heart, muscles, or bones as though they are machines or instruments that our minds or souls "use" to achieve our purposes, they actually are part and parcel of our human-

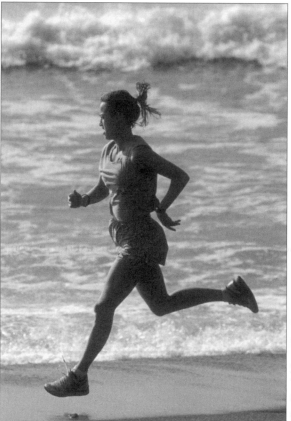

© Tom Devol / Gnass Photo Images

Although body movement is the core focus of kinesiology, the discipline also recognizes the holistic nature of humans.

ity. Regardless of the analogies we use to describe or refer to our bodies, we should never lose track of this important point.

🔑 Although kinesiology most often focuses on the bodily aspects of physical activity, it is important to remember that human beings are holistic creatures with interrelated cognitions, emotions, body, and soul.

The Active Body

Having said this, a good way to launch our study is to focus on the most obvious aspects of physical activity by reviewing briefly the amazing role our bodies play in enabling and supporting physical activity.

The Framework

Movement begins with the skeleton (see figure 1.4), a tower of bones put together with hinges and ball joints, so superbly rigged and balanced that humans can run 100 meters (109 yd) in less than 10 seconds; swim the English Channel; high jump over 2.4 meters (8 ft); and perform such amazing feats as jumping into the air, spinning three times, and landing on a quarter-inch-wide skate blade as they dance on the ice to Vivaldi's *Four Seasons*.

Our bodies have 206 bones that anchor our muscles and protect our vital organs (for example, the cranium covers our brain and the ribs shield our heart and lungs). Movement occurs at the joints where muscles and tendons exert their considerable forces. At the center of our structure is the vertebral column, made up of 25 bones that support our upright carriage and enable us to stand, walk, run, sit, and engage in all large-muscle movements. To get a glimpse of the complexity of your skeletal structure, examine one of its most intricate systems—your hands. They are an engineering marvel unmatched by most machines. Each contains 27 bones including an opposable thumb that gives us the dexterity required to use tools such as pliers, hammers, and screwdrivers; to perform brain surgery; or to play the piano. Your entire skeleton shows this same careful attention to detail that allows your bones

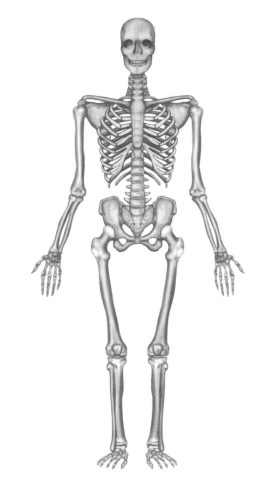

Figure 1.4 Movement occurs at the joints, which connect the 206 bones of the human skeleton.

and joints to work together to achieve a vast array of movements.

The Power

Movement is produced when a selected number of the over 600 muscles constituting 40% of your body weight shorten, thereby exerting a pull on the bones to which they are connected (see figure 1.5). When muscles contract, muscles on the reverse sides of the joints involved must relax if movement is to be produced. (Try contracting the muscles on the front side of your upper arm and the back side at the same time and you'll see how impossible it is to move without one side giving in to the forces generated on the other side.) To complicate matters even further, muscles usually do not produce movements by working individually, but rather by participating with as many as 20 or 30 other muscles, all contracting at just the right levels of force, and at just the right time, to pull on bones at just the right angle and for just the right duration to complete the intended movement.

The force that muscles are capable of generating is truly amazing. The world record for the clean and jerk (the "clean" is lifting a bar from the floor to the waist, and the "jerk" is pushing it overhead) is *three times* the lifter's body weight (Guinness Book of Records, 1999)! Equally amazing is the fact that muscles can continue to contract over a long period of time without fatiguing. For how long? Consider this: The world record for push-ups in a 24-hour period is 46,001 (Guinness Book of Records, 1999)! That's a long time for the triceps and other muscles of the back and chest to continue to work. But equally impressive is the ability of our muscles to contract in ways that permit us to perform precise and delicate movements, often at very high rates of speed. That a pianist can play as many as 20 notes

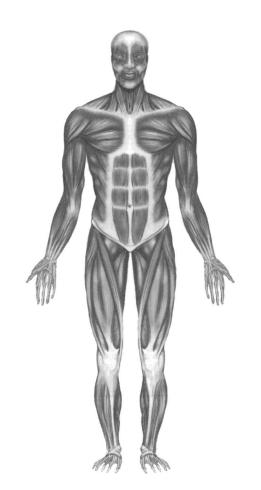

Figure 1.5   The human body has over 600 muscles that make up more than 40% of its total weight.

a second, striking precisely the correct keys with varying levels of force to interpret the musical score, is just as amazing as the human capacity to perform thousands of push-ups.

Physical activity is produced by the systematic contraction of muscles that exert forces on bones causing them to move in desired sequences and directions.

The Engine

The human heart performs like a pump that moves blood through an incredible pipeline that extends over 96,561 kilometers (60,000 mi), including microscopic capillaries. The heart beats about 100,000 times each day, pumping the 4.73 liters (10 pints) of blood in the average adult body through more than 1,000 complete circuits of the body. This circulatory system (see figure 1.6) is responsible for fueling the muscles and removing carbon dioxide and lactic acid (the by-products of energy production in the muscles). It also helps keep the body from overheating during physical activity, much like the water circulating around your car's engine keeps it from getting too hot.

Athletes who compete in endurance activities (e.g., marathons, cross-country races) develop very efficient circulatory systems. Whereas the resting heart rate of an untrained young adult is about 70 to 80 beats per minute (bpm), trained endurance athletes may have resting heart rates of 28 to 40 bpm. With training, the volume of blood pumped per beat can increase from between 80 and 110 milliliters to between 160 and 200 milliliters during maximal exercise; the amount of oxygen that is diffused into the blood can increase as much as three times (Wilmore & Costill, 1999). As our bodies become more active, the blood is automatically redistributed away from inactive body parts to those that really need it. For example, at rest 15% to 20% of the blood goes to the muscles; during exercise, the percentage rises to 80% or 85% (Wilmore & Costill, 1999).

The Energy

Our bodies need energy to fuel our muscles and maintain all of our other body systems (see figure 1.7). Energy production is the primary func-

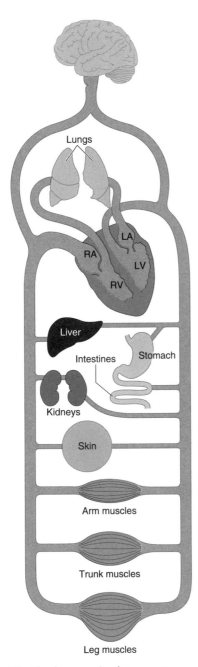

Figure 1.6 The human circulatory system moves blood completely through the body over 1,000 times each day.

tion of our viscera, the neatly packed organs of the respiratory, digestive, and urinary systems that fill our chest and abdominal cavities.

Energy comes from ingested food transformed by the digestive system into chemical energy through a complex metabolic process requiring oxygen (which comes from the respiratory system) for its completion. The primary source of energy for muscles is in the form of glycogen, a carbohydrate that the muscles store in limited quantities and which must be replaced if activity is maintained for a long time.

The minimally active person eats and uses about 2,000 calories per day; athletes who train at high levels typically consume 3,000 to 4,000 calories per day (see figure 1.8). These excessive calories are used to fuel the extraordinarily high level of physical activity required by training regimens. The recommended diet, for both active and inactive people, consists of 55% carbohydrates, 30% fat, and 15% protein. Complex carbohydrates, such as those found in pasta or potatoes, are widely considered to be the best fuel for people who engage in regular, vigorous physical activity. One of the pressing health problems in industrially developed countries is excessive consumption of calories and fat, coupled with physically inactive lifestyles.

Physical activity is made possible by the action of the heart as it moves blood through the circulatory system and by metabolic processes that convert food into energy.

The Control

The command center for movement is the nervous system, made up of the brain, the spinal cord, and a complex network of peripheral nerves (see figure 1.9). The nervous system coordinates all of the body's activities in response to signals from inside and outside the body. In the larger nerves, those signals can be transmitted at 500 impulses per second and travel at 100 meters (330 ft) per second.

When you move, whether it is to turn the pages of this book, play the saxophone, or water-ski, the action begins with a burst of electrical activity in your cerebral cortex. The command center in the front part of your cortex forms a plan for the movement. The plan is relayed to the motor center in your cerebellum where a final plan of action is determined taking into account the feedback from the various limbs about the movement that already is in progress. The plan is then put into action while signals are constantly returned to the command center to keep it informed about how the movements are progressing.

All of this happens at incredible speed. When a sprinter is set in the blocks, it takes 0.03 seconds for the sound of the gun to reach the

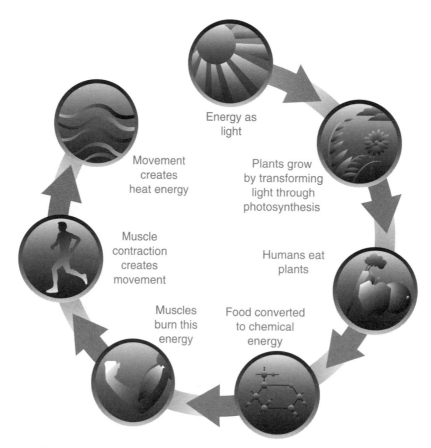

Figure 1.7   How energy for human movement is produced.

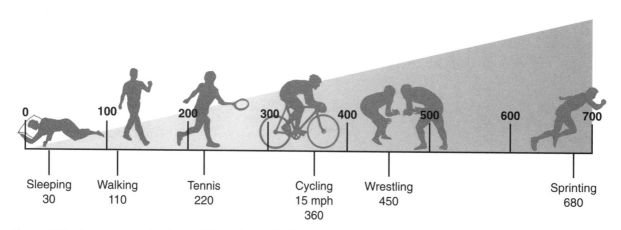

Figure 1.8   Energy expended by a 178-centimeter (5-ft, 10-in), 73-kilogram (160-lb) adult male in kilocalories per 30 minutes of exercise.

Data from Sharkey, B.J., 1997, *Fitness and health*, 4th ed., Champaign, IL: Human Kinetics, pp. 239-241.

runner's ears. In 0.01 seconds the ears transform the sound waves into nerve signals relayed to the cerebral cortex. The motor plan for the sprinter to blast out of the blocks is completed in 0.02 seconds, and the signal is sent to the leg muscles in another 0.02 seconds. The muscles explode to propel the sprinter forward in yet another 0.02 seconds. In total, it takes about one-tenth of a second for the sprinter to respond to the sound of the starting pistol.

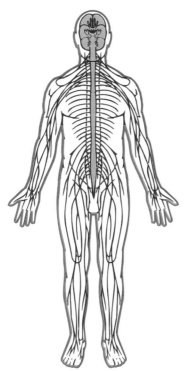

Figure 1.9 The human nervous system is made up of the brain, spinal cord, and a complex network of nerves.

🔑 Control of the action of the muscles is maintained by higher centers in the brain, although lower brain centers and the spinal cord facilitate the coordination of sensory input and motor output to produce skilled movement.

Anyone who aims at a career in the physical activity professions should know the basic facts about how the human body performs and responds to various types of physical activity. Much of your undergraduate program of studies in kinesiology will focus on this, and for good reason. But as we have noted, kinesiology is a holistic discipline that includes knowledge far beyond the physiological processes associated with movement. *Indeed, it may not be an exaggeration to say that no other discipline is so diverse in its aims, so interdisciplinary in its subject matter, or so complex in its organization.*

The three-dimensional analysis of physical activity offered in this book—experience, study, professional practice—is designed to help you organize your thinking about the discipline of kinesiology and the broader field of physical ac-

tivity. Not only will it help you develop a framework for understanding physical activity and the physical activity professions, but it will also help you understand the basis for your course work in kinesiology and assist you in planning and implementing career goals. Let's look briefly at each of the three dimensions.

Experiencing Physical Activity

By this point in your life, you have had literally millions of physical activity experiences (figure 1.10). You've learned to master thousands of complex motor skills including tying your shoelaces, brushing your teeth, driving your car, playing Frisbee, and maybe performing cartwheels. Many of these forms of physical activity are absolutely essential to living your life. Others, such as sports and leisure time pursuits, are discretionary—you choose to do them because they are fun. All of them offer the potential to teach you something about physical activity, yourself, and the world around you.

We *experience* physical activity when we perform it or watch it. Inevitably, performing or watching generates very personal sensations, emotions, thoughts, and feelings. Watching an Olympic gymnastics championship is likely to

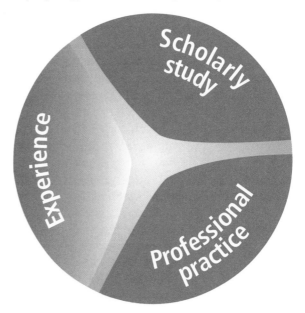

Figure 1.10 Experience and the other two sources of kinesiology knowledge.

Inventory of Personal Experiences With Physical Activity

1. What physical activity that you perform regularly requires the most skill?
2. What sport do you most enjoy performing?
3. What is the hardest physical work you have ever done?
4. What sport do you most enjoy watching?
5. What is the most dangerous physical activity you have ever performed?
6. What is the longest distance you have run?
7. What physical activity would you most like to learn to perform well?
8. What physical activity have you performed that you never want to perform again?
9. Briefly describe the emotion(s) you most commonly experience when doing exercise.
10. What have you learned about yourself as a result of performing your favorite physical activity?

produce very different feelings than watching a dance performance or a football game; digging a ditch is likely to induce different feelings than swinging a golf club. Precisely how we experience physical activity depends on the nature of the activity itself, the context in which it is performed, and our own peculiar sets of attitudes and past experiences.

Our past experiences have a significant influence on the meanings we attach to particular physical activities. They also influence our future decisions about engaging in a particular activity again. Obviously, some types of physical activity, such as those required in our work or those required to eat and maintain our personal hygiene, must be performed whether or not we enjoy them. But beyond this we have a great deal of discretion concerning which activities we will perform, with whom, under what conditions, and for how long. Ultimately, our decisions about such things as whether to spend our leisure moments playing basketball or playing hockey, running 5 miles or swimming 50 laps, taking the elevator or the stairs, mowing the yard or hiring someone else to do it, and seeking out physical activity or living the life of a couch potato will depend largely on the personal meanings we attach to physical activity experiences.

While classrooms, laboratories, and libraries offer kinesiological knowledge, direct participation in physical activity is an important source of

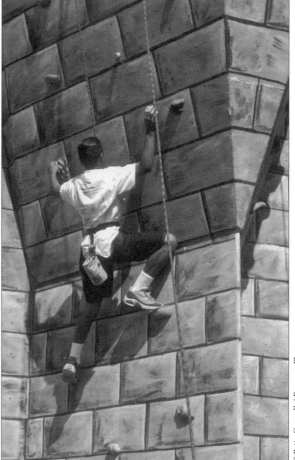

Direct participation in physical activity is an important source of kinesiological knowledge.

© Betty Crowell / Faraway Places

knowledge as well. By incorporating participation in physical activity as part of the formal course work, faculty in kinesiology departments add experiential knowledge to the overall body of knowledge that comprises the discipline of kinesiology.

When we participate in physical activities as part of the course work in kinesiology, we learn not only about the particular physical activities in which we're involved, but also about ourselves (and often others around us) as moving human beings. Climbing a rock face, skating on a frozen pond, or lifting weights can be the unique means by which we gain a greater understanding of how the activity is performed, knowledge of our own capacities and limitations, and knowledge about those around us. And performing certain types of physical activities such as surfing, hiking, or long-distance running offer unique opportunities for reflective and meditative thought not normally available in other aspects of our lives.

The Spheres of Physical Activity Experience

For most of us, physical activity has become such an ordinary aspect of our lives that we fail to recognize how often it intersects with our everyday experiences. We depend on physical activity when we work, play, cook our meals, drive our cars, type reports, or sign our names. As a student of kinesiology, it is very important that you understand the place of physical activity in each sphere or category of your life experiences. In this book, we refer to these various aspects of our everyday lives in which physical activity plays a distinct role as the spheres of physical activity experience (see figure 1.11).

We experience physical activity in a variety of spheres of our personal lives. Each opportunity to perform or watch physical activity represents a unique opportunity to learn about physical activity and our own (and sometimes others') interests and capacities and the meanings we attach to the activities.

Studying Physical Activity

Interest in formally studying and learning about physical activity (figure 1.12) is at an all-time peak that shows every indication of continuing well into the future. About 600 colleges and universities in the United States, and many more in other countries, have academic programs devoted to the study of physical activity. In addition, unknown numbers of institutes and centers outside of academe—from medical complexes, to military and space research programs, to industrial engineering centers—explore the various dimensions of physical activity. And judging from the numbers of books on sports, exercise, and fitness flooding popular bookstores, laypeople also have a keen interest in studying physical activity.

Faculty who design formal programs of study in colleges and universities pride themselves on organizing knowledge in ways that promote the fullest understanding. But, since physical activity is such a pervasive phenomenon—almost as

Self-Discovery

One way humans use physical activity to learn about themselves is to test their physical limits by attempting to improve upon records set by others. For example, it was long believed that people could not free dive (without assisted-breathing apparatuses) deeper than 30.5 meters (100 ft), but in 1956 two Italian divers set a record of 40.8 meters (134 ft). Twelve years later this record was shattered with a dive of 75 meters (247 ft) by Robert Croft, a U.S. Navy diver. Then, in the mid-1980s the record was shattered again by Jacques Mayol who dove to 109.7 meters (360 ft). And in 1996 Francisco Ferreras of Cuba stunned the diving world with a record-breaking 130-meter (428-ft) dive, an incredible feat given that Ferreras's body had to withstand 160 pounds of pressure per square inch—a total weight on his body in excess of 100 tons!

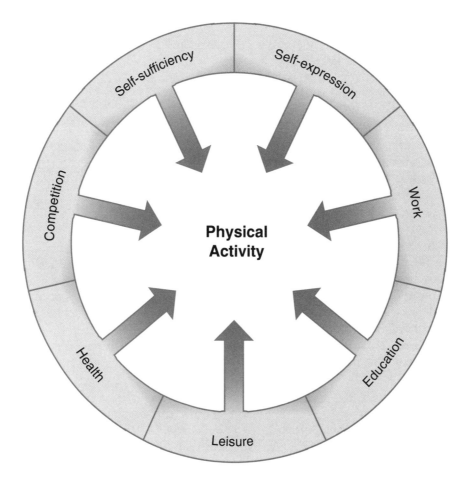

Figure 1.11   The spheres of physical activity experience. Physical activity plays an important role in every major sphere of our lives.

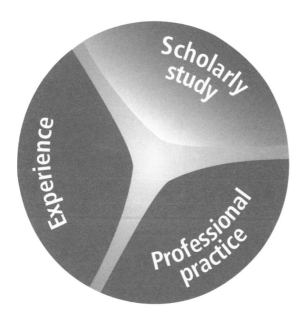

Figure 1.12   Scholarly study and the other two sources of kinesiology knowledge.

pervasive as human nature itself—it hasn't been easy for kinesiologists to organize knowledge about this phenomenon around a single framework that will help us study it systematically. In fact, debates continue about how the discipline of kinesiology should be organized (Newell, 1990b).

For the present, scholars have been content to divide the scholarly study of kinesiology into a number of subdisciplines. Each subdiscipline concentrates on the relationship of physical activity to some larger, older, and more established discipline such as psychology, physiology, sociology, biology, history, or philosophy. For instance, exercise physiology draws on basic concepts and theories from physiology, motor behavior draws on psychology, and philosophy of physical activity draws on philosophy. This means that kinesiology students must develop a working knowledge of the language and theo-

Growth of Interest in the Scholarly Study of Physical Activity

At least 10,000 scholars around the world study physical activity, either on a part- or full-time basis, spending an estimated $80 to $100 million annually to acquire knowledge in the field. The growth of interest in the scholarly study of physical activity can be seen in the increase in scholarly journals and academic societies over the last 35 years (see figure 1.13).

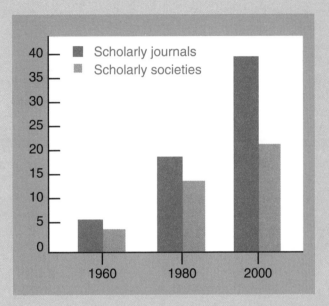

Figure 1.13   The increase in scholarly journals and scholarly societies in the physical activity field from 1960.

ries of a number of major disciplines and learn to apply them to physical activity. This, you will find, represents a formidable challenge!

Over the past four decades, the subdisciplines have developed into specialized areas of study, each with its own place in undergraduate and graduate curriculums in kinesiology, its own academic and professional societies, and its own scholarly journals. For example, members of the Association for the Advancement of Applied Sport Psychology meet annually to hear the latest research reports about the psychological aspects of sport and exercise. They keep abreast of developments in this subdiscipline by reading *The Sport Psychologist*, a journal devoted to applied psychological research in sport psychology, or the *Journal of Sport and Exercise Psychology*, a journal about more theoretical aspects of the subdiscipline. Many kinesiology departments now offer master's degrees and doctoral degrees in sport and exercise psychology. This same pattern

of specialization can be seen for exercise physiology, biomechanics, pedagogy of physical activity, motor learning and control, sociology of physical activity, history of physical activity, and philosophy of physical activity.

Most kinesiology professors have received in-depth education in one or two subdisciplines rather than in all of them. Your professors, for example, may identify themselves as biomechanists, exercise and sport psychologists, exercise physiologists, or some other title denoting their special expertise. This process of specialization has advanced our knowledge of kinesiology by permitting researchers/scholars to focus on very specific aspects of physical activity. The disadvantage is that communication among kinesiologists from the different subdisciplines is not always easy. Sometimes this hinders efforts to integrate all of the different kinds of knowledge and apply them to professional practice.

The Spheres of Scholarly Study of Physical Activity

Figure 1.14 shows the subdisciplines of kinesiology grouped into three general **spheres of scholarly study**: the sociocultural sphere, the behavioral sphere, and the biophysical sphere. Each sphere contains two or three subdisciplines. The subdisciplines are grouped into spheres on the basis of the types of research questions that are asked by scholars in the subdisciplines as well as the methods and techniques used to study physical activity. Subdisciplines within each sphere also tend to draw on concepts and theories from the same disciplines such as psychology, biology, or sociology. Knowing how these subdisciplines are related to each other and to the overall body of knowledge of kinesiology will help you understand their role and importance in your kinesiology curriculum.

The subdisciplines that have been included in the spheres are those that are most dominant right now. Because kinesiology is a dynamic discipline that is expanding rapidly, the subdisciplines that comprise it will likely expand also. In fact, some have already moved toward dividing into smaller, more specialized subfields. Biomechanics, for example, could be further separated into anatomical biomechanics and sport biomechanics. Sport psychology and exercise psychology are developing into separate subdisciplines. And exercise physiology, the oldest of the subdisciplines, may divide into such areas as sport physiology, work physiology, exercise epidemiology, exercise and nutrition, and others. This expansion of the boundaries of scholarly knowledge and the increased specialization that follows likely will continue for many years. This, of course, underscores the need for kinesiologists and physical activity professionals to continue to work to stay abreast of knowledge contained in the spheres of scholarly study.

In many departments, each subdiscipline is represented in the curriculum by a separate course (e.g., sport history, sport psychology, or

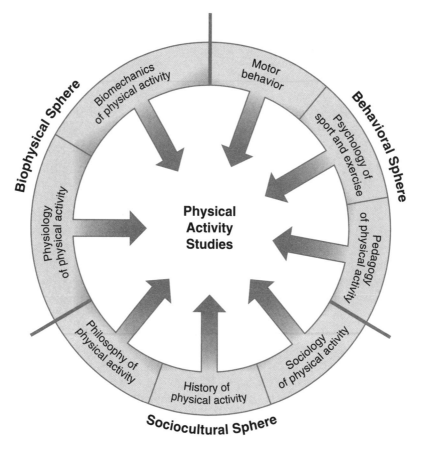

Figure 1.14   The spheres of scholarly study of physical activity.

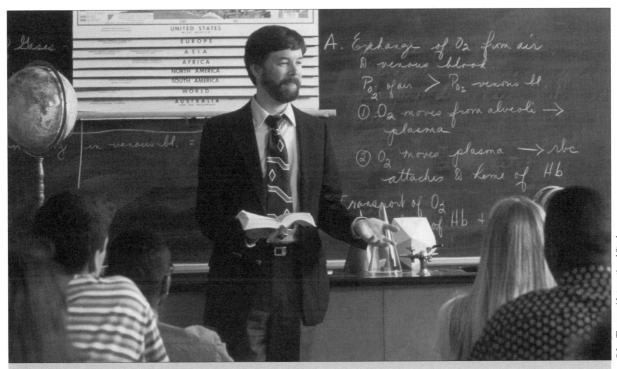

Kinesiology courses may be sociocultural, behavioral, or biophysical in nature.

© Jay Thomas / International Stock

motor learning). In some cases two or more subdisciplines may be combined in one course. For example, the sociocultural sphere includes the study of history of physical activity, sociology of physical activity, and philosophy of physical activity. In your department these three subdisciplines may be taught in a single course, or a separate course may be allocated to each of them. As kinesiology continues to flex its muscles, and the knowledge base expands, the number of courses devoted to the scholarly study of physical activity will probably expand.

As you dig into the material in section 2 of this book, remember that the subdisciplines and spheres of scholarly knowledge are merely frameworks to help us study and organize our thinking about physical activity. Mastery of the knowledge in each subdiscipline will require you to think in slightly different ways, to master different theories, and to use different terminology. But keep in mind that breaking the discipline up into these "little pieces" can lead to fragmentation in our thinking about physical activity and cause us to forget that kinesiology is one unified body of knowledge. For the present, this method of organizing the scholarly study of kinesiology seems to be the best way to approach it. As the disci-

pline evolves, however, students and professors who are best able to make connections between facts, concepts, and principles drawn from different subdisciplines and different spheres of scholarly study will be in the best position to make significant contributions to the discipline.

It is important to add one final note about the spheres of scholarly study. You can see that the diagram in figure 1.14 includes pedagogy of physical activity as a subdiscipline under the behavioral sphere. *Pedagogy* may be defined as the art and science of teaching. **Pedagogy of physical activity** is a subdiscipline that involves studying the teaching and learning of physical activity, a type of professional practice that is given a great deal of attention in the field of physical activity. Although teaching is a form of professional practice (the third component we will be exploring), the knowledge that kinesiologists have gathered through their research about teaching and learning constitutes a subdiscipline in the behavioral sphere. It is knowledge generated and learned through scholarly effort. For this reason, we have included information about teaching and learning physical activities in section 2 (as an area of scholarly study) and also in section 3 (as a professional career) in this book.

Examining physical activity through research and logical, systematic analyses constitutes the scholarly study of physical activity. Our scholarly knowledge about physical activity has been organized into subdisciplines, each providing a unique perspective from which to view the dynamics and processes of physical activity.

Practicing a Physical Activity Profession

Tammy Lawson lives to dance and perform gymnastics; eventually she wants to own a dance and gymnastics studio. Lavell Treen wasn't a football star, but he so much enjoys the game that his professional goal is to become a coach at the college level. Yvonne Singer was on the varsity basketball team in high school, but she spent most of her junior year undergoing rehabilitation for a knee injury. Now she's interested in a career as an athletic trainer or physical therapist. Darrick Gavin was overweight and unfit until a friend interested him in weight training and bodybuilding. Now he's a fit and confident young man who would like to become a personal trainer to help others discover what he has learned. Jane Drein completed an undergraduate degree in business and has returned to school to complete a baccalaureate degree in kinesiology. She hopes to enter sport management and eventually become a college athletic director or manager of a major sport arena/stadium complex.

Like most college students, you probably didn't decide to enroll in college simply to learn about physical activity. You (and probably your parents) hope your studies and your degree will lead eventually to a job, preferably a job in the physical activity field. But you probably have many questions. What types of jobs are available to kinesiology graduates? What do these jobs entail? What are their requirements? Is special certification or a graduate degree required? What types of certifications are appropriate? What social environments surround the workplace? Does your personality suit you for some types of work better than others? Is this a profession you can be happy in for the rest of your

life? What does the job pay? These and many more questions face students exploring careers in physical activity.

Section 3 of this book introduces you to the third dimension of kinesiology—professional practice (see figure 1.15). Professional practice may be envisioned as a process of putting knowledge to work, a specific type of work performed by most of those who graduate from kinesiology programs.

When we engage in professional practice, we learn new things about providing physical activity services to the public. For example, if you become a physical education teacher, as you pursue your career you will probably learn a lot that you were never taught in college classes about how to work productively and collaboratively with other teachers in your school. This knowledge gained on the job is different from knowledge acquired through research, and it is also different from knowledge acquired through your own direct experiences performing or watching physical activity. Some of this on-the-job knowledge eventually gets incorporated into classes by college and university faculty, and when this happens it becomes part of the discipline of kinesiology.

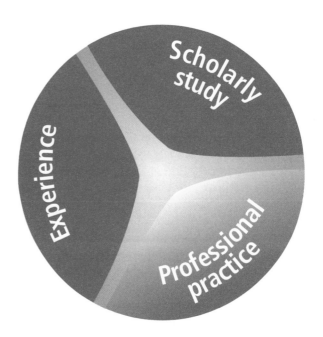

Figure 1.15 Professional practice and the other two sources of kinesiology knowledge.

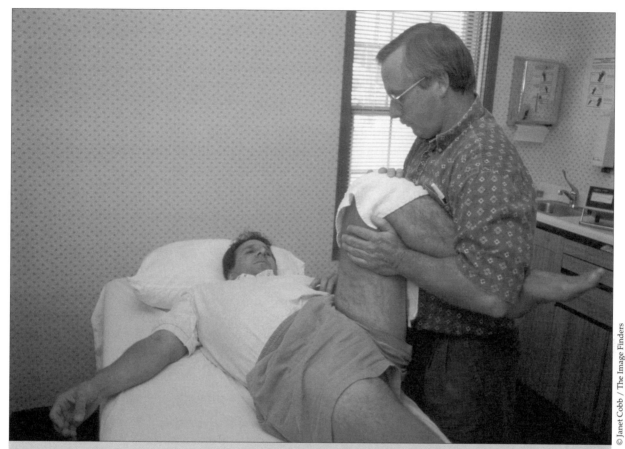

Graduates with kinesiology degrees are finding a wide range of career options open to them.

© Janet Cobb / The Image Finders

Becoming a Professional

Now let's turn to thinking about your career plans. One of the first decisions you will have to make is whether you really want to serve in a professional capacity. But what does it mean to be a professional? In chapter 13 you will learn that becoming a professional entails special responsibilities such as devoting yourself to serving others, giving priority to your clients' needs and interests, performing your duties in an ethical manner, and keeping abreast of developments in your field to ensure that your decisions are based on the best available evidence. Whereas those who specialize in scholarly study focus on knowledge and how to communicate it effectively to others, those who specialize in professional practice focus on enhancing the lives of those they serve.

Not all types of work qualify as professions. Truck drivers, small business owners, hairstylists, or television repairpeople are not profession-

als. This is primarily because the educational qualifications required to do the work do not involve mastery of a complex body of knowledge. In chapter 13 you will see how various types of work can be located on a continuum from strictly nonprofessional (e.g., common laborer) to strictly professional (e.g., surgeon). Most types of work are located between these two extremes. More important, you will learn about the expectations society holds for professionals, and you will be given an opportunity to decide whether you really want to pursue a professional career.

Careers in the Physical Activity Field

Once you have made a commitment to becoming a physical activity professional, *you* must take primary responsibility for developing your career. A career is a lifelong pursuit that may move through various stages as you progress from one type of employment to another. For example, a career in the teaching profession may begin at the public school level and wind up at the community college or university level. Or an entire teaching career may be spent at one institution. A career in the fitness industry may take you from a position as a personal trainer at a local commercial center, to a position in a corporate fitness program, and ultimately to the position of director of a hospital-linked wellness center. Career counselors now predict that young people graduating from college, on average, will change careers up to four times throughout their life spans. Of course, where you *finish* your career is not a pressing issue at this time. Getting a *good start* on a career is.

The Spheres of Professional Practice in Physical Activity

One of the exciting aspects of kinesiology is the diverse range of careers that may be developed from a solid undergraduate education. Unlike your friends who may be enrolled in education, nursing, or accounting programs that offer training tailored to specific careers, a degree in kinesiology offers many options. Figure 1.16 lists a number of different professions that often have their roots in a kinesiology degree. Obviously, each of these may have specialized requirements *within* a kinesiology curriculum, but all can be viewed as professional applications of kinesiology. Each of these various occupations can be assigned to one of the spheres of professional practice in physical activity displayed in figure 1.17.

Section 3 of this book not only provides you with information concerning these professions, but it will also help you get a start toward making yourself marketable as a professional. From this point forward in your college experience, you need to realize that you are involved in a competition. Whether you like to compete or not, you will be competing for grades on exams, papers,

Health and Fitness Promotion

Program Director of Corporate Fitness Center

Fitness Instructor or Program Director at Commercial Fitness Center

Personal Trainer—Private Practice

Exercise Leader/Nutrition Consultant at Weight Control Center

Exercise Leader/Consultant at Wellness/Disease Prevention Center

Exercise and Wellness Coordinator at Geriatric Center

Stress Management Clinic—Exercise and Stress Management Consultant

Exercise Physiologist—Various Exercise-Related Clinics and Programs

Fitness Programmer at YMCA, YWCA

Therapeutic Exercise

Athletic Trainer

Occupational Therapist

Physical Therapist

Cardiac Rehabilitation Specialist

Exercise Therapist at Orthopedic Clinic

Instruction

Sports Director at Resort

Professional Golf Instructor

Professional Ski Instructor

Professional Tennis Instructor

Professional Swimming Instructor

Varsity Coach at School or College

Physical Education Teacher at School or College

Adapted Physical Education Teacher

Strength and Conditioning Coach

Sport Psychologist/Performance Enhancement

Sport Management

Director of Youth Sport Programs

Director of Youth Camps

Leader in Community Recreation Program

Athletic Administration in School or College

Front Office Administration in Professional or Semi-Pro Sports

Sports Marketing

Sports Promotion, Information, and Media

Sports Officiating

Aquatics Director

Sports Facility Supervisor

Scholarly Study

Research Scientist in Human Performance Lab

Professor of Exercise Physiology

Professor of Sport History

Professor of Exercise and Sport Psychology

Figure 1.16   Possible careers in the physical activity professions.

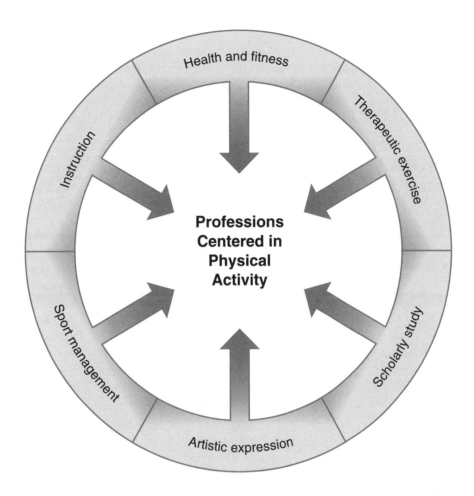

Figure 1.17   The spheres of professional practice centered in physical activity.

and projects. And when you graduate, you will continue to compete, vying with other kinesiology graduates for professional positions. In many ways, this is the most important competition you will enter. How should you prepare for this? If you were preparing to compete for a world championship in the marathon, you probably would commit yourself totally to planning and implementing a strategic training program that offers you the best chances for achieving victory. If preparation is important for an athletic competition, how much more important is it for your lifelong career!

Throughout this book you will be reminded again and again of this important point: *You and only you are responsible for preparing yourself for your chosen career.* It is your academic department's responsibility to offer you a well-sequenced, relevant curriculum. It is your professor's responsibility to offer competent advisement and teach-

ing. But it is *your* responsibility to take advantage of these resources to develop yourself into the best professional possible. From this point on, view yourself as a preprofessional, one who is not simply taking courses or majoring in a subject, but rather one who is a professional-in-training.

To become a marketable, sought-after professional, you must make choices about your experiences on and off campus. Obviously, committing yourself to mastering the material of your course work is the first step, but it is only the first step. Hours spent outside of the classroom in professionally relevant voluntary service work or summer employment are also critical. As a preprofessional you should show an interest in your profession that goes beyond excelling in course work. Becoming a student member of professional physical activity organizations is one way to demonstrate this early commitment. In the chapters that follow, you will be encouraged to think on your own and act on behalf of your own educational and professional development. It is never too early to take these vital steps.

For most students, the goal of pursuing a degree in kinesiology is to obtain a job in a physical activity profession. Those who identify with a profession very early and diligently pursue their course work as well as professionally related experiences outside the classroom will be the top competitors for jobs in physical activity professions.

Wrap-Up

Having read this introduction, you are now ready to explore physical activity as a form of human experience, an object of scholarly study, and a focal point for a professional career. Take some time now to review the key points of this chapter to prepare yourself for what lies ahead.

In the sections that follow we will explore each dimension of the physical activity field in greater detail. Section 1 will help you to appreciate the importance of experiencing physical activity as a source of enjoyment; as a means to health, education, and rehabilitation; and as a necessary ingredient of our lives at play and work. Section 2 contains an overview of the major facts, concepts, and theories in the subdisciplines that together comprise knowledge gained from the scholarly study of physical activity. Each chapter is a "minicourse" on a separate subdiscipline. This should give you a solid orientation for the more in-depth study of these subdisciplines you will undertake later in your program. Finally, section 3 focuses on professional practice centered in physical activity. The goals of this section are to introduce you to the most prominent physical activity professions and to point out ways in which undergraduate course work in kinesiology connects to these.

Study Questions

1. What is the technical definition of physical activity? Of movement? Give an instance in which human movement does not meet the technical definition of physical activity.

2. What is meant when kinesiology is described as a "holistic" discipline?

3. What two forms of physical activity receive the most attention in kinesiology?

4. What are the three sources of knowledge of kinesiology?

5. What anatomical/physiological functions related to the active body are suggested by the following: "the power," "the framework," "the engine," "the energy," "the control"?

6. List the spheres of physical activity experience, and give an example of a physical activity in each sphere.

7. List the spheres of scholarly study and the subdisciplines contained in each.

8. List the spheres of professional practice centered in physical activity, and give an example of a career in the physical activity professions for each sphere.

Experiencing Physical Activity

In this section . . .

Is it more important to perform and experience physical activity, to study it, or to center a professional practice around it? While you may never have to answer such a tough question, a good case could be made that experiencing physical activity is indeed the most important. What good would it do to study physical activity or design a professional practice around it if nobody ever performed it? In most cases we study and conduct research on physical activity in order to improve the performance capabilities, health, and enjoyment of others—benefits obtainable only through actually performing physical activity. Experiencing physical activity is where "the rubber meets the road" in kinesiology.

But physical activity experience has many different dimensions. Consider how each of the following questions focuses on a distinct aspect of the term *experience*. Why are physical activity experiences important and in what aspects of our lives do they intersect? How have your experiences in physical activity affected the development of your skill, training, and physical fitness? How do your experiences in physical activity affect your thoughts of, emotions about, and general impressions of physical activity?

The chapters in this section will help you answer these three related, but separate, questions. The first question directs your attention to the experience of doing physical activity. To help you answer it, chapter 2 surveys many ways in which physical activity penetrates our daily lives. You will be introduced to the seven spheres of physical activity experience—distinct aspects of our lives in which physical activity plays an important role, usually with distinctive purposes in mind.

Reading and *studying* this chapter will help you develop a new level of respect for the role of physical activity in your daily life, even though you have been immersed in it from the time you were born. You may have decided to major in kinesiology because of a particular interest in sport or exercise. If so, you are to be congratulated for having narrowed down your choice of a career so early in the game. But even if you are particularly attracted to one particular type or form of physical activity, as a kinesiology major you are expected to be—first and foremost—a student of physical activity. This means that physical activity experiences in all of their forms should hold a particular fascination for you.

The second question points toward the cumulative effects of experience on your physical capabilities. Knowing how physical experience can be manipulated to bring about specific changes in performance capacity or health is the subject of chapter 3. This ability to manipulate physical activity experiences intelligently is a distinctly human capacity. Kinesiologists are "physical activity experience experts." They understand the connections between types and amounts of physical activity experiences and specific outcomes, whether the goal is the development of skillful movement (skill); improved health (physical fitness); improved strength, endurance, and flexibility (conditioning); or merely enjoyment. Knowing the most efficient, most effective, and safest way to achieve physical activity goals is the kinesiologist's stock-in-trade.

Knowing how physical activity experiences affect our skill, endurance, strength, flexibility, health, fitness, or enjoyment is one thing; knowing and appreciating their effects on our inner lives is just as important. Chapter 4 introduces you to this third dimension of experience. After reading and *studying* this chapter, you will understand that physical activity is not only a physical experience; it is just as much an emotional, cognitive, and spiritual experience. The ways in which physical activity affects our thoughts and feelings, how these feelings may affect our future physical activity choices, and how we derive knowledge and meaning through physical activity are all part of what we call subjective physical activity experience. All of our involvement in physical activity ultimately has a bearing on this subjective domain.

By nature, these subjective experiences are difficult to describe, and sometimes they affect us in very personal ways. Because of this we sometimes ignore this profound interior world of human experience, choosing instead to focus on observable dimensions of experience such as our time in a 6K race, how much weight we lost during an exercise program, how many points we scored, or our rate of recovery from an injury. After reading this chapter, you will probably wonder why we even refer to it as *physical* activity. Clearly, it is *human* activity in its broadest sense!

Physical activity experience is so prevalent in our lives that we tend to take it for granted. Yet it is the very foundation of the study of kinesiology. In this section we invite you to view physical activity experience from an entirely new perspective beginning with the seven spheres of physical activity experience.

2

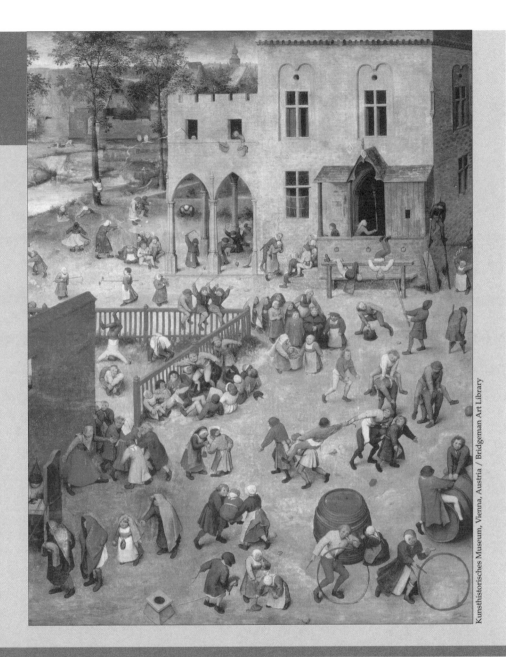

Kunsthistorisches Museum, Vienna, Austria / Bridgeman Art Library

The Spheres of Physical Activity Experience

Shirl J. Hoffman

In this chapter . . .

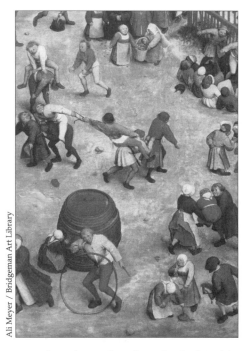

Ali Meyer / Bridgeman Art Library

Imagine that you are in a spaceship flying over planet earth and the technology on the craft enables you to see everybody on the face of the planet. As you look down, you see the village depicted in the painting in the opening photo. This painting is entitled *Children's Games,* and it was painted by the famous renaissance artist Pieter Brueghel. Although most of the people in the painting are engaged in various games, the scene shows a rich variety of physical activities and physical activity contexts. Can you find examples of each of the following in this painting?

- People performing physical activity as part of their normal daily lives
- People performing physical activity, either as a way of communicating or expressing emotions or personal feelings
- People performing physical activity in the context of work
- People performing physical activity as part of an educational experience
- People performing physical activity as a part of a leisure time experience
- People performing physical activity as a way of improving their health
- People competing in physical activities

You probably found it easy to identify physical activity being performed in the contexts of leisure and competition. In some cases physical activity appears in the context of work (women carrying a basket). And in many of the examples people are gesturing, and their body movements suggest that they are expressing their feelings through movement. Since

Brueghel's painting was about games, we do not see many people performing daily tasks, but we do see people simply walking—a form of physical activity done as part of our daily tasks. Do any of the activities appear to be carried out in the context of health maintenance and improvement? That depends on how vigorously each activity is performed. Perhaps you were more impressed by the fact that many of the activities seemed more likely to lead to bodily harm than health benefits!

How important is physical activity to your daily life? If you're like most people, you probably think seriously about the question only when your capacity for moving is limited due to disease or injury. For example, nothing makes us appreciate the importance of the ankle joint in walking quite like having a sprained ankle, or the importance of the thumb in grasping quite like having a broken thumb. Physical activity pervades our lives in thousands of ways and in countless forms and levels of intensity. Although kinesiologists traditionally have concerned themselves primarily with sport and exercise, they recognize that the field of physical activity and the boundaries of kinesiology extend beyond sport fields and fitness centers to the workplace, the rehabilitation center, the dance studio, and to many other activities we perform in everyday life.

This chapter is intended to get you thinking broadly about physical activity. It will lead you on an expedition of sorts through a vast expanse of different types of physical activities done for different reasons and in different settings. The purpose is to help you form a broad frame of reference for thinking about physical activity, and to help you understand how critically important the subject matter of kinesiology—physical activity—is to our daily lives.

 ## CHAPTER OBJECTIVES

In this chapter we will:

- Broaden your understanding of the universe of physical activities
- Familiarize you with the ways physical activity is experienced in different social compartments we call spheres
- Introduce you to some of the potential benefits and limitations of physical activity

One way to begin to appreciate the enormous variety of physical activities and the way they intersect your daily life is to ask yourself how often and in what ways you were physically active during the past week. To answer these questions you may first think about the various social situations you were in during the past week, and then the purposes served by physical activity in each situation. For example, you might think: I worked at the restaurant 20 hours last week. With this as a framework to guide your recall, you might then proceed to remember that you walked back and forth from tables to the kitchen approximately 200 times, poured approximately 400 cups of coffee, prepared 200 salads, and collected credit cards or made change at the cash register approximately 50 times. Or you might think: I played golf on Saturday. With the framework of playing golf to guide your thinking, you might recall that you walked about 4 miles and executed approximately 18 drives, 25 shots with mid-irons, 13 approach shots, and 30 putts.

The life experiences in which you perform physical activity tend to shape the purposes to be served by physical activity, which in turn determine the types and amount of physical activity in which you engage. This can serve as a convenient framework for surveying the importance of physical activity in your daily life. However, you can quickly become overwhelmed when you stop to think about the variety of your life experiences that are intersected by physical activity. For example, golf might be one context, work in the restaurant another, but during the week you also may have gone jogging, played tennis, worked at your second job at the local movie theater, brushed your teeth, walked to class, played the piano, typed at your computer, driven your car, or signed your name on a check. The purposes and contexts seem endless! Clearly, then, if we are to begin to get a handle on the importance of physical activity in our lives, some system of organizing our personal experiences with physical activity—some conceptual framework—is in order.

In chapter 1 we used the term *spheres of physical activity experience* as a way of classifying the different life experiences in which physical activity plays an important role (see figure 2.1). We defined spheres of physical activity experience as various dimensions of everyday life in which physical activity plays an important and distinctive role. Generally, the spheres identify different purposes for which we perform physical activity, usually, but not always, in different social contexts. For example, the work sphere includes all physical activity done in the workplace for the purpose of doing work. The education sphere includes physical activity that is carried out in educational settings, usually for the purpose of improving someone's capacity to perform physical activity.

Some spheres are less definitive in terms of social context. The self-sufficiency sphere, for example, includes physical activity carried out for the purpose of surviving and living an independent life. While most of these activities are carried out in the home, they also can be performed at work, at leisure, or in educational settings. Likewise, physical activity in the self-expression sphere may occur in a variety of social contexts, but always serves the purpose of allowing us to express our emotions.

Keep these three things in mind as you study the spheres:

1. The spheres are not intended to classify specific types of physical activities. Rather, they highlight the compartments or aspects of our life experiences in which physical activity plays an important part.

2. Some activities may be common to more than one sphere of experience. For example, if you run three miles each day, it may be something you do as part of the compartment of your life we call leisure (the leisure sphere), but the same activity may also be

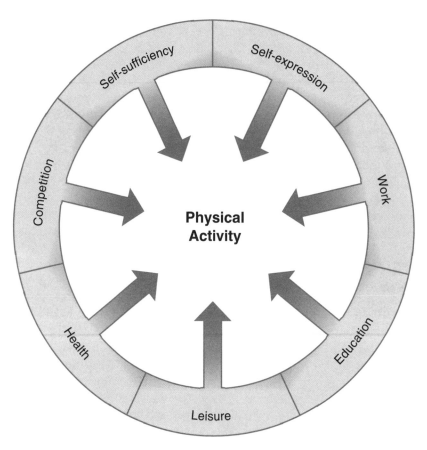

Figure 2.1 Spheres of physical activity experience.

part of your "health life" (the health sphere) or your "expressive life" (the self-expression sphere).

3. Remember, the purpose of this chapter is to provide you with a *general framework* for thinking about the importance and pervasiveness of physical activity in your life, not to compartmentalize the activities themselves.

In the sections that follow, we will explore each of the seven spheres of physical activity experience—self-sufficiency, self-expression, work, education, leisure, health, and competition—by defining them and examining some activities that comprise them. We will discuss both positive and negative issues related to the spheres and learn about professionals who specialize in addressing some of those issues. Keep in mind that these spheres serve merely to help you look at the many ways and contexts in which you experience physical activity. We hope this discussion will challenge you to think more deeply about the many levels of this field, levels that go far beyond the merely physical.

The Sphere of Self-Sufficiency

A significant part of our lives is devoted to taking care of ourselves, and physical activity is an important means by which we accomplish this (see figure 2.2). As you thought about the physical activities you engaged in last week, no doubt some of them were fairly menial tasks such as walking from your bed to the bathroom, feeding yourself, or brushing your teeth. Although menial, such tasks are absolutely critical to your ability to live independently or even survive. What would you do if you couldn't perform them? Obviously, you would be forced to rely on the help of others; you would have lost your self-sufficiency. You also may have thought of activities which, while not essential for your survival or independent living, do contribute to your self-sufficiency and personal comfort. These might include operating the vacuum cleaner, washing the dishes, ironing clothes, or washing your car.

Physical and occupational therapists work with people who, through injury or disease, have

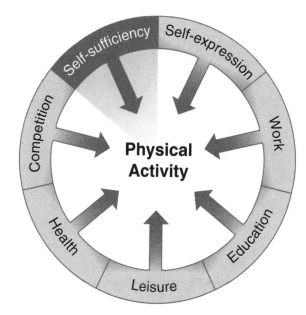

Figure 2.2 Self-sufficiency as a sphere of physical activity experience.

lost the ability to perform the important tasks of daily life. Typically, these therapists divide self-sufficient physical activity into two major categories: **activities of daily living (ADLs)** and **instrumental activities of daily living (IADLs)** (see table 2.1). The former includes more personal behaviors related to grooming, using the toilet, dressing, eating, or walking. People who require daily assistance in these tasks are usually disabled or frail as a result of age. Activities classified as IADLs include the less personal activities of telephoning, shopping, cooking, or doing laundry (Katz, Ford, Moskowitz, Jackson, & Jaffee, 1963). Generally, IADLs are more physically demanding than ADLs. Health insurance companies often use these classifications of physical activity in daily living to gauge the level of disability of patients and to determine the type of health support they require.

The physical activities we perform around our homes are often more complicated and demand more energy than typical ADLs and IADLs. Shoveling snow, fixing our automobiles, painting our apartments, repairing electrical fixtures, and similar tasks are examples of **home maintenance activities** that reflect our level of self-sufficiency. All require relatively high levels of energy or skill or both. Although many people hire others (e.g., gardeners, painters, automobile mechanics, plumbers) to perform home maintenance

TABLE 2.1
Examples of Activities of Daily Living (ADLs), Instrumental Activities of Daily Living (IADLs), and Home Maintenance Physical Activities

ADLs	IADLs	Home maintenance
Eating	Shopping	Painting house
Dressing	Cooking	Mowing lawn
Walking	Writing checks	Washing car
Using toilet	Washing clothes	Cleaning apartment

activities for them, the explosion of sales of do-it-yourself manuals and home improvement television shows suggests that more and more people are choosing to perform these household activities themselves. What home maintenance activity is most popular? Gardening. Nearly 30% of all adults over 18 years of age report having participated in gardening activities during the prior two weeks (U.S. Department of Health and Human Services [USDHHS], 1996).

🔑 In order to live functional, independent lives, we must perform ADLs and IADLs, the latter of which tend to be more physically demanding. We also become self-sufficient by performing physical activities intended to maintain or improve the home. These activities are called home maintenance activities.

Limitations in Self-Sufficiency Physical Activity

A variety of movements are required to carry out daily tasks such as housecleaning, doing laundry, bathing, cooking, opening jars, writing checks, and shopping for groceries. For example, using a vacuum cleaner includes the fundamental actions of walking, standing, grasping, reaching, pushing, and maintaining an upright posture. Remaining self-sufficient requires us to transport objects of different weights, ascend or descend stairways, or any number of fairly complex actions. When the movement systems that enable us to perform these activities are compromised through disease or injury, occupational and physical therapists are

often consulted to help people learn or relearn self-maintenance activities.

Before devising treatment plans or "interventions" for rehabilitating people with physical disabilities, physical and occupational therapists first must understand completely the physical activity requirements of each specific task. This usually requires a very thorough analysis of the movements a person must perform in order to carry out the task. Only then can the therapist decide which muscles need to be strengthened or movement patterns refined to restore the patient to self-sufficiency. These "activity analyses" can also help us to understand the amazing complexity of what at first may seem to be fairly simple tasks.

For example, an activity analysis of the relatively "simple" self-care task of standing up from a seated position, a major challenge to the victim of a cerebral stroke, reveals at least four critical phases: (1) the feet must be well placed on the floor in a position to receive weight evenly divided on both legs; (2) the trunk must be flexed forward at the waist while remaining extended; (3) the knees must move forward of the ankles; and finally, (4) the hips and knees must extend for final alignment (Carr & Shepherd, 1987).

🔑 Injury or disease can hinder a person's ability to perform daily physical activities. Physical therapists create therapeutic strategies based on activity analyses to help people recover their functioning within the limits of the disease or injury.

The illustration in figure 2.3 shows a stroke patient attempting to stand up from a seated position. Using the four-part analysis described earlier, the therapist can identify the patient's problem quickly. He is attempting to complete phase 4 (extend his knees for final alignment) before he has completed phases 2 and 3 (sufficiently flexed his trunk forward and moved his knees in front of his ankles). By skillfully matching the patient's movements against a model of correct performance, the therapist can design a training program to speed recovery in this ADL task.

Self-Sufficiency and Aging

You may not have given much thought to the importance of ADLs and IADLs in your life because you may have experienced little trouble performing them. But a substantial and growing proportion of the population require assistance in even these basic self-care tasks, a condition that deprives them of independence in their daily living. In 1990 an estimated 35 million people (one in every seven Americans) had a disabling condition that interfered with their performance of daily activities (LaPlante, 1990). These conditions were the result of such things as injury, chronic disease, congenital disability, and aging. Of these, the movement limitations associated with aging are a major focus of physical activity professionals because the population of aged people is growing rapidly. Currently, 13% of the population is 65 years of age or older, and it is anticipated to grow to 22% by 2030 (Howell, 1997).

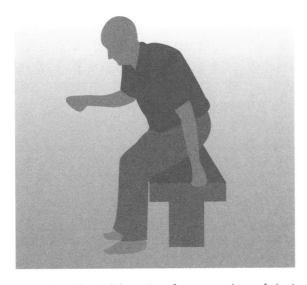

Figure 2.3 Physical therapists often use analyses of physical activity to help patients relearn basic skills.

Physical Activity Limitations Among the Elderly

It's difficult to exaggerate the severity of the problem of physical activity limitations in the elderly. Table 2.2 shows the percentage of adults reporting limitations in the performance of ADLs and IADLs. Impairments in ADLs range from 11.8% of the population of 55- to 64-year-olds to nearly 50% of the 85+ population! Among the very elderly, the large-muscle activities of bathing and dressing are most often impaired (21.7% and 13%, respectively), followed by moving (8.9%), toileting (8.2%), and eating (2.7%) (Dunkle, Kart, & Lockery, 1994). Twenty-four percent of adults aged 85 and older must have assistance in performing one or more of these ADLs (Cutler, 1994). Sixty percent of those 85 and older report limitations in performing IADLs.

Another fact evident from table 2.2 is that physical limitations are not shared equally across the spectrum of the elderly. Non-white, rural, elderly women earning less than $15,000 per year are most likely to report limitations. Thus, the effects of increasing age on physical activity can be traced to a number of critical social, as well as biological, factors.

Older people are often injured in their attempts to perform ADLs and IADLs. In fact, accidents suffered by the elderly account for 43% of all home fatalities. Common accidents include falling on stairways or in bathtubs or suffering burns or scalds. Most can be traced to movement limitations, but environmental factors such as poorly lit stairways, frayed rugs, and poorly maintained homes also play a part. Because older people realize that the risk of accidents around the home is high, many simply stop performing certain ADLs and IADLs. This results in a severely diminished quality of life (Czaja, 1997). When elders lose either the ability to perform self-care activities or confidence in their ability to perform them, it can be an emotionally devastating experience, depriving them of the satisfaction of being able to live up to their physical, mental, and emotional potential.

The prospects of a growing population of individuals who are dependent on others to carry out their daily tasks is also undesirable from an economic standpoint. When major segments of the population lose their ability to perform ADLs and IADLs, a heavy burden is placed on

TABLE 2.2
Percentage of Elderly Population Limited in ADLs and IADLs

	ADL* Number of limitations			IADL** Number of limitations		
	1	2+	Total	1	2+	Total
Age						
55–65	5.4	6.4	11.8	9.8	4.1	13.9
65–74	7.9	9.3	17.2	13.0	7.5	20.5
75–84	11.1	16.4	27.5	15.9	16.6	32.5
85+	12.7	36.8	49.5	14.9	44.8	59.5
Gender						
Male	7.6	8.6	16.2	7.5	6.0	13.5
Female	8.5	13.3	21.8	16.0	12.5	28.5
Family income						
< $15,000	10.7	14.8	25.5	16.5	13.2	29.7
> $15,000	5.6	7.5	13.1	9.3	6.3	15.6
Race						
White	8.0	11.0	19.0	12.5	9.5	22.0
Non-white	9.6	14.9	24.5	15.5	14.8	30.3
Residence						
City	8.5	12.2	20.7	12.7	11.2	23.9
Suburbs	7.1	9.8	16.9	11.3	8.7	20.0
Rural	9.0	12.5	21.5	14.3	10.3	24.6

*ADL includes bathing, dressing, getting into or out of bed or chair, walking, getting outside of the apartment or house, and eating.

**IADL includes preparing meals, shopping, managing money, using the telephone, and housework.

Adapted, by permission, from R.E. Dunkle, C.S. Kart, and S.A. Lockery, 1994, Self-caring. In *Functional performance in older adults*, edited by B.R. Bonder and M.B. Wagner (Philadelphia: F.A. Davis), 128.

the national health-care system. Although they account for only 13% of the population at present, the elderly account for 33% of health-care expenditures, largely because of their dependence on institutions (nursing homes) to provide self-care activities. Over the next 40 years nursing home costs are expected to increase from $84 to $134 billion (Kane, Ouslander, & Abrass, 1994).

These trends represent an awesome challenge to those in the physical activity profession who work with older populations. While an increase in the numbers of elderly people over the next few decades is inevitable, *an increase in the proportion of this population who are hampered by limitations of physical activity is not.* Many of those who suffer the most limitations in later years are those who failed to make physical activity a daily part of their normal lives—throughout their lives. Recreational activities and exercise programs designed and administered by physical activity professionals will play an increasingly larger role in preventing and rehabilitating these age-related disabilities.

Limitations in the performance of ADLs and IADLs among the elderly require them to depend on others or institutions to perform the tasks of daily living. This is a problem of great personal and economic importance.

Mobility and Driving Among the Elderly

Walking (mobility) is an especially important physical activity for the elderly since it forms the basis for many other ADLs and IADLs. Yet limitation in the ability to walk is one of the most pressing problems for the elderly (Dawson, Hendershot, & Fulton, 1987). Winograd and colleagues (1994) estimate that nearly 20% of people over the age of 65 have difficulty walking. In a sample of elders over age 85, more than 50% of women and 33% of men reported difficulty walking up ten steps.

Of course, in industrialized countries being fully mobile involves more than simply being able to walk. Being able to drive is a skill that is taken for granted in the modern age. Driving is essential to such IADLs as shopping, visiting the doctor, attending church, and visiting friends. Driving places heavy demands on both the perceptual and motor systems, therefore the declines in physical capacity that typically come with aging can make operating a vehicle a challenging physical activity.

Because the elderly are reluctant to give up their licenses, the average age of older drivers has increased from 65 to 69 years of age (Barr, 1991). In fact, older drivers represent the fastest growing segment of the population of drivers both in terms of the number of drivers and miles driven annually per year (Transportation Research Board, 1988). You won't be surprised to learn that this translates into a fairly high rate of driving accidents and fatalities for the elderly. Although older drivers do not have a disproportionately higher number of car accidents than the population of licensed drivers at large, they clearly have many more accidents *per mile driven*. In terms of miles driven, car accidents are the lowest among people in their late 20s until their mid-50s, but they increase sharply thereafter as a function of

age (Williams & Carsten, 1989). The consequences are serious. Although driving fatalities among the population of licensed drivers fell 20% during the 1980s, fatalities among older drivers rose 18% (Barr, 1991). Adding to the problem is the fact that older drivers are much more vulnerable to the trauma of a car crash than younger drivers. The seat belt that so effectively restrains a younger driver can fracture a rib, puncture a lung, or cause the death of a frail older driver.

Does this higher accident rate have anything to do with the declines in the capacity for physical activity in the elderly? Yes it does. Obviously, the ability to process visual information is also important in driving, and aging tends to bring declines in our ability to do this as well. For example, the "useful field of view" (UFOV)—the visual information a driver can effectively monitor during a single glance—is known to be a predictor of driving success, and UFOV tends to decline with age (Owsley, Ball, Sloane, Roenker, & Bruni, 1991), along with acuity under reduced illumination, motion perception, and dynamic visual acuity (Shinar & Schieber, 1991). These problems are compounded by the fact that older drivers tend not to notice that their vision is impaired and continue to drive until these problems are called to their attention by their physicians.

But declines in the capability for physical activity—especially the ability to perform the correct movement at the correct time—is also responsible for increased accidents among the elderly. Laboratory tests have shown older people to be slower at selecting and initiating a response to a stimulus, and to be at an even greater disadvantage when the complexity of the task increases. Older people move more slowly once a decision has been made to move, and they move with less force, putting them at a disadvantage when an abrupt stop is necessary. Furthermore, limitation in range of joint movement, a common impairment of the elderly, can put them at a disadvantage, particularly in performing such important actions as scanning mirrors and turning the head to monitor blind spots they can't see at the rear and side (Stelmach & Nahom, 1992).

Will physical activity programs help older drivers to forestall some of these deteriorating effects? Happily, some research suggests that declines in reaction time and movement time can be checked by practice, and that performance of activities that require rapid initiation and termination of movements, such as those required in driving a car, can be improved through exercise (Salthouse, 1988; Spirduso, MacRae, MacRae, Prewitt, & Osborne, 1988). Perhaps the full contribution of kinesiologists to the improved safety of elder drivers has yet to be investigated.

🔑 Driving a car involves integrating visual information with motor responses, a process known to deteriorate progressively among adults beyond the age of 55. The result is that deaths due to highway accidents are more common in this age category than in younger age groups. Evidence suggests that training programs may help forestall the deterioration in driving performance.

The Sphere of Self-Expression

The urge to express our inner feelings is one of the most basic human instincts. All of us would like to demonstrate, in one way or another, what is unique about us, what makes us special. Obviously, we are limited in the ways we can do this. People often hesitate to express themselves in speech, and few possess the talents of poets,

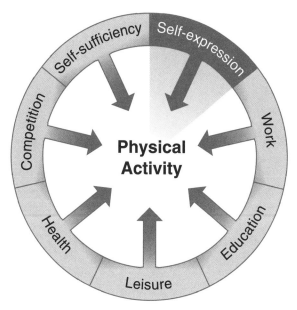

Figure 2.4   Self-expression as a sphere of physical activity experience.

songwriters, or artists. One way we can give outlet to our inner feelings is by moving our bodies (see figure 2.4).

Have you ever stopped to consider how often we express our feelings and other messages in our body movements and postures? We walk rapidly and with a spring in our step when we feel happy, and in a slow, plodding manner when we feel sad. We jump up and down for joy, stretch our arms overhead in elation, hang our heads in sorrow, and clap our hands in appreciation. If you're like most people, you use body movements, often unconsciously, to express your inner emotional state. In all of these instances our body movements seem to be "wired directly" to our emotions, so that changes in our movements occur without voluntary effort on our part. While interesting aspects of our human identities, these examples do not meet our technical definition of physical activity because they do not involve deliberate or voluntary movement directed toward a goal.

Many times, however, we *deliberately* use movements to express feelings and moods and to convey other messages. Have you ever thought about how much you depend on physical activity to help you communicate when you are talking? By using gestures, hand signals, and changes in body posture, we can deliberately and intentionally emphasize such verbal messages as describing shapes and showing directions. We also use physical activity intentionally to express our feelings and emotions in dance, religious liturgy, and various ceremonies. Actually, a case could be argued that we express something about ourselves every time we move, whether it's shooting a jump shot, running a race, or diving from a platform into a pool. Let's examine some ways in which we use physical activity to express ourselves.

Gestures

Gestures are movements of our hands, fingers, or other body parts used to communicate our intentions to others. We use them in place of or in conjunction with talking. Beckoning someone to approach us by flexing and extending our index finger with our palm up, or holding up our hand with palm away from us to signal someone to stop are examples of gestures. Scientists who study nonverbal communication distinguish among three types of intentional gestures: emblems, illustrators, and regulators.

Emblems

Emblems are body movements, usually hand movements, that can be directly translated into words easily understood by those in the culture or subculture in which they are used (Morris, 1994). They may be used with or without accompanying words, but even when used without words, emblems convey a great deal of information (see figure 2.5). For example, they can be used to communicate at a distance or in environments in which verbal communication is difficult or impossible such as in construction settings where crane operators receive messages from ground workers, or in noisy athletic arenas where coaches must send signals to players on the court. A referee at a football game uses the emblem of hacking his left arm with his right hand as a way of

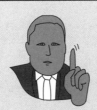

Finger wag

This means "No" or "Don't do that." When used with children, it might be accompanied by the verbal message: "Naughty, naughty." The finger wag is a variation of the side-to-side head shake.

Temple circle

This means that the person who is talking, or the person to whom one might point after the gesture, is "crazy," "nuts," or "off their rocker." Apparently it signifies that the brain is turning around, out of control.

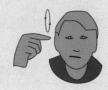

High five slap

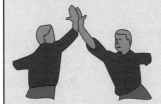

This gesture, commonly but not necessarily limited to sport settings, signifies "well done" or "congratulations." Apparently, it had its origins in American football; in its most extreme form, participants reach as high overhead as possible, occasionally while their feet are off the ground.

Foot tap

This gesture sends the message: "I'm getting impatient." The same message is sometimes sent with the fingers strum and foot jiggle gestures. It is thought to have derived from the foot making movements of running away.

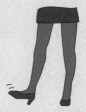

Arm raise with elbow flexed to 90 degrees

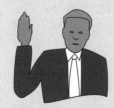

Signifies "I swear." It is used when the performer is "taking an oath."

Figure 2.5 Emblems used for sending messages.

From BODYTALK: THE MEANING OF HUMAN GESTURES by Desmond Morris. Copyright © 1994 by Desmond Morris. Reprinted by permission of Crown Publishers, a division of Random House, Inc.

telling everyone in the stadium that a team has been charged with "unnecessary roughness." Scuba divers also communicate underwater using an elaborate system of emblems.

Illustrators

Illustrators are gestures that we use to illustrate or complement what is being said. When you talk about yourself, you may point to yourself, or you may point to someone else in the room when you are talking about him or her. Illustrators are used to describe the motion of objects. If you were to tell someone about the path of a foul ball that narrowly missed your head when you were sitting along the third base line at the baseball park, you might use an illustrator gesture to describe it. Illustrators can also convey a particular tone in a verbal message. When a coach pounds the fist of his right hand into the palm of his left while talking, he is adding a sense of determination and seriousness to his verbal message.

Regulators

Regulators are body movements used to guide the flow of conversation. Hand and body movements used in greetings (shaking hands, waving, nodding) and in partings (waving, shaking hands, hugging, etc.) are examples of regulators. Regulators also are used by one party to signal to another party or parties that he or she is finished with the conversation. These signals include shifting weight from one foot to the other or turning toward the door. Hand gestures, shifts in gaze, and head movements all may be used in conversations to signal to the other person that you have not yet finished talking or, conversely, that it is his or her turn to talk.

Cross–Cultural Differences in Gestures

A gesture's meaning is usually specific to a particular culture (see figure 2.6). For example, to some Americans, a "cheek–screw," in which a straightened forefinger is pressed against the center of the actor's cheek and rotated, may mean "cute"; to others it may mean nothing. But in Italy it is regarded as a token of praise. Some of the most culturally specific gestures are regulators, especially those used for greetings. If you were to meet an acquaintance in America and he folded his arms across his chest when you extended your

hand to shake his, you might think him rude, but this movement indicates a very respectful greeting in Malaysia. In Eskimo country, a hit on the shoulder doesn't mean you are being challenged to a fight. It means "hello" (Argyle, 1988). Even within cultures, the meanings attached to gestures can change over time. Thirty years ago, if you saw two Americans raising their right hands over their heads and slapping each other's palms, you might think it some form of secret greeting. Today, giving each other a "high five" has become a popular form of greeting, and in sport it is a gesture of congratulations. Can you think of other relatively recent innovations in American gestures?

We use physical activity as a form of communication and expression in combination with or in place of words. Gestures can supplement or substitute for spoken words.

Gestures and Gender Differences

Do women express themselves differently from men in their movements? Have you ever heard someone say that a woman throwing a ball in an advanced, mature, overarm pattern was "throwing like a man"? Or maybe you've heard a man with an inept running style described as "running like a girl." Although the people saying such things usually don't realize it, such descriptions tend to be insulting to women by implying that it is somehow natural for women to throw and run in an inefficient, incorrect manner, a premise that is easily proven false. With sufficient practice, both men and women can learn to throw and run in a correct manner.

Having said this, it is interesting to note that researchers have observed some gender differences in movements used to communicate nonverbally. Many of these gender-related bodily movements (termed "gender identification signals" by pioneer researcher Ray Birdwhistell [1971]) are learned through socialization, and some may be genetically based.

For example, males tend to exhibit more expansive movements than females and demonstrate more restlessness by fidgeting and, when sitting, moving their legs and feet more and by changing body position more often. Females typi-

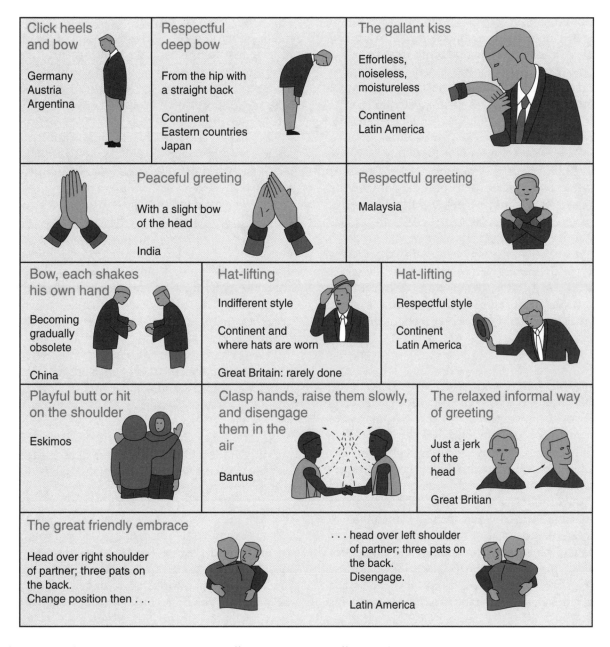

Figure 2.6 Physical activity is used to send different greetings in different cultures.

Adapted, by permission, from T. Brun, 1969, *The international dictionary of sign language* (London: Wolfe).

cally use more gestures to express themselves; engage in more self-touching; and use finer movements with hands, feet, and head. Men and women college students differ in the way they carry their books with women wrapping both arms around the books in a hugging fashion while males carry them at their side using only one arm (Jenni & Jenni, 1976). What is the basis for these differences? While both genetics and socialization may contribute to differences in self-

expressive physical activity, it seems likely that the social influence is primarily responsible.

Dance and Ritual

Often, we express our feelings in the way we execute physical activity. The expressive elements are combined with the movement used to accomplish specific tasks. For example, we may not run, swim, or lift weights *specifically* to express something about ourselves, but often we cannot help it. The manner in which a basketball player bounces the ball before shooting free throws or the movements she selects to propel the ball toward the basket include **instrumental movements**—those critical movements required to attain the goal of the activity—as well as **expressive movements**—idiosyncratic movements not required for goal attainment but which express something about the individual. It may be impossible to separate instrumental movements from expressive movements in such athletic performances as a twisting layup, a run around the bases, or a marathon run.

Sometimes, however, we do employ physical activity deliberately to express sentiment and emotion with no instrumental goal in mind. In dance and in ritual, physical activity serves the express purpose of conveying feelings and symbolic meaning.

Dance

Dance has a long and interesting history. From the earliest periods of recorded time physical activity has been employed to express human emotion and meaning symbolically. Why dance? Why couldn't these meanings have been conveyed through speech or writing? Because the vehicle of human movement enables us to communicate complex thoughts and feelings that are difficult or impossible to transmit verbally. Much the way painters use color and form, sculptors use texture and shape, and musicians use tones and rhythm, dancers use the mediums of force, time, and sequencing of movements to express aesthetic messages. The shape and dimensions of our bodies also affect the aesthetic characteristics of our dance. A leap by a tall, slender dancer will evoke much different emotions in observers than the same leap executed by a short, overweight dancer. In either case, the moving body can tell a story that is inexpressible in word or song.

The physical requirements of dance can be as exacting as—or even more exacting than—the most strenuous sport or exercise routines. Muscular and cardiorespiratory endurance, flexibility, strength, balance, agility, and coordination all are critical to dancing. Long and arduous practice and conditioning regimens are required to learn to achieve the standard body positions and movements required in ballet, for example. Likewise, the free-flowing, creative routines of mod-

ern dance, in which the dancer may be given more freedom in interpreting the notations of the choreographer, require intense training and conditioning. Regardless of the form of dance performed, the end result is the same: "the presentation of a significant emotional concept through formal movement materials . . ." (Phenix, 1964).

Sometimes we dance not to communicate our feelings to others but simply to give outlet to our feelings, even when we are alone. Certainly, an audience, a partner, or a band are not required in order to enjoy dancing! Did you ever dance to the music on the radio when no one else was in the room? Sometimes we dance spontaneously, merely to express joy and jubilation, as, for example, when football players dance in the end zone after scoring a touchdown. Sometimes we dance simply because we feel like it, to enjoy the good feelings that come from moving our bodies in rhythm to music.

Do you like to dance at parties? If so, why? It may be because social dances such as swing, hip-hop, tango, electric slide, or country line dancing are simply enjoyable, or it may be that you like to demonstrate your skill in moving your body in relation to a partner and/or to the beat of the music. On the other hand, social dance may allow you to express a part of yourself that is difficult to express any other way.

Rituals

Physical activity also is an important part of rituals associated with civic and religious ceremonies. What do we mean by "rituals"? **Rituals** are physical actions performed to express symbolically some experience, truth, or value held deeply by a particular group. Rituals usually involve fairly specific movements; that is, they must be performed in a way prescribed by the religious or ceremonial occasion. For example, Americans signal devotion to their country by placing their right (not their left) hands over their hearts when they repeat the pledge of allegiance (a civic ceremony). Attorneys stand and face the judge when he or she enters the courtroom as a way of symbolically expressing their faith in the judicial system. Religious rituals may be performed by priests, ministers, and rabbis, as well as by worshippers. Standing, kneeling, raising arms, and making the sign of the cross are examples of using physical activity to express symbolically religious beliefs and traditions. The use of physical

Reading Body Positions

We send a range of different messages concerning the way we feel or what we are doing by the way we position our bodies. Indicate which body position signifies the following messages or actions by placing the letter corresponding to the posture in the appropriate blank.

___Affected
___Searching
___Welcoming
___Puzzled
___Curious
___Thinking
___Determined
___Stealthy
___Suspicious
___Watching
___Excited
___Shy
___Self-satisfied
___Indifferent
___Sneaking
___Rejecting
___Attentive
___Violent anger
___Searching

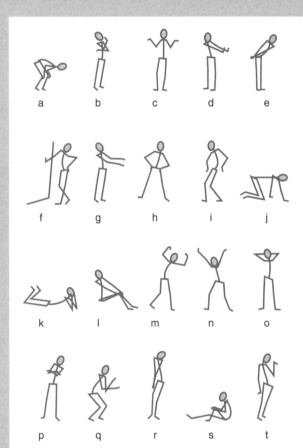

Answers: (a) curious; (b) puzzled; (c) indifferent; (d) rejecting; (e) watching; (f) self-satisfied; (g) welcoming; (h) determined; (i) stealthy; (j) searching; (k) watching; (l) attentive; (m) violent anger; (n) excited; (o) stretching; (p) surprised, dominating, suspicious; (q) sneaking; (r) shy; (s) thinking; (t) affected

Adapted, by permission, from G.B. Rosenberg and J. Langer, 1965, "A study of postural-gestural communication," *Journal of Personality and Social Psychology* 2: 593–597.

activity in rituals is not limited to civic or religious ceremonies. Ritual pervades spectator sports as well. If you have ever participated in "the wave" during a football game you have been engaged in a sporting ritual.

Dance is an art form that uses physical activity to express attitudes and feelings that may be difficult or impossible to express in normal verbal communication. Rituals often employ physical activity to express symbolically sacred values or beliefs.

The Sphere of Work

Work constitutes a significant portion of the total life experiences of most of us, and work almost always involves physical activity (see figure 2.7). What different kinds of work have you done in your life? Have you worked as a construction laborer, a truck loader for a shipping company, a lawn maintenance technician, a pizza delivery person, a housepainter, a server at a restaurant, a kitchen worker for a fast-food chain, an office assistant, or a check-out attendant at a grocery store? If so, what kinds of physical activity have these different jobs required?

In thinking about the answer to this question, it probably occurred to you that the type and intensity of physical activity can vary enormously from job to job. The check-out attendant at the grocery store and the construction laborer both are engaged in physical activity, but they are not physically active in the same ways. Also, although you may have easily recognized the importance of physical activity to the work of the pizza delivery person or truck loader, you may not have appreciated the equal importance of physical activity (though of a different kind) in the work of secretaries, accountants, computer consultants, and graphic artists. The physical actions of typing, filing, and operating an adding machine, while not strenuous, require precise positioning of the limbs and fingers, movements that are essential to the satisfactory execution of these jobs.

Throughout recorded history societies have tended to associate manual labor, with its high physical activity demands, with lower status, while according higher status to managerial and supervisory jobs requiring little physical demands. Yet, jobs requiring high levels of physical activity may offer a "health bonus" for workers. Increased levels of some forms of physical activity may ward off certain diseases associated with physical inactivity (sometimes called hypokinetic diseases or "low-movement diseases"). For example, researchers have found that moderate levels of physical activity, whether engaged in at work or leisure, promote good health and longevity. An early, classic study comparing incidences of heart attacks among drivers and conductors of English double-decker buses revealed that drivers, who were mostly sedentary (and had the easiest, higher-status job), had higher incidences of heart disease than conductors (lower-status workers), who were constantly in motion walking up and down stairs (Morris et al., 1953). This suggests that the types of work that may be attractive to us (those with low amounts and intensities of physical activity) may not be conducive to good health.

As the workplace in the United States increasingly adopts technological innovation, and the nature of work shifts from activity-intensive manufacturing, agriculture, and construction to service and professional occupations, the amount of physical activity required to perform work will continue to decrease. Table 2.3 shows projected employment for five types of work. While only modest increases are projected for physically active occupations (maintenance, packagers), the projected increases for sedentary types of work (computer engineers, occupational therapists, human services workers) are relatively significant. As a result, we may expect workers to be placed at increased risk for diseases associated with reduced physical activity, unless they increase their levels of activity during leisure (nonwork) times.

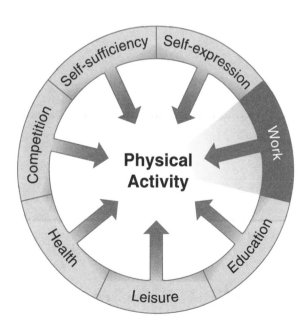

Figure 2.7 Work as a sphere of physical activity experience.

As technology continues to shape the character of work, the amount of physical activity required on the job is likely to decrease, placing workers at higher risk for diseases brought on by physical inactivity.

TABLE 2.3
Employment Trends

Type of employment	Number of workers		
	1996	2006	% increase
Occupational therapists	57,000	95,000	66
Human services workers	178,000	276,000	55
Computer engineers, systems managers	343,000	498,000	45
Hand packers and packagers	986,000	1,208,000	23
Maintenance repairers	1,362,000	1,608,000	18

Data from U.S. Department of Commerce, 1996a, Employment projections, by occupation: 1996 and 2006. *Statistical abstract of the United States 1996*, p. 420. Washington, D.C.: Government Printing Office.

Physical Activity, Efficiency, and Injury in the Workplace

We can view work as a process in which workers trade physical activity for compensation. Employers, in turn, translate workers' physical activity into the production of goods or services. The more efficient this production is, the greater the profit enjoyed by the employer will be. Thus, workers' physical activity is the foundation on which the commercial enterprise rests.

Businesses can increase the efficiency of production in two ways. The first is to replace inefficient physical activity with lower-cost technology. For example, machines and robots now allow car manufacturers to produce many more cars per day at lower costs than when all of the assembly was done by manual labor. But technology cannot replace all physical activity; in many jobs, the movements of workers remain critical to the efficient production of goods or services. In these cases increases in production are sought by improving the efficiency and safety of workers' movements and working conditions. For example, assembly line workers packaging television sets in boxes, picking fruit from trees or vegetables from fields, or operating machines in furniture and textile factories can be made more efficient and safer by changing workers' movements, redesigning the machines with which they do work, or reconfiguring the surroundings in which work is performed.

The physical activity professionals who specialize in improving the efficiency, safety, and well-being of workers are called ergonomists or human factors engineers. Although experts continue to discuss the differences between the roles of these specialists (some believe human factors is more theoretical and relies more heavily on psychology and that ergonomics is more practical and relies more on anatomy and physiology), the trend is for these terms to be used synonymously (Kroemer, Kroemer, & Kroemer-Elbert, 1994).

Ergonomists or human factors engineers apply their knowledge of exercise physiology, psychology, anatomy, and biomechanics in studying the demands of various jobs. They then make recommendations regarding changes in movements used to perform the task, changes in the work environment, or changes in programs for training workers. Often, simply rearranging the location of objects to be assembled, adjusting the height of workers' chairs or tables, redesigning the shape of workstations as shown in figure 2.8, or modifying the order in which components are grasped in the assembly process can result in a marked improvement in worker efficiency. Obviously, a thorough knowledge of the structure of the body as well as a complete understanding of how the body moves are essential to the work of ergonomists.

Productivity in the workplace suffers its greatest decline when workers are injured and miss

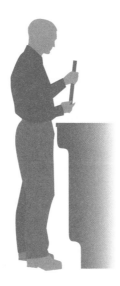

If work is done while standing at a bench, added toe space cut out of the lower part of the bench can allow the worker to step closer to the workstation. The cutout should be high enough to accommodate the worker wearing thick soles but shallow enough so that the worker does not hit the edge of the cutout with the front or instep of the foot.

Figure 2.8 The design of workstations can affect worker efficiency.

From ERGONOMICS: How to Design for Ease & Efficiency by Kroemer/ Kroemer/Kroemer-Elbert, © 1994. Reprinted by permission of Prentice-Hall Inc., Upper Saddle River, NJ.

edly flexing their wrists through a large range of motion while hammering. By carefully analyzing the wrist movements of the carpenter, ergonomists have redesigned the hammer to limit the amount of wrist flexion required (see figure 2.9).

Some forms of work require repetitive physical activity that, over long periods of time, can damage muscles, tendons, and nerves. Such injuries usually require rehabilitation by physical and occupational therapists. To prevent such injuries, corporations often hire consultants called ergonomists or human factors specialists to redesign the characteristics of the jobs to make them more efficient and less hazardous.

work. This is especially troublesome when the injuries occur directly as a result of performing the physical activity required to carry out the job. By this we do not mean workplace accidents (which remain a serious problem), but rather injuries caused by the physical activity a job requires. These injuries, known as **cumulative trauma disorders,** result from repeated physical stress to joints and muscles, which in turn damages tendons and nerves. Assembly line workers packaging items reproduce the same arm, hand, finger, and trunk movements several hundred, even thousand, times each day. Although our bodies are remarkably durable and adaptable, sometimes work asks too much of them, and they suffer deterioration or collapse.

Carpal tunnel syndrome, a painful injury to the wrist as the result of repetitive movements, may be the most widely recognized cumulative trauma disorder in the workplace. The many tasks that can cause this injury include manual assembling, packing, typing, driving, lifting, hammering, or simply sitting at a desk for long periods of time performing clerical work. One way ergonomic specialists attempt to reduce the likelihood of this disorder is to redesign the tools or workspace.

Carpenters are among those particularly prone to carpal tunnel syndrome brought on by repeat-

0 degree hammer

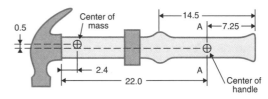

20 degree hammer

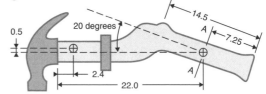

40 degree hammer

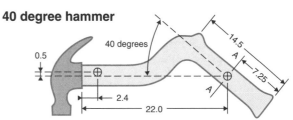

Figure 2.9 Human factors engineers often redesign equipment to increase the efficiency of work and prevent injury. Here hammers with angled handles of 20 and 40 degrees have been designed as a way of reducing repetitive motion injury suffered by carpenters.

Reprinted with permission from *Human Factors*, vol. 31, issue no. 4, 1989. Copyright 1989 by the Human Factors and Ergonomics Society. All rights reserved.

Physical Demands and Psychological Stress of Occupations

Rank the following occupations according to the physical demands and psychological stress demands placed on workers. In this case, a ranking of 1 means high physical demand or high stress (Kranz, 1995). Then compare your order with that listed at the end of the table.

Occupation	Physical demands	Psychological stress demands
Firefighter		
Minister		
Janitor		
Stockbroker		
Corrections officer		
Sport instructor		
Carpenter		
Truck driver		
Flight attendant		
Butcher		
Race car driver (Indy style)		
Garbage collector		

Answers (in order of highest to lowest): **Physical demands:** firefighter, garbage collector, race car driver, carpenter, truck driver, butcher, janitor, sport instructor, corrections officer, flight attendant, stockbroker, minister. **Psychological stress demands:** firefighter, race car driver, stockbroker, corrections officer, truck driver, carpenter, garbage collector, butcher, minister, sport instructor, flight attendant, janitor.

Physical and Psychological Demands of Work

What types of work do you think require the most physically demanding forms of physical activity? This is an important question, not only to employers but also to labor unions, insurance companies, and employees, as well as to ergonomists. To determine physical demands of work, the Bureau of Labor Statistics takes into account the amount of weight a person is normally required to lift on the job. The bureau identifies five distinct categories of physical demands (Kranz, 1995):

1. *Sedentary work,* which requires the occasional lifting of 10 pounds (4.53 kg) or less

2. *Light work,* which requires the lifting of a maximum of 20 pounds (9.1 kg)

3. *Medium work,* which includes tasks in which loads of up to 50 pounds (22.7 kg) are lifted, with frequent lifting of objects up to 25 pounds (11.3 kg)

4. *Heavy work,* which requires lifting up to 100 pounds (45.4 kg)

5. *Very heavy work,* which requires lifting of loads in excess of 100 pounds (45.4 kg), and

frequent carrying of objects weighing 5 pounds (2.3 kg) or more.

Using the classification system of the Bureau of Labor Statistics, along with other factors such as whether a job requires kneeling, bending, climbing, or balancing, and the number of hours required per day, *Jobs Rated Almanac* (Kranz, 1995) calculates a total physical demand score for each of 250 occupations. A low score signals relatively low amounts of physical activity. Although the ratings suggest that high-status jobs such as managerial jobs and professionals require relatively low levels of physical activity, this is not always the case. Some types of low-prestige work are fairly sedentary, while many high-prestige jobs have high physical activity demands. For example, veterinarians, surgeons, basketball coaches (NCAA), and undertakers have an average rating of 183, while the less-prestigious jobs of bus driver, office machine repairer, corrections officer, precision assembler, and forklift operator have a mean rating of 151.

From a total health perspective, we are also interested in the psychological stresses placed on workers by various jobs. Our experience in the workplace might suggest that high-prestige jobs that tend to require less physical activity may also be the most stressful. Are high-prestige jobs always the most psychologically stressful? *Jobs Rated Almanac* (Kranz, 1995) also includes a ranking of jobs on the basis of the stress levels they induce. These rankings are based on such considerations as whether the worker faces deadlines, is in competition with others, encounters physical hazards or uncomfortable environmental conditions, is expected to perform precise movements, or whether the life of another is determined by the worker's actions.

Of the jobs rated, the five least stressful (high score indicates high stress) were medical records technician (15.49), janitor, forklift operator, musical instrument repairer, and florist. The five jobs rated highest in stress were taxi driver, race car driver, corporate executive, firefighter, and the most stressful of all, president of the United States (176.55). Although the highest levels of stress are not always experienced by managers, supervisors, and professional workers, generally the types of employment most likely to raise stress levels often tend to be the jobs requiring low levels of physical activity. Thus, certain classes of

workers—usually those responsible for making the major decisions for institutions and corporations—find themselves in a potentially health-threatening situation, subjected to this "double-whammy" of high stress and low physical activity. These individuals may be especially vulnerable to heart attacks, hypertension, and strokes unless, of course, exercise is pursued outside of work.

The loss of key personnel due to death or disease is potentially devastating to businesses. In order to combat the health-eroding effects of high-prestige work and to ensure a vigorous and energetic workforce, many companies offer physical activity and fitness programs. In fact, between 1985 and 1992 the number of such programs increased from 14% to 33% in companies employing 50 to 99 workers, and from 54% to 83% in companies employing 750 or more workers (USDHHS, 1995). Directorships of such programs are attractive employment options for those in the physical activity professions.

With the advent of industrialization and technology, the physical activity requirements of work have diminished. The result has been the creation of jobs that threaten workers with higher levels of stress and lower levels of physical activity. Businesses have attempted to solve the problem by sponsoring exercise and sport programs for employees.

The Sphere of Education

Physical activity also plays an important role in the sphere of education (see figure 2.10). Education is essential, both for the preservation of cultural traditions and for providing the knowledge and skills that enable society to progress. Physical activity is involved in all phases of education, from the eye movements required in reading and the wrist, finger, and arm movements required in writing, to the more expansive forms of physical activity required in learning how to play a musical instrument or operate a power saw in vocational arts class. In almost every form of educational program, the end result is to change the behavior of those being instructed, and physical

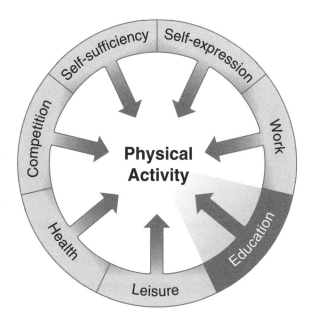

Figure 2.10   Education as a sphere of physical activity experience.

activity is essential for demonstrating these behavioral changes.

Although we will be most interested in educational programs in sport, exercise, and recreation, these are only the tip of the instructional iceberg. Look around and you will see physical activity instruction occurring everywhere! Physical therapists are teaching patients how to walk, dental and medical school faculty are teaching students how to perform the intricate movements required in surgery, fathers and mothers are teaching their children how to dribble a soccer ball, industrial psychologists are training employees in new techniques for assembling TVs or stereos on the production line, American Red Cross staff are teaching would-be lifeguards how to rescue endangered swimmers, senior automobile mechanics are training younger mechanics how to use tools at the local garage, and instructors at business schools are teaching secretaries-in-training how to operate word processors. Anywhere physical activity is important you will find some form of instruction, whether formal or informal, nearby. Instruction in physical activity may be as universal as physical activity itself!

🔑 The education sphere includes that aspect of our lives in which we set out to learn new skills or knowledge. Almost always, physi-

cal activity plays an important role in this sphere, whether it be in connection with learning cognitive material or learning to perform physical skills.

Instruction in Sport and Exercise

Not long ago, instruction in sport and exercise was limited largely to public schools, college physical education programs, municipal recreation programs, and the military. Today, sport and fitness centers; resorts; corporations; hospitals; and tennis, golf, and swimming clubs are also in the sport and fitness instruction business. Millions of young kids are taught how to play sports by their fathers or mothers or older siblings as well as youth sport team coaches. Adults, mindful of the adage "you can't teach an old dog new tricks," used to shy away from instruction in sport activities, but now they seek it out, often paying as much as $75 to $100 per hour for lessons from top skiing, scuba, fencing, squash, or fitness training specialists.

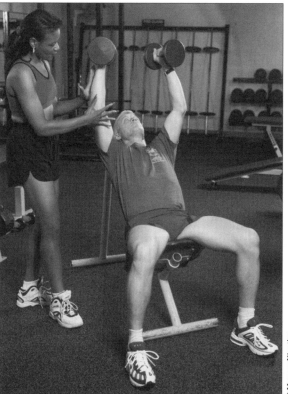

Physical activity instruction occurs in many arenas, not just in the traditional physical education class.

Private clubs and commercial spas, gyms, ice rinks, riding stables, dance studios, and martial arts centers now compete with school-based programs in the instruction business. Many large corporations offer recreation programs for their employees as a perk, and many of these include basic instruction in sports and exercise. Instruction through the media has also become a huge business. Television's Golf Academy Channel offers instruction in golf on a 24-hour basis. How-to books on every conceivable sport line the shelves of the mega-bookstores, and sport specialty magazines include regular instructional features.

Coupled with this interest in learning to perform sports and exercise is a growing demand for knowledge about how to live a healthful lifestyle. Corporate managers, keenly aware of the economic advantages of a healthy workforce, are making instructional programs available at the worksite, often in collaboration with their HMOs or health insurers. Typically, these classes use a variety of methodologies to integrate theoretical information about exercise, nutrition, and body mechanics with practical experiences in the exercise room.

The explosion of interest in learning about sports and exercise has led to an expansion of instruction beyond the walls of schools and colleges.

Physical Education

Although instruction in sport, fitness, and exercise occurs in a myriad of formal and informal settings, it is most visible and accessible in physical education classes offered as part of the school curriculum. Our educational system is based on the belief that it is in the best interest of a democracy to make available to its citizens a free and accessible program of education. Instruction in sport, exercise, and fundamental movements has long been viewed as an integral component of the educational enterprise.

In this section we will focus on the life experience you probably knew as "phys ed" or "gym class," and what physical activity professionals more appropriately call "physical education." Because these programs have such enormous

potential for influencing the physical activity patterns of large segments of the population, they have attracted the attention of all physical activity professionals, not simply those who are planning careers in teaching. For this reason it is important that you—as a future physical activity professional—appreciate this potential as well as some of the problems associated with school-based physical activity programs.

Chances are that a significant part of your public school education experience was spent in physical education class. In fact, 94% of all public school programs in the country require at least some course work in physical education. But even though most of us have attended physical education class, we have not all shared the same experience. School districts do not all teach the same program of physical activities. Sometimes teachers within the same school district or even within the same school teach different subject matter and use different methodologies. Perhaps you were fortunate enough to have had a competent and enthusiastic teacher who offered carefully structured and sequenced classes. If so, you probably learned much about physical activity. On the other hand, you may have had a bored or unimaginative teacher who "threw out the ball" and offered little in the way of instruction. If this was your physical education experience, you probably learned less than your colleagues who attended classes taught by more competent and energetic teachers.

Your conception of physical education will be influenced by your own personal experiences in the subject. What are your recollections? Was it a good experience for you or a bad one? Were the outcomes you and your classmates experienced worth the money your school district paid to support the program, or should it have been abolished? Each reader will have different answers to these questions. In any case, it is important that you recognize that your own experience—whether favorable or unfavorable—may not be an accurate reflection of what physical education is like in most schools.

Physical education is the curriculum that teaches children how to perform sport and exercise. It is a part of almost all public school educational programs.

Objectives of Physical Education Programs

Effective educational programs begin with clearly stated objectives. Objectives are vital maps for educators. They point teachers toward the ends that are to be achieved in their lessons. They determine what teachers will teach and the methods they will use to do so. Students should also understand the objectives that are guiding the teachers' actions. When you think back to your experiences in physical education classes, you may realize that the teachers' objectives were not always clear to you. Sometimes it may have seemed that the objective was developing fitness. At other times learning sport skills seemed to be the goal, while at other times the teacher may have seemed most interested in the students developing a sense of fair play. What then, *are* the objectives of physical education?

School superintendents, principals, classroom teachers, parents, physical education teachers, and students all may have slightly different views concerning the objectives of physical education. Physical educators even disagree among themselves concerning the most important objectives to be achieved by school physical education programs. This lack of agreement concerning the objectives of physical education programs has probably deterred the improvement of physical education in some schools. Because physical educators have been unable to agree on objectives, public school programs differ widely in content and methodology. As a result, experts have been unable to come to a universal agreement concerning what constitutes "a physically educated person." In an effort to bring the factions closer together, the National Association for Sport and

A physically educated person:

1. demonstrates competency in many movement forms and proficiency in a few movement forms.
2. applies movement concepts and principles to the learning and development of motor skills.
3. exhibits a physically active lifestyle.
4. achieves and maintains a health-enhancing level of physical fitness.
5. demonstrates responsible personal and social behavior in physical activity settings.
6. demonstrates an understanding and respect for differences among people in physical activity settings.
7. understands that physical activity provides opportunities for enjoyment, challenge, self-expression, and social interaction.

Figure 2.11   The objectives of physical education.

Reprinted from *Moving Into the Future: National Physical Education Standards: A Guide to Content and Assessment*, with permission from the National Association for Sport and Physical Education (NASPE), 1900 Association Drive, Reston, VA 20191.

Physical Education (NASPE), working hand in hand with public school teachers and university professors, published a list of content standards for physical education programs. They are presented in the form of behaviors (see figure 2.11) that should be demonstrated by a physically educated person (NASPE, 1995).

Although developing physical fitness probably is at the top of most teachers' lists of objectives for physical education, only two of the seven NASPE standards focus on fitness and achieving

Are You a Physically Educated Person?

On the basis of the NASPE standards and objectives for physical education listed in figure 2.11, do you consider yourself to be a "physically educated person"? Think back over your elementary and high school physical education experiences. How often did you have physical education class? Was it a required subject in your school? Were you taught mostly lifetime sport activities (e.g., tennis, golf, archery) or team sports? Was physical fitness emphasized? Were you taught the health benefits of a physically active lifestyle? Did your classes increase or decrease your sensitivities to the needs and problems of others? Did you enjoy physical education class? What factors made it enjoyable? What, if any, factors tended to discourage you from participating in class?

a physically active lifestyle. Others emphasize the need to attain competency in a diverse number of activities, to experience social and psychological growth, to learn concepts about motor skills, and to have an opportunity for fun and self-expression. You can begin to see the problem. Even this "narrowed" list of standards leaves a great deal of room for diversity in objectives, instructional approaches, and content. For the time being, school physical education programs will likely continue to aim at a cluster of different objectives, each requiring slightly different approaches and content. Individual teachers will also likely continue to emphasize those objectives that most closely align with their personal philosophies of physical education.

Fitness and Social Responsibility as Objectives of Physical Education

What physical education teachers emphasize in their classes tends to be influenced by trends, events, and forces in society at large. For example, a strong feeling on the part of society that its citizens should be exposed to sport skills during the school years is responsible for the emphasis given to skill instruction in most programs. Sometimes the physical education program is influenced by widespread perceptions of social problems. Two such problems have been very much in the national spotlight in recent years:

- The health risks confronting young people who appear to be living increasingly inactive lives

- The rising number of children who, because of poverty, disintegrating families, drugs, and violence, lack the requisite social skills to take part in society as constructive citizens

Let's examine each of these problems briefly and consider how physical education could contribute to their solutions.

Physical Fitness. Health officials have become alarmed at the overall poor fitness and sedentary lifestyles of children (USDHHS, 1996). The population of "couch potatoes" (in the case of Internet addicts, they are now called "cyber-potatoes") is growing, and many of them are children that haven't yet reached middle school. How many hours of TV do you watch? You might be surprised to learn that elementary schoolchildren spend more time watching television than they do performing any other activity except for sleeping (Dietz, 1990). If you were like most children, by the time you graduated from high school, you had spent 15,000 to 18,000 hours watching television, compared to 12,000 hours spent in school (Strasburger, 1992)!

As a way of combating this sedentary lifestyle in children, a national health report entitled *Healthy People 2000* (USDHHS, 1990) recommended that schools increase the amount of time students spend in physical education classes. One goal was to increase the percentage of students in grades 1 through 12 who participate in daily physical education to 50% by the year 2000. Unfortunately, the rhetoric of health leaders is far ahead of what actually takes place in public schools. Look at the alarming figures in table 2.4. Although a fairly large percentage of students are enrolled in physical education classes, very low percentages attend physical education on a daily basis, and the percentage enrolled in daily physical education classes drops steadily from grade 9 to grade 12.

Is this better or worse than it used to be? The situation appears to have grown worse. Although total enrollment in high school physical education classes remained unchanged from 1991 to 1995, *daily* requirements for such classes declined from 42% to 25% during the first half of the decade! Even where physical education is required daily, best estimates are that only 19% of students in these classes are physically active for 20 minutes or more during each class (USDHHS, 1996).

Developing physically fit students is an important objective, but the challenge to physical education extends far beyond this. If students do not develop good habits of exercise by learning to incorporate moderate to intense forms of physical activity into their lifestyles for the remainder of their lives, little will have been achieved by making students fit while they are in school. What good will we have done if we create a population of fit young people who eventually all slip into sedentary lifestyles after they graduate? Coupled with this is the need to develop competency in these lifetime sport skills. People who have confidence in their abilities to swim, play tennis, golf, rollerblade, or play squash are more likely to engage in these sports throughout their lives. Unless physical education classes are scheduled on a daily basis, teachers will have little

TABLE 2.4
Percentage of Students (Grades 9–12) in USA Enrolled in Physical Education

Group	Enrolled (%)	Attend daily (%)
Overall	59.6	25.4
Sex		
Males	62.2	27.0
Females	56.8	23.5
Race/ethnicity		
White/non-Hispanic	62.9	21.7
Black/non-Hispanic	50.2	33.8
Grade level		
Males		
9	80.5	42.1
10	72.6	34.8
11	51.5	17.4
12	45.4	14.8
Females		
9	80.8	39.7
10	71.4	33.8
11	41.2	12.3
12	39.1	11.1

Adapted from U.S. Department of Health and Human Services, 1996, *Physical activity and health: A report of the Surgeon General* (Pittsburgh: Superintendent of Documents), 198.

sports, continue to dominate the American public school physical education curriculum. Clearly, much work needs to be done if physical education classes are ever to realize their potential for increasing the levels of physical activity of the general population.

The development of physical fitness in students, especially during their adult years when the threat of becoming physically inactive is greatest, is an important objective of physical education. Surveys suggest that

TABLE 2.5
Percentage of All Physical Education Courses in Which More Than One Class Period Was Devoted to Each Activity in 1994

Activity	Percentage of all courses
Basketball	86.8
Volleyball	82.3
Baseball/softball	81.5
Flag/touch football (American)	68.5
Soccer	65.2
Jogging	46.5*
Weight training	37.3*
Tennis	30.3*
Aerobic dance	29.6*
Walking quickly	14.7*
Swimming	13.6*
Handball	13.2*
Racquetball	4.9*
Hiking/backpacking	3.0*
Bicycling	1.3*

*Indicates lifetime activity.

Adapted from U.S. Department of Health and Human Services, 1996, *Physical activity and health: A report of the Surgeon General* (Pittsburgh: Superintendent of Documents), 237.

chance to develop skill competencies in their students.

Because of this emphasis on lifelong patterns of physical activity, high school physical education programs should include a heavy concentration of lifetime activities such as tennis, golf, handball, or racquetball, rather than team sports, which people are less likely to play following graduation. Yet, in spite of health and education leaders' emphasis on the importance of featuring lifetime sports in the curriculum, the data in table 2.5 suggest that team sports, not lifetime children do not receive physical education frequently enough to produce fitness gains or to develop competency in sport skills, and that public school programs give insufficient emphasis to lifetime sport activities.

Social Responsibility and At-Risk Kids. A second problem confronting society is the growing population of children "at risk" for social marginalization, poverty, crime, neglect, and violence, and what some have termed "socially toxic environments" (Lawson, Briar-Lawson, & Larson, 1997). In America it is estimated that every 8 seconds a child drops out of school, every 15 seconds a child is arrested, every 60 seconds a child is born to a teenage mother, and every 4 minutes a child is arrested for drug abuse (Children's Defense Fund, 1997).

Can educational programs of physical activity help to stem this tide of social devastation? Some experts believe they can. By designing school-based physical education programs outside of the normal class day, often in conjunction with physical education departments of colleges and universities located in urban centers, physical educators have launched imaginative and effective programs for combating the influences of toxic social environments. Some of these programs are operated in the summer.

Professor Don Hellison is one of the country's most prominent scholar-practitioners in this area. Hellison has spent his lifetime as a university professor developing, testing, and refining physical activity programs designed to develop social responsibility in at-risk children, usually those from urban environments. Hellison hopes that such programs might help children to withstand the forces that work against their social and emotional development in their home and neighborhood lives (Hellison, 1996). He has also been at the forefront of efforts to train teachers for this type of work.

Physical activity programs for developing social responsibility must be planned and implemented carefully to achieve this very specific educational objective. Children taught by Hellison and his students spend approximately 70% of their time in planned physical activities designed specifically to develop personal and social responsibility. The remainder of the time is spent learning and being involved in physical activity for the fun of it. As a result of such programs students become proficient in sport skills and develop physical fitness, but these objectives are incidental to the principal objective of developing the attitudes and skills that will enable them to live constructive lives as members of their communities.

Why physical education? Couldn't other kinds of programs such as work, art, or music be just as effective? What special properties does physical education have that makes it especially suitable for developing social responsibility? First, physical education has the advantage of being a popular school subject. Second, the essential nature of sport lends itself to teaching about fairness, freedom, and responsibility (Miller, Bredemeier, & Shields, 1997). Of course, organized community youth sport programs also are attractive to young people, but the context of physical education classes seems more suitable for developing social responsibility. For one thing, children are subject to less pressures than usually is the case in highly competitive sport programs. Also, teachers are freer to de-emphasize competition and winning and establish an atmosphere of cooperation, a climate conducive to developing social responsibility. Although the effects have yet to be well documented by research, the experience of those working in such programs strongly suggests that a well-taught, regularly offered program of physical education specifically planned to teach students the attitudes and behaviors essential for satisfying and productive lives can help children resist social forces and conditions that threaten their social, emotional, and material security.

Carefully planned programs of physical activity often have the added benefit of helping children who are at risk for many personal and social problems develop social responsibility.

The Sphere of Leisure

Another area of our lives in which physical activity takes place is leisure (see figure 2.12). What do you do in your free time—play sports, exer-

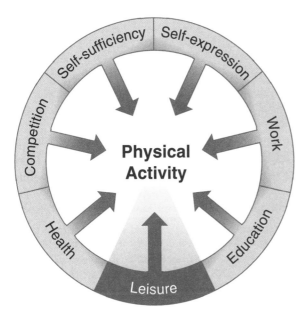

Figure 2.12 Leisure as a sphere of physical activity experience.

cise, read, attend concerts, watch television, hike? If you're like most people, much of your free time is spent engaged in physical activity, and you tend to associate leisure with play. In fact the term *leisure pursuits* is often used synonymously with *play* or *recreation*. But sometimes we choose to work in our free time. Have you ever given up an opportunity to spend a summer weekend (free time) camping or at the beach, volunteering instead to work an extra shift at work? If so, was what you did in your free time "leisure"?

As you can see, the terms *leisure* and *free time* are a bit more ambiguous than they first appear. Can you really work in your leisure time? You might have noticed that some people play softball or soccer with an intensity that seems to be anything but "leisurely." Or conversely, can some people play (be at leisure) while they work? Perhaps. Artists, novelists, and professors sometimes seem to approach their work almost as if it were a leisure experience. Thus, a good place to start in our examination of the leisure sphere of physical activity experience is to clarify what we mean by free time and leisure.

Distinguishing Leisure From Free Time

When we are able to disengage from our everyday lives and participate in activities that really interest us, we often refer to this as **free time**. We are free from our everyday routines, free to do what we want to do, when, where, and with whom we want. While we often use the terms *free time* and *leisure* synonymously, experts distinguish between the two.

Leisure theorists describe **leisure**, not as free time, but as "a state of being" (De Grazia, 1962). Philosophers, beginning with the ancient Greeks, have struggled to describe this state, but none have done so entirely satisfactorily. In its purest state, leisure is a feeling that all is well with the world, a feeling of supreme contentment. It can provoke feelings of celebration and wonder, creativity and discovery, excitement and reflection. Pieper (1962) described leisure as the "basis of culture," the psychological and spiritual disposition that is the fundamental prerequisite for the great works of art, music, theater, and philosophy.

How do we achieve this state of being called leisure? Sometimes we find it while engaged in sedentary activities such as sitting beside a gurgling stream, reading a novel, or listening to

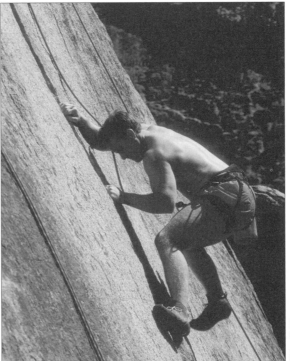

Physical activity can help us achieve a state of leisure—where we are freed from the obligations and stresses of our everyday lives and gain a greater understanding of who we really are.

© Mary E. Messenger

music. At other times, we can achieve the state of leisure through large-muscle activities such as running, hiking, surfing, or skiing. Precisely what this state of being is or how it comes about may never be explained fully. One thing seems clear. It has the effect of clarifying to ourselves and others who we truly are when we are freed from the sense of obligation, anxiety, and pressure that can confront us in our everyday lives.

In order to use our free time to achieve a state of leisure, we must be able to divorce ourselves psychologically from other aspects of our lives, a challenging task for many people. In addition, we must be sure to choose an activity that is conducive to a state of leisure. While many of us choose to watch television during our free time, a study of teenagers showed that they do not find it a very satisfying experience (Csikszentmihalyi, 1990b). Hollow free time experiences are not leisure experiences. They don't challenge us, stimulate our imaginations, or help us reveal our identities the way true leisure experiences do. Thus, if free time is to be converted into leisure time, it must be used for participating in activities that tend to nourish and maintain the state of being known as leisure.

🔑 Leisure is a state of being, and free time activities can help us attain this state. Large-muscle physical activities such as sport and exercise have the potential for nourishing and maintaining a leisure disposition.

Physical Activity as Leisure Activity

The entire range of leisure pursuits—from sedentary activities such as chess or reading to large-muscle activities such as water skiing or softball—is the focus of study in the discipline known as leisure studies or recreation. Kinesiology concerns itself primarily with the large-muscle forms of leisure pursuits in which substantial physical activity is required. If this leads you to wonder if the interests of kinesiologists overlap with those of leisure professionals, the answer is yes. Both faculty and students in departments of leisure studies and in kinesiology view sport and exercise as a legitimate part of their fields of study. While it might seem that this blurring of the boundaries of the two disciplines would be prob-

lematic, it has existed for several decades and has not deterred the continuing expansion and refinement of each of these exciting areas of study.

Activities such as golf, community theater, softball, hiking, long runs in the park, and boating have great potential for putting us at leisure. But even these can be approached in ways that make such a leisurely disposition impossible. For example, becoming upset over an official's call, cheating, intentionally injuring an opponent, or exercising under the compulsive stimulus of anorexia nervosa are not compatible with a leisure state. The context in which the activity takes place is also important. Is it possible for athletes to attain a state of leisure when 80,000 spectators are sending up a deafening roar from the stadium? In the final analysis, whether or not a sport or exercise is truly a leisure pursuit depends on its nature, the context in which it is pursued, and the motivations and attitudes participants bring to the activity. Professionals in the leisure industry try to help people make choices about their free time that increase the state of being known as leisure.

🔑 At the very best, free time activities of sport and exercise offer us only the potential for achieving the state of leisure. Whether or not a physical activity is truly a leisure pursuit depends on the nature of the activity and the context in which it is pursued. The challenge of the physical activity professions is to teach people to participate in free time physical activity pursuits in ways that nourish the disposition known as leisure.

Since your future as a physical activity professional will likely be affected by participation trends in large-muscle leisure activities, it is worth taking the time to examine the most popular forms of this type of leisure physical activity. (Although competitive sports clearly fit under the leisure activity umbrella, we will look at their popularity under the competition sphere and focus here on large-muscle, noncompetitive forms of leisure activities.) As you can see in table 2.6, swimming and riding bicycles (with 61 and 56 million participants, respectively) are among the most popular of these activities. These figures do

TABLE 2.6
Participation in Selected Noncompetitive Leisure Activities

Activity	In millions			% change '85–'95	% change '90–'95
	1985	1990	1995		
Swimming	73.3	67.5	61.5	–16.3	–8.0
Bike riding	50.7	55.3	56.3	11.0	1.8
Camping	46.4	46.2	42.8	–7.0	–7.3
Billiards	23.0	28.1	31.1	35.0	9.4
Hiking	21.1	22.0	25.0	18.0	13.6
Boating/sailing	31.3	33.5	28.7	–8.0	–14.3
In-line skating	N/A	3.6	23.9	N/A	560.0
Dart throwing	9.4	16.4	19.4	106.0	18.0
Backpacking	10.2	10.8	10.2	0	–5.5
Skiing (alpine)	9.4	11.4	9.3	1.0	–18.4
Skiing (cross-country)	5.5	5.1	3.4	–38.0	–33.3
Canoeing	7.9	8.9	7.2	–8.8	–19.1
Water skiing	12.9	10.5	6.9	–47.0	–34.2
Windsurfing	1.2	0.9	0.5	–60.0	–44.0

Reprinted, by permission, from National Sporting Goods Association, *Research* (May 1996), 36.

not include exercise walking, which was pursued by over 70 million people (National Sporting Goods Association [NSGA], 1996), or gardening, which was pursued by people in approximately 74% of all households (U.S. Department of Commerce [USDC], 1996g).

Outdoor activities such as hunting and fishing continue to attract large numbers each year (35 million and 14 million, respectively) (USDC, 1996f), and increasing numbers of people are spending their leisure time hiking. Visits to the national parks are skyrocketing, growing from 100 million in 1963 to 271 million in 1977 and estimated to reach half a billion by 2010 (Satchell, 1997). Unfortunately, these data do not distinguish between visitors who remain mostly sedentary while in the park and those who scale mountain peaks, climb rocks, and take physically demanding hikes into wilderness areas.

Since surveys of physical activity tend to vary widely, both in terms of the questions asked and the populations polled, research on leisure time physical activities is, at best, an inexact science. With this caveat in mind, the data suggest that our preferences for leisure time physical activity may be shifting away from more physically demanding types to more sedentary types such as movies, sound recordings, surfing the internet, travel, gambling, and television. The data in table 2.6 show that, aside from modest increases from 1985 to 1995 in bike riding and hiking and an enormous increase in recent years in the numbers of people participating in in-line skating (projected to be the fastest growing recreational activity through 2001 ["Fitnews," (1995)]), participation in noncompetitive leisure physical activity from 1990 to 1995 has stabilized or declined. Unfortunately, the trend is especially noticeable in the more vigorous forms of physical activity.

Concurrent with this decrease in vigorous physical activity in leisure is an increase in attendance at cultural events, tourist attractions, movies, and other sporting amusements that do not involve significant amounts of physical activity (USDC, 1996d). Although these data may not represent the full picture of our leisure activity participation, they could be indications of a troubling trend. Physical activity professionals would do well to continue to monitor these trends carefully over the next few years.

🔑 Although participation in recreational leisure time activities involving moderate to intense physical activity remains high, the rate of growth appears to have slowed and in some cases declined, while participation in more sedentary activities appears to be on the rise.

Sports Watching

One form of sedentary leisure activity clearly on the rise is sports watching. In excess of one billion dollars is spent on tickets to professional and amateur sporting events each year, approximately the same amount spent on all movies, and 60% of the total spent on all theater, opera, and nonathletic entertainment sponsored by nonprofit organizations. Over 190 million spectators attended professional and college baseball, basketball, football, and professional hockey games in 1994, up from approximately 150 million in 1985 (see table 2.7). Annual spectator attendance has more than doubled in women's college basketball since 1985 (USDC, 1996e). Attendance at figure skating is not included in table 2.7. It is the fastest growing spectator sport with 7% of the population ranking it as their favorite, a 75% increase from 1994 ("Figure Skating Jumps in Fan Vote," 1997).

Such data don't give the complete picture, however. The figures in table 2.7 do not take into account the millions who watch high school sports, youth sport teams, and other amateur sports. Nor do they include the millions who watch sports on television. It is estimated that television sets in American homes are each tuned to sports for an average of 180 hours each year ("Game Plans," 1994).

TABLE 2.7
Attendance at the Most Popular Spectator Sports

Sport	In millions		
	1985	1990	1994
Baseball			
Major League	47.7	55.5	71.2*
Basketball			
NCAA men's	26.6	28.7	28.3
NCAA women's	2.1	2.8	4.6
Professional	11.5	18.5	19.3
Football (American)			
NCAA	34.9	35.3	36.5
Professional	14.0	17.6	14.8
Hockey			
Professional	11.6	12.3	15.7

*Data is for attendance in 1993.

Adapted from U.S. Department of Commerce, 1996e, Selected Spectator Sports: 1985 to 1994. *Statistical abstract of the United States 1996*, 61. Washington, DC: Government Printing Office.

The growth in sport spectatorism represents something of a dilemma for the physical activity profession. On one hand, the jobs of many physical activity professionals—coaches, athletes, athletic trainers, and physical activity instructors—depend on sport retaining its viability as mass entertainment. Sport management, an increasingly popular career option for physical activity professionals, consists of specialists who plan, market, stage, publicize, and supervise mass spectator sport events. In a nutshell, their job is to make sports watching a profitable enterprise by increasing the number of people watching sport events. At the same time, the rise in mass spectatorism, a largely sedentary activity, works at cross-purposes to the profession's efforts to increase physical activity in the general population.

Of additional concern to physical activity professionals is whether sports watching constitutes a viable leisure pursuit. Does it promise to nourish the psychological/spiritual state called leisure? Some believe that it can. Michael Novak's popular book *The Joy of Sport* (1976) and Fred Exley's *A Fan's Notes* (1968) are eloquent testimonies to the fact that sports watching may add to the quality of our leisure lives. On the other hand, an obsessive preoccupation with the fortunes of one's favorite sport team can be socially unhealthy, especially when it leads to neglect of more important things such as human relationships. As enthusiasm for watching sports continues to grow, the profession will be challenged to differentiate between healthy, constructive spectatorship and addictive, destructive preoccupation.

Although participation in many sports appears to have stabilized, and perhaps declined, interest in watching sports continues to grow, abetted by a thriving commercial and television market. This trend toward mass watching as opposed to mass participation may not be compatible with national health efforts to increase the physical activity participation levels of the population at large.

Aging and Leisure Activities

Not long ago, the majority of the population believed that life essentially ended at 65. The elderly faced the problem of finding sedentary ways to "fill up" their free time until they died. Thanks to advances in health maintenance and the growth of the field of gerontology, we now know that people over 65 have enormous potential to learn new skills, explore new vistas, and engage in forms of physical activity that most elderly people wouldn't have dreamed of engaging in 20 years ago.

Table 2.8 presents the combined results of seven surveys of the leisure physical activities of people in four different age groups. Notice how many are large-muscle physical activities! While it isn't possible to compare participation across all age groups since the data in each column were culled from different surveys, we can make a number of interesting observations. Particularly interesting is the relatively slight fall off in participation in leisure activities by the 65- to 74-year-old group compared to younger groups. In fact, this age category showed a slight increase over younger groups in participation rates of walking. More than 12 million people 65 years of age or older engage in exercise walking (NSGA, 1996). Although the 75+ age category shows a noticeable drop-off in leisure physical activity, particularly in sport-related activities, older populations are clearly continuing to involve themselves in physical activity throughout their lives. The fact that nearly half of this older group continues to walk for fitness and that 10% swim is an encouraging finding and is likely to rise over the next few years. This trend represents a new and

When Sports Watching Gets Out of Hand

When fascination with a sport team becomes obsessive, it can cause people to do strange things.

In October, 1973, a Colorado man shot himself in the head one Sunday evening. He left a suicide note that referred to his favorite team, the Denver Broncos. The Broncos had fumbled seven times that day in their loss to the Chicago Bears. Although the identity of the fan was not disclosed, the sheriff did disclose the contents of the note. It read: "I have been a Broncos fan since the Broncos were first organized, and I can't stand their fumbling anymore." Fortunately, his aim wasn't any better than that of the Broncos' quarterback. He survived.

From Michael Roberts, 1976, *Fans* (Washington, DC: New Republic Book).

Connie Scramlin, 58, loved the Detroit Tigers. She underscored her devotion to the team by arranging her own funeral as a tribute. She was dressed in a Tigers' uniform, placed in a coffin lined with tiger lilies, trimmed in midnight blue and orange, and emblazoned with the Tigers' emblem. "Take Me Out to the Ballgame" was played at the funeral.

Reprinted, by permission, from Associated Press Wire Service, June 21, 1991.

TABLE 2.8
Leisure Activities of the 65+ Population

% participating	45–54 age group	Activity days	% participating	55-64 age group	Activity days
64.7	Jogging/walking for fitness	96.7	64.7	Sightseeing	18.2
64.4	Sightseeing	17.0	60.3	Jogging/walking for fitness	82.6
62.8	Picnicking	7.3	54.0	Picnicking	4.5
53.4	Swimming	12.0	34.9	Swimming	8.6
41.9	Hiking	14.1	34.9	Hiking	15.4
34.5	Bicycling	14.0	22.3	Bird watching	39.3
27.2	Fishing	6.1	20.5	Bicycling	11.6
26.6	Boating	—	19.2	Fishing	4.3
21.7	Bird watching	35.5	16.3	Boating	—
15.0	Hunting	2.9	13.6	Hunting	2.2
14.8	Camping	2.7	13.0	Golf	3.2
13.6	Golf	4.0	12.3	Camping	1.6
11.3	Baseball/softball	1.8	4.4	Tennis	1.2
7.4	Basketball	1.3	4.2	Baseball/softball	0.6
7.4	Tennis	1.9	3.9	Basketball	0.7
6.5	Snow skiing	0.6	2.8	Snow skiing	0.3
6.3	ORRVs	1.7	2.5	Ice skating	0.1
4.7	Horseback riding	1.4	2.2	ORRVs	0.1
4.4	Ice skating	0.1	1.1	Horseback riding	0.1
0.3	Football/soccer	0.1	1.1	Football/soccer	0.1
Mean = 24.4		Total = 225.2	Mean = 19.4		Total = 197.6

exciting population that can benefit from the services of physical activity professionals.

The Sphere of Health

Attending to our personal and community health needs consumes a large part of our normal daily experiences. We bathe, dispose of our garbage, ensure that we drink clean water, eat proper foods, visit physicians when we are ill, and so forth, in order to maintain our health, which in turn enables us to be productive citizens and enjoy life. All of these health-related activities involve physical activity in varying degrees. We can't, for example, brush our teeth, bathe ourselves, or carry out the garbage without performing physical activity. But there is a much more direct way that physical activity intersects with this sphere. We now possess hard, scientific evi-

% participating	65-74 age group	Activity days	% participating	75+ age group	Activity days
65.9	Sightseeing	26.0	48.5	Jogging/walking for fitness	74.8
62.3	Jogging/walking for fitness	97.6	45.9	Sightseeing	25.8
59.8	Picnicking	4.6	38.5	Picnicking	2.0
31.7	Hiking	22.7	21.5	Bird watching	44.3
26.6	Swimming	12.5	17.8	Hiking	10.5
26.0	Bird watching	45.6	9.6	Swimming	4.1
18.9	Bicycling	10.7	6.7	Bicycling	3.6
18.3	Fishing	4.9	5.9	Boating	—
13.8	Boating	—	5.2	Fishing	0.4
10.5	Hunting	3.0	4.5	Camping	0.4
8.1	Camping	2.2	3.7	Golf	2.8
3.9	Baseball/softball	0.4	1.5	Baseball/softball	0.1
2.7	ORRVs	0.5	1.5	Basketball	0.1
2.4	Snow skiing	0.4	0.7	Tennis	0.7
2.1	Tennis	0.7	0.7	Hunting	0.1
2.1	Ice skating	0.1	0.0	Football/soccer	0.0
2.1	Basketball	1.3	0.0	Horseback riding	0.0
1.5	Horseback riding	0.8	0.0	ORRVs	0.0
0.3	Football/soccer	0.1	0.0	Snow skiing	0.0
			0.0	Snow skiing	0.0
Mean = 18.6		Total = 242.6	Mean = 10.6		Total = 170.0

Adapted, by permission, from F.A. McGuire, R.K. Boyd, and R.E. Tedrick, 1999, *Ulyssean living in later life*, 2d ed. (Champaign, IL: Sagamore Publishing).

dence that physical activity performed in the right amounts and with sufficient frequency contributes to our health in many important ways (see figure 2.13).

We now know that moderate to vigorous levels of physical activity performed regularly and at safe levels almost always result in health benefits. We also know that the payoffs aren't limited to workouts or painful exercise routines performed specifically to "get in shape" or become fit. Physical activity performed as part of work, sport participation, or another leisure pursuit also reaps benefits. At the same time, it seems equally clear that the safest, most effective, and most efficient routes to attaining health benefits from physical activity are carefully designed programs supervised by exercise professionals well versed in the science of physical activity. As the public

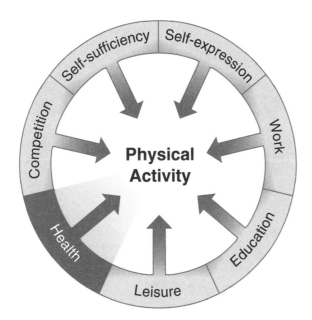

Figure 2.13 Health as a sphere of physical activity experience.

comes more and more to understand this, the demand for highly trained fitness leaders and consultants will continue to increase.

Physical Activity and the National Interest

Why is it important to the national interest that Americans maintain and improve their health through physical activity? For one thing, it is important to the national economy. A sick population not only incurs medical expenses, but also drains the economy through lost productivity. Consider this: The United States spends a greater proportion of its gross domestic product on health care than any other industrialized nation. In 1992 health care in the United States represented 13.6% of its gross domestic product compared with 10.3% in Canada, 8.7% in Germany, and 6.9% in Japan. The deaths of over 500,000 people each year due to cardiovascular disease costs the nation over $135 billion annually. Approximately 600,000 people suffer strokes each year, over one-third of the U.S. population is overweight, 23% suffer from hypertension—46% of 45- to 54-year-olds—and approximately 35% of 45- to 54-year-olds have cholesterol levels above 240 (USDHHS, 1995). All of these diseases can be prevented or modulated in their effects by programs of regular physical activity.

The economic impact of a population whose health is impaired by illnesses should not overshadow the personal impact. Each incidence of illness brought on by lack of physical activity represents one individual who has been robbed of his or her potential for living an active, productive, enjoyable life. In response to the previously stated and other epidemiological data, the U.S. Department of Health and Human Services developed a list of health objectives to be attained by the millennium. These objectives were published in a book entitled *Healthy People 2000* (USDHHS, 1990). Increasing the physical activity levels of the American people is the first objective listed in this document. A portion of these physical activity and fitness objectives are shown in figure 2.14. Though the objectives listed in this document were set in the 1990s, many were not achieved by the year 2000, but they remain worthwhile goals for the nation.

The reason physical activity figures so prominently in the nation's health objectives is that it has been shown to effectively prevent and help rehabilitate the costly diseases described earlier. In addition, physical activity has been associated with a reduced risk of colon cancer and appears to help lower the risk of developing non-insulin-dependent diabetes mellitus. Regular physical activity may enable the elderly to live independently for a longer period of time and prevent falls and other injuries among this population. Regular exercise also lowers the risk of mortality for both younger and older adults (USDHHS, 1996). Clearly, the profession of kinesiology is well positioned to make a significant contribution to the attainment of national health goals.

The failure to make physical activity a part of our daily lives has led to a health crisis of critical proportions. The response of U.S. health agencies was to draft a list of national health objectives for the year 2000, which included recommendations for increasing the level of the nation's physical activity.

Physical Activity as Prevention and Therapy

Exercise also plays an important role in therapeutic medicine. Through regular, supervised physi-

Risk-Reduction Objectives By the Year 2000

1.0   Increase to at least 30% the proportion of people aged 6 and older who engage regularly, preferably daily, in light to moderate physical activity for at least 30 minutes per day.
(Baseline: 22% of people aged 18 and older were active for at least 30 minutes 5 or more times per week, and 12% were active 7 or more times per week in 1985.)

2.0   Increase to at least 20% the proportion of people aged 18 and older and to at least 75% the proportion of children and adolescents aged 6 through 17 who engage in vigorous physical activity that promotes the development and maintenance of cardiorespiratory fitness 3 or more days per week for 20 minutes per occasion.
(Baseline: 12% for people aged 18 and older in 1985; 66% for youth aged 10 through 17 in 1984.)

3.0   Reduce to no more than 15% the proportion of people aged 6 and older who engage in no leisure-time physical activity.
(Baseline: 24% for people aged 18 and older in 1985.)

4.0   Increase to at least 40% the proportion of people aged 6 and older who regularly perform physical activities that enhance and maintain muscular strength, muscular endurance, and flexibility.
(No baseline data.)

5.0   Increase to at least 50% the proportion of overweight people aged 12 and older who have adopted sound dietary practices combined with regular physical activity to attain an appropriate body weight.
(Baseline: 30% of overweight women and 25% of overweight men for people aged 18 and older in 1985.)

6.0   Increase to at least 50% the proportion of primary care providers who routinely assess and counsel their patients regarding the frequency, duration, type, and intensity of each patient's physical activity practices.
(Baseline: Physicians provided exercise counseling for about 30% of sedentary patients in 1988.)

Figure 2.14   Selected objectives from *Healthy People 2000*.

Adapted from U.S. Department of Health and Human Services, 1990, *Healthy People 2000* (DHHS Pub. No. [PHS] 91-50213) (Hyattsville, MD: Public Health Service).

cal activity patients can regain the use of limbs that have been rendered useless due to strokes, injuries, or disease. Physical activity programs increase the strength, range of motion, and endurance in limbs that have been immobilized in casts. A particularly effective form of exercise therapy is cardiac rehabilitation, in which supervised programs of physical activity are designed and implemented specifically for those who have suffered heart attacks. Activity programs designed to reduce weight represent another form of therapeutic exercise. Obviously, it is difficult to draw a clear line that distinguishes between preventive and therapeutic or rehabilitative exercise; when we engage in an exercise for its therapeutic effects, we also gain a measure of prevention.

How Do We Exercise?

What are the most common kinds of health-related physical activity? We noted earlier that exercise walking, with 70 million participants in 1995, is the most popular form of health-related exercise. This is down slightly from the 71 million participants in 1990, but it is considerably more than the 41 million who participated in 1985 (NSGA, 1996). Is participation in exercise increasing or decreasing? Look at table 2.9. Here participation rates are compared across a 10-year period for exercise walking, exercising with equipment, aerobics, running/jogging, and calisthenics. What do these data tell us?

For one thing, the data suggest that aerobics, largely an activity of the 18- to 44-year-old female segment of the population, may have reached a plateau in popularity between 1985 and 1995 (NSGA, 1996). We can also see that participation in jogging/running, and particularly calisthenics, has declined. On the other hand, exercising with equipment (stair-climbing equipment, stationary bicycles, etc.) has seen a dramatic increase. This may be because technology makes exercise more convenient, more accessible, and

TABLE 2.9
Changes in Exercise Patterns Between 1985 and 1995

Type of exercise	In millions		
	1985	1990	1995
Exercise walking	41.5	71.4	70.3
Exercising with equipment	32.1	35.3	44.3
Aerobics	23.9	23.3	23.1
Running/jogging	26.3	23.8	20.6
Calisthenics	26.1	13.2	9.3

Reprinted, by permission, from National Sporting Goods Association, *Research* (May 1996), 36.

usually less dependent on the weather. We may expect this application of technology to exercise to continue. No doubt future exercise leaders will be faced with the need to update constantly their knowledge about the "machine–exerciser interface" and the effects of various machines on physiological processes.

Psychological Effects of Exercise

Healthful living includes psychological as well as physical well-being, and a wealth of evidence suggests that regular physical activity can contribute to an enhanced sense of well-being, whether by increasing the secretion of mood-altering hormones, adjusting participants' levels of psychological arousal, or reducing reactions to stress. Feelings of well-being also may come about as a result of reductions in fatigue, enhanced body image, or even as a result of social contacts encountered in physical activity contexts (Kircaldy & Shephard, 1990).

Sometimes exercise is lauded as a means of preventing mental health disorders, largely on the strength of evidence showing that acute (short-term) bouts of exercise can effectively reduce anxiety in anxiety-prone individuals. Evidence also suggests that chronic exercise (regular exercise over the long term) can reduce symptoms of depression and possibly even reduce the risk of developing depression, although much more research is needed on this topic (USDHHS, 1996).

Exercise, along with cognitive skills training, meditation, yoga, and other methods, also can help alleviate stress. Practitioners should not, however, recommend physical activity as a means of overall mental illness prevention. As one scholar observed: "For the present, it is probably safest to assume that highly active, fit individuals may at some point in their lifetimes be prone to the same reactive mood disorders and mental health problems as are less active, unfit individuals" (Brown, 1990).

Detriments of Physical Activity

It might be good at this point to take a reality check. Obviously, physical activity can be a valuable adjunct to healthy living. But it is not an unqualified "good." Just because some physical activity is good, it doesn't necessarily follow that more is better. The modern physical activity professional must be acutely aware that physical activity can also bring about detrimental physical and psychological effects.

Overexercise, whether in the form of weight training, running, aerobics, or repetitive motions in work settings, can result in stress fractures, strained muscles, inflamed tendons, and psychological staleness. We have already noted that carpal tunnel syndrome, a painful and debilitating injury to the hand and wrist brought on by repeating the same hand motions day after day as in typing and assembly tasks, plagues thousands of workers. Sport participation and vigorous exercise brings, with all of its enjoyment and excitement, the dark side of injury and damage brought on by long-term wear and tear. Injured knees, fingers, wrists, hips, and backs take their toll on athletes, not only in the weeks and months following the injury, but in later years as well. Years of pitching a baseball can lead to rotator cuff injuries; stress fractures are common to gymnasts.

Some forms of contact sports such as American football have such alarming injury rates that we may well question whether the injuries incurred are really accidents. Indeed, we have come to expect them to occur, as evidenced by regulations in many states requiring high school football teams to have a physician on the sideline and an ambulance waiting in the vicinity of the field.

Habitual physical activity is also detrimental when people develop an unhealthy emotional

Tennis Injuries Plague Junior Players

Seena Hamilton, director of the Easter Bowl, an event that attracts the top junior tennis players to Miami each spring, became alarmed about the potentially damaging effects of the sport when out of more than 100 players, 25 were forced to withdraw as a result of injuries sustained at the 1996 tournament. In a survey she commissioned of 429 junior players (their mean age was 14.7 years), 62% reported having had at least one injury that required a doctor's visit or prevented them from playing for more than three days. The most common injuries were to joints: 32% reported having injured their ankles, 31% their shoulders, 30% their knees, 26% their backs, and 20% their wrists. The injurious effects of playing appear to accumulate over time. Sixty-eight percent of girls in the 10- to 12-year-old group played without injury; only 28% of those in the 17- to 18-year-old group were injury-free. Among the 17- to 18-year-old boys, only 2% played injury-free.

Hamilton believes that the juniors are playing and training too much. A fellow director of a large tennis club agreed. "I've been coaching kids for 18 years," he said, "and what I see is that the parents don't believe the kids. The junior player says he is hurting, and the parent thinks he is trying to get out of practice. The best thing for everyone is to take your child's word for it" (Stevenson, 1997, p. Y27)

dependence on exercise. Physical activity addiction is characterized by a single-minded focus on an activity to the extent that daily obligations, important for a healthy and well-balanced life, are neglected. When does devotion to an activity such as running or golf become addictive and harmful? There are no clear boundaries separating healthy from unhealthy exercise, but eyebrows might be raised when physical activity interferes with work or harms important personal relationships. Another signal is when emotional disorders are brought on when the opportunity to engage in the activity is taken away. Many avid runners, for example, experience acute bouts of depression when they are injured and unable to run. High school wrestlers who must "make weight" in order to compete within a specific weight category often engage in harmful practices. Young women interested in gymnastics or figure skating can become preoccupied with weight loss and continue to exercise when body mass is already minimal. As with most other activities in our daily lives, the best prescription for a happy, healthful, and balanced life is to pursue physical activity with a sense of dedication and commitment, but in moderation.

When pursued in moderation with an eye toward a balanced life, physical activity is desirable. When it is performed under circumstances that put the integrity of the body at risk, or induce questionable behavior patterns and psychological states, it is undesirable.

The Sphere of Competition

Do you like to compete against others? Does the chance to compete with classmates for the highest grade, to compete with coworkers for the "worker of the month award," or to compete against others for the league championship heighten your interest in the activity? Chances are that competition plays an important role in some part of your life. And there is a good chance that physical activity figures prominently in whatever form that competition takes (see figure 2.15).

Competition is not an activity in and of itself but rather is an organizing principle for activity. Not only can it add to the enjoyment of an activity, but it also often leads to an increase in the level of performance. Skipping stones on a pond can be an exciting experience for children; when they decide to see who can skip a stone the farthest, it becomes even more exciting, and their

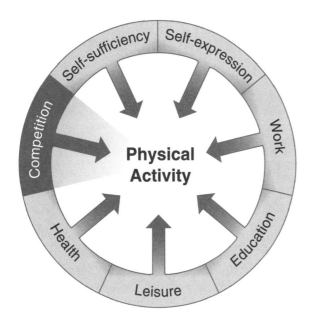

Figure 2.15 Competition as a sphere of physical activity experience.

stone-skipping performances may also improve. Some people thoroughly enjoy shooting baskets alone on the playground, or playing golf by themselves or in leisurely social contexts with friends. Others seek the peculiar kind of excitement that can only come from competition.

Nature of Competition

Competition is derived from the Greek word meaning "to strive together," but most of us think of it as "striving against." We compete *against* opponents. But if you think about it, competition between teams or individuals really does require an element of cooperation or striving *together*. Cooperation is necessary to hold the game together. Opponents who play their best help us to play our best. When players become spoilsports or give up, or when they cheat, the game falls apart.

When most people think of competitive physical activity, they think immediately of sports, physical activities that place a premium on skill, strength, endurance, or other physical qualities and in which one's performance is assessed in relation to a standard or the performance of others. One sport sociologist defines sports as "institutionalized competitive activities that involve vigorous physical exertion or the use of relatively complex physical skills . . ." (Coakley, 1998, p.

19). Unlike physical activity in the other spheres of experience, sports depend entirely on the organizing principle of competition. Extract competition from sports and you are left with a goalless, aimless physical activity. For this reason we have designated a separate sphere for competition.

Competition can be added to physical activity in different ways. In **side-by-side competitive activities** such as golf, swimming, running, bowling, shotputting, or cycling, no direct interaction takes place between competitors. Competitors do not interfere with each others' chances of succeeding; in fact, doing so is against the rules. In **face-to-face noncontact activities** such as volleyball, baseball, tennis, or racquetball, competitors interact by trying to maximize their own chances and decrease their opponents' chances of winning. In this form of competition, players deliberately attempt to thwart the efforts of their opponents and take advantage of their competitive weaknesses, although no direct contact between opposing players is permitted by the rules. In **face-to-face contact activities** such as football, rugby, hockey, or wrestling (and increasingly soccer and basketball), players thwart the efforts of opponents by direct physical manipulation (blocks, tackles, checks, etc.). Finally, **impersonal competition** occurs when participants "compete" against records set by others. Trying to set a new record for the time taken to swim the English Channel, or trying to climb a mountain by a route never before taken, are activities in which one's competitors (holders of the record) are not present. In fact, they may not even be alive!

One problem with adding competition to activities is that it can become more than an organizing principle to increase our enjoyment or push us to better performances. Often it becomes an end in itself. When coaches and players elevate the goal of winning a contest above the sheer enjoyment of the activity or the basic values of friendship, caring, and cooperation, they are converting competition into an end rather than a means to an end. Mihalyi Csikszentmihalyi, a psychologist who has taught us much about sport, says, "The challenges of competition can be stimulating and enjoyable. But when beating the opponents takes precedence in the mind over performing as well as possible, enjoyment tends to disappear. Competition is enjoyable only when it is a means to perfect one's skills: when it becomes an end in itself, it ceases to be fun" (Csikszentmihalyi, 1990b).

🔑 Competition is a spice added to physical activity to make it fun and to push us to higher performance levels. We are intrinsically fascinated by matching our talents with those of others, or against impersonal standards. When competition becomes an end in itself rather than a means to an end, however, it may no longer be fun, and in some cases it can be harmful.

Popular Competitive Pursuits

Many people begin playing sports at an early age and continue to play throughout childhood. Recent estimates are that half of all children in grades 9 through 12 are members of at least one sport team run by a school or other organization (USDHHS, 1996). In many cases this early contact results in a lifetime commitment to a sport. This accounts at least partly for the fact that more

than 200 million people aged seven and older participate in at least one sport more than once a year (USDC, 1996b). Everywhere we look we see sports being played—on playgrounds, on high school and college athletic fields, and especially on television. More people participate in sports than in artistic activities *combined*, including playing classical music (4 million), participating in modern dance (8 million), creating pottery (8 million), painting (10 million), or creative writing (7 million) (USDC, 1996c). This pervasiveness of sports often leads people to conclude that participation in sports is on the rise. But is it?

A survey of reported sport participation rates of those seven years old or older in the ten-year span from 1985 to 1995 (see table 2.10) presents a very mixed picture. Although participation increased dramatically over this decade for bowling, basketball, golf, baseball, soccer, and hockey, participation rates in softball, badminton, tennis, racquetball, and volleyball plunged severely (NSGA, 1996). So severe has been the plummet in tennis participation that the International Health, Racquet and Sportsclub Association, in cooperation with the Tennis Industry Association,

TABLE 2.10
Changes in Participation Rates in Sport Activities Between 1985 and 1995

Activity	In millions*			% change '85–'95	% change '90–'95
	1985	1990	1995		
Bowling	35.7	40.1	41.9	+17	+4.4
Basketball	19.5	26.3	30.1	+57	+12.6
Golf	18.5	23.0	24.0	+30	+4.3
Volleyball	20.1	23.2	18.0	–10	–22.4
Softball	21.6	20.1	17.6	–34	–14.2
Baseball	12.8	15.6	15.7	+23	+0.01
Tennis	19.0	18.4	12.6	–34	–31.5
Badminton	11.4	9.3	5.8	–50	–37.6
Racquetball	7.9	8.1	4.7	–41	–41.9
Hockey	1.0	1.9	2.5	+150	+31.0

*Individuals, seven years of age or older, who participated in the activity more than once a year.
Reprinted, by permission, from National Sporting Goods Association, *Research* (May 1996), 36.

How Much Time Do You Spend Playing and Watching Sports?

Keep a diary of your sports and sports watching activities over the next two weeks. Keep daily tallies for each category listed here and record the totals in the blanks that follow.

1. Total number of hours spent playing sports: _____
   a. Of this total, approximately _____ hours were in connection with a varsity team.
   b. Of this total, approximately _____ hours were in an individual sport.
   c. Of this total, approximately _____ hours were in a team sport.
   d. Of this total, approximately _____ hours were in a coed competition.
   e. Of this total, approximately _____ hours were enjoyable.
   f. Do you wish you had played more? What factors tended to weigh against your participating more?_____

2. Total number of hours spent watching sports: _____
   a. Of this total, approximately _____ hours were spent watching sports on television.
   b. Of this total, approximately _____ hours were spent watching sports alone.
   c. What sport activities did you watch and what percentage of time was spent watching each?

Sport	%		Sport	%
_____	___		_____	___
_____	___		_____	___
_____	___		_____	___

   d. Generally, do you prefer watching sports live or on television? _____

ran a three-year campaign to "make tennis hot again" ("Sports Looking to Change Image," 1995). In a separate action, the U.S. Tennis Association announced a program to pump $31.4 million into a national effort to attract 800,000 new players by 2002 (Price, 1997). Ektelon, a maker of racquetball products and accessories, launched a number of programs designed to increase the appeal of racquetball, which also has experienced an astounding downward slide in participation.

The solid gains in hockey participation are encouraging, although the absolute number of participants in this sport are relatively small (2.5 million). As you might expect, young people are more likely than older people to participate in sports, although some recent evidence suggests that the growth in basketball participation by 12- to 17-year-olds is occurring at a slower rate than

it is among adults. The same trend is evident in soccer where the declining rate of participation by 12- to 17-year-olds stands in sharp contrast to the huge increase in adult participation ("Industry May Hinge on Kids Exercising," 1995).

Age, Socioeconomic Factors, and Competition

Age and socioeconomic factors have a major influence on sport participation rates. As we have seen, older people are less likely to engage in sports than younger people: whereas 59 million people between the ages of 18 and 24 participate, only 18 million of participants are between the ages of 65 and 74. Still, more than 7 million people in the United States between the ages of 75 and 96 continue to engage in sports, many of them competing in state and national masters championships!

Household income also has a dramatic effect on participation rates in almost all sport activities, but especially in golf and skiing where nearly seven times as many people in the $50,000 to $74,900 family income group participate as people in families earning less than $15,000. As you might expect, income has a much smaller effect on participation in more accessible and less expensive types of physical activity such as bicycle riding, swimming, and bowling (USDC, 1996b).

🔑 Increases in some forms of sport participation have slowed dramatically in recent years, and in many sports, participation has decreased. This is most apparent in participation by adolescents, which shows a sharp drop following high school graduation.

Wrap-Up

We have covered a lot of ground in this chapter. We began by emphasizing the importance of physical activity in our daily lives. We underscored its importance by showing how physical activity intersects our lives in almost every dimension of human experience. As a way of helping you to appreciate this, we divided life into various dimensions or spheres and showed how physical activity plays a critical role in each.

We saw that physical activity is essential to performing the daily tasks that allow us to live independently (the self-sufficiency sphere), a problem that becomes acute when we are disabled from injury, disease, or old age. Sometimes we use physical activity to communicate our intentions to others through gestures, postures, or other movements (the self-expression sphere). At other times we purposely perform physical activities in dance and rituals as a way of expressing our emotions, attitudes, and creative impulses.

Physical activity is central to our work (the work sphere), but we saw that different jobs require different types and amounts of physical activity. For example, some high-status, high-paying jobs require very little physical activity while inducing a great deal of stress and creating health hazards for people in these positions.

Almost all of our formal educational programs set aside time for systematic instruction in physical activity, usually sports and exercise (the education sphere). We noted the variability in quality of these programs and questioned whether the time devoted to physical education and the activities normally included in such classes were sufficient to meet physical activity goals published by public health officials.

Although our free time can be used for a variety of purposes, we often engage in activities and contexts that help us achieve a leisure state (the leisure sphere). We saw that large-muscle physical activity, properly structured and performed in conducive contexts, can be an excellent means to leisure. We also reviewed evidence that suggests a national trend toward less physically demanding leisure activities, one of which is sports watching.

Physical activity is also an important part of our efforts to maintain and improve our health (the health sphere). We reviewed the major health benefits of regular physical activity and tracked the trends in the types of exercise people pursue to experience these benefits. Finally, we looked at physical activity in competitive contexts, primarily sports (the competition sphere). We saw that in some circumstances, competition can make physical activity more fun and challenging and motivate us to perform better. When competition becomes an end in itself, however, it can detract from the very best that physical activity has to offer.

In examining the spheres of physical activity experience, it becomes apparent that we rely on physical activity every day, not only to survive, but also to live full and rich lives. Surely it has many practical benefits. Yet it would be misleading to leave you with the impression that physical activity is important only because it is useful to achieving some external ends. Physical activity may be just as important to us for the special types of personal experiences it offers as for any benefits we derive from participating. We will explore this personal or subjective side of physical activity in chapter 4. But first let's take a detour to underscore the vital importance of physical activity *as* physical activity, and to learn more about its important characteristics and varieties.

Study Questions

1. What are ADLs and IADLs, and why are they important to independent daily living?

2. What type of physical activity professionals are likely to be involved with treatment of an individual with carpal tunnel syndrome? What professional is likely to be involved in redesigning the workplace so that the risk of carpal tunnel syndrome is reduced?

3. What are gestures, and what purposes do they serve in our daily living?

4. Why is public school physical education important? What objectives do physical education teachers pursue?

5. List three health benefits of regular physical activity.

6. What does the element of competition add to physical activity? When is this helpful, and when might it be harmful?

7. Describe a situation in which physical activity may help nourish and maintain a state of leisure. Describe a situation in which physical activity may diminish the possibility that a state of leisure will be attained.

3

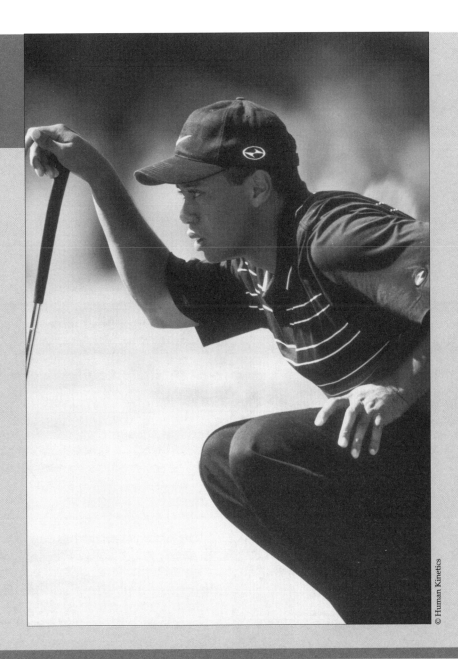

© Human Kinetics

The Importance of Physical Activity Experiences

Shirl J. Hoffman

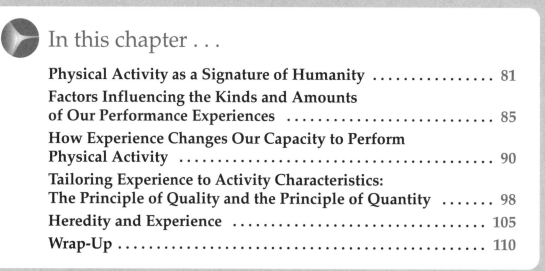

In this chapter . . .

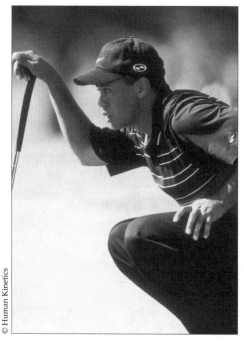

© Human Kinetics

To those who follow golf, Tiger Woods is an authentic phenomenon—"an extremely unusual or extraordinary thing" (Neufeldt, 1988, p. 1013). After only a few years on the professional tour, his accomplishments already rival some of the greatest who have played the game. His booming 350-yard drives, pinpoint accuracy from the fairway to the greens, and his deft putting skills, all executed in the pressure-packed atmosphere of the PGA tour, combine to produce performances never dreamed possible. How do we begin to explain Tiger Woods' sensational mastery of the game of golf?

As a start, consider this: Before Tiger could walk, his father, Earl, would take him to the garage in their home and strap him into a high chair while Earl methodically hit ball after ball into an indoor practice net. It wasn't so much that Earl wanted to practice, it was his way of modeling the golf swing to Tiger, and, to his way of thinking, the first step he took toward developing his son into the world's best golfer. From that point on, golf was to consume most of Tiger's life. This wasn't because his father made him do it, but because he loved it, from those very first sessions in which he watched his father hit balls. Before Tiger entered kindergarten he was winning golf tournaments. At age 3 he won a Pitch, Putt, and Drive competition against 10- and 11-year-olds. At age 6 his father had him listen to tapes designed to help him deal with the psychological stresses of the game. By age 10 he had won two Junior World 10-and-under championships in San Diego. At age 12 he began to take lessons from a teaching pro, and at 13, Tiger had begun working with a sports psychologist and won his first national tournament. By age 14 he had traveled to Paris to play in the Southern California/France Junior Cup, and in the pro-junior event at a tournament in Fort Worth, Tiger shot a score of 69, beating or tying 18 of the touring pros. At age 17 he played in his first PGA tournament (while an amateur), and of course went on to join the PGA tour, winning a host of tournaments, including two majors, during his first few years of competition (Rosaforte, 1997).

How did Tiger become an elite golfer? Giving the question some thought, you may have come to the conclusion that Tiger possesses innate abilities and inherited traits that are perfectly suited to the game. Certainly innate ability and maturation have made their contributions, (a point considered later in this chapter), but a more likely explanation is his extensive experience with the game. From the first year of his life golf has been the significant physical activity in his life. He has been engaged in the kinds and amounts of physical activity experiences that inevitably lead to improvement in performance of this particular skill. Has anyone ever played more golf over his or her life span than Woods? It's hard to believe that's possible! In this chapter we will explore in a very general way how our experiences with physical activity can transform our performances, health, and our physical appearances.

The word *experience* is defined in many different ways so it might be a good idea to clarify precisely how we will be using the term in this chapter. One definition is "individual reaction to events, feelings, etc." (Neufeldt, 1988, p. 478). In this sense we may "experience" sadness, joy, beauty, and a host of other impressions. These experiences are within us. This version of experience, termed **subjective experience,** will be explored in the next chapter. In this chapter we will be concerned with experience defined as any "*activity* [italics added] that includes training, observation of practice, and personal participation" (Neufeldt, 1988, p. 478). This form of experience called **activity experience** refers to our actual performances or observations of physical activity. If you are *experienced* as opposed to *inexperienced* in skiing, you will have performed it on many occasions in many different contexts and probably with many different people. Tiger Woods, for example, has a tremendous depth of activity experience with golf. In real life, our activity experiences are always accompanied by subjective experiences, but here we pretend that they can be separated, merely to make it more convenient to study them.

As you move through this chapter, you will be reminded again and again of the critical importance of experience in our efforts to expand our capacities to perform physical activity and to improve health and psychological well-being.

 ## CHAPTER OBJECTIVES

In this chapter we will:

- Help you gain an appreciation for physical activity as it contributes to and expresses the signature of humanity

- Encourage your appreciation for the various ways experience can expand the human potential for physical activity

- Help you develop insights into factors to be taken into account in prescribing physical activity experiences

- Explain some basic principles governing the relationships among skill, practice, and learning and among physical performance capacity, training, and conditioning

- Discuss the relationship between physical activity experience and physical fitness

- Discuss how the effects of experience may be modified by heredity and other factors

As central as physical activity is to human life, we do not come into the world readily equipped to do it. Birth innately endows us with an ability to move, but performance experience is required in order to develop control over our movements—to convert sheer movement into physical activity. Newborn humans spend a lot of time kicking their legs and waving their arms. These are aimless and spontaneous movements that occur without prompting or encouragement from their parents. Infants also move automatically in response to external stimuli. For example, holding a newborn in the prone position over water may elicit swimming-like movements of the arms and legs, applying pressure to the sole of the foot elicits a crawling pattern, and turning the head of a supine infant to one side causes the arm and leg on the same side to extend. These reflexes, along with spontaneous movements of the arms and legs, are important to the development of the infant's motor system, but because they are neither voluntary nor goal-directed, they do not constitute physical activity as it is defined in this text. Much experience and maturation are required for these movements to blossom into what we know as physical activity.

Physical activity experience refers to our history of participation, training, practice, or observation of any particular physical activity. It is differentiated from subjective physical activity experiences, which are our reactions, feelings, and thoughts about physical activity.

Physical activity experiences are important because they are the essential means by which we increase our capacities to perform physical activity. Think about the changes that came about as a result of your earliest experiences with physical activity. You probably don't remember the rough-and-tumble experience of learning to walk, but if you have ever watched infants try to master the skill, you can appreciate the role your early experiences played in the development of this important skill. The transition from the primitive to the mature pattern displayed in figure 3.1 happens only as the infant accumulates the physical activity experiences of walking. Many of these efforts will be colossal failures, yet even infants learn from failure. With experience, the short stride and high "guard arm" position, the toeing out to maximize balance, and the tendency to swing the arms in conjunction with the legs rather than in opposition to the legs will give rise to the well-timed locomotor movements depicted in the last picture in figure 3.1.

From the moment of birth, physical activity experiences enable us to become increasingly proficient in physical activity. The amount of experience people accumulate in a particular activity varies considerably, beginning at the earliest years.

Almost everybody engaged in physical activities wants to be able to perform them faster, more forcefully, for a longer period of time, or more skillfully. The only way to do this is to expose ourselves systematically to more and more *appropriate* physical activity experiences. Such experiences enable people enrolled in fitness programs to become stronger or to increase their cardiovascular endurance. Physical activity experiences also improve the skills of athletes, dancers, factory workers, military personnel, and stroke recovery patients.

Physical activity experiences also are important because they are the means by which we achieve the expected health and psychological benefits of physical activity. These benefits usually go hand in hand with an increased capacity for performing physical activity, but not always. As we will see, physical activity often leads to reductions in body weight and percent body fat and decreased stress levels, but it also is possible to achieve these changes without significantly improving your physical activity performance, or for that matter, without engaging in physical activity at all.

In section 2 of this text you will study the scientific bases for the effects of experience by learning how physiological systems respond to repeated performances of activities. This will help you appreciate at a deeper level why your capacity for running a mile in a shorter time is improved by training experiences that stress the cardiovascular system, or why your capacity for lifting heavier weight is improved by progressively increasing the resistance your muscles are made to work against. You will also come to understand why we become better tango dancers or gymnasts by immersing ourselves in well-organized practice and conditioning routines.

Obviously, not all types of physical activity experiences induce positive changes. Poorly planned training or practice programs, for example, may not help you achieve your goals. In

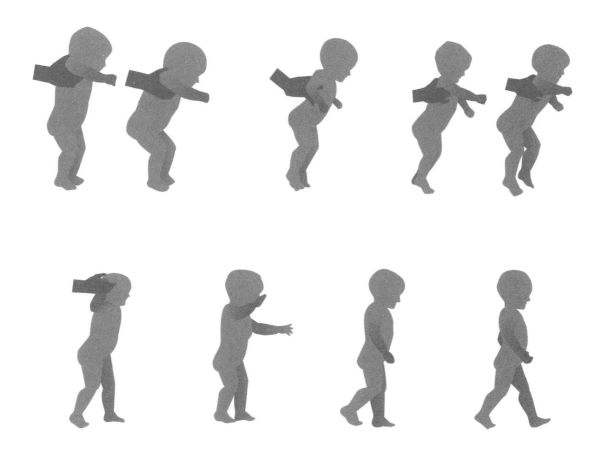

Figure 3.1 Physical activity experience is essential to the normal development of motor patterns such as walking.

Adapted, by permission, from M.B. McGraw, 1943, *The neuromuscular maturation of the human infant*. (New York: Columbia University Press).

fact, they may be wasteful or your time and energy or, worse, retard progress toward your goals by causing injury or exposing you to unnecessary harm. This is why trained physical activity specialists are so important. Professionals such as physical therapists, coaches, physical education teachers, and personal trainers specialize in the "physical activity experience business." *Their professional expertise lies in the systematic manipulation of physical activity experiences based on scientific principles, for the purposes of improving the skill, performance levels, and health and well-being of those they serve.* Scholars and researchers in kinesiology also are in the experience business; through their work they discover procedures that professionals can use to plan and direct physical activity experiences. Many of the courses required for kinesiology majors center on specific ways physical activity experiences can safely and efficiently be manipulated to bring about intended changes in clients' capacities for physical activity.

The central concern of all kinesiologists and physical activity professionals is the systematic manipulation of physical activity experiences based on sound scientific principles in order to bring about improvement in skill, performance, health, and well-being.

Physical Activity as a Signature of Humanity

Although it is tempting to think of physical activity experience as merely the mundane repetition of muscular activity, such a limited view wouldn't do justice to this far-reaching and important concept. Actually, physical activity draws on those aspects of humanity that help define us as the highest order of living creatures, and were

Comparing Humans and Robots

Robotic engineering has enabled the construction of machines that are able to accomplish many tasks more efficiently and effectively than humans can. Robots have been particularly effective in carrying out assembly tasks in the automobile and other industries. Does this robotic physical activity differ from human physical activity, and if so, in what ways? Consider how the human performance of each of the following physical activities would differ from a robot's performance. (You may find it helpful to review the definition of physical activity in chapter 1.)

1. Golf: A robotic "golfer" is able to drive the ball 400 yards (366 m) consistently.
2. Dance: A robotic "dancer" is able to accompany a partner by moving in the proper directions and in time to the music.
3. Weightlifting: A robotic lifter is able to lift a 336-kilogram (900-lb) weight from the floor.
4. Marathon running: A robotic runner is programmed to run a marathon at a consistent pace of 24 kilometers (15 mi) per hour, enabling it to break the world record.
5. Keyboarding: A robotic word processor is able to type a 100-page manuscript in 10 minutes without error.

it not for this, physical activity experience would not be able to work its marvelous effects. Let's step back from the topic of experience for a moment to explore how physical activity helps define our humanity and how our innately human capacities enable us to develop our physical activity capacities through experience.

What characteristics set humans apart from animals or machines? Your first thought might be that we possess souls or a moral sense, or that we are able to engage in complex forms of social communication, or that we possess a capacity for high-level reasoning that animals and machines can never replicate. Good cases can be made for each of these arguments. What you probably didn't think about, however, is that our extraordinary capacity to translate complex mental concepts into precise and creative physical actions is also a defining human characteristic.

Can you imagine what the future of people might be if they became robots: able to execute stronger, faster, and more expansive movements than humans, but lacking the intelligence to plan and guide their movements? Or could you imagine people who are the converse of robots: able to think thoughts as deeply as Einstein, feel emotion as keenly as Mozart or with moral conviction as strong as that of Mother Theresa, but with no way of converting these essentially human

traits into physical actions? The robots would be doomed because their amazing capacity to move was controlled by forces external to themselves. The second group would also be doomed because they could never get anything done—their enormous thoughts and feelings would have no way of being expressed in human movement. Neither group would be able to advance the cause of society.

🔑 A unique capacity for performing physical activity is one of the major features that contribute to the distinctive character of the human race.

But what about animals? Don't animals have this capacity to link movements with intentions and to plan their physical movements; can't they perform physical activity? (Remember that only movement that is voluntary and intended to accomplish a goal meets the technical definition of physical activity.) All evidence suggests that some animals actually do engage in goal-oriented, voluntary movements. Chimpanzees in West Africa, for example, use small stones as tools to crack palm nuts using the same motor patterns as the villagers from whom they (apparently) learned the technique (Kordtlandt, 1989). Even relatively small-brained birds seem to be able to match movements with intentions. Some years ago, a species in the British Isles learned to rip open the cardboard tops of milk cartons and drink the cream, forcing milk companies in the region to redesign the containers that are delivered on people's porches. Small ground finches can uncover food by pushing aside stones weighing 14 times their body weight with their feet (equivalent to a 75-kilogram [200-lb] human moving a 1,360-kilogram [1.5-ton] rock!) by bracing their head against a large rock for leverage (Gill, 1989). Yet, amazing as these examples might seem, it can be argued that the human capacity for physical activity far exceeds that of these and other lower animals. This is an important assertion; let's look at it more carefully.

Human and Animal Physical Activity Compared

Recall that physical activity is movement that is intentional, voluntary, and directed toward achieving an identifiable goal. Understanding the technical definition of physical activity is essential to understanding the discussion that follows. Having reviewed the definition, you are now ready to consider four ways in which physical activity may be considered unique to the human species.

Intelligence-Based Physical Activity

First, because we are big-brained, highly intelligent creatures, our physical activity tends to be rooted in more intricate plans and directed toward more sophisticated goals than is the case with lower animals. Motor plans or mental images serve as dynamic maps to guide our movements in skills as simple as a standing long jump or in more complex skills such as piloting an airplane, performing brain surgery, or catching a Frisbee. Animals, by comparison, entertain relatively simple plans. A cheetah, for example, will easily outrun a human in a contest in which the goal is simply to run as fast as possible, but, being unable to formulate a clear understanding of the goal and the constraints imposed by the rules, a cheetah will not be able to adapt its extraordinary running skill to the complexities of an Olympic relay race or to the rule-bound game of soccer.

Ethically and Aesthetically Based Physical Activity

Because humans are essentially spiritual creatures possessing unique moral and aesthetic senses, we can use our movements to express our imagination and moral reasoning. Our movements can be used to express beauty, joy, wonder, and other deep and complex moods. This isn't to deny that other animals also have

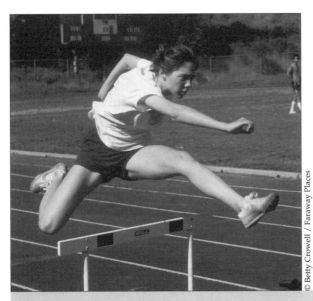

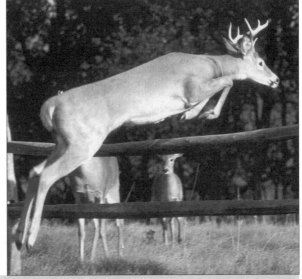

Humans link physical activity to more sophisticated cognitive plans than animals do.

emotional lives. Chimps, for example, can become so depressed when their mothers die that they sometimes die too (Heltne, 1989). Although some chimps can use sign language to express emotions and create basic paintings, rarely have animal emotions been translated through muscular actions into symbolic works of art or other elaborate expressions of sorrow, joy, or wonder. If thousands of chimpanzees were each given a hammer and chisel, by mere chance one of them might be able to create a recognizable work of art, but never something as profound as Michelangelo's *David* or Rodin's *The Thinker*. Animals may engage in elaborate mating dances, but the choreography is the product of instincts, not intentional expression of mood in movement as occurs, for example, in *Swan Lake*.

Flexibility and Adaptability of Physical Activity

Human physical activity is distinguished from that of other animals by virtue of the unique com-

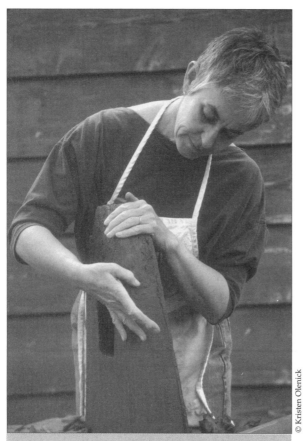

Humans are able to connect physical activity to complex aesthetic sensibilities.

© Kristen Olenick

binations of movements permitted by our anatomy. At first, this may seem to be an exaggeration. After all, elephants are equipped for performing far more forceful movements than humans, and greyhounds can surpass us in speed, dolphins in swimming, and monkeys in agility. In what ways, then, can we say that humans hold a movement advantage?

Two properties of our anatomies give us a great advantage in moving. First, with our upright posture and bipedal gait we are the only animals whose forelimbs have been totally freed from assisting with walking, flying, brachiating, or swimming. With a foot specially constructed to bear weight and give leverage to the leg, a pelvis specifically designed for attaching strong muscles needed to help maintain bipedal balance, and thigh bones to permit long strides in walking, our ability to walk on two feet has been described as "the most spectacular physical trait of human beings" (LaBarre, 1963, p. 73).

Second, humans have available a dexterity of movement made possible by a unique complex of hands, arms, shoulders, and stereoscopic vision. The human hand possesses a true opposable thumb, a much more beneficial construction than the typical primate hand with its five fingers all operating more or less on the same plane. This arrangement allows us to perform delicate grasping, manipulating, and adjusting movements not possible by others in the animal kingdom. But this is not the only advantage. Our hands are positioned at the end of a series of long arm bones, joined to an amazingly moveable shoulder girdle that a dog or cat would die for! (Imagine a dog, cat, or horse being able to scratch its back with its forelimb!) This moveable shoulder girdle enables us to position our hands through an enormously large path in space. This upper-arm advantage is complemented by a facility for stereoscopic vision (lacking in many animals) that not only gives us advantages in depth perception but also allows us to perform most of our movements in our field of vision.

Ability to Improve Performance Through Planned Experience

The fourth—and perhaps the most significant—characteristic that distinguishes humans is the ability to improve the capacity for physical activity through planned, systematic practice and training. Only humans possess the intelligence that allows them to use physical activity in planned, systematic, and scientifically verifiable ways as a means of improving their health, performance, or skill, or as a means of physical rehabilitation. Obviously, the cardiovascular efficiency of the young lion or eagle improves as its hunting range expands, but the driving force of its activity is hunger and survival, not a systematic conditioning plan to improve the physiological functioning of its body. Also, while some species of animals teach their young methods of hunting and fishing, the methods are relatively primitive, lacking the sophistication of human plans.

In summary, the capacity to link physical activity to complex plans and deep moral and aesthetic sentiments, an anatomy that permits these sophisticated thoughts and feelings to be played out in complex sequences of skeletal movements, and a highly developed ability to systematically plan and implement activity experiences to improve physical performance, have contributed immensely to the advance of civilization. In this sense, physical activity enables us to explore, test, and manifest our humanity. Two physical therapists have described it this way:

> Humanization, becoming part of human society . . . [is] the process whereby the individual, beginning life as a biologic organism, becomes a person whose primitive [physical] *actions* are gradually transformed into behavior that . . . satisfies needs . . . [and] contributes to societal development [italics added] (Fidler & Fidler, 1978).

Human physical activity is distinguished from that of lower animals by four characteristics. Humans are able to match their movements to sophisticated plans to produce more intricate activities, are able to express deep emotion through physical actions that produce works of art, have unique anatomical characteristics that give them an extraordinary degree of flexibility and adaptation in moving, and are able to systematically plan experiences that lead to improvement in their performance.

Our rational capacity for systematically manipulating physical activity experience has given rise to the need for kinesiology, a discipline devoted to the intelligent application of experience to the solution of physical activity problems.

Factors Influencing the Kinds and Amounts of Our Performance Experiences

Because our potential for physical activity helps us to express what is unique about our humanity, it might seem that each of us naturally would maximize opportunities to engage in it and to incorporate it into our lives. However, although it is natural for us to engage in physical activity, as we saw in the last chapter and can see in the following box, relatively few of us are inclined to do so, at least in its more vigorous forms. Neither are most of us inclined to tap our full potential for developing our skill in a wide variety of activities. It is probably fair to say that average adults perform most motor skills at levels far below their capabilities.

Why this paradox? Why is it that something so fundamental to our human nature and so beneficial to us is not explored to its fullest potential? This is one of the most pressing questions confronting the physical activity professions today, and as you will see when you study chapter 9, it is an area of study central to exercise psychology. Unfortunately, there is no simple answer. A multitude of factors intervene in our lives to encourage and discourage us from exploring physical activity. If you think back over the events of the past three days, you could probably easily identify factors that influenced you to be active and those that influenced you to be sedentary. Let's take a quick look at how three categories of factors might affect the type and extent of our physical activity experiences: the social environment, individual circumstances, and personal attributes (see figure 3.2).

Although we posses a unique facility for performing, planning, and implementing physical activity experiences to improve our performance of physical activity, most of us are not inclined to explore this potential to the fullest.

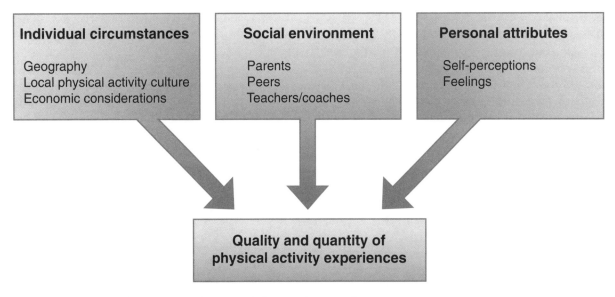

Figure 3.2   Our physical activity experiences are influenced by many factors.

Our Disinclination to Engage in Vigorous Physical Activity

According to the U.S. Department of Health and Human Services:

- More than 60% of U.S. adults are not regularly active.

- Approximately 25% of U.S. adults do not engage in any leisure time physical activity five or more times per week.

- Only 22% of adults engage in at least 30 minutes of light to moderate leisure time physical activity at least three times per week.

- Only 15% report engaging in at least 20 minutes of vigorous leisure time physical activity at least three times per week.

- In spite of a wealth of scientific evidence suggesting that regular physical activity contributes to health and well-being, data suggest that participation in leisure time physical activity did not increase appreciably between the mid-1980s and mid-1990s.

- About 50% of Americans between the ages of 12 and 21 regularly participate in physical activity. Nearly 25% engage in no vigorous physical activity of any kind.

- About 14% of young people report engaging in no vigorous, moderate, or light physical activity of any kind.

Social Environment

The people with whom you interact on a regular basis can have a significant effect on the types and amounts of physical activity experiences you pursue, both as a child and as an adult. As a child you may have received a substantial amount of social support to engage in physical activity, which caused you to be physically active in your younger years. Friendships and social alliances have been shown to have a strong influence on the amount of vigorous exercise undertaken by both young and middle-aged men and women (King et al., 1992; Sallis & Hovell, 1990). If your girlfriend or boyfriend has a physically active lifestyle, it probably encourages you to do the same. If your boss plays tennis or racquetball, you might be attracted to the game also. Although each of us ultimately is responsible for our own decisions regarding physical activity, our dispositions toward it can be affected by those with whom we associate.

Parents

When you were a child did your parents lead a physically active life, or were they largely sedentary? If they modeled an active lifestyle, took you with them to their workouts at an exercise facility, took a daily run in your neighborhood, or were avid tennis or squash players, they can take some credit for the fact that you are an active person too. If, on the other hand, they were couch potatoes who avoided sport, exercise, and other physical activity, you may have had to resist their adverse influence. The extent to which preschoolers, middle school children, and adolescents become involved in physical activity seems largely related to the extent of their parents' involvement in physical activity. Parents who encourage their children—especially preschoolers and adolescents—to engage in physical activity experiences are more likely to have active children. It is a good point for future parents to keep in mind. In fact, merely showing support for your children's physical activity by transporting them to physical activity settings or assisting with the organization of the activity (e.g., serving as a Little League coach or sponsor of the cheerleading squad) can increase the probability that your children will be physically active (U.S. Department of Health and Human Services [USDHHS], 1996).

How likely is it that our early childhood experiences will have an impact on our physical activity patterns later in life? Interestingly, researchers have not been able to discover a strong link between the amount of physical activity engaged in during youth and the amount engaged in during adulthood. There is reason to believe, however, that the *types* of activities engaged in during younger years may set a course for the selection of activities in later years. For example, one study found that adolescents and adults who participated regularly in sports had become active participants by age eight (Snyder & Spreitzer, 1976). Another study showed that the best predictor of the sport experiences we will pursue as adults are those we pursued as children (Greendorfer, 1979).

Having said this, you should recognize that a strong relationship between the extent of sport participation in youth and the extent of physical activity participation in adulthood has not been established. For example, participating in school or college sports does not appear to influence the amount of physical activity one engages in as an adult (Brill, Burkhaulter, Kohl, Blair, & Goodyear, 1989; Cauley, Donfield, LaPorte, & Warhaftig, 1991; Dishman & Sallis, 1994). You are probably familiar with some individuals who were star athletes in college and became physically inactive following graduation just as you can probably think of individuals who did not lead physically active lives as children but who became avid adherents of exercise and sport in later years. Obviously, we have much to learn about this connection. However, until a more complete picture emerges, it seems best to ensure that constructive physical activity experiences are integrated into the early years of development.

Peers

The extent of your friends' involvement in physical activity also may have influenced your physical activity decisions. Do you hang around people who like to be physically active? If so, there is a good chance you are physically active too. For example, some researchers believe that the physical activity patterns of your peers may be as important as those of your family in determining whether you become involved in sport (Lewko & Greendorfer, 1988). When we move beyond sport to consider the influence of peers on patterns of general (nonsport) physical activity, the precise influence of peers is less clear, although it appears to be an important determinant (Dishman, Sallis, & Orenstein, 1985).

As you grew older, did you come into contact with more physically active peers, or did those around you become more inactive? Unfortunately, the statistical probability is that your peer group became less rather than more active as you grew older. For example, a national survey revealed that at age 15, only 6–10% of school students reported not being engaged in vigorous physical activity during the 7 days preceding the study. At age 18, the figure was 18–19% (USDHHS, 1996)!

What leisure time or competitive physical activities did you participate in as a child? Did you play Little League or soccer or football? Did you take dance or gymnastics lessons? Did you ride bikes, climb trees, or roller-skate with your friends in the neighborhood? How do these match the physical activities you do now? Are they the same or different? Do you see similarities in the general types of physical activities you pursued as a young child and those you pursue now? What factors have contributed to your continuing (or discontinuing) to engage in these activities?

If your peer group is immersed in watching MTV, playing video games, or other sedentary pursuits, it is quite likely that you will lead an inactive lifestyle too, rather than allowing various types of vigorous physical activity to form the nucleus of your social life. As you grow older, peer groups may continue to affect your physical activity decisions. If you are married, your spouse and your spouse's friends are likely to influence your decisions to participate or not participate in physical activity (Loy, McPherson, & Kenyon, 1978). It is likely that your relatives', friends', and social groups' predispositions toward physical activity, indirectly but predictably, will continue to influence your decisions throughout life.

Teachers and Coaches

If you were an athlete in high school, there is a good possibility that your coaches—youth sport teams, junior high school, high school varsity—had a significant impact on your physical activity decisions. Athletes, for example, tend to associate their participation in sports with the earlier influence of coaches, especially during adolescence (Ebihara, Ideda, & Myiashita, 1983). Physical education teachers and coaches are influential because they are in a position to confirm or disconfirm a young person's competency in an activity. To have your father or mother remark that you performed well in a soccer game will probably encourage you to continue to develop your skills in that sport, but a similar remark from the coach is likely to be even more influential.

Obviously, physical education teachers and coaches also can create social environments that discourage young people from seeking out physical activity experiences. In this sense, teachers and coaches may act as gatekeepers to the physically active life for thousands of children each year. Thus, it is not an exaggeration to say that the be-haviors of a teacher or coach may have profound and lifelong effects on a student's physical activity experience.

The people closest to you, including your parents, peers, coaches, and teachers, are major influences on the kind and amount of experience you have with a particular physical activity, especially when you are young.

Individual Circumstances

Various circumstances, such as the availability and accessibility of facilities and play spaces, can determine the amount and kinds of people's physical activity experiences (Garcia, Broda, Frenn, Coviak, Pender, & Ronis, 1995; Zakarian, Hovell, Hofstettere, Sallis, & Keating, 1994). Geography is another important factor. Those living in northern climates are more likely to develop competency in skiing, skating, and outdoor activities such as hunting, hiking, and fishing than in swimming or golf, simply because the weather dictates the availability of appropriate sport environments. Temperate climates with warm, sunny days tend to encourage jogging, rollerblading, and walking. Sometimes local cultural traditions emphasize particular sports. High school football is particularly important in Western Pennsylvania and Texas; boys' wrestling and girls' basketball are very popular in Iowa. The game of the inner city is basketball, a cultural tradition that owes at least partly to the fact that space isn't available for other sports such as baseball or football.

Economic considerations can also dictate activity preferences. Generally, highly educated people in higher income brackets with high-status jobs tend to be more active than their poorer, less educated counterparts. Part of the reason is that economic considerations often limit opportunities for participation in physical activities to those with higher income levels. For example, table 3.1 shows that skiers are six times more likely to be from upper than lower income levels. Five times as many people at upper income levels participate in golf, over twice as many play tennis, and half again as many participate in swimming. These sports involve expensive equipment, high admission fees, or, in cases such as swimming, transportation or admission to fee-based private clubs. Although the differences in participation rates are relatively small for exercise walking (an inexpensive activity), those at the highest income levels are two-and-a-half times more likely to exercise with equipment, probably at health spas that require fees that low-income populations cannot afford. In contrast, income level has a negligible effect on participation rates in the relatively inexpensive sports of hunting and fishing.

Often, our physical activity experiences—and consequently, those in which we develop proficiency—are determined by factors that lie outside of our control, such as climate, regional cultures, and economic considerations.

Personal Attributes

As we have noted, decisions to become involved in physical activities are largely personal matters; certainly they are not *entirely* determined by factors outside your control. Your own perceptions, feelings, and decisions play a major part in the process. For example, a decision to prepare yourself for a marathon or train for bodybuilding competition may have to do with your personal attraction to certain characteristics of these activities. If you participate in hang gliding, it may have something to do with your willingness to take risks, the exhilaration you feel from heights, and your perceived ability to keep the

TABLE 3.1
Influence of Income on Participation in Selected Sport Activities

Sport activity	Household income		
	< 15,000	25,000–35,000	50,000–75,000
Bowling	6,684	6,487	9,084
Bicycle riding	6,897	6,685	10,393
Exercise walking	10,491	9,807	13,593
Exercise with equipment	3,915	4,639	9,412
Fishing (fresh water)	8,891	7,158	9,251
Football	2,457	2,263	3,105
Golf	1,439	2,668	7,342
Hunting	3,234	3,555	3,473
Skiing (Alpine)	552	930	3,365
Swimming	8,545	8,817	14,284
Tennis	1,669	1,752	3,758

Participants in thousands (e.g., 26,000 = 26 million).

Data from Statistical Abstracts, 1996.

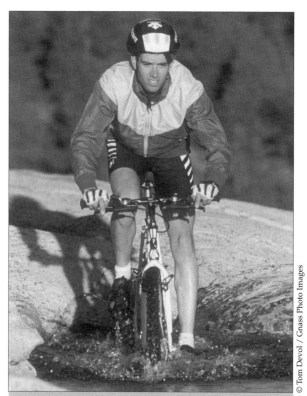

The physical activities we engage in may be influenced by economics, geography, culture, others' influences, and even our own personal attributes.

future physical activity professional you will need to pay careful attention not only to the developing research in this area but also to the particular needs, desires, and attributes of the individuals who will be seeking your services.

Let's stop and retrace the path we've taken to arrive at this juncture. We've seen that the capacity to elaborate plans and actions into complex movements is a unique characteristic of humans. Coincidental to this is our remarkable capacity to use experience to our advantage to learn motor skills; to increase our strength, endurance, and flexibility; and to improve our health. Yet evidence suggests that most of us do not come close to exploring the limits of our physical activity potential. This led us to consider in a very general way some factors that affect our decisions to incorporate physical activity into our lives. These included the effects of parents, peers, and teachers and coaches, as well as individual circumstances such as geographical region, cultural traditions, and economic considerations, not to mention our own attitudes and dispositions. Now we've arrived at a point from which we can explore some specific ways in which experience changes our capabilities of performing physical activity.

🔑 After we have accounted for all of the factors in our social and ecological environments that affect our decisions about physical activity, we are left to consider the indeterminable factors lying within us, such as our perceptions of ourselves, our competency in the activity, and the activity itself, that also may affect our decisions about physical activity.

glider in the air. As we will see in chapter 4, we tend to involve ourselves in activities we enjoy, and it is very difficult to pin down precisely those factors that cause us to enjoy some activities and shun others. Available evidence does allow us to suggest that decisions to become involved in or avoid physical activities may have to do with our feelings of self-esteem and our perceptions of our competence in the activities. Nevertheless, an almost endless number of personal factors can affect these perceptions.

In the end, it may be as difficult to determine precisely why one individual chooses to exercise regularly while another chooses to avoid it, or why one chooses to play tennis while another prefers water skiing, as it is to determine why some people like broccoli and some can't tolerate it, or why some people like heavy metal music and others prefer classical. We have seen that physical activity reflects something of our humanity. It also seems to be the case that our physical activity preferences may reflect something about our uniqueness as individuals. Thus, as a

How Experience Changes Our Capacity to Perform Physical Activity

As a student who is considering majoring in kinesiology, it is vital that you become familiar with the processes and mechanisms by which performance experience results in improvements in our capacities to perform physical activity. In courses such as biomechanics, exercise physiology, motor learning, development and control, and sport psychology you will learn about theories and research that consider such information in detail. Before you begin this advanced study, however, you will find it helpful to step back and look at the effects of physical activity experience in much more general terms. This will provide you with a conceptual framework on which more specialized knowledge of the scientific bases of physical activity can be constructed. In this section we direct your attention to such a general framework in hopes that you will begin to think more broadly and comprehensively not only about the effects of experience but also about the diverse nature of physical activity and the contexts in which it is performed.

Think back to a particular form of physical activity in which you have had a special interest. How did your experience with this activity affect your ability to execute it on successive occasions? If it was a skill such as volleyball, the effects of your accumulated experiences probably were most evident in changes in your ability to execute the sequences of movements associated with serving, setting, or spiking. If the activity was cardiovascular training, the effects of your accumulated experiences may have been evident not so much in changes in the nature of your movements but in your improved capacity to perform the activity over longer periods of time at increasing levels of intensity. These represent two very different effects of experience: (1) improvement in skill through practice, which is called learning, and (2) improvement in physical performance through training, which is called conditioning (see figure 3.3).

Skill, Practice, and Learning

Earlier we saw that infants face a lifetime challenge of recombining and refining their primi-

tive motor responses into goal-directed voluntary actions to meet the demands of daily life. Throughout life we continue to be confronted with the challenges of assembling sequences of movements and body positions in order to accomplish specific tasks. Activities in which performers attempt to attain specific goals by executing efficient, coordinated motor responses are called **motor skills**. Threading a needle, performing a cartwheel, and typing a letter are all motor skills, even though each activity places distinctly different demands on our perceptual and motor processing systems.

Becoming a skilled mover is a never-ending process of gaining more and more control over our motor systems by gradually refining the nerve and muscle systems through performance experience. The type of performance experience engaged in for the express purpose of refining motor control function in order to improve skill is known as **practice**. Laypersons tend to think of practice as merely an endless repetition of the same movements over and over by rote, but that isn't really how practice works. Practice of motor skills actually involves a lot of cognition. It involves higher brain function and integration of spinal neural activity as well as muscular action. (In fact, muscular action is merely the result of these higher cognitive processes.) Practice is a deliberate effort to "get it right" by remembering how we moved on earlier attempts and revising our cognitive plans for moving on the next trial. On each practice trial we vary the level of force or direction of our movements, adopt new strategies, and analyze feedback from our movements so that we may, for example, throw a ball farther or more accurately. This is why one scientist called practice "a particular type of repetition without repetition" (Bernstein, 1967, p. 134).

Sometimes we refer to practicing as a process of "acquiring" experience, implying that we can

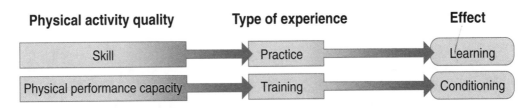

Figure 3.3 The nature of improvements in physical activity depends on the types of physical activity experience.

collect and store our practice experiences. This is a helpful metaphor. If we were unable to store memories of past physical activity experiences, we wouldn't be able to learn new skills. Each trial would be like our first. We would be like people who have lost their short-term memory due to damages to an area of the brain known as the basal ganglia. Because such people can't store information about their previous response in memory, successive repetitions of a skill usually do not bring about learning. They may have played the piano 100 times, but each time they attempt it, it is an entirely new experience. With a normally functioning brain, however, we can benefit from memories of our past experiences and gradually reshape our motor responses in ways that allow us to attain skill goals more and more accurately and with greater efficiency.

The refinements in the nervous system that result from practice are referred to as **learning**. Although much has yet to be discovered about learning, scientists agree that learning is a "central" rather than a "peripheral" phenomenon. This is another way of saying that learning is a result of a "rewiring" of neural circuits in the brain and spinal cord rather than changes in peripheral organs such as bone or muscle. We also know that these changes tend to be relatively permanent. If, after having played many years of tennis you do not return to the court again for several years, the level of your play will deteriorate, but with a little practice you will regain it rapidly. Amazing, isn't it?

When you learn a motor skill, you actually remap the neural routes in your central nervous system. Neurologically speaking, after you learn to serve a tennis ball, you are a different person than you were before you mastered the skill. You know from your own experience that this remapping doesn't happen overnight. Depending on the skill, it may take weeks, years, or even decades to master. Obviously, the extent to which changes in skill become permanent depends a great deal on how much you practice the skill.

The type of experience necessary to bring about changes in skill is called practice. The relatively permanent effects of practice are called learning.

Physical Performance Capacity, Training, and Conditioning

Experience with an activity can bring about another type of change in our performance, which, while just as predictable, is much different from learning. Improvements in physical activities sometimes have little to do with skill. Refining the accuracy or timing of movements or coordinating them with features of the environment may be much less important than improving your capacity to exert greater amounts of force, or improving the range of motion of your joints or the length of time you can sustain an activity. These are not elements of skill as much as they are elements of **physical performance capacity**.

Consider the case of Melinda and Theresa, lacrosse players both of whom had devoted long hours of practice to the sport, and both of whom had played in competitive leagues. Each had developed approximately the same level of skill in lacrosse, evident by their equal proficiency in passing, catching, shooting, and guarding opponents. Then Melinda—a perceptive kinesiology major—began to supplement her practice with a

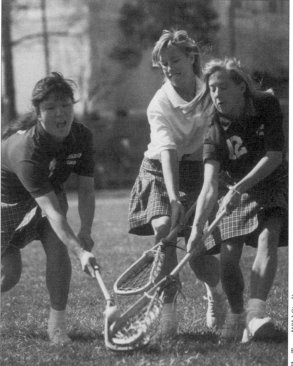

Training can improve a person's muscular strength, muscular endurance, cardiorespiratory endurance, and flexibility.

The Terry Wild Studio

rigorous training program designed to increase her physical capacity through development of muscular strength, muscular endurance, cardiorespiratory endurance, and flexibility, all of which she believed to be important in the sport of lacrosse. As a result, Melinda's lacrosse proficiency improved more than Theresa's. Although both players had learned the *skills* of lacrosse to the same level, Melinda ended up the better player because she also developed other performance qualities that also were important in the sport.

The supplemental types of experiences that Melinda arranged (in this case we may presume weightlifting and endurance and flexibility exercises) are called **training**, not practice, and the changes brought about by these experiences are known as **conditioning**, not learning. Training is physical activity experience designed to improve muscular strength, endurance, cardiovascular endurance, flexibility, and other aspects of performance that serve to condition the performer. Whereas practice brings about improvement in

skill as a result of our learning to coordinate the accuracy and timing of movements, training brings about improvements in physical performance capacity through conditioning, increasing our capacity to move our bodies more forcefully (strength), over longer durations (endurance), and in more flexible ways (flexibility). Generally, the experiences of practice that lead to learning are studied in depth in courses in motor behavior while the experiences of training that lead to conditioning are studied in courses in physiology of physical activity.

Practice Versus Training

Table 3.2 outlines some basic differences between practice and training. Practice produces effects on memory, cognition, perception, and other central nervous system processes associated with problem solving. Training produces effects that are largely peripheral to the central nervous system, usually on muscle, bone, soft tissue, and the

TABLE 3.2 Differences Between Practice and Training	
Practice	**Training**
Practice increases our capacity for organizing movement patterns in complex ways to accomplish specific goals, usually measured in terms of the accuracy or timing of movements of limbs or body parts.	Training increases our ability to produce greater quantities of physical activity such as maximal force over a short period of time (lifting a weight) or more moderate levels of force over longer periods of time (hiking long distances or running marathons), or to move our bodies through larger ranges of motion.
Practice is a cognitive process that leads to a reorganization of the nervous system. Practice is an attempt to solve a problem, the problem being to discover ways of moving our bodies in order to accomplish skill goals.	Training usually involves relatively simple, well-learned movements. Training is not intended to discover the best way to move but is intended to overcome limitations in strength, endurance, or flexibility.
Practice proceeds by systematically varying successive movements based on error information furnished by feedback.	Training usually involves repeating the same movements over and over; changes usually are in terms of the quantity of movements (time, resistance, etc.) rather than the quality of movements.
Practice leads to relatively permanent changes. Even after a long layoff of riding a bicycle or keyboarding, you can return quickly to your original skill level.	Changes induced by training tend to dissipate relatively quickly if appropriate physical activities are not performed.
Practice usually is not aimed at inducing health benefits. Practice may lead to improvement in the skills of archery, bowling, or Frisbee catching without any accompanying increase in fitness.	The changes brought about through training usually confer certain health benefits. For example, running long distances is excellent conditioning for soccer, basketball, or European handball. It also reduces the risk of heart disease, reduces percent body fat, and maintains flexibility in joints.

cardiovascular system. Practice requires deliberate effort and intention by the performer to modify performance, but training per se generally requires little in the way of deliberate attention or problem solving. In fact, conditioning is often an unintended by-product of performing skills such as chopping wood or shoveling snow. Quite simply, if you repeat movements that appropriately stress muscles, tendons, and bones; elevate the heart rate to certain predetermined levels; or move your joints through large ranges of motion, some level of conditioning is inevitable, whether you intended for it to happen or not. On the other hand, mindlessly practicing a skill is not likely to lead to learning.

Physical activity experiences known as training are employed to develop such performance capacities as muscle strength and endurance, cardiovascular endurance, or flexibility. The state of having developed these capacities is known as conditioning.

Whether practice or training is the most appropriate experience for improving your performance in a particular activity depends on the relative importance of skill or physical performance capacity to success in the activity. Even at this early stage you should be able to determine the extent to which an activity depends mostly on skill or physical performance capacity. Activities in which success depends primarily on learning

precise and coordinated sequences of movements are located at the right end of the continuum in figure 3.4. Improvement in these activities is largely a product of practice. At the extreme left end of the continuum are activities that require little in the way of skill but depend heavily on factors such as strength, endurance, and/or flexibility. These are improved primarily by training experiences. Figure 3.4 shows how some activities might be located on the training/conditioning to practice/learning continuum. Look closely at the activities placed on the continuum. Do you agree with their placement?

A few examples should help you grasp this important concept. An athlete's recovery from a postoperative rehabilitation program following knee surgery is largely dependent on developing strength rather than skill. The movements at the knee have not been forgotten ("unlearned"); rather, they have been weakened by the reduced capacity of the muscles. Power lifting includes an element of skill but is largely dependent on strength. Training is clearly the appropriate experience in such activities. In rifle shooting or driving a car, however, success depends almost exclusively on learning to coordinate the limbs with visual information. Archery requires some strength to create tension in the bowstring, but it too is largely dependent on learning coordinated sequences of movements. Practice is the appropriate experience in these situations.

Because most physical activities incorporate both physical performance capacity and skill elements, improvement often requires both prac-

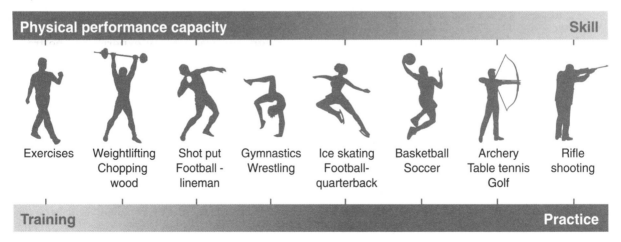

Figure 3.4 Emphasis given to practice or training depends on the relative importance of skill or physical capacity factors in the activity.

tice and training experiences. Rehabilitation programs designed to help individuals learn to walk following a stroke, or regimens designed to improve athletes' javelin or shot put throws or pole vaulting or gymnastics skills all aim at helping people achieve accurate and well-timed movements. At the same time, however, they also aim at developing well-conditioned bodies.

If your goal was to become a member of the varsity soccer team, much of your preparation would involve practicing the various skills of dribbling, tackling, and passing the ball. But because the game also requires you to run continuously, training would also be required, especially running sprints and long distances in order to develop cardiorespiratory endurance. You also might train with weights, especially with your legs, to increase kicking force. Like so many sports, soccer requires attention to both practice and training experiences.

 Generally, practice without training, or training without practice, are incomplete elements in the formula for developing excellence in most physical activities.

In which physical activities would you most like to excel? Is the best route to improvement through experiences that emphasize practice or conditioning or both? Describe the types of experiences you think would be most effective in improving your performance.

Performance Experience and Physical Fitness

Training experiences are important not only for developing proficiency in a particular sport or rehabilitation activity, but also for increasing our overall capacity to perform activities of daily living. The term we use to describe this capacity is **physical fitness**. As we learned in chapter 1, the type of training specifically intended to improve fitness is called exercise.

A physically fit person is one who has developed through exercise a capacity to perform the essential activities of daily living at a high level, has sufficient energy remaining to pursue an active leisure life, and is still able to meet unexpected physical demands that may be imposed by emergencies. For example, our conception of a physically fit person is one who is physically able to carry out the demands of his or her job; play tennis, racquetball, or other sports on the weekend; and still be able to run downstairs in case of a fire, walk five miles on the interstate to get help when his or her automobile breaks down, or shovel snow from the driveway after a big storm.

Because this type of fitness is reflected in a capacity to *perform* physical activities, it is called **motor performance fitness**, which has been defined as "the ability to perform daily activities with vigor" (Pate, 1988, p. 177). Motor performance fitness may be reflected in how many sit-ups or push-ups you can do, how long it takes you to run/walk a mile, or other activities that rely on strength, endurance, or flexibility. Because qualities such as balance, agility, coordination, quickness of response, and similar factors are also important in performing daily activities, some kinesiologists regard these as additional indicators of motor performance fitness. This is especially so for those working with elderly populations. Unlike motor performances that depend upon strength, endurance, or flexibility these latter factors would seem to be developed more by practice than exercise.

A second type of physical fitness, generally regarded by those in the health-related professions to be more significant than motor performance fitness, is **health-related fitness**. This type of physical fitness refers to having developed, through physical activity experience, the traits and capacities normally associated with a healthy body, specifically in relation to diseases known to result from a physically inactive lifestyle (often called **hypokinetic diseases**). Heart disease is one type of hypokinetic disease; high cholesterol, high blood pressure, and obesity also may be associated directly with an inactive lifestyle. Health-related fitness may be assessed directly using various technologies without actually assessing motor performance. Using a skin-fold caliper to measure percent body fat is one example. In other cases, health-related fitness may be assessed while the subject actually engages in motor performances. For example, recording an electrocardiogram, heart and respiration rates, and blood pressure while a person exercises can give kinesiologists a fairly clear picture of an individual's health in relation to cardiovascular-related hypokinetic diseases.

Measuring Physical Fitness

Most physical activity professionals, whether working in gymnasiums, clinics, fitness testing laboratories, fitness centers, or athletic conditioning programs, are faced with the task of assessing the fitness of their clients. Because of this, knowing how to assess physical fitness is as important as knowing how to define it; in fact, how you decide to measure physical fitness is a pretty clear reflection of how you define it! How would you go about measuring fitness in a population of college students? If you approached this task by recording the number of sit-ups they could perform in a minute, timing them on a 100-meter (109-yd) dash and in an agility test, or measuring range of motion of their spines or at their hip and shoulder joints, your conception of fitness is probably closely related to motor performance fitness.

If, on the other hand, you decided to test for fitness by having subjects run on a treadmill for a specified period of time during which you monitored heart rate, blood pressure, oxygen consumption, and an electrocardiogram, and followed this up with a test of blood cholesterol level and skin-fold measurements to determine body fat, your definition seems much more associated with health-related fitness.

Table 3.3 lists the various components assessed by motor and health-related fitness tests. As you can see, some of the motor fitness measures bear little relation to the health of the individual. Could an individual with a very diseased cardiovascular system score highly on a balance, strength, or agility test? It is quite likely. Table 3.3 shows that some components of fitness are assessed by both motor and health-related tests. Flexibility tests, for example, are a measure of motor performance capacity but also reflect something about the health of the joints. (Regular physical activity guards against the onset of diseases that limit motion, just as regular vigorous activity guards against diseases that destroy the circulatory system.)

Which type of physical fitness should physical activity professionals be most concerned

TABLE 3.3
Components of Physical Fitness

Component	Motor performance	Health-related fitness
Anaerobic power	✓	
Speed	✓	
Muscular strength	✓	✓
Muscular endurance	✓	✓
Cardiorespiratory endurance	✓	✓
Flexibility	✓	✓
Body composition		✓
Agility	✓	

✓ indicates that the test measures this particular component of physical fitness.

Adapted, by permission, from R.R. Pate, 1988, "The evolving definition of physical fitness," *Quest* 40: 178.

about? Generally, health-related fitness is the measure of most interest to those in the medical community and, increasingly, to those in kinesiology. Given the growing interest among public health officials in the role of physical activity in disease prevention, the emphasis on health-related fitness is likely to continue. At the same time, it is not unreasonable to continue to conceive of physically fit persons as those who can effectively carry out their daily activities. This will become increasingly important as our population grows older. In light of this, assessment of both motor performance and health-related fitness would seem to be in order for most populations.

Training experiences undertaken specifically to improve our general capacity for performing daily activities and prevent disease processes associated with low levels of physical activity are known as fitness activities.

Depth or Breadth of Experience: Generalists Versus Specialists

Physical activity causes our bodies to respond in ways that are fairly specific to the types of practice and training experiences we pursue. Thus, limiting our physical activity experiences to a single type or narrow range of types will tend to increase our depth of capacity in those limited activities in which we have engaged. On the other hand, exposing ourselves to a broad range of different practice and training experiences is likely to result in an increase in our breadth of capacity for physical activity. Given the fact that we have a finite amount of time and energy to devote to physical activity, those who focus on breadth tend not to gain the practice and train-

ing needed to develop excellence in any one activity. By the same token, those who concentrate on developing depth of capacity often do not have time to develop even moderate levels of competence in other activities.

The person with breadth of experience is known as a physical activity generalist. Have you ever known someone who isn't particularly outstanding in any single activity, but is able to perform respectably in a variety of different activities? An individual who has developed low-average to above-average competency in,

In-Depth Experiences Can Take Us to Very High Levels of Physical Activity

- Water skiing is a leisurely sport, but probably not when skiing at the fastest recorded speed of 230.22 kph (143.08 mph).

- Johann Hurlinger of Austria walked the 1,400 kilometers (870 mi) between Vienna and Paris *on his hands*, and Shin Don-mok of Korea has sprinted 50 meters (54 yd) on his hands in 17.11 seconds!

- Putting a golf ball into a 11.4-centimeter (4.5-in) diameter hole from 9 meters (30 ft) is a remarkable demonstration of body–eye coordination, but two golfers (Jack Nicklaus and Nick Price) have sunk putts from a distance of 33.5 meters (110 ft). Impressive though this is, it pales in comparison to Shaun Lynch's hole-in-one from the tee on a 496-yard "dogleg" at a course in England in 1995!

- Sometimes disabled people are challenged to test the limits of their physical activity potential. Rick Hansen of Canada did it after he became a paraplegic following a car accident. Hansen wheeled his chair 40,074 kilometers (24,901 mi) through four continents and 34 countries, a journey that took him over two years!

- Ski jumper Espen Bredesen traveled through the air a distance that reached over twice the length of an American football field (209 meters [686 ft]) in 1994.

- An Englishmen by the name of Geoff Capes threw a standard 2.27-kilogram (5-lb) building brick a distance of 44.5 meters (146 ft). The longest distance a human has thrown an object (a ring) without any velocity-aiding feature is 383 meters (1,257 ft) (over four American football fields).

- In 1994 a man ran the marathon *backwards* in a time of 3 hours and 53 minutes.

- The cliff divers of Acapulco, Mexico, regularly dive from a height of 26.7 meters (87.5 ft) into 3.66 meters (12 ft) of water. In order to clear the rocks below, their dive must carry them 8.2 meters (27 ft) out into the water.

- One of the most exacting motor skills is billiards, which requires precise positioning and movement of the arms and torso. In 1995 Paul Sullivan sunk all 15 balls in 32.72 seconds.

- A Canadian ice skater holds the record for barrel jumping: 18 barrels, or a distance of 8.96 meters (29.4 ft).

- Perhaps nothing amazes us as much as outstanding feats of endurance. Thomas Godwin cycled every day during 1939 (before advanced cycle technology) and covered over 120,701 kilometers (75,000 mi), or an average of 330 kilometers (205 mi) per day!

Data from M.C. Young, 1997, *The Guinness book of world records*. (New York: Guinness Media).

say, rock climbing, wrestling, ice skating, football, and baseball is an example of a generalist. Competency in this broad range of activities was possible only because the individual sought out an extraordinarily large range of physical activity experiences. The advantage that accrues to generalists is the enjoyment and satisfaction that comes from being able to take advantage of opportunities to engage in a wide variety of activities, although not necessarily at a high level.

Physical activity specialists are those who devote themselves to developing depth of capacity in a single or narrow range of activities. Not only does this require much time and effort, but it also usually leaves little time for gaining experience in other activities. The young girl who wants to become an Olympic gymnast must commit herself to training, practicing, and competitive schedules; she is unlikely to be found on the tennis court, golf course, or swimming pool on a regular basis. Tiger Woods is extraordinarily skilled in golf, but apparently is not a very good dancer. The advantages that accrue to specialists are the pride and satisfaction that come from being able to do one or a small number of activities at an above-average level.

Concentrating efforts on a single physical activity can result in remarkable proficiencies, as anyone who watches national- or international-class athletes can appreciate. For example, weekend golfers count themselves fortunate if they manage to drive the ball 183 meters (200 yd), but professional golfers now regularly drive the ball more than 274 meters (300 yd), and at least one golfer (Mike Austin) was able to drive the ball a full 471 meters (515 yd)! It's a marvel that we are able to balance on a bicycle at all let alone propel one at speeds up to 268.671 kph (166.944 mph), as Fred Rompelberg did in 1995. You might wonder why they would want to, but by immersing themselves in in-depth physical activity experiences, Anthony Thornton developed the capacity to walk a distance of 153 kilometers (95 mi) in 24 hours . . . *backwards*, Chris Gibson developed the capacity to perform 3,025 consecutive somersaults on a trampoline, and Amaresh Jha was able to balance on one foot consecutively for 71 hours and 40 minutes (Young, 1997). These examples, along with those in the box on page 97, are striking testimony to the way in-depth experience can improve the sophisticated nerve-muscle-cardiorespiratory systems that allow us to perform.

Within the span of the seven spheres discussed in chapter 2 most of us tend to be generalists, possessing a more or less wide range of skills and performance capacities that enable us to negotiate the physical challenges encountered in many different aspects of life. When occasions arise, however, we are able to focus more exclusively on a specific activity, for example, embarking on an in-depth rehabilitation program as a result of injuries, or deciding to improve our golf or tennis game. Whether it is better to trade off the advantages of being moderately competent in a number of physical activities in order to become a specialist in one is something only you can decide.

Given an opportunity to become a national-class or international-class athlete in one sport at the cost of having limited experiences with other sports, would you do it?

Whether to be a generalist who seeks out a variety of physical activity experiences or a specialist who focuses more intensely on one or two activities is a choice only the individual can make. Such choices are best made, however, when one understands the advantages and limitations of each.

Tailoring Experience to Activity Characteristics: The Principle of Quality and the Principle of Quantity

By now it should be clear that the route to improving your skill or physical capacity is by selecting appropriate practice and training experiences. Merely engaging in random physical activity experiences is unlikely to bring about your goals for improvement or health enhancement. It would be silly, for example, to think that cardiovascular endurance for running could be developed by training in flexibility, or that skill in kicking a football could be developed by practicing juggling. The type of physical activity experience must be matched appropriately with the desired performance improvement in order to bring about the intended effects. Thus, knowing how to match physical activity experiences with physical activity goals is an important competency that must be mastered by practicing kinesiologists.

By studying exercise science, you will develop a clear understanding of the types of experiences and their underlying rationales. Here your attention is directed to two very general principles that can serve to guide your thinking about the relationship between experience and physical activity; these are the principle of quality and the principle of quantity.

The **principle of quality** states that experiences that engage us in the most critical components of an activity are most likely to lead to increases in our capacity to perform that activity. It might be helpful to think of **critical components** as that which is most important for an individual to possess in order to perform the activity at a high level. Ask yourself what an individual must possess in order to lift a heavy weight or to serve a tennis ball. In the first case your answer was probably "strong arm muscles" or (more appropriately) "strength in the large muscles of the entire body." In the second case you may have answered "good form" or "the correct movements," or (more appropriately) "a coordinated pattern of muscle action that brings the hip, trunk, shoulder, and wrist joints into play at precisely the correct times in order to propel the ball forcefully into the opposite service court."

This principle suggests that if you want to be a weight lifter, your physical activity experiences must engage you in training exercises that focus on the critical component (strength-related activities). If you want to learn to serve a tennis ball, your physical activity experiences must engage you in practice that focuses on the movement pattern to be learned. Running four miles a day is not an appropriate training experience for developing weight lifters because it fails to take into account the critical component of strength, just as pitching horseshoes is an inappropriate practice experience for developing the tennis serve because it involves a different movement pattern and skill goal.

According to the **principle of quantity**, when all other factors are equal, increasing the frequency of our engagement with the critical components of an activity leads to increases in our capacity to perform that activity. Generally, the person who has performed the *critical components* of an activity the *most often* becomes most competent in that activity. It is important to remember that the principle of quantity incorporates the principle of quality. Extensive experience—whether practice or training—that does not engage us in the most critical aspects of the activity is unlikely to result in substantial improvement in performance.

A volleyball coach devoted much of each practice session to having his players jump sideways over benches, jump rope, and toss medicine balls. Do these seem like appropriate training experiences for volleyball players? What critical components might not have been taken into account in preparing these volleyball players for competition?

This means that whether your client is a postcardiac patient, an athlete recovering from injury, a teenager embarking on an exercise program to lose weight, a student in a physical education class, or an older adult hoping to improve her capacity for performing activities of daily living, *your attention as a physical activity professional must first be directed to the critical components underlying the performance of the activity.* The process of systematically identifying the critical components of an activity is called **task analysis**.

Let's take these concepts into the workplace. If Fred, a marathoner embarking on a training program to lower his time in the 42.2 km (26-mile, 385-yard) event, asked you to help plan training experiences that would help him achieve his goal, your first challenge would be to conduct a task analysis of the activity in order to identify its critical components. This, coupled with your scientific and clinical knowledge as a kinesiologist, would enable you to plan appropriate training experiences. Based on such an analysis and your understanding of the science of exercise, you would come to the conclusion that muscular endurance is required if he is to run for over two hours without fatiguing the muscles in his legs, and that cardiovascular endurance is required if his circulatory system is to develop the capacity for delivering large amounts of oxygenated blood to the working muscles. Thus, training activities that emphasize these components would assume a priority in the training plan.

Experience will result in an improvement of physical activity capacity only if it engages us in the essential aspects or components of the activity (principle of quality). Generally, the more often our training or practice focuses on these components the greater will be our performance of the activity (principle of quantity).

When you begin to study kinesiology in depth, you will discover that the general principles of quality and quantity are subject to many qualifications. You also will discover that identifying the critical aspects of various physical activities and determining the appropriate types of practice or training experiences are not easy tasks. For example, what are the critical elements in batting a pitched ball? Is skill or physical capacity the primary consideration, or are both important? Is watching the ball the most important element? Developing force with the arms? Developing limb–target accuracy? Developing force with the hips and trunk? What are the critical elements that must be mastered by a patient learning to walk following a stroke, or the components of a throwing motion that must be rehabilitated in a pitcher following surgery? How much and what kinds of practice and training experience does each case require? Your competence as a physical activity specialist will depend a great deal on your skill at carrying out such analyses and using the results to plan appropriate practice or training experiences.

Kinesiologists, physical education teachers, and coaches are constantly conducting task analyses in order to identify the critical components of physical activities; this information is used to design appropriate practice and training experiences.

Identifying Critical Components of a Physical Activity

How do physical activity specialists go about zeroing in on the critical components of an activity? In many, perhaps most, instances professionals use informal, intuitive task analyses developed over many years of practice. Like veteran physicians diagnosing patient ailments, experienced physical activity professionals can identify the critical elements of a task quickly without resorting to a checklist or other formal system. For beginners, however, a general framework is usually recommended. What follows are some examples of basic frameworks for conducting task analyses of physical activities.

The first thing to consider when deciding what types of experiences are appropriate for bringing about improvement in an activity is whether skill or physical performance capacity plays a central role in the activity. If the activity is located more toward the skill-practice-learning end of the continuum displayed in figure 3.4, the focus of the experience will be on elements of skill. In this case the goal of your analysis will be to identify aspects of the performance that can be learned and that need to be manipulated in carefully constructed practices. If the activity is located near the physical performance capacity-training-conditioning end of the continuum, your focus will be on aspects that should be taken into account in planning training experiences in order to promote conditioning.

Determining Skill Components Critical for Learning

If the physical activity in question falls near the skill-practice-learning end of the continuum in figure 3.4, the analyst's first task is to identify components of the activity that must be practiced in order to maximize learning.

In making such important decisions, physical activity professionals often refer to **motor skill taxonomies,** classification systems that categorize skills according to their common critical elements. Obviously, there are many ways to classify motor skills. We could, for example, classify them according to whether they required large movements or small movements, whether they are performed in the water or on land, whether they involve fast movements or very slow movements, or whether or not they require equipment. But it is doubtful any of these factors could be considered "critical" because they do not appear to have direct implications for how practice experiences should be planned. Remember, if a taxonomy is to be useful, it must at least supply us with hints about how practice experiences should be designed.

One of the most illuminating classification systems designed for analyzing motor skills in the past 40 years is a simple scheme that locates skills on a continuum from closed to open skills, as shown in figure 3.5 (Poulton, 1957). The classification is based on the presumption that a critical component of all skills is the predictability of the environmental events to which performers must adapt their movements. In this view, performing a motor skill essentially is a matter of adapting one's movements to objects, persons, or environments (Gentile, 1972). For example, in order to execute the rather simple task of picking up a pencil, performers must move toward the pencil, reach out their hands in the direction of the pencil, and move their hands and fingers in such a way as to grasp the pencil. Moving their arms or hands away from the pencil or keeping their fingers in a stiff and extended position will not allow them to accomplish the goal. In this sense, then, the location and shape of the pencil control or "regulate" the movements of the performer.

If the pencil to be picked up is resting on a table, its position is fully predictable before and throughout the movement. This means that the movements to be executed to achieve the goal are predictable also. Motor skills that are per-

formed in highly predictable environments and that require highly predictable movements are called closed skills. Learning this closed skill is a matter of developing a stereotypical and consistent movement pattern that moves the arm, hands, and fingers to the same place on each trial. Also, because the pencil is stationary, performers need not be concerned about coordinating the timing of their movements to coincide with changes in the environment. In this sense, performers are free to execute the movements "in their own time."

If the task were changed by rolling the pencil across the table, the goal being to pick it up before it reached the edge, performers could no longer plan and execute their responses in their own time. Now what was originally a closed skill has been converted to an open skill. The skill is "open" in the sense that it requires performers to monitor a constantly changing environment so that they can adjust their movements accordingly.

In our example we can see that when the skill is "opened up," the pencil not only controls the direction and location of performers' movements but also effectively controls *when* the movements should be initiated. And if the velocity and the direction in which the pencil moves in each trial is changed, performers are faced with an even more complex challenge. Since the pencil might roll at high speeds or low speeds and in any direction, it could well topple over the edge of the table before the performer has time to decide on a response and execute it.

And consider this: Because the velocity and direction of the pencil's movements may require

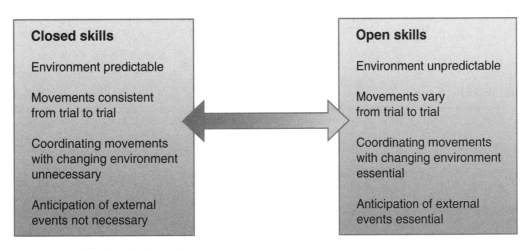

Figure 3.5 The open skill–closed skill continuum.

trial-to-trial variations in the performers' movements, the stereotypical response that worked so well when the pencil was stationary wouldn't work well in this situation. That is, rather than learning to perform a single, consistent, "grooved" response, performers must learn a variety of responses, one for each of the different directions in which, and speeds at which, the pencil might be moved. Moreover, since the velocity and direction of the pencil is unknown beforehand, performers are forced to anticipate which response might be required if they are to have sufficient time to prepare and execute it before the pencil has rolled off the edge of the table. Learning such skills may involve perceptual analysis of the pencil's movements as much as it does learning how to move the body.

Thus, open skills present performers with very unpredictable environments. This simple change in the structure of the task—creating a moving rather than a stationary environment to which performers must adapt their movements—*creates fundamental changes in the challenges of the task.* In other words, whether the skill is performed in an open or closed environment is one critical component of the task and therefore must be taken into account in planning practice experiences.

The determining factor for locating any skill on the open skill–closed skill continuum is the predictability of the movements required to attain the goal. Figure 3.6 shows how some skills might be located on the continuum. Remember, skills near the closed end are performed in highly predictable environments. Thus, the movements required for successful execution are also highly predictable. Gymnastics, sewing, or hitting a softball from a batting tee are examples of closed skills.

Along the span of the continuum are skills in which the movements to be executed are less predictable because the environmental events to which performers must adapt change their location as the skill is being performed. Skills such as a tennis serve, hitting a softball pitched at a very slow speed, or dancing with a partner involve moderate amounts of unpredictability in the environment and consequently moderately unpredictable movements.

At the extreme open end of the continuum are activities in which the movements required are very unpredictable since the location of the environmental objects to which performers must adapt change position in a very irregular way. Note that skiing down a mountain has been placed near the open end of the continuum even though the environment (the terrain, trees, moguls, etc.) remains stationary. In such skills, especially skills in which the body is moving swiftly, the *relative motion* between the performer and the environment creates the same element of unpredictability as when the performer is stationary and the environment is moving.

The types of practice experiences essential for bringing about improvements in skills vary depending on the location of the skill on the continuum. For example, skills near the closed end of the continuum are best practiced in situations in which the environment is structured the same on each trial. Emphasis would be placed on "grooving in" a theoretically correct technique that could be repeated trial after trial. Learning golf involves developing such a stereotypical pattern of movement. Practice regimens for skills near the open end would involve structuring the environment in various ways on each trial so that the direction and velocity of movement of the

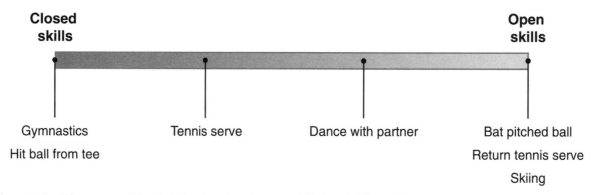

Figure 3.6 Where some skills might be placed on the open skill–closed skill continuum.

relevant objects, persons, or environment change on each trial. Thus, the goal of practice with open skills is to develop a flexible technique that allows one to adapt to a wide variety of environmental stimuli. Also, practice for open skills is likely to concentrate on developing strategies for anticipating changes in the environment that are likely to occur. Baseball batters often do this when facing pitchers they have studied or watched on video. This provides performers with more time to plan and execute their responses. Obviously, skills located near the center of the continuum will require appropriate application of all of these practice strategies.

It's important to remember that the open skill–closed skill continuum focuses on only one critical component of motor skills. There may be other critical components as well. At this early stage in your acquaintance with the theory of motor skills, merely recognizing whether a skill is predominately open or closed will go a long way toward helping you understand not only the enormous complexities of skills but also how to determine appropriate experiences for bringing about improvement. Chapter 8 will introduce you to many other considerations that must be taken into account in planning practice experiences for skills.

Skills may be located on a continuum anchored at one end by skills in which performers must adapt their movements to fixed and therefore highly predictable environments (closed skills) and at the other by skills in which performers must adapt their movements to changing and highly unpredictable environments (open skills).

Determining Experiences Appropriate for Training

Having considered how to determine the types of *practice* experiences essential for learning skills, how can we determine the types of *training* experiences likely to lead to the conditioning essential for improving physical performance capacity? Remember, unlike skill, physical performance capacity depends on training experiences involving such critical components as muscular endurance, cardiorespiratory endurance, strength, and flexibility. Knowing the critical components that underlie a particular ac-

tivity permits you to plan training strategies for developing them.

If you were confronted with the problem of developing training programs for a young woman who wanted to improve her competitive performance in bicycling and a young man who wanted to improve his performance in golf, how would you go about determining what types of physical activity experiences to recommend? In other words, the important question is, What are the critical components of bicycling and golf? You might approach the problem by locating the two activities on the continuum depicted in figure 3.4. It should be clear to you immediately that the key to successful performance in golf is primarily *learning* to perform a coordinated sequence of movements, and that *practice* experiences are probably more important than training experiences for the golfer. This is not to say that strength, endurance, and flexibility are not important in golf, only to say that they are less important than skill in this case. It will also be clear to you that while success in bicycling is probably related to the development of a coordinated sequence of efficient movements, it is primarily determined by factors such as cardiovascular and muscular endurance. Let's call these critical components related to performance (rather than skill) "performance components." The question you should ask yourself at this point is, What are the critical performance components underlying these two tasks?

You can approach this question in two ways. One is to consult experts you have reason to believe are knowledgeable in such matters. Let's assume you consulted seven exercise physiologists and asked each of them to rate the importance of each of a selected number of general performance components on a scale of 0 to 3. You could total the ratings for each component and derive a table such as that presented in table 3.4 (this table actually was constructed by consulting experts). Examining the table we can see that four of the five physical capacity components listed were judged to be critical to bicycling, suggesting that any training regimen should focus on each of these. In the opinion of the experts, none of the components figured prominently in golf performance, something that won't surprise you. Although golf performance may be improved somewhat through strength and endurance training, it is predominately a game of skill,

TABLE 3.4
Ratings by Experts of Physical Capacity Elements

Physical fitness	Jogging	Bicycling	Swimming	Handball/ squash	Skiing (alpine)	Basketball	Tennis	Calisthenics	Golf	Softball
Cardiorespiratory endurance (stamina)	21	19	21	19	16	19	16	10	8	6
Muscular endurance	20	18	20	18	18	17	16	13	8	8
Muscular strength	17	16	14	15	15	15	14	16	9	7
Flexibility	9	9	15	15	14	13	14	19	9	9
Balance	17	18	17	17	21	16	16	15	8	7

Seven experts weighted degree to which each sport activity developed cardiorespiratory endurance, muscular endurance, muscular strength, flexibility, and balance on a scale of 0–3. Ratings were combined for all seven judges (21 = highest score). A sport receiving a high rating for developing muscular strength is an indication that muscular strength is a critical component for that activity.

Adapted, by permission, from D.J. Anspaugh, M.H. Hamrick, and F.D. Rosato, 1991, *Wellness.* (St. Louis: Mosby Year Book), 165.

hence more effectively improved through practice. In addition, an analysis of the predictability of movements required in golf would show that it is a closed skill, and this consideration would guide the planning of practice experiences.

> One way to identify the critical performance components underlying any physical activity is to ask experts to rate how important selected components are in the successful performance of the activity.

A second approach to determining critical performance components is to answer a series of questions about the activity based on your knowledge of the activity and your understanding of kinesiology. Binary decision trees such as that depicted in figure 3.7 are often used by physicians when diagnosing diseases or by electricians when they troubleshoot a circuit defect. They are helpful in focusing your attention on the most important questions. Binary decision trees also can help you approach task analyses in a clearheaded and systematic way.

Begin with the question in the upper left-hand corner and follow the path of your answers to arrive at the critical performance component. The path your questioning takes is determined by your yes/no answers. Obviously, figure 3.7 is not intended to be an exhaustive analysis of all of the critical performance factors that might be important in an activity. Even though this is a very general taxonomic model, it will help you appreciate the many critical components underlying physical activities. It will also lay the groundwork for learning in a more detailed fashion all that goes into determining how to match performance experiences with critical performance components.

> Binary decision trees that focus your attention on the most important questions to ask about a performance often can help identify the critical performance components underlying the task.

Think back to the case of Tiger Woods. Can we say that the *only* thing that separated him from most of the other professional golfers is the fact that he has played so much golf? He has a body build that lends itself to developing power in the swing, and he is able to move his hip, trunk, shoulder, and wrist joints at an astoundingly high rate of speed. These qualities probably have more to do with his genetic makeup than what he has gained from practice. All of this raises the question: Does the depth of our physical activity experiences—in and of itself—determine how proficient we will become in a sport, exercise, or other physical activity? Not at all. Although experience may account for most of the differences in proficiency between individuals, this shouldn't cause us to ignore the fact that heredity makes a contribution too, and this, of course, has nothing to do with physical activity experience. Although it is a bit of a digression, let's take a brief side trip to explore the way heredity can influence our physical activity experiences.

Heredity and Experience

You and a friend may both have had about the same amount of competitive basketball practice and both may have adhered to rigorous conditioning programs to improve your jumping ability and overall strength, but you may be a much better player than your friend. Why? Perhaps because you were more dedicated and more highly motivated to succeed. You also may have had the benefit of superior coaching. But part of the answer may also be that you were lucky enough to have inherited a greater proportion of the abilities required to play basketball. For example, you may be taller, a faster runner, more agile, or you may have what seems to be a natural facility for changing direction, jumping, or coordinating the movements of your arms and legs, all of which are important to success in basketball. Most of these may be modified somewhat through practice, but the genetic contribution of your parents may have played at least as important a role. Before we close the cover on this study of the role of experience, then, let's briefly consider ways in which the effects of experience might be modified by the effects of heredity.

Abilities as Building Blocks for Experience

Genetic predispositions that advantage or disadvantage us for particular activities are called

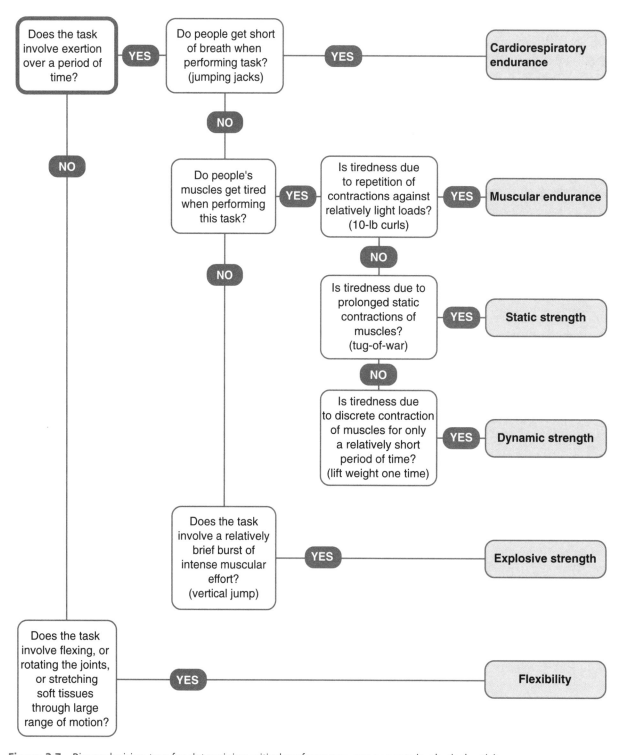

Figure 3.7   Binary decision tree for determining critical performance components in physical activity.
Concept from Fleishman and Stephenson, 1970.

abilities. Abilities are still not well understood by physical activity scientists. They are thought to be genetically endowed perceptual, cognitive, motor, metabolic, and personality traits that are susceptible to little or no modification by practice or training. For example, batting a baseball requires special visual abilities, surfing requires certain balance abilities, and orienteering requires spatial ability. People who possess great amounts of the unique abilities required for a particular activity have a greater potential for success in that activity than those who did not inherit these abilities. Notice that we said these individuals have a greater "potential." Usually, potential by itself is not sufficient for achieving high levels of skill or performance. The key to exploiting and eventually realizing potential is engagement in appropriate physical activity experiences.

Think of abilities as the foundation on which our experiences are constructed. Those with greater amounts of the abilities required in an activity have a potential for higher achievement, but that potential will not be realized unless the individual also capitalizes on opportunities for improving performance through practice and training. Thus, the highest level of competency you are able to achieve in a particular activity is determined by the sum of your abilities and your practice and training experiences. Sometimes, people inherit the abilities required by an activity but fail to exploit those abilities through practice and training (underachievers). Others appear to have little "natural" ability for an activity, but they compensate for this by unusually ambitious practicing and training schedules (overachievers). Figure 3.8 shows how various combinations

of ability, practice, and training theoretically may result in various levels of physical activity performance. Obviously, this model greatly simplifies what is really a very complex interaction of physical activity experiences and abilities.

Our body proportions, skeletal size, bone mass, limb length, limb circumference, and distribution of muscle and fat are also influenced by genetic factors, and they clearly have a bearing on our capacity to perform various physical activities. If you inherited a small frame, you probably won't excel in American football, rugby, or sumo wrestling no matter how much you practice and train. On the other hand, if you inherited a very large frame, don't expect to make the Olympic team in gymnastics, ice skating, or diving in which a compact body configuration is essential to rapid twisting and turning. Figure 3.9 shows some theoretically "ideal" body proportions for some selected sport activities. Keep in mind that while inherited body characteristics may be a limiting factor for those aspiring to elite status as highly specialized performers, for most individuals this is not an important consideration. For those hoping to achieve moderate levels of performance that will enable them to participate at a recreational or social level, training and practice will be sufficient stimuli to achieve these goals.

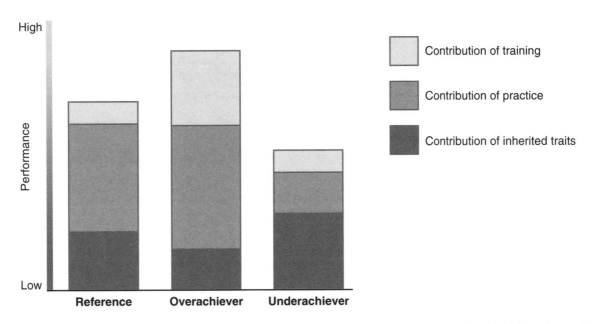

Figure 3.8 Hypothetical example of contributions of practice and training to improvement in physical activity performance.

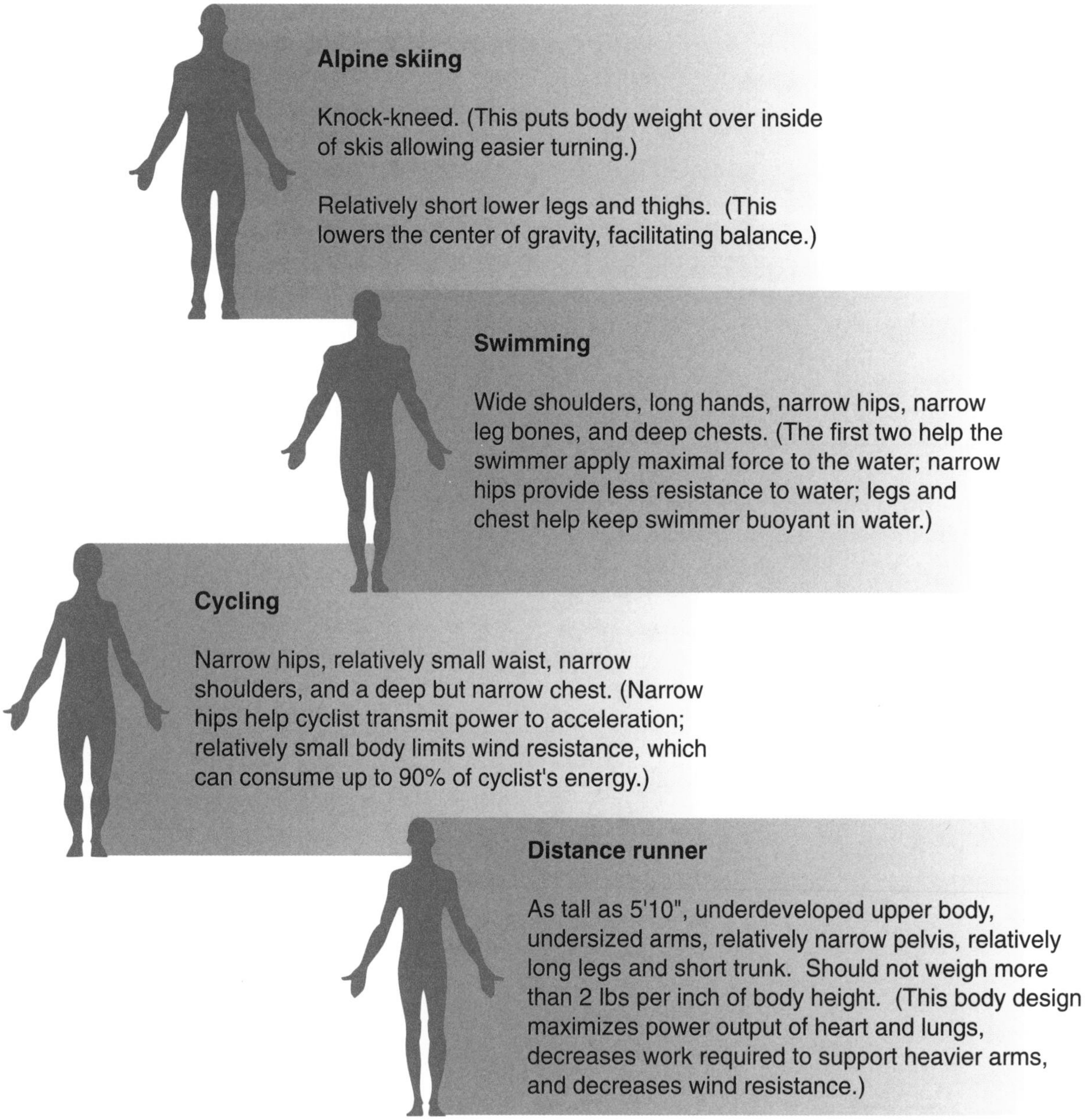

Alpine skiing

Knock-kneed. (This puts body weight over inside of skis allowing easier turning.)

Relatively short lower legs and thighs. (This lowers the center of gravity, facilitating balance.)

Swimming

Wide shoulders, long hands, narrow hips, narrow leg bones, and deep chests. (The first two help the swimmer apply maximal force to the water; narrow hips provide less resistance to water; legs and chest help keep swimmer buoyant in water.)

Cycling

Narrow hips, relatively small waist, narrow shoulders, and a deep but narrow chest. (Narrow hips help cyclist transmit power to acceleration; relatively small body limits wind resistance, which can consume up to 90% of cyclist's energy.)

Distance runner

As tall as 5'10", underdeveloped upper body, undersized arms, relatively narrow pelvis, relatively long legs and short trunk. Should not weigh more than 2 lbs per inch of body height. (This body design maximizes power output of heart and lungs, decreases work required to support heavier arms, and decreases wind resistance.)

Figure 3.9   Ideal body proportions for selected sports.

Adapted, by permission, from R.B. Arnot and C.L. Gaines, 1984, *Sportselection* (New York: Viking Press).

🔑 Ultimately, how well we are able to perform an activity is determined both by our physical activity experiences and our abilities.

Interaction of Experience and Abilities

As we mentioned earlier, the contribution of inherited abilities to the performance of physical activity is much more complicated than the simple diagram in figure 3.8 suggests. For example, genetics may not only supply us with the abilities required to perform certain activities (movement speed, hand–eye coordination, explosiveness, etc.), but also determine how our bodies respond to experience. Because we each inherit a different amount of the ability that allows us to profit from experience, we do not all respond in the same way to a given amount and kind of experience.

Have you ever known an underachiever? An overachiever? What aspect of his or her behavior leads you to place him or her in this category? Is there a physical activity in which you would describe yourself as an underachiever? An overachiever? Why? Why do you think some athletes are underachievers? Why do you think some athletes are overachievers?

As a case in point consider long-distance running, in which performance is largely determined by a runner's ability to deliver oxygen to the muscles (and use it) and to eliminate carbon dioxide, a phenomenon known as maximal oxygen uptake. Endurance training generally increases runners' maximal oxygen uptake, but it doesn't affect everyone in the same way. A standard bout of conditioning may result in improvements in endurance performance of 16% for some individuals and 97% for others (Lortie, Simoneau, Hamel, Boulan, Landry, & Bouchard, 1984). Why this wide variability of physiological response to training? Part of the reason may be that experience, in this case endurance training, interacts with various genetic traits. Thus, those lucky enough to have inherited this "training response–ability" will probably show greater improvement as a result of a standard bout of training than those who lack it.

Like the effects of training on conditioning, the effects of practice on learning may also be modified by inherited abilities, although the process appears to operate somewhat differently. Theoretically, each motor skill requires the application of certain motor abilities, which are distributed unevenly among the population. If you are fortunate enough to have inherited the "speed of response" ability, you will likely perform well in tasks that require this ability (e.g., sprinting or batting). If you inherited an ability called "mechanical reasoning," you may do well in motor tasks that require this ability (e.g., the operation of complex equipment).

But the problem becomes more complicated when we look at the contribution of abilities to skills when they are practiced for long periods of time. Practicing skills usually leads to higher lev-

els of performance, but scientists have discovered that the abilities required to be successful at very low levels of performance may actually be different from those required to perform at very high levels. For example, cognitive abilities such as mechanical reasoning and spatial ability may be important in some skills during the initial stages of learning but not during later stages. On the other hand, motor abilities such as speed of movement or reaction time might not be important in early stages but are critical at higher stages of learning (Fleishman & Hempel, 1955). Thus, the effects of practice, like the effects of training, interact with the influence of inherited traits. If you have inherited a large capacity for mechanical reasoning, you may develop skill very rapidly during initial practice trials. If, however, you lack the same large capacity for speed of movement (and, if speed of movement is a critical component of the task), you will proceed very slowly during later practice trials.

It's probably not wise for the average person to base his or her decision to engage in a particular activity solely on whether he or she seems to possess large amounts of requisite abilities for that activity. Conceivably, this could be a legitimate concern for the young person who envisions competing in the Olympics someday, but for most of us, our collection of inherited abilities—whatever they may be—coupled with practice and instruction will enable us to play most sports at an adequate level. Besides, none of us can ever know for sure what all of our abilities are. Consequently, you should indulge in the physical activities you enjoy, realizing that, regardless of your abilities, the only avenue to achievement will be through experience. And in most cases, the greater the quantity of high-quality experience you have with an activity, the better your performance will be.

The upper limits of learning and conditioning are determined by both our physical activity experiences and inherited factors called abilities. Since experience is the only variable over which we have control, the best strategy for achieving excellence is to avail ourselves of the highest-quality physical activity experiences possible.

Wrap-Up

We began this chapter by making the obvious observation that the key to improving our physical activity performances is to accumulate physical activity experiences. Thus, it is critical that we engage ourselves and those whom we serve in experiences of the right quality and quantity. Knowing the specific types of experiences essential for learning skills or improving physical capacity in any activity or for developing physical fitness is a key element in the expertise of physical activity professionals. Although you will not be able to appreciate fully all of the variables that come into play in prescribing physical activity experiences for clients until after you have completed your study of kinesiology, this chapter introduced you to a number of general factors that must be taken into account. These include considering whether the activity consisted of skills that must be learned through practice, or whether the activity consisted of physical performance capacities that must be conditioned through training. We also saw that any practice or training regimen must focus on the critical elements of the activity and provide in-depth experiences if performance is to improve. Finally, we looked briefly at the traits we inherit as factors that interact with experience to bring about performance changes across individuals.

Study Questions

1. List four unique characteristics of human physical activity.

2. What factors influence our decisions regarding what physical activities we will engage in and how physically active we will be?

3. What type of activity is improved by practicing? What do we call the improvement brought about through practice?

4. What is the principle of quality? What is the principle of quantity? Give an example in which each would be used by a physical activity professional to design an appropriate physical activity experience.

5. What is meant by an "ability"? In what way might abilities limit the level of proficiency we attain in a physical activity?

4

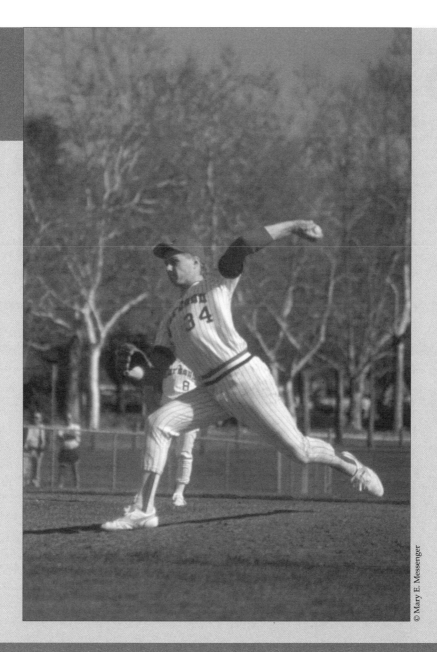

© Mary E. Messenger

The Importance of Subjective Experiences in Physical Activity

Shirl J. Hoffman

In this chapter . . .

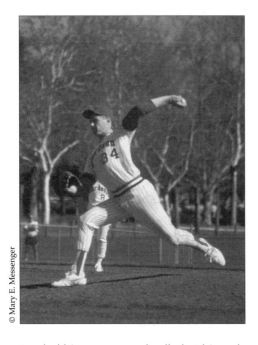

© Mary E. Messenger

"Ryan Jaroncyk (not the player pictured here) was an outstanding high school baseball player, so good in fact that he was drafted in the first round by the New York Mets and signed a contract for $850,000. In addition, he was given a $100,000 college scholarship. The baseball scouts felt that he had the talent to be an outstanding shortstop in big-league baseball. His future was to be fame, fortune, and fun.

There was a big problem, however, that most people didn't know about. Ryan hated baseball. In fact, he can't remember ever liking it. "I always thought it was boring," he said. Even though he was a star early on in Little League, he got tired of waiting for the next at bat; there wasn't enough action for him. Why, then, did he continue to play baseball? Partly because he was very good at it. Also because his father wanted him to. His father pushed him hard, attended his games, and yelled at him when he would make mistakes. It was quite an effective way to develop Ryan's talent in baseball, but Ryan did not find it a pleasant experience.

Shortly after signing with the Mets, he announced that he was quitting. When some pressure was applied by his father and others, he reconsidered and played for a few months in the minor leagues. Not long after this, he quit baseball for good. As a way of signaling the finality of his decision, he gathered all of his baseball equipment together—gloves, hats, and his bats from Little League and high school—drove to a nearby town and put them in a dumpster. 'I feel very happy,' he said." ("The Kid Had It All, But Just Didn't Like Baseball," 1997)

If you're like Ryan's parents and friends, you're probably wondering what in the world happened to this fellow. Was he crazy? Why give up all those years of hard work and success? Can you imagine making the same decision?

Ryan's story is important because it shows how easily we can be fooled by looking only at outward activity experiences. Examining physical activity in terms of performance characteristics or health benefits actually tells us little about what is happening inside the performer. In order to become enthusiastic about a particular form of physical activity—whether sport, aerobics, weight training, or taekwando—something in the activity must contact our innermost selves in a way that causes us to return again and again to the activity. This relationship between physical activity and our inner lives—our thoughts and feelings—is the subject of this chapter.

 ## CHAPTER OBJECTIVES

In this chapter we will:

- Discuss four commonly overlooked truths about physical activity
- Describe the nature of subjective experience and its place in physical activity
- Explain factors that influence our personal experiences of physical activity—what makes some activities enjoyable, some boring, and some frustrating
- Discuss how our individual preferences, tastes, dispositions, activity history, and personal circumstances contribute to our subjective experiences in physical activity
- Describe the subjective experience of watching sports and how various factors affect us as spectators

You will notice that this chapter focuses primarily on physical activity experiences that revolve around sport and exercise. There are two reasons for this. First, we pursue many of the physical activities we do in the competition and health spheres expressly for the way they make us feel. In sport, for example, we often produce very little for our effort except the fun we have while we are engaged in it and the memories that linger after we have finished. Second, we focus on activities in these spheres because traditionally they have formed the centerpiece of kinesiology. Kinesiologists are interested in physical activity of all kinds, but they are especially interested in sport and exercise.

Before you continue reading, answer the following questions:

1. Do you exercise regularly? Do you like to exercise? What is it about exercise that you find enjoyable? What, if anything, about exercise do you find unenjoyable?
2. Do you play sports, and if so, why? If you don't play sports, is it because something about the experience "turns you off"? Explain.
3. How would you feel if federal laws were enacted to prohibit you from exercising or from participating in sports? How likely would you be to break the law?
4. If you were to be given a contract that paid you $100,000 a year, but you had to dig ditches in hard ground for 10 hours each day, five days a week, would you take the job? If an alternative job was to play sports for 10 hours a day, five days a week, or work out in a modern fitness center for the same amount of time, would you be more likely to do this than to dig ditches? Why?
5. In your experience, are the feelings associated with exhaustion in sport or exercise somehow different from the tiredness you feel when you do hard physical work? If so, why do you think this is?

Four Truths About Sport and Exercise

Ryan's story underscores four fascinating truths about sport and exercise.

Physical Activity Is Always Accompanied by Subjective Experiences

The first truth is that physical activity is always accompanied by subjective experiences that are every bit as important as its objective or physical experiences discussed in chapter 3. When we consider our experience with a particular activity, our thoughts usually turn to activity experience. For example, we think of an *experienced* runner as one who has spent much time on the track, streets, and country trails, running. In this sense, experience refers primarily to performing. The reason we so naturally equate experience with performing the activity is that the sheer physicality of human movement rivets our attention. When Michael Jordan (perhaps the top basketball player of the 1980s and 1990s) glided effortlessly through the air and slammed the ball down through the hoop, his movements represented a concrete image, a tangible event that we can observe.

But experiencing an activity means more than just performing it. *Experiencing* running is not just putting one foot ahead of the other in a mindless repetition of movements. It also involves feeling your racing pulse and the warmth of your body, the sense of energy being released in your muscles, the pain of fatigue. It includes the memories the experience leaves with you and the changes in the way you think and feel about the act of running and about yourself as a result of the run.

Anyone who has watched Michael Jordan play basketball knows that his performance could generate some dramatic emotions—amazement, awe, even disbelief come to mind. But Jordan's performances also affected his own subjective state. His play did not involve robotic movements executed with little feeling or emotion. After making an outstanding shot or pass, he would raise his fist in triumph, leap in the air, or laugh. These gestures are external signals that physical activity also involves subjective experiences and that performing activities can touch us at a deep emotional level.

We often underestimate the importance of these subjective aspects, perhaps because physical activity has been linked historically to the scientific fields of biology and medicine. These are areas that are more objective than the humanities or social and behavioral sciences, which deal with intangible qualities such as values, feelings, and cognitions. Even those working in the biological or health-related fields now recognize that a complete understanding of physical activity must take into account the response of the entire person—the intellectual, emotional, and spiritual capacities as well as those of the physiological systems. It might help you to think of the physical features of activity as merely setting the stage for our subjective experiences. George Sheehan, a cardiologist who has written extensively about the spiritual side of running, described it this way: "The first half hour of my run is for my body. The last half hour is for my soul. In the beginning the road is a miracle of solitude and escape. In the end it is a miracle of discovery and joy" (1978, p. 225).

Subjective experience refers to the entire range of emotional and cognitive reactions, dispositions, knowledges, and meanings we derive from physical activity. Obviously, Ryan Jaroncyk didn't have the same subjective experiences playing baseball that Sheehan had running. Sheehan's experiences led him again and again to the tracks and trails where he ran throughout his adult life into old age. Jaroncyk's experiences led him to stop playing baseball when he was still a teenager. This isn't to say that Sheehan's reaction was correct or that Jaroncyk's reaction was wrong. The stories merely illustrate the fact that how physical activity makes us feel is a very personal matter, and that the feelings we associate with physical activity often determine whether we will continue to engage in it.

The interior and sometimes mysterious aspect of our lives, where we collect, recall, and reflect on the feelings and meanings physical activity has for us, is the realm of subjective experience.

The Subjective Experiences of Physical Activity Are Unique

The second truth about physical activity is that its subjective experiences, particularly those of sport and exercise, are unique. Whether physical activity is associated with work, education, or some other sphere of physical activity experience, the subjective experience of merely moving our bodies is different from that of sitting or lying motionless. So, too, the subjective experiences of sport and exercise are different from those that accompany self-expressive or self-sufficient physical activity. We usually feel better when we run on a treadmill or play racquetball than when we paint our apartment or wash the kitchen floor, even though both require physical activity. It is precisely because the subjective experiences of sport and exercise are different from most of our daily activities that we engage in them. Would you work out in the gym, play sports, swim five miles each day, or run cross-country if these activities provided essentially the same human experiences as brushing your teeth, driving your car, or taking a final exam? Probably not.

One of the primary reasons we seek out exercise and sport is that they supply us with unique forms of human experience unavailable to us in our everyday lives.

We Might Perform Physical Activities Without Understanding Why

A third truth about physical activity is that we can sometimes engage in a particular form of physical activity over time without ever pausing to ask ourselves what feelings the activity generates in us, what we get out of it, or how it fits within the larger scheme of our life's meaning. Sometimes we become so involved in the competition or in achieving our goals that we lose sight of the activity's subjective aspects, even though these aspects can be our main reason for doing the activity. When we focus so much on the competition in sports, for example, or in the case of exercise on achieving our workout goals, then the important subjective aspect of the activity gets relegated to the background. Think back to the questions in the box on page 113. Did you have to think much to come up with answers, or had you thought about these questions before? If not, why not?

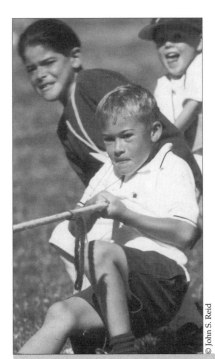
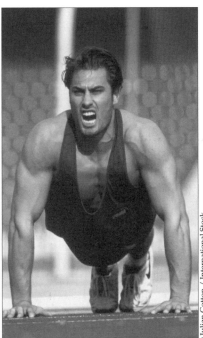
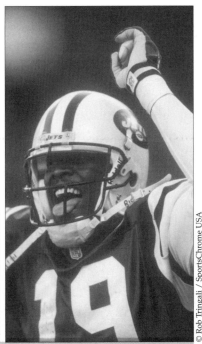

Often the subjective experiences of physical activity are revealed in the expressions on our faces.

© John S. Reid

© Julian Cotton / International Stock

© Rob Tringali / SportsChrome USA

Physical Activity Will Not Be Meaningful Unless We Enjoy It

Finally, a fourth truth about physical activity is that unless we are attracted to the subjective aspects of physical activity—unless we discover something enjoyable in it—it is unlikely to become personally meaningful to us. As we saw with Jaroncyk, accolades, money, recognition, prestige, and other factors external to the activity cannot fill the void. If the thoughts and feelings that accompany your engagement in physical activity don't spark you to invest it with the deepest resources of your mind and will, the experience can ultimately be hollow.

The physical, tangible side of physical activity provides the raw material for the experience, but it's the subjective experience that keeps us coming back for more. If you have ever ice-skated in solitude on a frozen pond or cycled along country roads on a brisk fall morning, you have probably enjoyed the subjective pleasures physical activity can bring. The same subjective pleasures may come to you when you're struggling through a difficult wrestling practice in a hot and humid room or when your lungs are bursting in the final stages of a tough aerobics workout. Engaging in physical activity can touch us emotionally, mentally, and spiritually. When we allow this to happen, our physical activity experiences are more meaningful.

Although it is easy to overlook the subjective side of physical activity, unless you allow yourself to be touched emotionally, mentally, and spiritually by the activity, it is unlikely to become personally meaningful to you.

Why Subjective Experiences Are Important

Learning about subjective experiences in physical activity is important for several reasons. For one, they can help clarify the bases of your career choices. You may be planning a career as a personal trainer or exercise consultant because you want others to know the kind of self-confidence you have experienced as a result of participating in a conditioning program. Or perhaps you have decided to become a physical education teacher or coach because of the good feelings you experienced when participating in sports in high school.

Learning about subjective experiences can also help to develop your skills as a physical activity professional. Sport psychologists, for instance, can appreciate more fully how physical activity programs affect the thoughts and feelings of their clients, students, or patients if they have studied the subjective aspects of physical activity. Such knowledge can be helpful in designing programs and interventions that help people understand their own subjective experiences and meanings in physical activity.

But the most important reason to study and learn about subjective experiences is that how we feel and what we think before, during, and after

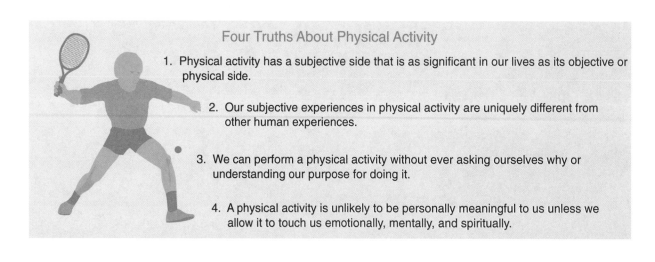

Four Truths About Physical Activity

1. Physical activity has a subjective side that is as significant in our lives as its objective or physical side.

2. Our subjective experiences in physical activity are uniquely different from other human experiences.

3. We can perform a physical activity without ever asking ourselves why or understanding our purpose for doing it.

4. A physical activity is unlikely to be personally meaningful to us unless we allow it to touch us emotionally, mentally, and spiritually.

Rating Your Feelings About Physical Activity

For each physical activity in the left-hand column ask yourself how strongly you are likely to experience each of the feelings listed across the top. Rate the intensity of each feeling on a scale of 1 to 5, where a rating of 5 indicates that you would strongly experience the feeling and a rating of 1 indicates that you would not experience the feeling at all.

	Feelings						
	Joy	Pain	Boredom	Anxiety	Embarrassment	Enthusiasm	Freedom
Activity							
Mow yard on hot summer day							
Do 50 push-ups by yourself							
Do 50 push-ups in competition with friends							
Run for 30 minutes through park with friend							
Walk in the rain on warm summer day							
Exercise your knee on weight machine to rehabilitate it following surgery							
Play favorite sport because you want to							
Play favorite sport because your roommate wants you to							
Ride a bicycle through park							
Ride a stationary bike at fitness center							

we engage in a physical activity largely determines our decisions to participate or not participate in it. Being attracted to mountain climbing rather than canoeing, aerobics rather than running, baseball rather than track and field all may be traced in some part to the subjective experiences these activities evoke. This chapter explores how physical activity affects us in ways that are not measured by stop clocks, strength gauges, or competitive points: the focus is on internal dynamics rather than external performance.

The Nature of Subjective Experiences

Imagine . . . that you have just shot a 6-meter (20-ft) jump shot at the buzzer to win a close game against your team's arch rival . . . that after an extremely tough practice you are sitting on a bench in the locker room, tired beyond belief but also surprised at how good it felt to endure the pain and pressure of that practice . . . that 10 years after graduating you return to your school for an alumni game, and as you sit on the same bench in the same locker room, you reflect back on what being a member of the team meant to you and how the experience has influenced your attitudes about the sport, about others, even about yourself.

These three short scenarios probably stimulate distinctly different feelings within you. In the first, your thoughts and feelings are likely to be intense and sharply focused on your game-winning shot. These thoughts and feelings are *immediate* in that you live the experience during and/or shortly after performing the activity. The sensations of jumping and having the ball leave the hand, and the image of the ball arching toward the basket are all indelibly etched in your mind's eye. You feel a deep sense of pride because you came through when the chips were down. You may also feel instant elation over contributing to a win for your team.

In the second scenario, you may again feel pride for gutting it out and finishing the practice, but you might also think that you learned a valuable lesson about yourself. While these thoughts and feelings are less immediate than those evoked by the first scenario, they are still in part a direct response to the activity just performed.

In the third scenario, your thoughts and feelings are nostalgic and mellow and far removed from any specific activity. You could not have experienced this sense of meaning without having been deeply involved in the activity, but neither could you have discovered it without the time that has passed since.

These scenarios illustrate how multifaceted subjective experiences can be—they can be intense and immediate, or they can be past experiences that you relive time and time again. We'll discuss each of these two kinds of experiences in the following sections.

Immediate Subjective Experiences

It may be impossible to engage in physical activity without our movements creating an immediate emotional and cognitive impression on us. This is because our bodies are equipped with "movement sensors" called proprioceptors, sensory devices in tendons, ligaments, muscles, and in the inner ear that are stimulated by physical actions; they provide us with information about the body's movements and position in space. Obviously, we pick up a virtually unending array of visual and auditory information when we move. Another sensory apparatus in the circulatory system picks up biochemical changes in the blood that affect our perceptions of fatigue and effort. Thus, each time we engage in physical activity, our nervous system is flooded with complex sensory signals that not only help us perform the activity but are transformed by our brains into perceptions, feelings, and knowledge. Of course, we can choose to ignore many of these sensations, just as we can ignore the vast array of subtle colors in a beautiful painting or the nuances of sound in a symphony recording. Recognizing that this sensory information is "there" is the first step toward appreciating the subjective side of physical activity.

But recognizing this isn't always easy, especially for novices who are concentrating on completing a demanding set of exercises, absorbed in the details of learning a new skill such as golf, or overcome by fatigue or pain. When learning a new aerobics routine or attempting to use an exercise machine we haven't used before, our attention must initially be directed to performing the movements of the activity. After we have become familiar with the activity, however, the movements can be executed without conscious attention, freeing our minds to think more deeply about the subjective aspects of performance. No doubt this is why experienced performers tend to give the richest and most elaborate accounts of subjective experiences in physical activity.

All physical activity is accompanied by sensations that can be converted to perceptions, emotions, and knowledge. To get the full experience of a physical activity, we must be open to the emotional and cognitive impressions the activity provides.

Along with experience level, the type of activity also affects how much we can attend to our subjective impressions. Activities we can do alone such as running, swimming, white-water rafting, rock climbing, or working out on a machine don't require much interaction with our social environment, leaving us more opportunity to reflect on the feelings brought on by the activity. Group aerobics, team sports such as basketball or volleyball, or individual sports such as wrestling require constant monitoring of our social surroundings. In aerobics we must coordinate our movements with the music and actions of the leader; in team sports we must constantly move in rela-

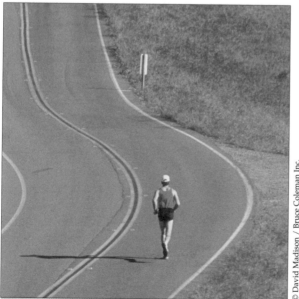

Some forms of physical activity lend themselves naturally to concentrating on subjective experiences.

© David Madison / Bruce Coleman Inc.

tion to balls, opponents, and teammates, leaving little sustained thought or reflection *while the activity is ongoing*. Because of the solitary nature of running and the automatic, repetitive movements it entails, long-distance runners have been extraordinarily conscious of the feelings and meanings brought on by their physical activity.

Replayed Subjective Experiences

Simply because an attention-demanding activity prevents you from concentrating on your subjective experiences while performing doesn't mean that it hasn't made a distinct impression on you. Subjective experiences often endure in memory for months, years, or even a lifetime. In one of the scenarios that opened this section, a basketball player returned years later to a memory-laden locker room and, perhaps for the first time, thought really hard about what playing high school basketball had meant to him. The same feelings might be experienced by a person who thinks back to the day she earned a fitness award, or to the early-morning high school exercise program that taught her how to control her weight and eat nutritious meals. This process by which we reexperience the subjectiveness of physical activity is called **self-reflection**. When we reflect in this way, it is as though we replay a videotape of past experiences, only the videotape includes not only visual but also kinesthetic, auditory, and other impressions from an earlier time. Because of the passage of time, self-reflection often enables us to place specific subjective experiences within a framework that makes them more meaningful.

Reflecting on our experiences in physical activity can be done in various ways and for different reasons. Reflecting might be a means of summing up our total experience with the activity, accumulated over many years, in order to determine its overall value or worth to our lives. We might also replay experiences at times of anxiety in order to calm ourselves or give us a boost in confidence. A tennis player, for instance, after losing the first set in a two-out-of-three match and then quickly falling behind in the second set, might replay previous successes she has had under similar circumstances. If she can relive the feelings of the previous experience, she might be able to attain some of the same mental focus that led to her earlier victories.

The subjective experiences that accompany physical activity may have a profound effect on us during and immediately after our performances. Reflecting on our past experiences with an activity following the passage of time often helps us put them into a more comprehensive and meaningful frame of reference.

The Components of Subjective Experience

When exploring a territory as broad and expansive as subjective experience, it's helpful to move slowly and break the area down into its various components. In the following sections, we'll discuss sensations and perceptions, emotions and emotional responses, and various ways in which knowledge is gained through subjective experience.

Sensations and Perceptions

Sensations are raw, uninterpreted data collected through sensory organs. Our past experiences help us interpret these raw sensations into meaningful constructs or perceptions. Physical activity automatically stimulates a barrage of sensations. These include the feelings of contracting our muscles and moving our bodies, as well as feelings of an increased heart rate, breathlessness, or muscle fatigue. If we attend to them, these sensations provide us with an "on-line" report of our inner states. Organized into meaningful information by the process of perception, these sensations can be used to make ongoing corrections in our physical activity. For instance, our decision about when to stop an exercise usually is made on the basis of some perceptions of fatigue or discomfort, as are judgments about how forcefully we are moving, how much resistance our movements are encountering, or, in the case of divers and gymnasts, how our bodies are oriented to the ground.

Sensations from outside our bodies also become part of the subjective experience. What we see or hear when we perform, even what we smell, are all welded into a cohesive subjective experience. It isn't unusual for football or soccer players who spend much time in contact with the ground to reflect automatically on their playing experiences whenever they smell wet earth. The sound of waves may trigger past visions of riding the waves for surfers, or the clang of a bell may cause boxers to think back on their experiences in the ring.

Emotions and Emotional Responses

Our perceptions during physical activity can elicit from us many different reactions. Sometimes physical activity will increase our level of excitement and motivation; at other times it may dampen it. We might become angry, annoyed, surprised, pleased, disappointed, enthusiastic, and so on. Such reactions can stem from the feelings of an activity, our impressions about the quality of our performance, or the outcome of a particular event. We call such subjective reactions emotions; they differ depending on the person and situation. For example, achieving a personal goal or performing an activity well may result in the emotion of elation or joy; failing to achieve a goal or performing poorly may prompt such emotions as disappointment or shame. Psychologists have identified over 200 different emotions and have yet to agree as to precisely how to define them. What seems clear is that they involve a complex combination of psychological processes including perception, memory, reasoning, and action (Willis & Campbell, 1992).

One way of understanding emotions is to consider them the result of disruptions in bodily states. Changes in our body chemistry, such as those resulting from the release of endorphins during vigorous physical activity, the release of adrenaline during panic, or the consumption of coffee or alcohol, are usually accompanied by a change in our emotions. Often, the changes in our body chemistry and our emotional states are too subtle for us to detect. We might feel the end-result emotion without being aware of the changes that brought us there. For instance, a gradual change in our body chemistry might trigger a gradual change in our emotional state that goes unrecognized until it peaks out as elation or bottoms out as depression.

Emotions also can be detected from changes in our physical activity. The emotion of fear, for example, can make us tremble, or anxiety or excitement can cause us to perform movements forcefully and rapidly, even in situations in which forceful and rapid movements may not be desired. (We don't want our surgeons to be too excited in the middle of an operation!) This tendency to reveal something about our emotional state in our physical activity is called **emotional expression**. Emotional expressions are external manifestations of internal emotional states.

Physical activity is always accompanied by the internal sensations of moving our limbs and bodies; changes in our physiological functioning; and sensations from outside our bodies including vision, sound, touch, and smell. When organized into perceptions, they can give rise to emotions that we associate with particular physical activities.

Knowledge Gained Through Subjective Experience

When someone mentions knowledge, what comes into your mind? Facts learned in history or science? Mathematical formulas? Story themes from great works of literature? These represent a very specific type of knowledge derived from logic, reason, and analysis. It is called **rational knowledge**. You'll rely on this type of knowledge as you study the theoretical aspects of physical activity such as exercise physiology, biomechanics, or sport history, or when you read this book.

But a different type of knowledge—**intuitive knowledge**—derived from our subjective experiences in physical activity is equally important. Intuition is a process by which we come to know something without conscious reasoning. Usually it is difficult to describe this type of knowledge or to know precisely how we mastered it. Intuitive knowledge gained from subjective experiences usually is personal in that it is knowledge about ourselves rather than about the exercise, the skill, or other people. Philosopher Drew Hyland (1990) identified three types of self-knowledge associated with participating in physical activity: psychoanalytic self-knowledge, Zen self-knowledge (mystical knowledge), and Socratic self-knowledge (see figure 4.1). Since

knowledge gained through subjective experience is closely associated with our reasons for participating in physical activity, we'll discuss each of these in detail.

Psychoanalytic Self-Knowledge

Psychoanalytic self-knowledge is knowledge about our deep-seated desires, motivations, and behavior. It relates primarily to the types of activities we choose to participate in and the manner in which we pursue them. For example, when a young woman with an impoverished, disadvantaged background chooses to participate in a sport such as polo, golf, or squash, her choice may be a commendable effort to transcend social barriers. On the other hand, it may represent a less commendable attempt to deny her social roots. When a young man chooses contact sports over noncontact sports, it may reveal a love of competition and physical contact—or it could represent "a precariously controlled desire to physically dominate or even hurt others" (Hyland, 1990, p. 74).

Psychoanalytic self-knowledge may also be revealed in the manner in which we choose to participate. Exercisers who are so concerned about the times of their runs or so intent on improving their performance that they can't enjoy the participation may have developed a narrow, single-focused pattern of behavior that may not serve them well in ordinary life, where many different responsibilities must be met. When a

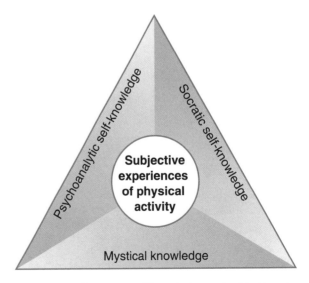

Figure 4.1   Three types of knowledge embedded in subjective experiences of physical activity.

softball player is a "poor loser," it may be because she has invested an inordinate amount of her self-worth in the game; the same may be true for a winner who "rubs it in" after the game is over. On the other side, someone who can't get serious about an exercise program or a sport competition may be reflecting a fear of failure. By not taking the game seriously, failure need not be taken seriously either. By carefully examining the activities we choose to engage in, as well as our styles of involvement, we can learn a great deal about ourselves.

Mystical Knowledge

Mystical knowledge, termed "Zen self-knowledge" by Hyland, refers to subjective experiences available to experienced performers only in rare and special circumstances. Mystical knowledge is knowledge of a dimension not experienced in ordinary life. Some would call the experiences that give rise to this type of knowledge "transcendent" to suggest the experiences took them out of the real world. These subjective experiences can be so powerful that memories of them remain with performers for years, sometimes for a lifetime. The most common type of mystical experience during physical activity is called **peak experience**. Research suggests that peak experiences tend to come involuntarily and unexpectedly (Ravizza, 1984). Time usually seems to slow down and sometimes specific features of the environment stand out in sharp contrast to

the background. Almost always, athletes report being "totally absorbed" in the activity.

Peak experiences provide no specific knowledge of their own. In some cases they may be windows through which performers claim to have a more extensive and inclusive world opened to them. Sometimes peak experiences may provide not so much knowledge as a feeling of awe and reverence to which a religious or philosophical interpretation may be attached. In other cases performers may claim to have gained new insights into themselves as beings connected to an all-encompassing universe.

Socratic Self-Knowledge

Socratic self-knowledge is realizing the difference between what we know and what we don't know. We may translate this into the realm of exercise and sport as knowledge of what we can and cannot do. Knowing our performance limits can help us to operate within the confines of our skills and abilities. When coaches refer to the importance of athletes "playing within themselves," they are giving testimony to the importance of Socratic self-knowledge.

Ignoring personal limits can lead to disastrous performances and even injury. At the same time, as we saw in chapter 3, we must test these personal limits or we'll never improve. This is the purpose of practice and training: to expand the range of our performance limits systematically and gradually, thereby not only improving the

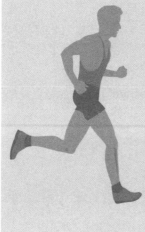

Replaying a Peak Performance

Mike Spino, a former top collegiate distance runner, wrote this penetrating account of his subjective experience during a training run on the back roads of upstate New York:

"Furiously I ran: time lost all semblance of meaning. Distance, time, motion were all one. . . . My running was a pouring feeling. . . . I kept on running. I could have run and run. Perhaps I had experienced a physiological change, but whatever, it was magic. I came to the side of the road and gazed, with a sort of bewilderment, at my friends. I sat on the side of the road and cried tears of joy and sorrow. Joy at being alive, sorrow for a vague feeling of temporalness, and a knowledge of the impossibility of giving this experience to anyone" (Spino, 1971, pp. 224-225).

Have you ever had a similar peak experience like this while participating in sport or exercise? In what ways was the experience similar to or different from that reported by Spino?

quality of our performance but also reorienting our perceptions of our own self-limits, taking into account our newly developed ability to perform. One of the important roles of the personal trainer, coach, physical education teacher, physical therapist, or exercise leader is to help performers set realistic goals that will allow them to test the limits of their performances in a safe and productive manner.

🔑 Performing physical activities can be a source of knowledge, including knowledge about our motivations for engaging in activity, knowledge about different dimensions of reality, and knowledge of our personal performance capabilities.

Communicating Subjective Experiences

Subjective experiences, by nature, are private experiences. And because they can be affected by many factors—including our success or failure in the activity; the conditions surrounding our participation; and the meaning given to the activity by our parents, personal trainers, coaches, or the media—it is unlikely that two individuals participating in the same activity will have exactly the same subjective experiences. You cannot know precisely what the person riding the stationary bicycle next to you is experiencing; neither can he know what you are experiencing.

Because subjective experiences are interior by nature, the only way to compare our experiences with those of others is by talking about them. Some people have been able to describe their experiences quite eloquently. For example, Bill Bradley described his experiences with the New York Knicks this way:

> In those moments on a basketball court I feel as a child and know as an adult. Experience rushes through my pores as if sucked by a strong vacuum. I feel the power of imagination and the sense of mystery and wonder I accepted in my childhood before life hardened. (1977, p. 57)

Roger Bannister, the first person to break the four-minute mile, described his subjective experience of that historic race this way: "No pain, only a great unity of movement and aim. The world seemed to stand still, or did not exist. . . . " (Bannister, 1955, pp. 213–214). We have no reason to suspect that Bradley and Bannister are exaggerating or fabricating their experiences, but it is impossible to validate their accounts. We can only know for certain what we experience; we cannot have the same certainty about the experiences of others.

If you've never before talked about your subjective experiences in physical activity, you may find it difficult at first. Most people are hesitant to share their deepest feelings—not only about physical activity, but also about anything of a personal nature—with others, especially those they don't know well. You may worry that what you have to say about your subjective experiences will be misunderstood or will cause others to laugh. Such feelings are normal, since most of us have had very little practice in sharing such information, nor have we been encouraged to do so. Generally, coaches and aerobics instructors tend to care much more about the physical aspects of human performances than the subjective aspects, and rarely encourage students to talk about them.

Yet, even when we overcome our natural reluctance to talk about our subjective experiences, it is not always easy to find the right words to describe our feelings. Sport philosopher Scott Kretchmar suggested that words may never adequately describe what we feel about physical activity. He pointed out that "the 'medium of exchange' in sport is 'feel,'" and noted that "any meaningful distinctions in this realm typically outrun any verbal ability to refer to them" (1985, p. 101).

Be that as it may, words remain our primary medium for communicating our subjective experiences. Furthermore, struggling to put our feelings into words may help us come to grips with the deeper meanings physical activity has for us. Sy Kleinman, a philosopher particularly sensitive to the meanings of physical movements, would agree: "Engagement in game, sport, or art, and a *description* of this kind of engagement enable us to know what game, sport, or art is on a level that adds another dimension to our knowing . . ." [italics added] (1968, p. 31). Although you may feel inarticulate in describing your physical activity experiences, such descriptions can be an important way to clarify to yourself why you engage in activity and what it means to you.

> Replay a notable physical activity experience in your mind. What thoughts and feelings do you associate with the experience? Can you describe it in *one* word? Could you describe it in one sentence? In five sentences?

In attempting to communicate our subjective experiences in sport and exercise to others, it usually is difficult to find the correct words to express our feelings. This is an important activity, however, as it helps us better understand the meanings we find in physical activity.

Intrinsic and Extrinsic Approaches to Physical Activity

By now it should be apparent to you that how you feel when and after you engage in a physical activity can determine whether or not you return to it in the future. But our subjective experiences are not the only factor that motivates us to participate. One of the most often cited reasons for participating is the benefits physical activity offers. Perhaps you recall listening to a lecture by your physical education or health teacher that outlined these benefits and encouraged you to "exercise for the health of it." Maybe you recall listening to your coach's speech at the athletic banquet suggesting that sport is important because it "builds character." The physical activity you perform at work is probably motivated by the promise of a paycheck; patients who adhere to a grueling program of therapeutic physical activity are motivated by the promise of returning to normal functioning.

These are examples of **extrinsic approaches to physical activity**. One who has an extrinsic orientation to exercise professes to engage in it pri-

marily because of the physical or psychological payoffs it offers. The physical education teacher who argues for her program because it develops fundamental skills in young children, or a recreational therapist who justifies shuffleboard as a means of psychological relaxation, are portraying sport in an extrinsic manner, as is the businessman who works out at the fitness center with his boss as a way of impressing him and boosting his chances for a promotion. When we approach an activity from an extrinsic standpoint, we do not value it primarily for its subjective experiences; we value it because we believe it contributes in some way to a more important end.

Having an extrinsic approach to physical activity makes a great deal of sense in many instances. We perform self-sufficiency activities for a very practical (extrinsic) reason: to complete tasks around the house. We perform physical activity at work in order to earn a paycheck. We move in physical education class in order to learn a skill and meet the course requirements. However, in the leisure, competition, and self-expression spheres, and often in the health sphere, an intrinsic rather than an extrinsic approach may make more sense. Intrinsic reasons for performing physical activities may be what keep us interested over the long term.

Running or playing golf or swimming or doing high-impact aerobics simply because we enjoy the experience of the activity are illustrations of having an **intrinsic approach to physical activity**. This approach also is called autotelic (*auto* = self, *telic* = end or goal) to illustrate that the goal of the activity is discovered within the activity itself. When we approach weight training or mountain biking or any other activity as an end in itself, we are displaying an autotelic or intrinsic disposition toward the activities.

Physical activity brings many extrinsic benefits to participants, but we should never presume that the mere *fact* of these benefits makes them the primary reason for engaging in the activity. To a large extent the physiological benefits of physical activity are inescapable. When you pursue the subjective experiences of mountain climbing, for example, you automatically reap the benefits of increased muscular endurance and strength.

One way to think about the physiological, psychological, or sociological benefits of physical activity is to compare them to the nutritional benefits we might receive after eating a meal at a four-star gourmet restaurant. Although a nutritionist could demonstrate that the meal we eat at the restaurant supplies us with a significant percentage of our daily dietary requirements, nutritional benefits are not the primary reason we go to such places. We are attracted not by the promise of improved health but by the unique subjective experience of eating at a nice restaurant. The nutritional benefits are merely icing on the cake. So too we may think of many of the extrinsic benefits of physical activity—for example, health or character or new friendships—as merely icing on the cake. Physical activity, especially sport, exercise, and dance, is much more likely to become meaningful to us if we develop an attraction to its intrinsic qualities. Having said this, it is important to recognize that few people probably approach any activity entirely in an intrinsic or extrinsic manner; with most of us it's usually a combination of the two.

Physical activity usually is accompanied by external benefits whether in the form of health benefits from exercise, developing friendships through sports, or earning a salary through physical activity at work. Nevertheless, activities—especially those connected with sport and exercise—are more likely to become personally meaningful to us if we are attracted to the subjective experiences of the activity itself.

It might seem obvious that most of us are attracted to sport because of its intrinsic benefits, but this is not always the case. The questionnaire on page 126 is the Task and Ego Orientation in Sport Questionnaire (TEOSQ) (Duda, 1992), an instrument used by researchers to determine the extent to which respondents approach sport with primarily an intrinsic or extrinsic orientation. You may find it useful to measure your own orientations to sport by indicating for each item whether you strongly disagree (1) to strongly agree (5) with each statement. As a reference point for interpreting your score, it may help to know that the mean scores for 56 male and 67 female high school basketball players from a Midwestern community were as follows: 4.16 and 2.81 for males and 4.49 and 2.37 for females, on the task

and ego orientation scales, respectively (Duda, Olson, & Templin, 1991).

How do you interpret your score on the TEOSQ? If you scored relatively high on task orientation, you likely define competence in a competitive physical activity on the basis of how well you improve your performance, and you probably approach the sport from an intrinsic orientation. On the other hand, if you scored relatively high on ego orientation, you likely define competence in an activity by comparing your performance to that of others. Individuals with a high ego orientation are more likely to adopt an extrinsic approach to sports; they usually value participation as a means to an external end rather than valuing it as a subjective experience in itself. In evaluating your own motivations, it's important to keep in mind that a low score on one type of orientation does not necessarily mean that you will have a high score on the other. You may be relatively high or low on each, or high on one and low on the other.

Intrinsic Approaches to Exercise for Health

People generally find it easier to appreciate the importance of subjective experiences in sport than in exercise. "We play sports for fun; we exercise for health," so the thinking goes. It is difficult to imagine that we could be attracted to exercise by its subjective experience when it is the subjective experiences associated with exercise that seem to be so aversive. Wouldn't most of us prefer to take the improved strength, endurance, flexibility, longevity, and other benefits of exercise and dispense with the pain and discomfort required to attain them? Some of us might, but certainly not all. As curious as it may seem, the discomfort produced by physical exertion is not always interpreted as a negative feeling by exercisers. In many cases, the subjective experience of performing rigorous exercise is an algebraic summation of both pleasure and pain that results in an overall sense of satisfaction and well-being. This point was made by psychologist Csikszentmihalyi ("Cheek-sent-ma-hi") (1990a) in talking about the agony endured by a swimmer: "The swimmer's muscles might have ached during his most memorable race, his lungs might have felt like exploding, and he might have been dizzy with

The Task and Ego Orientation in Sport Questionnaire

Attitudes Toward Sport

Directions: Answer each of the following statements and indicate how much you personally agree with each statement by circling the response—strongly agree (5) to strongly disagree (1)—that best expresses your feeling.

When do you feel most successful in sport? In other words, when do you feel a sport activity has gone really good for you? *I feel most successful in sport when . . .*

		Strongly disagree				Strongly agree
Item A	I'm the only one who can do the skill.	1	2	3	4	5
Item B	I learn a new skill and it makes me want to practice more.	1	2	3	4	5
Item C	I can do better than my friends.	1	2	3	4	5
Item D	Others can't do as well as me.	1	2	3	4	5
Item E	I learn something that is fun to do.	1	2	3	4	5
Item F	Others mess up and I don't.	1	2	3	4	5
Item G	I learn a new skill by trying hard.	1	2	3	4	5
Item H	I work really hard.	1	2	3	4	5
Item I	I score the most points.	1	2	3	4	5
Item J	Something I learn makes me want to go and practice.	1	2	3	4	5
Item K	I'm the best.	1	2	3	4	5
Item L	A skill I learn really feels right.	1	2	3	4	5
Item M	I do my very best.	1	2	3	4	5

Scoring instructions: Add up the total point values for ego items (A, C, D, F, I, K) and divide by 6 to obtain your score on the ego orientation scale. Add up the total point values for task orientation items (B, E, G, H, J, L, M) and divide by 7 to obtain your score on the task orientation.

Reprinted, by permission, from J.L. Duda, 1992, Motivation in sports settings: A goal perspective approach. In *Motivation in sport and exercise*, edited by G.G. Roberts (Champaign, IL: Human Kinetics), 57-91.

fatigue—yet these could have been the best moments of his life" (p. 4).

But how do we know that subjective experiences of exercise are important to us? Two lines of evidence suggest this. The first is that, while extrinsic factors may be the principal reason for undertaking an exercise program, intrinsic factors of subjective experience often come to be dominant over time. For instance, when people become committed to long-distance running, the prospective health benefits that may have

prompted them to run in the first place often take a back seat to experiential outcomes such as feelings of achievement and self-development (Clough, Shepherd, & Maughan, 1989). This was reflected in psychologist Michael Sachs' description of his feelings about running when he noted: "Running has become much more than a means to the end of getting in shape; it has become the end itself" (Sachs, 1981, p. 118).

The second line of evidence can be observed in our everyday lives in the way we make qualitative distinctions between the subjective experiences of strenuous work and strenuous exercise. If health and fitness are the primary reasons for exercising, then we shouldn't care whether the exercise comes in the form of a Stairmaster, a treadmill, a stationary bike, a brisk walk behind a wheelbarrow, digging a ditch, or moving heavy stones. (In fact it would make more sense to get our exercise through work since at the conclusion we would have actually accomplished something!) But most of us *do* care! We make important distinctions between these forms of activity, and these distinctions are reflected in our decisions. Have you known someone who hires out the jobs of painting the house, mowing the lawn, or raking leaves and at the same time pays dues to a local fitness center for the privilege of doing even more grueling forms of exercise there? Measured from a purely physiological standpoint the physical activity of work may have the same healthful benefit as the physical activity of exercise, yet the former tends to be avoided, the latter eagerly sought out.

🔑 Even though exercise provides participants with many health benefits, there is reason to believe that many people engage in it because of the unique subjective experiences it offers.

Clearly, then, the subjective experiences gained from exercising appear to be unique, different from work, and influential in our decisions to engage in it. Scientists have yet to identify precisely how the subjective aspects of exercise differ from those of work. How does exercising make you feel? One way to assess your subjective responses to exercise is by completing the Subjective Exercise Experience Scale (SEES) (McAuley & Courneya, 1994) on page 128.

Internalization of Physical Activity

Have you ever decided to participate in an activity merely to please a friend or meet a class requirement? If so, the subjective experiences of the activity at first were probably incidental to your participation. But with time, your attitude toward the activity may have changed. Eventually, your decision to participate may have begun to center around something in the activity itself rather than

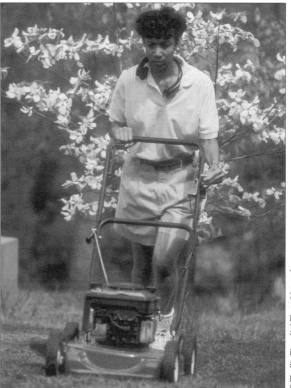

© Phyllis Picardi / Photo Network

If you hire someone to cut your grass, that person's getting not only your money but also the health benefits you could be getting from the physical activity.

extrinsic factors. Psychologists frequently use the term **internalization** to refer to the gradual process by which something takes on intrinsic value, or passes from "a level of bare awareness to a position of some power to guide or control the behavior of a person" (Krawthwohl, Bloom, & Masia, 1964, p. 27).

The process of internalization can be summarized in five stages (see figure 4.2). The first time you watched Major League Baseball, hiked up a mountain trail, embarked on a weight training program, or went fly fishing, you were probably merely *aware* of the new stimuli and physical activity that surrounded you. Later, after doing the activity many more times, you may have *responded* to the activity with positive feelings. Eventually, you might have come to value the activity to the point of *going out of your way* to seek it out. With continued involvement you may have begun to *conceptualize* and *organize* the importance of the activity by talking about the characteristics of the activity you found most attractive. If you were further attracted to the activity,

The Subjective Exercise Experience Scale

This questionnaire was developed by McAuley and Courneya (1994) to assess psychological responses to exercise. Circle a number on the scale next to each item to indicate the degree to which you are experiencing each feeling now, at this point in time. Record your scores on the scale prior to exercise and fill out the questionnaire again after a vigorous exercise bout. Record the before- and after-exercise differences in your score for the three main factors described (at the end of the questionnaire). Did your scores for positive well-being, psychological distress, and feelings of fatigue change as a result of the exercise bout?

I feel:

1. **Great**
    1 2 3 4 5 6 7
    Not at all   *Moderately*   *Very much so*

2. **Awful**
    1 2 3 4 5 6 7
    Not at all   *Moderately*   *Very much so*

3. **Drained**
    1 2 3 4 5 6 7
    Not at all   *Moderately*   *Very much so*

4. **Positive**
    1 2 3 4 5 6 7
    Not at all   *Moderately*   *Very much so*

5. **Crummy**
    1 2 3 4 5 6 7
    Not at all   *Moderately*   *Very much so*

6. **Exhausted**
    1 2 3 4 5 6 7
    Not at all   *Moderately*   *Very much so*

7. **Strong**
    1 2 3 4 5 6 7
    Not at all   *Moderately*   *Very much so*

8. **Discouraged**
    1 2 3 4 5 6 7
    Not at all   *Moderately*   *Very much so*

9. **Fatigued**
    1 2 3 4 5 6 7
    Not at all   *Moderately*   *Very much so*

10. **Terrific**
    1 2 3 4 5 6 7
    Not at all   *Moderately*   *Very much so*

11. **Miserable**
    1 2 3 4 5 6 7
    Not at all   *Moderately*   *Very much so*

12. **Tired**
    1 2 3 4 5 6 7
    Not at all   *Moderately*   *Very much so*

Sum items 1, 4, 7, and 10 to derive your score for overall experience of positive well-being; sum items 2, 5, 8, and 11 for overall experience of psychological distress; sum items 3, 6, 9, and 12 for overall experience of fatigue.

As a point of reference for interpreting your scores, it may help you to know the mean pre- and postexercise scores for a group of 51 middle-aged males and females (McAuley & Courneya, 1994): Positive well-being = 19.55 preexercise, 20.37 postexercise, +1.23 change; psychological distress = 6.63 preexercise, 5.39 postexercise, –.96 change; fatigue = 8.80 preexercise, 9.98 postexercise, +1.18 change.

Adapted, by permission, from E. McAuley and K.S. Courneya, 1994, "The subjective exercise experience scale," *Journal of Sport and Exercise Psychology* 16 (2): 163-177.

Low ↑

A. Becoming Aware of Badminton

1. You attend a badminton lesson because it is a requirement for a college degree program.
2. You agree (unenthusiastically) to watch your friend play in a badminton tournament.
3. You decide to take lessons privately from a friend who plays competitive badminton. Most of your shots are weak and misplaced, but two or three times you hit the shuttle well and find it satisfying.

B. Responding Positively to Badminton

1. When your friend forgets to meet you for your lesson one week, you call him the day before your next week's lesson as a reminder. You find yourself looking forward to each week's lesson.
2. You decide (with some prompting from a friend or teacher) to participate in a local tournament for novices.
3. Your skills have improved considerably and you find yourself looking forward to the lesson and to the opportunity to competively challenge your teacher/friend.

C. Going Out of Your Way to Participate in Badminton

1. You join the local badminton club.
2. The local badminton club is forced to move its sessions from the gymnasium near your house to one in the next community ten miles away, but you continue to attend.
3. You actively seek out other badminton players, encourage your non-badminton-playing friends to try the game, and arrange to play against others at various times during the week.

D. Conceptualizing Badminton Into a Value System

1. Given a limited time for recreation sport, you decide to discontinue your weekly game of racquetball in order to have more time for badminton.
2. You begin to discriminate among competitors, selecting those with sufficient talent to test your abilities.
3. You evaluate different strategic approaches to the game, and make finer discriminations about badminton equipment, training programs, and techniques.

E. Participation in Badminton Becomes Internalized

1. Playing badminton becomes part of your "normal" life. You now play several times each week. You now have an identity among those who know you as "a badminton player."
2. You make significant financial sacrifices to purchase the best equipment and to travel to tournaments.
3. All personal decisions regarding investment of time, energy, and money, center around their effects on your opportunities to play badminton.

High ↓ (Internalization)

Figure 4.2 Internalizing the game of badminton.

you reached the final stage, *internalization*. This occurs when your behaviors demonstrate a commitment to the activity and you are able to integrate your beliefs and attitudes about the activity into a comprehensive philosophy or worldview.

As we progress from merely enjoying an activity to becoming engrossed in it, the activity can develop deep meaning for us, so deep that it can become incorporated into our beliefs, attitudes, and personal identity. When this happens, we have *internalized* the activity.

Factors Affecting Our Enjoyment of Physical Activity

It is not altogether clear how internalizing an activity is different from learning to enjoy it. Perhaps the first thing that comes to your mind when asked why you work out regularly at the fitness club, go rollerblading, or play lacrosse is that you enjoy it. This sounds simplistic, but the concept of enjoyment is fairly complex. Let's focus briefly on this concept in order to better understand it and, in turn, understand what factors affect our enjoyment of physical activity.

There is probably a long list of factors; here we'll focus on three general categories, including (1) factors related to the activity, (2) factors related to the performer, and (3) factors related to the social context in which the activity is performed.

Factors Related to the Activity

If you reflect on the physical activities you enjoy and ask yourself why you enjoy them, the first things that come to mind are probably specific characteristics of the activities. For instance, you might enjoy tennis because you prefer individual over team sports and like a game that makes you concentrate. You might prefer aerobics to running because you enjoy moving your body to music. In both of these examples the enjoyment comes from a specific quality of the activity itself. Csikszentmihalyi (1990b) identified several characteristics of activities (those that involve physical activity and those that do not) that make them enjoyable. The three we'll discuss here involve (1) balance between the challenges of the activity and the abilities of the performer, (2) whether the activity provides clear goals and feedback, and (3) whether the activity is competitive.

Challenges of the Task Are Evenly Matched With Performer's Ability

Imagine that two students have designed strength development programs using free weights. The first selects a weight that is very easy to lift (13.6 kg [30 lb]), and each day he lifts this weight 10 times, never increasing the weight nor the repetitions. Soon he becomes bored, realizes that he's not enjoying the activity, and quits. The second student decides to begin his weight training program by trying to lift 90.7 kilograms (200 lb). Each day he comes to the gym, pulls with all of his might, but is unable to lift the weight off the ground. Soon he becomes frustrated and, like the first student, realizes he's not enjoying this; he also quits.

The diagram in figure 4.3 shows that when our skills and abilities go far beyond the challenges of the activity, we usually experience boredom. On the other hand, when success in the activity requires skills and abilities we lack, we often experience frustration or anxiety. Csikszentmihalyi

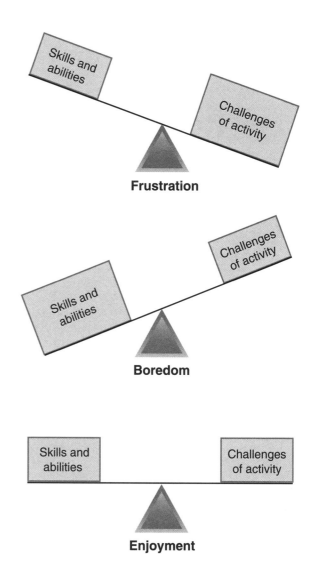

Figure 4.3 We are more likely to enjoy a physical activity when its challenges are balanced by our skills and abilities.

claims that "enjoyment appears at the boundary between boredom and anxiety" (1990b), another way of saying that enjoyment requires a delicate balance between the challenges of the activity and the skills and abilities of the performer.

The Activity Provides Clear Goals and Clear Feedback About the Results of Performers' Efforts

Part of the fun we get from playing sports results from testing our skills and abilities against the challenges of the game. Shooting the ball in the basket or putting the ball in the cup are goals that we try to accomplish by executing a series of coordinated movements. Enjoyment stems not so much from the goal being accomplished (e.g., the golf ball being in the cup) as it does from our having *attempted and caused* the ball to go into the cup. Unsurprisingly, the enjoyment of attaining goals is greatest when the goals are difficult to attain. If we attained the goal at every attempt, our enjoyment would soon vanish.

If attempting to attain the goal of an activity is central to our enjoyment of it, it makes sense that lack of a clear idea of what that goal is can detract from our enjoyment. This can happen when we find ourselves in a game—say cricket—in which we don't understand the rules or purpose of the game. Exercising on a piece of equipment about which we know very little may be unenjoyable because we don't have a clear sense of what it is we are supposed to be doing.

Some degree of feedback is also central to our enjoyment of physical activity. Imagine yourself shooting free throws. You may have a clear idea of the goal, but each time the ball leaves your hands, the lights go out and you never know whether the ball went through the hoop. At first, the novelty of the situation might make it fun, but soon it would become very dull. Knowing how we're doing relative to the activity goal is an important component of enjoyment. Activities such as table tennis or squash provide a lot of immediate feedback; others such as marathon running, in which the final outcome occurs more than two hours after the gun has been fired, provide much less.

Teachers, coaches, and trainers can play an important role in providing feedback to learners. After each trial or group of trials, the teacher usually provides a commentary on the major mistakes performers made, along with recommendations for correcting them. This information, when coupled with encouragement, can affect performers' subjective experiences. For example, age-group swimmers are more likely to enjoy swimming when they perceive their coach as one who gives informative feedback along with encouragement following unsuccessful performances (Black & Weiss, 1992).

The Activity Is Competitive

According to Csikszentmihalyi (1990a), competition often heightens enjoyment of physical activity, something we have already noted in chapter 2. **Competition** is not an activity per se, but an organizing principle that frames physical activity within a larger purpose. It enables us to compare our performances against a standard such as par on a golf course or a time on a race course, or with another person or group of persons, such as in basketball, football, or baseball. Just as poetry can be added to language, color to art, or melody to sound to make them more enjoyable, competition can be added to physical activity to make it more enjoyable.

One problem with adding competition to activities is that it can become an end in itself. When coaches and players value winning above enjoyment of the activity or the basic individual and social values of friendship, caring, and cooperation, they are elevating competition to an end rather than a means. Csikszentmihalyi says, "The challenges of competition can be stimulating and enjoyable. But when beating the opponent takes precedence in the mind over performing as well as possible, enjoyment tends to disappear. Competition is enjoyable only when it is a means to perfect one's skills; when it becomes an end in itself, it ceases to be fun" (1990a, p. 50).

Jack Nicklaus on Competition

Widely regarded as the best golfer to have played the game, Jack Nicklaus, winner of 16 major championships including the Masters, the British Open, the U.S. Open, and the PGA Championship, was a fierce competitor who always managed to remember that competition was a way of increasing his enjoyment of physical activity, not an end in itself. He said: "My strongest motivation through all my best years wasn't the championships I won and the golfers I defeated, but those who beat me. Losing to them simply increased the challenge, pushed me to practice and play harder. But my perspective on it all never changed. Win or lose, golf was a game and nothing more."

Quote, from J. Potter, 1998, "Hip problems force Jack Nicklaus to end streak," *USA Today*, July 9, p. 11c.

We are more likely to enjoy physical activities when the challenges of the activity match our abilities, when the activity has clear goals and feedback, and when the activity is arranged in a competitive framework.

Factors Related to the Performer

The second category of factors that influence our enjoyment of physical activities concern those that lie within ourselves. Whether we enjoy a particular type of physical activity depends a great deal on our dispositions and attitudes. **Dispositions** may be thought of as short-term, highly variable psychological states that may be affected by a host of external factors. **Attitudes** are relatively stable mind-sets toward concrete objects that may be favorable or unfavorable.

Dispositions That Affect Enjoyment of Physical Activity

Three dispositions identified by Csikszentmihalyi (1990b) are particularly relevant in physical activities: (1) how competent we feel in performing the activity, (2) the extent to which we are able to become absorbed in the activity, and (3) how much control we feel we have over the activity. We'll describe each briefly.

Perceived Competency. As a rule we enjoy activities we do well more than those that make us feel incompetent. Psychologists use the term **self-efficacy** to refer to how adequate we feel to perform a task. Research has shown that people who feel competent in exercise are more likely to adhere to rehabilitative exercises (Dishman, 1990), are more likely to engage in higher levels of intensity when participating in physical activities (Sallis et al., 1986), and will be more faithful in attending exercise programs (McAuley & Jacobson, 1991). One study showed that aerobic dancers with higher ratings of self-efficacy reported enjoying the activity more, and they exerted more effort than those with low ratings of self-efficacy (McAuley, Wraith, & Duncan, 1991).

Absorption. We all remember times when we were deeply engrossed in an exercise or sport, and other times when we simply "went through the motions." When we surrender to an activity and become absorbed in it, we lose consciousness of ourselves as distinct entities apart from the activity. Csikszentmihalyi (1990b) found that when people lose a sense of themselves while performing an activity, feelings of enjoyment increase. One reason is that when we are self-conscious, we tend to engage in evaluations of our performances. Because most of us have higher expectations for our own performances

than we are able to achieve, self-evaluation is likely to result in negative feedback, which is not enjoyable.

Perceived Control. Experiencing a sense of mastery or control over our environment is inherently enjoyable. Knowing that we can master a tough cross-country course; control the basketball when dribbling, passing, or shooting it; control our opponent in a wrestling match; or control our bodies in a difficult gymnastics skill adds to our sense of enjoyment of these activities.

At first glance, people who pursue **sensation-seeking activities** such as hang gliding, parachute jumping, ski jumping, and rock climbing, in which so many factors are uncontrollable, would seem to argue against this principle. Yet, strange as it might seem, a sense of control is one of the factors that draws people to such high-risk sports (McIntyre, 1992). In such activities enjoyment appears to stem not from the presence of threatening forces but from feelings of being able to control these forces through elaborate preparation and training and by painstaking adherence to safety procedures. After all, if we had complete control of our bodies and the surrounding environment, sports of all kinds would be pretty boring because we could always accomplish our goals. A degree of risk and uncertainty is fundamental to our enjoyment.

Each of us has within us certain temporary dispositions that affect our enjoyment of physical activity. Our enjoyment tends to increase when we feel competent in the activity, when we become absorbed or "lost" in the activity, and when we feel we have control over our bodies and the environment.

Attitudes That Affect Enjoyment of Physical Activity

Along with temporary dispositional factors, more stable and enduring attitudes also can affect our enjoyment of physical activity. Just as variability in individual preferences, tastes, and attitudes toward food, movies, clothes, friends, cars, and the like, vary widely, so do attitudes toward different activities. In the late 1960s Gerald Kenyon (1968) and his associates designed and field tested a scale for assessing attitudes toward physical activity. By surveying individuals' preferences for a wide range of activities—either as participants or observers—Kenyon was able to identify six categories of attitudes toward physical activity. Each of these represents a distinct preference for a particular form of physical activity based on "sources of satisfaction" that accrue to performers.

Physical Activity as a Social Experience. Some forms of physical activity, such as team sports or group exercises, are intrinsically social events. That is, they normally take place in active social environments and involve interacting with other people. Team sports are the most social of sport activities, as are team aerobics or exercises done in health clubs where others are present. Other forms of physical activity such as rock climbing, surfing, or long-distance running incorporate less social interaction, although even these activities may provide opportunities for social engagement before, during, and after participation. Social aspects of physical activities are consistently identified by participants as positive experiences (Neulinger & Raps, 1972), and youngsters engaged in youth sports (Wankel & Krissel, 1985) as well as elite ice skaters (Scanlan, Stein, & Ravizza, 1988) have indicated that developing friendships and experiencing social relationships are an important source of enjoyment. Thus, individuals who enjoy high levels of social interaction are more likely to seek out physical activities that maximize such experiences.

People who have a natural affinity for social experiences are likely to seek out physical activities that provide opportunities for social interaction.

Physical Activity for Health and Fitness. In his survey, Kenyon (1968) discovered that some people valued physical activity for the contribution it made to their health and fitness. Surely many people *do* possess this extrinsic orientation to exercise. "Feeling in shape"—knowing that you can meet any physical demand likely to be presented to you in the course of a day—can give you a sense of confidence and well-being that adds immensely to your quality of life. But, as we have seen, it also is the case that many people simply enjoy engaging in the activities that lead to the development of fitness. The unique sensations that accompany the physiological response to vigorous and sustained exercise cause many people to return again and again to the running trails and gymnasiums.

Some people are attracted to activities requiring a great deal of strength and endurance, possibly because of the health benefits such activities bring or because they enjoy pushing their bodies to the physiological limits.

Physical Activity as the Pursuit of Vertigo. Some people are attracted to a certain category of physical activity that presents an element of risk or thrill, usually through the medium of "speed, acceleration, sudden change of direction, or exposure to dangerous situations, with the participant usually remaining in control" (Kenyon, 1968, p. 100). The thrill that comes from disorientation of the body in such activities is called vertigo. Vertigo is pursued in sensation-seeking activities that reorient the body with respect to gravity, such as in amusement park rides, free-fall parachuting, bungee jumping, downhill skiing, ski jumping, or any other activity that creates a sense of danger, thrill, and intense excitement.

It is not known why some individuals seek out such activities while others, just as deliberately, steer clear of them. Petrie (1967) suggested that those who pursue vertigo may tend habitually to reduce perceptual input so that a specific event is experienced at a lower level of intensity than it would be by someone who habitually augments (exaggerates) perceptual input. It also may be that involvement in vertiginous activities represents an attempt to compensate for tedious experiences in the workplace (Martin & Berry, 1974), is a form of stimulus addiction (Ogilvie, 1973), or is the result of complex sociocultural factors (Donnelly, 1977). Whatever the cause, our interest in such activities, both as participants and spectators, clearly shows no indication of declining.

Physical Activity as an Aesthetic Experience. We normally associate aesthetic experiences in physical activities with dance, but sport—and to

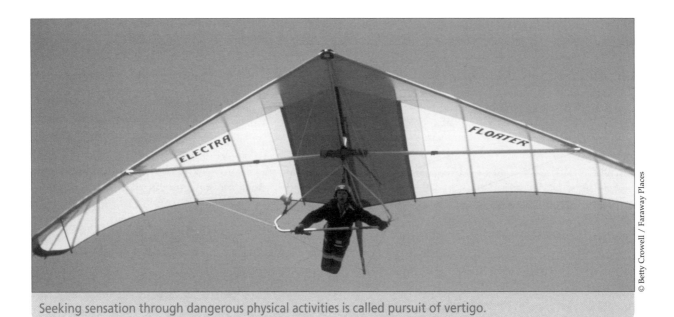

© Betty Crowell / Faraway Places

Seeking sensation through dangerous physical activities is called pursuit of vertigo.

a lesser extent, exercise—also is perceived by some individuals as providing certain artistic or aesthetic experiences, either to participants or spectators (Thomas, 1983).

This is especially the case in gymnastics, diving, ice skating, and other sports in which grace and beauty of movement are primary considerations in awarding scores to competitors. The aesthetic element is less apparent in sports in which the outcome is usually viewed as being more important than the manner in which the athlete moves (e.g., football, basketball, or baseball). Nevertheless, it is common to hear sport broadcasters refer to the well-choreographed football play or the dancelike characteristics of a basketball player leaping through the air, or even describe the movements of a tennis player as "art in motion."

Exercise seems less likely to be a source of this type of subjective experience, although dance aerobics clearly contains a strong aesthetic component. Outdoor activities such as hiking, mountain climbing, or kayaking bring participants in contact with the beauty of the natural environment, and this can add to the aesthetic experience of the activity. Women are more likely than men to engage in physical activities for the aesthetic experiences they provide, while men are more likely to value activities for their vertiginous, ascetic, and cathartic experiences (Smoll & Schutz, 1980; Zaichowsky, 1975).

People who find enjoyment in sensation-seeking activities also are attracted by the challenge of controlling the uncontrollable; people who find enjoyment in the aesthetic side of physical activity are likely to engage in gymnastics, diving, skating, and other movement forms that emphasize grace and beauty of motion.

Physical Activity as a Cathartic Experience. Catharsis refers to a purging or venting of pent-up hostilities and frustrations, either through attacking an enemy or some inanimate surrogate (object) in an aggressive fashion, or by watching an aggressive event. This concept has long been questioned by scientists (Berkowitz, 1969) and is no longer viewed as a credible hypothesis. It seems clear, for example, that watching aggressive sport contests is as likely to elevate feelings of aggression as it is to reduce them (Goldstein & Arms, 1971).

But physical activity can be viewed as cathartic in another way. As discussed in chapter 2, scientists have discovered that a vigorous bout of physical activity can lower anxiety (Morgan, 1982), thereby inducing a sense of relaxation and calm (but not necessarily reducing pent-up hostilities). Leisure theorists have long pointed to the value of leisure activities (including sports) in

Yoga: New Interest in an Old Cathartic Exercise

Once viewed as strictly for the far-out from la-la land, yoga has become a mainstream exercise. What many describe as a yoga revolution has been sweeping large cities such as New York and Los Angeles and is now fanning out into other parts of the country. Classes are attracting hundreds not only to yoga centers and community recreation facilities but also to fitness centers where yoga is becoming one of the most popular new offerings.

Yoga is an ancient exercise, some forms of which (such as Kundalini) involve little movement (some describe it as slow-motion calisthenics). Other forms such as Ashtanga yoga involve challenging physical actions as participants move quickly from one posture to the next. Obviously, it is not an exercise intended to improve cardiovascular functioning. Although yoga leads to remarkable gains in flexibility, usually the emphasis is on mind–body awareness. Through quiet, deliberate, slow movements; breath control; and meditation, participants experience a sense of calm and peacefulness that some call a spiritual form of fitness. As such, yoga may be the ultimate physical activity for those seeking a cathartic experience.

promoting feelings of rest and relaxation. Sports and exercise are novel activities that provide us with a change of pace. This change may, in itself, "recharge our batteries" by shifting our attention from problems and worries. Thus, the noon-time racquetball player may derive a sense of enjoyment, relaxation, and calm simply because his energies have been directed toward a new task and he has become absorbed in its features, not because "hostilities have been purged."

🔑 Participating in sports and exercise will not purge us of hostilities and aggression but may calm, relax, and refresh us.

Physical Activity as an Ascetic Experience. Physical fitness and training programs often require us to undergo pain, sacrifice, self-denial, and delayed gratification. These are sometimes referred to as **ascetic experiences**. Elite athletes are accustomed to ascetic experiences—torturous training regimens intended to improve their capacity for performance. Asceticism is also familiar to recreational athletes. Occasionally, you may see a runner, who by her attire and running style is obviously a novice, wheezing and groaning as she runs. Fitness clubs specialize in ascetic experiences; patrons with pained faces struggle to complete their exercise routines while a personal trainer shouts encouragement as they work through the pain.

You may be surprised to learn that not everybody interprets the ascetic experiences of breath-

lessness, fatigue, and muscle soreness as unpleasant. For example, in one study, 12- and 13-year-old soccer players told investigators that they enjoyed not only winning, learning new skills, and playing with teammates, but also "working hard" and "feeling tired after practice" (Shi & Ewing, 1993). In another study (Wankel, 1985), exercisers who did *not* drop out of the exercise program reported experiencing physical discomfort more frequently than those who *did* drop out. In this study, middle-aged men who reported experiencing fatigue as a result of vigorous exercise also reported *decreased* feelings of distress and *increased* feelings of psychological well-being as a result of the exercise. Thus, for some people, the discomfort of physical activity is attractive rather than repulsive.

So, it is important to distinguish between the raw sensations of physical exertion and participants' interpretations of those sensations. One system used to collect reports from individuals concerning their perceptions of the effort required to maintain a given level of exercise is the **Borg Scale** (see figure 4.4). Using this scale, exercisers are able to report orally the effort they feel in quantitative terms (called "ratings of perceived exertion" [RPE]) while they are exercising. Usually, as the intensity of the workload increases, so do oral reports of the perception of effort.

While you might be tempted to think that the higher the RPE the less the individual is enjoying the exercise, this isn't the case. Researchers have found that two individuals may rate a standard exercise bout as being "very hard," yet one

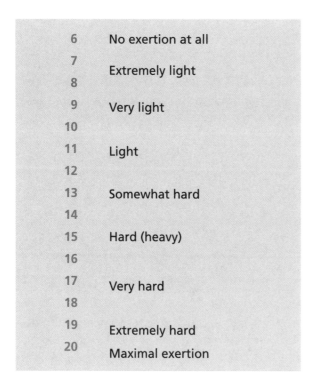

6	No exertion at all
7	Extremely light
8	
9	Very light
10	
11	Light
12	
13	Somewhat hard
14	
15	Hard (heavy)
16	
17	Very hard
18	
19	Extremely hard
20	Maximal exertion

Figure 4.4   The Borg Scale of Perceived Exertion (Borg, 1998).

Reprinted, by permission, from G. Borg, 1998, *Borg's perceived exertion and pain scales* (Champaign, IL: Human Kinetics), 31. Borg RPE scale © Gunnar Borg, 1970, 1985, 1994, 1998.

others they are unpleasant. Thus, how effortful an individual perceives a physical activity to be may not be as important in determining whether he or she continues to participate in the exercise program as how pleasant (or enjoyable) the individual finds the experience to be (Dishman, 1990).

Sometimes participating in exercise and sport can be painful and uncomfortable. These sensations are not always interpreted by participants in a negative light and, indeed, may be a source of attraction.

Factors Related to the Social Context

The third category of factors that can affect our enjoyment of physical activity concerns the nature of the social context in which the activity occurs. Have you ever competed in a very important sport contest with a large crowd looking on? How did that compare with your subjective experiences of playing the same sport on the playground or in intramurals? Do you feel differently when you work out in a fitness center with many onlookers than you do when you work out alone? Most people find these experiences profoundly different. It isn't that one is any "better" than the other; they are simply different.

may describe it as "a good feeling" and another may describe it as "a bad feeling." To some people the sensations of exercise, even those normally associated with discomfort, are pleasant while to

The Agony of the Long-Distance Swimmer

Several years ago Sally Friedman, a middle-aged artist from New York City, was training to swim the English Channel in the 58 °F waters of Schroon Lake, deep in the Adirondack Mountains of upstate New York. In talking about the agony of her training swims, she pointed to the curious way the ascetic experiences of those early-morning swims formed part of a subjective experience that became very important to her.

> While swimming usually brings out all that is graceful in me, that day I fought to free my arms from the water lest they be frozen in place. Each stroke shattered the brittle surface, every breath became a gasp. I just thought, "Okay, I'll make it to the next half hour and then I'll get out." But then the hot chocolate would fool me with the illusion of warmth and I'd think, "Okay, maybe I'll just go a little further. . . ." I would imagine that there are a fair number of people who wonder, "Why would any sane person put herself through such an ordeal?" There is a certain pleasure in thinking, "I have accomplished this. . . . I have done something beyond the realm of normal life, out of the ordinary, unexpected." It becomes a secret source of confidence, a private wellspring of originality.

Copyright © 1994 by the New York Times Co. Reprinted by permission.

What Are Your Attitudes Toward Physical Activity?

Rank the following experiences in terms of how well they define the primary reasons you like physical activity. A ranking of 1 indicates that the statement *best* describes your attraction to physical activity; a ranking of 6 indicates that the statement *least* describes your attraction to physical activity. After you have ranked each phrase, evaluate your top three rankings in relation to Kenyon's list of attitudes (see pages 133-135). Do your responses suggest that you value physical activity primarily as a social experience, for health and fitness, as a pursuit of vertigo, as an aesthetic experience, as a catharsis, or as an ascetic experience? Compare and discuss your responses with a classmate.

Ranking

1. I am attracted to the beauty of sport and exercise and/or to physical activity experiences that put me in touch with the beauty of the environment.   _____

2. I prefer activities that tax my body to the fullest, even though they often bring me pain.   _____

3. I like physical activities that disorient me, make me dizzy, and/or involve a certain degree of danger.   _____

4. I am most attracted to physical activities that promise to improve my health and fitness.   _____

5. The most important factor about exercise and sports is that they relax me and help me to relieve stress.   _____

6. I especially like physical activities that bring me in contact with other people, especially my friends.   _____

How participants feel when they are engaged in physical activity may depend as much or more on the social conditions surrounding the activity as on the activity itself. The presence of parents, friends, strangers; the "hype" that has preceded the contest; the feelings toward and your relationship with an opponent; and the way a particular game is interpreted to players by the media or coaches all can affect how the sport is experienced by the players. Running on a treadmill offers a different subjective experience than running through a park. Running when it is cold, dark, and raining offers a different subjective experience than running on a bright, warm summer day. Adding people to your exercise group changes the subjective experience of exercising just as adding competitors can change the social climate and the subjective experience of playing a game. Whether these changes add or subtract to your enjoyment depends on your individual preferences.

Another way the social context can affect our enjoyment is by affecting our sense of perceived freedom. As we mentioned in chapter 2, leisure theorists have long known that we enjoy activities more when we are free to choose them than when we feel obligated to do them. In fact, Bart Giamatti, former president of Yale University and, at the time of his death, the commissioner of Major League Baseball, described leisure activity as "... that form of non-work activity *felt to be chosen, not imposed*" [italics added] (1989, p. 22). This sense of freedom to participate is not simply a matter of being free from actual coercion; it is feeling free from any subtle coercive forces that instill a sense of obligation. Getting up early on Saturday morning to lift weights with a friend because she has been begging you for weeks robs you of your sense of freedom, and it can make for quite a different subjective experience than when you lift weights because you want to. Any social condition that creates within you a sense of obligation to engage in physical activity or to remain engaged in an activity can erode your enjoyment of it (although it doesn't have to).

🔑 Physical activities are never performed in a vacuum, and the social context that surrounds them can affect our sense of enjoyment. An example of this is when we feel forced to engage in an activity rather than when we freely choose to do it.

Spectatorship as a Subjective Experience

One of the most influential people in the development of modern physical education theory was Jesse Feiring Williams, a medical doctor-turned-professor who devoted his life to preparing generations of physical education teachers, coaches, and professors. Like many other scholars of his generation, Williams (1964) had a skeptical view of sport spectatorship because he believed it demanded only "simple sensory responses" and did not require "expressive, cooperative skill activity" that could be related to the purposes of education. The rise of spectatorship that worried Williams in 1927 has, as we saw in chapter 2, shown no sign of stalling as we discover more sports to watch and more ways to watch them. Good or bad, sports watching is a source of very vivid subjective experiences for wide segments of the human community. Because of its connection to the physical activity professions, it is important that we examine, if only briefly, the factors that affect our enjoyment of and attraction to sports watching.

Watching a sport contest on the local playground is unlikely to evoke the subjective experiences that are evoked in a sport spectacle, such as the Olympic Games, and neither may evoke the same subjective experiences that come from watching sports on television. Although we often watch our peers play sports in informal settings, sport spectacles attract most of our attention. Sport spectacles are staged competitions designed and promoted for audiences and intended to evoke an entire range of human emotions by virtue of their grandeur, scale, and drama. Unlike pickup games on the playground, they are entertainment first and foremost.

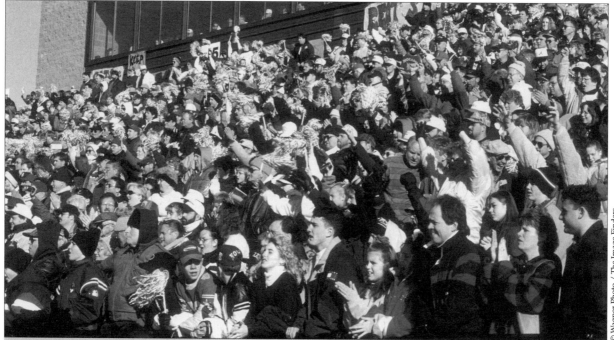

Sport spectacles are productions designed to attract viewers; contests often offer spectators a chance to participate in the spectacle.

© Wagner Photo / The Image Finders

Usually, we reserve the term *sport spectacle* for professional, collegiate, or international events that attract large numbers of spectators and supporting casts of cheerleaders, bands, majorettes, officials, and the media. In spectacles, both players and spectators play defined roles; the players take on various roles associated with the competition, and the spectators take on various roles as consumers, supporters, or detractors. Thus, when spectators cheer, boo, do the wave, or sing the alma mater, they are participating in a spectacle, of which the sport contest is only one aspect.

Ways of Watching Sports

We can engage in spectatorship in many different ways, ranging from aligning ourselves with a team's performance and suffering extreme disappointment when the team loses or jubilation when it wins, to the other extreme of watching in a completely disinterested fashion.

Vicarious Participation

Vicarious participation is a form of watching in which observers "participate" in the contest through the powers of imagination. If, while watching a sport event, you notice yourself tensing your muscles or adjusting your body position in accordance with an athlete's movements, it is probably because you are vicariously participating in the activity. Usually, vicarious participators are **fans** who identify with a particular player or team and have a vested interest in the contest's outcome. The word *fan* is rooted in *fanum*, the Greek word for temple, which underscores a metaphoric link between religious zeal and the enthusiasm fans often have for their favorite teams and players. When their team wins, it is as though they have won; when their team loses, they experience profound disappointment.

🗝 Vicarious participation in sport occurs when spectators imagine themselves performing the same activities as the athletes they are watching.

Disinterested Spectatorship

Sometimes we watch sport events without great emotional investment, a phenomenon known as **disinterested spectatorship**. We are likely to watch games in this manner when we care little about

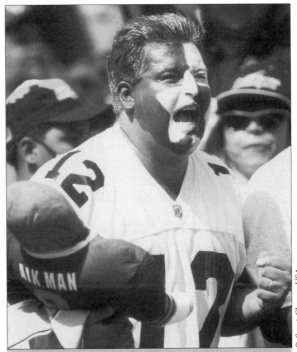

Sport fans often participate in sports vicariously through their favorite teams.

© SportsChrome USA

the outcome of the contest. Watching a contest between two teams with whom we are not familiar or watching a game that we have attended only because a friend invited us may result in disinterested spectatorship. Those who watch sports as part of their employment, such as reporters, referees, hot dog vendors, and sometimes coaches, often do so in a disinterested fashion.

Nevertheless, it would be a mistake to assume that disinterested spectators derive no pleasure from watching contests. For example, coaches who watch competitions between teams other than their own tend to observe athletes' performances in a detached, objective manner, yet may enjoy and admire the performances of those athletes. In these cases, spectators watch in much the same manner as audiences watch a symphony or a ballet: enjoyment comes not from the drama of competition but from watching the skillful actions of the performers.

Factors Affecting Enjoyment of Sports Watching

If someone were to ask you if you like to watch sports events, you might answer: sometimes yes, sometimes no. It depends on a number of different factors. Few people enjoy watching their favorite team being trounced, and fewer yet are likely to enjoy watching a game that they know very little about. Americans are unlikely to get excited about watching cricket or Australian rules football for the same reason that Australians and citizens of the United Kingdom are unlikely to enjoy American baseball. Our familiarity with sports and their importance in our culture often influences our attitudes toward them. Three factors play a major role in determining how much enjoyment we are likely to experience when watching a sports event: our knowledge of the game being played, our feelings toward the competing teams and players, and the extent to which the game entails a sense of drama, suspense, and uncertainty. Let's look a bit more closely at these factors.

Game Spectator Knowledge

Think about the sports you most like to watch. These are probably sports you know the most about. Knowledge about the game, what sport philosopher Scott Kretchmar (1994) calls "game spectator knowledge," often determines our enjoyment as spectators. Game spectator knowledge is knowing about the game, including players, strategies, and competitive tactics. Only by having a comprehensive knowledge of the activity can we fully appreciate the quality and significance of the athletes' performances. Such knowledge may come from reading about, watching, or playing an activity, although it is not necessary to have played a sport to enjoy watching it. An individual who knows little about the game of lacrosse may enjoy watching a game without knowing the game's history, strategies, rules, or personalities. But it is unlikely that this person's enjoyment of the game will be as robust as that of the lacrosse fan who understands precisely what the players and teams are trying to do at every turn of the game.

Spectators' Feelings Toward the Competing Teams and Players

Think of the last time you watched a contest in which one of your favorite teams was competing against an opponent that, for one reason or another, you had come to dislike. What turn of events added to your enjoyment of the experience? Probably, you enjoyed the experience more when good things happened to your favorite

team (they played well and scored points). Your enjoyment quotient probably also was elevated when bad things happened to the team you disliked (they played poorly, failed to score, or even suffered injuries). You probably experienced the highest level of enjoyment if your favorite team defeated the other team, and, conversely, you probably experienced the least enjoyment if your favorite team was defeated by the opposing team.

These connections between enjoyment and feelings about the competing teams are the focal point of the dispositional theory of enjoyment that has been the subject of considerable research (Zillman, Bryant, & Sapolsky, 1979) involving football, tennis, and basketball spectators. For example, researchers have discovered that failed plays of the disliked team were applauded almost as much as were successful plays of the favorite team. Comparing reports by those who watched the Minnesota Vikings defeat the St. Louis Cardinals in a professional football game, they found that those who both liked the Vikings and disliked the Cardinals reported maximal enjoyment, while those who both disliked the Vikings and liked the Cardinals reported maximal disappointment (Zillman & Cantor, 1976).

More recent research has shown that those who identify with a particular team are more likely to experience what researchers call the "bask in glory" feeling, expressing greater personal joy when their team wins than those who have identified with the team to a lesser degree (Madrigal, 1995). Enjoyment also tends to increase when spectators' favorite team defeats an opponent of high rather than low quality. In addition, fans tend to bask in glory and enjoy the game more when their team plays much better than they had originally expected it to (Madrigal, 1995).

Having a comprehensive knowledge of the players, rules, and competitive strategies adds to our enjoyment of watching sports, as do the feelings we harbor toward the participating teams.

Human Drama of Sports Competition

The sense of drama, suspense, and uncertainty that often accompany sport contests also enhance our enjoyment of them. Usually, this sense of drama requires that the competing teams be

Reflecting on Your Subjective Experiences as a Spectator

One way to examine your own experiences in watching sports is to interrupt your viewing of an event periodically to record your feelings at that moment. This is done easiest at home watching sports on television, but it also is possible to do in your seat at the stadium. Set a timer or wristwatch alarm for 10-minute intervals. Each time the alarm sounds, quickly jot down what you are feeling, why you think you are feeling as you are, and what is happening in the sport event that contributes to your feelings. You might also briefly note any effects you think the social environment (people you are watching the game with at home, or the stadium crowd) might have on your feelings.

After the contest is over, take time to review your notes and reflect on the total experience. How would you describe its emotional impact? What kind of knowledge, if any, did you gain from the experience? Would you describe the time you spent watching the event as "meaningful"? Have you gained insight into the effects sports watching has on you? How would you evaluate these effects—largely desirable or largely undesirable?

equally matched in talent and ability, although some of the best drama in sports occurs when the underdog overcomes great odds to defeat a heavily favored opponent. Games in which one team far outplays the other (such as in the typical Super Bowl game) tend to be less enjoyable, even when teams are evenly matched.

Enjoyment also is related to the extent to which the contest is perceived by spectators to involve human conflict. Research by Zillman and his associates (Zillman, Bryant, & Sapolsky, 1979) showed that when identical sport telecasts were viewed in the presence of broadcaster commentary that described the game as involving either bitter rivals who felt intense hatred for each other or friendly opponents, the former condition elevated spectators' enjoyment. Also, rough and aggressive play has also been found to increase spectator enjoyment, presumably because it demonstrates that players are sincere in their efforts to win.

In spite of the enormity of the sport spectator business, we know relatively little about the subjective effects of sports watching on the nation's collective psyche. Is watching sports a constructive use of our time? When the game is over, do we feel good about having watched it? Is it possible that it is a culturally hollow experience, little more than junk food for the human spirit? What conditions make sport spectating an ennobling

human experience? What conditions make it a debasing experience? These are important questions we need to ask and important topics for research by future kinesiologists.

Wrap-Up

Let's take stock of what we have learned about physical activity in this chapter. The theme of the chapter is that physical activity involves more than moving our bones and muscles or increasing the flow of blood through our circulatory systems. When we move our bodies, unique sensations arising from internal and external sources give rise to emotions, thoughts, and other inner states. These sensations, along with our interpretations of their meanings, constitute the subjective experience of physical activity. Subjective experiences of physical activity are important, not only because they play a significant role in determining our activity preferences, but also because, for many, they constitute the primary reason for engaging in physical activity in the first place. They also are keys to helping us learn about ourselves in physical activity environments.

The goal of most physical activity professionals is to help people develop an intrinsic orientation to sport and exercise, although in most cases participants' extrinsic orientation also plays a part. One way to think about an intrinsic orientation is as enjoyment. Anything that we value for its intrinsic qualities usually constitutes an enjoyable experience for us. Many factors can make sports and exercise more or less enjoyable, including those that lie within the structure of the activities themselves, those related to the dispositions and attitudes of the performers, and those associated with the social context in which physical activity is performed.

Finally, we examined briefly the subjective experiences associated with watching sports and saw that there are different ways of watching. Our subjective experience is affected by our knowledge of the game, our feelings about the competitors, and the drama of the competition, including its description by sport broadcasters. As yet, research concerning the benefit or harm of extensive sports watching has been limited. Be-

cause a significant part of our profession (sports management, athletic coaching, and administration) focuses on preparation of personnel for sports watching, we need to monitor carefully its long-term effects.

This brings to a conclusion our study of what it means to experience physical activity through performance and spectatorship. You are now ready to proceed with an in-depth study of the research knowledge about physical activity. As you become engrossed in the basic concepts of the scholarly subdisciplines of our field, do not forget that performing physical activity is an important source of knowledge. Both scholarly and experiential knowledge are essential for grounding you in the discipline of kinesiology and helping you to consider the different types of professions to which these knowledges can be applied.

Study Questions

1. Give an example of how an individual may *internalize* a daily run through the park.

2. List and describe three types of knowledge available to us from subjective experiences in physical activity.

3. What evidence exists to refute the notion that people don't like the sensations that accompany the hard physical effort required to exercise vigorously?

4. What types of physical activities might a person who values physical activity as an aesthetic experience engage in? A person who values physical activity as an ascetic experience? A social experience?

5. Differentiate between an ego and task orientation to sport participation. Which orientation is most likely to be associated with an intrinsic orientation to participation?

Scholarly Study of Physical Activity

In this section . . .

Although learning through physical activity experiences is an essential part of becoming a kinesiologist, the defining mark is mastery of a complex body of knowledge about physical activity. You may encounter many people who have been exposed to a wide variety of physical activity experiences and, through their exposure, have learned much about physical activity and themselves.

But it is unusual to encounter people who know about the theoretical aspects of physical activity, including its sociocultural, behavioral, and biophysical dimensions, beyond those who have successfully negotiated a formal course of study in kinesiology. Some people who haven't formally studied kinesiology may *think* they know much about physical activity (and some, of course, may), but often their knowledge is incomplete, out of date, or simply untrue. As a kinesiology major you, more than the typical person on the street, and more than your friends who might be studying biology, chemistry, history, or some other discipline, will be grounded in a solid knowledge base about physical activity.

In this section you will be introduced to philosophy, history, and sociology of sport; the neurophysiological bases of skilled movements; the interaction of psychological states and human performance; the conditions that promote the learning of skilled movement; the mechanics of movements; the physiological basis of exercise and its effects on the body; and the way movements develop and are affected by aging. Together, this knowledge and the thousands of concepts, theories, and principles embedded in it constitute the discipline of kinesiology.

You may already have recognized that the organization of the discipline of kinesiology mimics the typical organization of liberal studies. In fact, the three spheres of scholarly study of physical activity—the sociocultural sphere, the behavioral sphere, and the biophysical sphere—bear a general similarity to the way much of the general liberal education requirements are organized at most colleges and universities.

Each of the spheres in section 2 is broken down into smaller units called scholarly subdisciplines, and each chapter in this section is based on a separate subdiscipline. The eight subdisciplines are the way the leaders of the field have chosen to organize the scholarly study of physical activity. But you should remember that, in the final analysis, they are merely organizational frameworks intended to simplify the study of what is really a very complex phenomenon.

For the most part the subdisciplines within the sphere of scholarly study focus on knowledge *about* physical activity, such as its effects on the body, the physiological mechanisms that underlie it, how physical activity performance is increased, the social and psychological contexts in which physical activity takes place, and so forth. But it is also possible to engage in the scholarly study of professional practice, and this form of scholarly study is also an important part of kinesiology.

Scholarly study of professional practice focuses to some extent on knowledge accumulated through systematic research, although at this point in the development of the discipline, research in kinesiology has been directed much more at learning about physical activity than it has been directed toward learning how to use it. A growing body of scholarly knowledge is developing in sport management, athletic training, therapeutic exercise, and fitness management, but none is as developed as the rich body of scholarly knowledge concerning pedagogy of physical activity (teaching and instruction in physical activity). Most of this knowledge concerns the conditions that promote and hinder learning of physical activity in physical education classes and other instructional settings. Much of it is as relevant to fitness instructors or rehabilitation specialists as it is to teachers and coaches. Because it is vitally important to many who study kinesiology it is included here as one of the areas of scholarly study. No doubt in the years ahead, research concerning professional practice in sport management, athletic training, therapeutic exercise, fitness management, and other physical activity professions will have accumulated to the point where they too become part of the spheres of scholarly study in kinesiology.

Because each subdiscipline is to some extent an extension of another older discipline (e.g., psychology, sociology, biology, history), your past experiences with these disciplines will help you in understanding the theories and terminology used in the subdisciplines. As you embark on your study, you may wonder at times if what you are studying is really kinesiology or merely a collection of bits and pieces of theory from these older established parent disciplines.

This can be a troubling thought for those who prefer to think that kinesiology is an exclusive science that contains its own theories, concepts, and principles. The precise relationship between kinesiology and the parent disciplines and the precise way it should be organized are subjects of ongoing debate among kinesiologists. Viewed in its most optimistic light, kinesiology consists of unique knowledge about physical activity drawn from other disciplines, knowledge that had largely been ignored by those disciplines. If biologists, for example, had concentrated on studying and teaching about the effects of exercise, perhaps the subdiscipline of exercise physiology would not have evolved. If philosophers, historians, and sociologists had focused their energies on sport and exercise, the subdisciplines of philosophy of physical activity, history of physical activity, and sociology of physical activity may not have evolved. Because knowledge about physical activity was judged to be important, and because it was ignored by other disciplines, the 1960s witnessed the rise of the discipline of kinesiology. From its beginning it has consisted of knowledge about physical activity gleaned from all of the traditional disciplines, but combined and integrated into a coherent discipline in its own right—the discipline of kinesiology. In addition, of course, the discipline of kinesiology includes unique knowledge gained from experiencing physical activity (see section 1) and professional practice centered in physical activity (see section 3).

This section is intended to allow you to "get your feet wet" in the scholarly subdisciplines. When you finish reading and *studying* these chapters, you will not have mastered the subdisciplines. You will, however, have gotten a glimpse of what lies ahead of you in your program of studies, when you will have a chance to delve into each of these subdisciplines in greater depth.

PART I

SOCIOCULTURAL SPHERE

In this part . . .

5

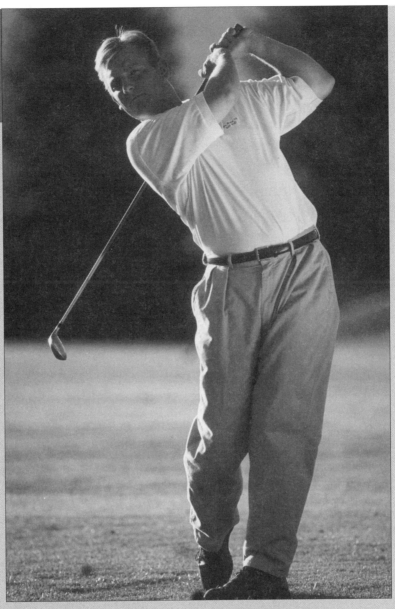

The Terry Wild Studio

Philosophy of Physical Activity

Janet C. Harris

In this chapter . . .

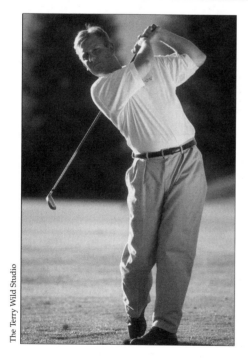

The Terry Wild Studio

You're competing in your city's annual golf tournament, which local players like you consider to be the most important golf event of the year. The champion is usually viewed as the best player in town and is given a lot of respect. Several times you have come close to winning the tournament, but someone has always managed to defeat you. All the top players have entered again this year, but you're confident because you've been playing well. You think this might be your year to go all the way. After playing very well the first two days, including a sudden-death victory in the second round, you lead your closest opponent by three strokes, and you're feeling good about your chances going into the final round. After the front nine, your opponent is playing exceptionally well and has cut your lead to one stroke. You too are playing well, near the top of your game, and you're enjoying the thrill of the competition. The two of you progress together through the back nine, matching birdies and pars on some very difficult holes. But then, on hole 16, your opponent becomes noticeably shaky and misses par for the first time all day. The 17th hole also goes poorly for your rival, and you start to wonder what happened. By the 18th hole, you've extended your lead to three strokes, and you make par to win the championship. Afterward, you learn that your opponent began to feel nauseous just before the 16th hole. Suddenly you feel let down. You've finally achieved a long-sought goal, but you don't feel the satisfaction you expected. Somehow, your victory is a bit tarnished. Why? What crucial aspect of sport was missing during the last three holes?

Why Philosophy of Physical Activity?

We humans depend heavily on ideas and thinking. We make sense of our world by using our highly developed brains to process much of the information we take in. For example, as youths most of us probably learned about sports through a variety of experiences: participation; interaction with parents, friends, coaches, and teachers; watching TV and playing video games; and reading newspapers and magazines. Maybe you watched *Monday Night Football* with your family, rode bikes after school with your friends, played on a high school varsity team, or collected and traded baseball cards. Your involvement in such activities probably led you to develop a general idea about what sport is. You most likely learned about other physical activities in much the same way.

Even though all of us spend a lot of time thinking, most of us probably haven't consciously considered concepts such as "sport" or "exercise," deliberately looking from different angles at the phenomena to which these words refer, in order to develop a more detailed understanding. Nor have we examined the complexities of the relationship between our minds and our bodies, a fascinating subject that philosophers have explored for over two thousand years. The mind–body relationship is an important aspect of philosophy of physical activity because our bodies are especially prominent when we move. Mental activity doesn't require visible bodily movement, but physical activities such as doing chin-ups or playing soccer require mental processes. Does this mean that your mind and body are separate? Does it mean that your mind is more important than your body? When we consider issues such as these, we are entering into the realm of philosophy of physical activity. Philosophical thinking requires that we sharpen our ability to think systematically and logically in order to develop coherent, general views of physical activity. It also requires us to be inquisitive about ongoing events around us that most people ordinarily take for granted. Philosophy of physical activity offers us new vantage points from which we can take a fresh look at activities such as sport, play, games, exercise, and dance, as well as the mind–body relationship.

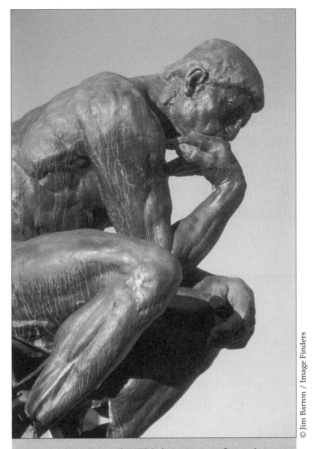

© Jim Barron / Image Finders

Auguste Rodin's *The Thinker*. How often do you pause for careful reflection?

Let's return to the scenario at the beginning of the chapter. Do you know why your golf victory was tarnished? Have you ever experienced a situation in which an opponent wasn't able to compete as well as usual, so you weren't tested by his or her full capabilities? A kinesiologist who has an understanding of philosophy of physical activity would point out that a good sport contest involves opponents who elicit the highest possible excellence from one another—they share a sense of distinction and thrive on competing at their outer limits (Delattre, 1975; Fraleigh, 1984, pp. 83–92; Osterhoudt, 1991, pp. 61–68, 118–120). When you don't have to play your best to win, victory is not worth as much. Although you'll probably be respected for the win anyway, especially after time passes and people forget the circumstances, you may always feel that the victory was not quite legitimate or complete. Situations similar to the one just described, but on a larger scale, occurred when the United States boycotted the Moscow Olympics in 1980, and then again when the Soviet Union boycotted the Los Angeles Olympics in 1984. Many athletes weren't able to test themselves against the full set of top international competitors.

 Philosophy of physical activity involves systematic, logical thinking that leads to coherent, general views of physical activity.

CHAPTER OBJECTIVES

In this chapter we will focus on these key topics:

▌ What background knowledge you already have about philosophy of physical activity

▌ What a philosopher of physical activity does

▌ The goals of philosophy of physical activity

▌ How philosophy of physical activity emerged and grew

▌ How research is conducted in philosophy of physical activity

▌ What research tells us about the nature of the human mind–body relationship, the nature of sport and its relationships to work and play, and ethical values and sport

What Background Knowledge Do I Already Have?

You've probably already walked down philosophical pathways without even knowing it! Recall that our knowledge of physical activity comes through three sources—experience, scholarly study, and professional practice. Through prior physical activity *experiences*, you may have tackled such issues as these: If you scored a run in softball but didn't touch second base, and the official didn't notice, was it okay to keep quiet about it? What about falsifying the address of a player you know at school so that she could be added to the roster of your neighborhood youth basketball

You can use insights from philosophy of physical activity in considering the following scenarios. Take a few moments to think about how you would address these. Share your answers with others in class.

• A high school football coach enjoys the hard work of getting ready for games and the excitement of competition. Football is a big deal at his school. At times, however, he thinks football is frivolous compared to things such as poverty, health care, and the availability of good jobs. How can football be both serious and frivolous?

• A school district is considering cutting back on physical education classes; the main argument is that physical activity isn't as central to education as academic subjects such as English or biology.

• A 17-year-old works out at a YMCA every day, and sometimes twice a day. She talks about a couple of her friends who developed serious elbow and foot injuries when they pushed themselves extra hard in workouts. She's not worried, however, because she's confident that physicians can do miraculous things to fix injured body parts.

• A fan is impressed with the sensuous grace and style of professional basketball players when they go up for a dunk—especially when he sees the slow-motion replays. He wonders whether the videos should be put on exhibit in an art museum.

• During practice rounds on the golf course, one of your friends sometimes moves her ball an inch or two so her shots will be easier. Her handicap is higher than yours, but it doesn't seem fair to compare your scores to hers since you prefer to play the ball from where it lands.

• An international cycling competitor knows that several of his opponents have been taking banned drugs in hopes of improving their performance. He hasn't been taking drugs, but he's competing with a brand new bike secretly engineered to be more efficient. He wonders whether drug-taking is any different from building a better machine as a means of improving performance.

team, thus giving your team the minimum number of players needed to join a local league? Situations such as these may have brought you face to face with moral dilemmas that are ripe for philosophical analysis. Even if you haven't had to do some soul-searching about a moral or ethical issue, occasionally you may have encountered a situation that made you stop and take notice. When this happened, you probably examined the issues more carefully and perhaps even discussed them with your friends, coaches, or parents. You were doing a bit of philosophy!

Were you ever fascinated by the grace and beauty of a long pass in American football, an aerobics routine at your local health club, or the drive of a golf pro on the PGA tour? You may have spent time thinking about what made these human actions seem beautiful. If so, you were standing on the brink of philosophical analysis!

You may have some background knowledge from related areas of *scholarly study*. Perhaps you have taken courses or participated in class discussions on ethics—a key area of philosophy of physical activity. Or perhaps you have studied the discipline of philosophy and will now see how what you learned relates to physical activity.

Even your observations of *professional practice* may have given you philosophical insights. Did you ever wonder why students with poor physical activity skills were sometimes given the same top grades in high school physical education classes that highly skilled students received? You may have just ignored this if it was a fairly regular occurrence, but if you at least raised the question in your mind, you took the first step toward doing a philosophical analysis.

Although there is much overlap among the subdisciplines, you can see from figure 5.1 that philosophy of physical activity is one of several subdisciplines in the sociocultural sphere of scholarly study. Along with history and sociology, philosophy of physical activity examines the social and cultural aspects of physical activity, whereas subdisciplines in other spheres focus on biophysical and behavioral aspects.

What Does a Philosopher of Physical Activity Do?

Philosophers who study physical activity usually hold a faculty position in a college or university.

They teach classes, do research, and engage in a variety of professionally oriented service activities. Their classes include general overviews of philosophy of physical activity, as well as more specialized offerings on topics such as ethics in sport; aesthetics of sport; values of physical activity; the mind–body relationship; and the nature of play, games, and sport. Their professional service might include organizing panel discussions in local high schools about ethics in sport; developing statements about the values of physical activity to help make sure that physical education is included in statewide curriculum guides; and appearing in a television special to discuss the aesthetic dimensions of the Olympic Games.

Scholars in this subdiscipline engage in research that involves asking philosophical questions about physical activity and then developing answers through careful, precise thinking. In many cases, they formulate questions by studying already-completed analyses, paying sharp attention to gaps or weaknesses that could be explored by further thinking. In addition, questions sometimes arise from life events such as those mentioned earlier in the chapter.

Because these investigators' thought processes are central to their research, philosophers of physical activity spend a lot of time doing their own analyses. They don't have laboratories where trained assistants carry out preplanned studies. They sometimes apply for small monetary grants to help them devote more of their time to their research. When writing a grant proposal, they must state clearly the main topic of the investigation, what makes it important, the process they plan to use to answer their main research questions, how much money they need, and what they will buy with it. They have to persuade those from whom they want money that their project is worthwhile and that they have the proper scholarly training to carry it out. In most cases, the end products of philosophical analyses are scholarly papers and books.

Philosophers of physical activity usually teach in colleges or universities, engage in professional service, and do philosophical research on various forms of physical activity and the human mind–body relationship.

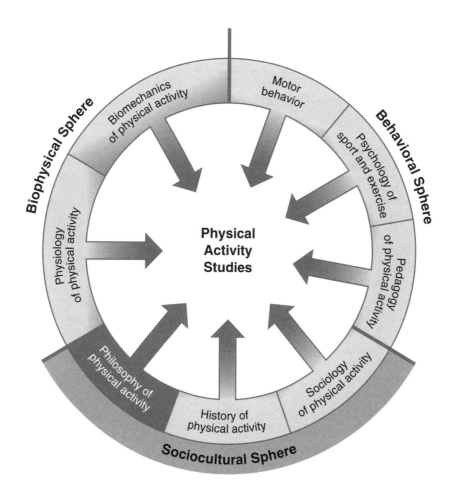

Figure 5.1   Philosophy of physical activity and the other scholarly subdisciplines.

Goals of Philosophy of Physical Activity

There are two major goals of philosophy of physical activity. The first is *to clarify thinking about forms of physical activity such as sport, play, games, exercise, and dance, as well as to clarify thinking about the mind–body relationship.* The aim here is to examine such phenomena for their broad, general features rather than to look at specific details. With respect to this goal, philosophers of physical activity have examined three main topics:

- *The relationship of physical activity to the human condition.* When you examine the nature of these physical activities, your primary focus is on the general human condition—the overall nature of each distinct form of physical activity, and the mind–body relationship—rather than on the details of daily life at your favorite tennis center, the bodybuilding gym in your neighborhood, or your campus fitness center. Your broader beliefs about being human may influence your conceptions of life at the tennis center or the gym, and you may use these specific slices of life as examples in philosophical investigations, but it is beliefs about the broader nature of things that philosophers seek to clarify.

- *Knowledge and physical activity.* In exploring the nature of knowledge of physical activity, philosophers include knowledge gained from all three sources: experience, study, and professional practice. So far, the focus has been mostly on knowledge people acquire through the first two: direct participation in physical activity (especially sport) and scholarly study of physical activity (in the various academic subdisciplines). You learned a bit about the former in chapters 3 and 4. Another way philosophers gain knowledge is by studying the nature of knowledge about physical activity produced by researchers in the other scholarly subdisciplines.

- *Values connected with physical activities and the mind–body relationship.* Values tell you about the significance or importance of things. For example, is it more desirable to win an Olympic gold medal, or to drop out of training early because you know your body will be permanently injured due to excessive overuse? Exploring a question such as this one involves studying values. Major topics in the study of values include ethics (the study of right and wrong actions), aesthetics (the study of beauty, taste, and art), and politics (the study of political and economic arrangements that best support the public interest by producing the most good for all). Philosophical studies of values are not concerned with how people *actually* live their lives, but rather with how they *should* live so that everyone can get the most out of life.

The second goal of philosophy of physical activity is *to encourage people to use their insights about physical activities and the mind–body relationship to make positive changes in people's lives* (Kretchmar, 1994, p. 177). Clarified thinking—the first goal—is likely to expand your understanding of your own physical activities as well as those of your family and friends. These broader insights may, in themselves, enhance your quality of life. They may also encourage you to change your behavior in ways that would make physical activity a more valuable experience for you as well as others. For example, you might decide to encourage adult recreational leagues to adopt policies making competition more playlike and less worklike. Some scholars believe that this enhances the quality of life for those who take part. Philosophical knowledge may also help practicing professionals argue persuasively for additional resources to expand physical activity programs, critique and change existing programs, and design new and better programs in the future. This is likely to improve the quality of life of the people they serve.

Goals of Philosophy of Physical Activity

1. To clarify thinking about forms of physical activity such as sport, play, games, exercise, and dance, as well as to clarify thinking about the mind–body relationship
2. To encourage people to use their insights about physical activities and the mind–body relationship to make positive changes in people's lives

History of Philosophy of Physical Activity

Occasional philosophical studies of physical activity were carried out in the United States as early as the late 19th century, but this research remained intermittent and isolated until the 1960s. Prominent philosopher George Santayana wrote "Philosophy on the Bleachers" in 1894, one of the earliest studies in North America. Well known for his thinking on aesthetics, he identified sport as a fundamental human expressive form (Osterhoudt, 1991). For Santayana, sport was almost the same as art—a dramatic physical performance brought alive by top athletes for the delight and enjoyment of spectators. Elite athletes, he thought, had playful freedom to create beautiful things for public display. The notion that sport and art are very similar is an extreme position. In later years many investigators softened their opinions, considering sport to be aesthetic (it is beautiful, harmonious, graceful) but not artistic (the primary goal of sport is not to create something beautiful).

At the turn of the century, Graves (1900) offered an early philosophical definition of the nature of sport. The following elements were crucial in his definition: amateurism, competition, well-matched opponents, and physical exercise. Graves considered sport to be primarily recreational and believed that commercialization and financial profit seriously tarnished it. Not all later scholars made use of this early work, but the characteristics of sport discussed by Graves appeared in many of their subsequent analyses.

Philosophical efforts to define sport continued throughout the 20th century.

During the first half of the 20th century, leading physical educators emphasized the importance of physical activity in education, and their ideas were very influential in shaping the field. Some of the most notable were Rosalind Cassidy, Clark Hetherington, Charles McCloy, Jay Bryan Nash, Jesse Feiring Williams, and Thomas Wood (Kretchmar, 1997).

The thinking of these early physical educators was situated in educational philosophies of the period emphasizing social growth, responsible citizenship in a democracy, human holism, a balanced life, and respect for individual differences. They argued that physical education classes focused on activities such as dance, play, games, and sport fostered the type of student learning that was congruent with the educational philosophies of the day. They thought, for example, that these activities could enhance students' social growth while at the same time honoring their individual differences. They were physical educators with an educational mission, and although they included a bit of philosophy in their work, they did not seek to develop a full-fledged philosophy of physical activity (Kretchmar, 1997).

Several well-known European scholars produced important studies in the middle decades of the 20th century that proved to be highly influential on Americans who later studied philosophy of physical activity. A number of prominent French philosophers explored the concept of the unity of mind and body. They opposed centuries of philosophical thought in which mind and body were considered to be separate, with the mind viewed as more influential on human functioning than the body. Examples include Gabriel Marcel's *Metaphysical Journal* (1927/1952), Jean-Paul Sartre's *Being and Nothingness* (1943/1956), and Maurice Merleau-Ponty's *Phenomenology of Perception* (1945/1962). Later in this chapter you'll learn that a society's views on the mind–body relationship have important implications for the field of physical activity.

Dutch historian Johan Huizinga's *Homo Ludens: A Study of the Play-Element in Culture* (1944/1950) was also highly influential on American philosophers of physical activity. His thought-provoking work was a major effort to define the nature of play, games, and sport. For Huizinga, play is a form of experience that is free, vacillates between frivolity and ecstasy, is separate from ordinary life, has no material gain, has its own time and space boundaries, and involves social interaction among people. In addition, play is also either a representation of something (e.g., exhibition, display) or a contest for something (but where no money or goods are at stake). He considered games and sport to be formalized aspects of play. When sport becomes commercialized, however, he believed that its playfulness gets corrupted.

Huizinga's research was an important point of departure for many scholars. For example, in France, Roger Caillois wrote *Man, Play, and Games* (1958/1961) in which he defined four types of activities: make-believe play; contests; games of chance; and disorienting, dizzying play and games. Both Huizinga and Caillois did extensive analyses of the relationships that play and games have with the larger cultures in which they are embedded. Many later philosophers of physical activity, however, were primarily interested in the general conceptualizations of play, games, and sport.

American investigations of philosophy of physical activity were sporadic before the 1960s. During this early period, leading physical educators examined the importance of physical education for furthering overall educational goals, and numerous European scholars produced important work on the mind–body relationship and on the nature of play, games, and sport.

Identifying the Subdiscipline

By the 1960s American physical educators studying philosophy of physical activity were pursuing new directions. Some were still interested in demonstrating that physical education can make important contributions to the broader mission of schooling in the United States, but they changed their focus. Influenced by newer works in philosophy of education, they systematically explored physical education from the standpoint of various traditional lines of philosophical thought (e.g., naturalism, idealism, realism, pragmatism, existentialism). Examples include Elwood Craig Davis's *The Philosophic Process in*

Historical Time Line

1894–1910	Beginnings of U.S. philosophical analyses of play, games, and sport.
1910–1950	Major U.S. physical educators emphasize the educational value of physical activity.
1920–1950	Prominent European philosophers examine unity of mind and body.
1940–1960	Prominent European scholars examine the nature of play, games, and sport.
1961–1964	U.S. physical educators explore physical education from various traditional philosophic standpoints.
1965–1969	Several U.S. physical educators shift away from philosophic studies of physical education to philosophic studies of sport and other forms of physical activity.
1970–present	The subdiscipline expands with philosophic analyses of a wide variety of topics concerning sport and other physical activities, play, games, and the mind–body relationship.
1972	Ellen Gerber edits *Sport and the Body: A Philosophical Symposium*, which became the standard undergraduate text in the subdiscipline.
1972	The Philosophic Society for the Study of Sport is established.
1974	The *Journal of the Philosophy of Sport* begins publication.
1994	Scott Kretchmar writes *Practical Philosophy of Sport*, a leading undergraduate text designed to engage students in "doing" philosophy.

Physical Education (1961) and *Philosophies Fashion Physical Education* (1963), and Earle Zeigler's *Philosophical Foundations for Physical, Health, and Recreation Education* (1964). The most common strategy of these early philosophers of physical activity was to compare prominent philosophers or philosophical schools of thought, and then point out the implications of using these ideas in shaping physical education curriculums. Readers were encouraged to think about their own views on physical education and decide which line of philosophical thought best matched their beliefs. Although these volumes were more philosophically oriented than earlier ones, they were still focused almost entirely on physical education as an educational enterprise (Kretchmar, 1997).

Other physical educators took a different tack, distancing themselves from educational philosophy and instead using philosophical techniques to produce new insights about physical activity itself—especially sport. This approach attracted a few scholars in other disciplines as well. The two most important physical educators in this vanguard were Eleanor Metheny (*Connotations of Movement in Sport and Dance*, 1965; *Movement and Meaning*, 1968) and Howard Slusher (*Man, Sport and Existence: A Critical Analysis*, 1967). Philosopher Paul Weiss's *Sport: A Philosophic Inquiry* (1969) was also at the forefront.

Metheny conceptualized movement as a source of insight and meaning for individuals. She focused on movement, especially in dance, as a way that a person can gain broad knowledge and understanding. Slusher used existential perspectives to examine ways that sport enhances our authenticity as human beings as well as our freedom and responsibility. Weiss was concerned with excellence in sport. Written before the upsurge in competitive sports for girls and women in the 1970s, he set his sights on men. He believed that men are so strongly attracted to sports because sports offer them the most promising route to excellence (Kretchmar, 1997).

Along with Howard Slusher, Metheny guided some of the first doctoral students in philosophy of physical activity at the University of Southern California. Altogether, she mentored 72 doctoral

In Profile

Eleanor Metheny

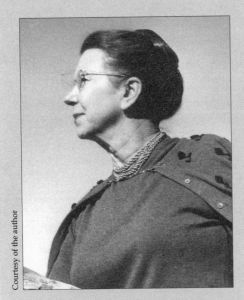

Courtesy of the author

A faculty member in the Department of Physical Education at the University of Southern California from 1942 through 1971, Eleanor Metheny contributed in important ways to philosophical research concerning the human body and physical activity. Portions of her works were translated into at least eight other languages. Three of her most prominent pieces are *Connotations of Movement in Sport and Dance* (1965), *Movement and Meaning* (1968), and *Moving and Knowing in Sport, Dance, Physical Education* (1975). Symbolic forms of movement fascinated Metheny. She frequently explored symbolism in the Olympic Games, as well as images of girls and women participating in sports.

Metheny earned an undergraduate degree in mathematics from the University of Chicago, and she also had a long-term interest in literature and poetry. In 1934 Metheny took a job as secretary and assistant to Professor Charles H. McCloy, a scientifically oriented physical educator at the State University of Iowa. McCloy later convinced her to enter graduate study, and she completed her doctoral degree in 1940 under his tutelage with a doctoral dissertation titled *Breathing Capacity and Grip Strength of Preschool Children.*

During World War II Metheny found time to ride in a cavalry unit in Griffith Park in Los Angeles that was established to defend and give aid in case of Japanese attack. Her frequent international travel included many trips to Greece to study the ancient Olympic Games. She became a travel consultant after her retirement from the University of Southern California in 1971, and she continued to travel and write until her death in 1982.

students, many of whom went on to become prominent college and university faculty members in the fields of history and philosophy of physical activity.

Halfway across the country, physical educator Earle Zeigler mentored another group at the University of Illinois. Weiss had other interests in philosophy and remained active in philosophy of sport for only a few years. Another important center of doctoral education developed at Ohio State University under the leadership of physical educator Seymour Kleinman. He focused on philosophic analyses of movement, dance, and the bodily dimensions of being human.

The Philosophic Society for the Study of Sport (now called the International Association for the Philosophy of Sport), a scholarly association to support the subdiscipline, was formed in 1972 following discussions among Paul Weiss, American physical educator Warren Fraleigh, and German philosopher Hans Lenk at the Olympic Scientific Congress in Munich, Germany. Fraleigh was the key organizer of the association, and he continued to be centrally involved as it developed. Weiss brought the new subdiscipline to the attention of philosophers, and over the years a number of excellent scholars from philosophy have pursued research in this area. Nevertheless, the roots of most investigators in the subdiscipline remain in kinesiology. The PSSS almost immediately set about developing a scholarly publication for the subdiscipline, and the first issue of the *Journal of the Philosophy of Sport* appeared in 1974.

The subdiscipline began to take shape when several scholars moved beyond educational philosophy to focus on philosophy of physical activity itself—especially sport—and soon a scholarly association and research journal were established

Expanding the Subdiscipline

Since the 1970s the subdiscipline has grown more organized and sophisticated. Researchers have conducted studies on a wide variety of topics, mostly focusing on sport or the mind–body relationship. In 1972 Ellen Gerber, who completed her doctorate under Eleanor Metheny, edited an important anthology of scholarly papers titled *Sport and the Body: A Philosophical Symposium*. It quickly became the standard text in the subdiscipline. Its section headings show which topics were most important at the time:

• The Nature of Sport • Sport and Metaphysical Speculations • The Body and Being • Sport as a Meaningful Experience • Sport and Value-Oriented Concerns • Sport and Aesthetics

By 1995 the major anthology was William Morgan and Klaus Meier's *Philosophic Inquiry in Sport*, then in its second edition. If you compare the section headings in this volume with the ones from 23 years earlier, you'll see that there was a broader range of topics in the later text:

• The Nature of Play, Sport, and Games • Embodiment and Sport • Play, Sport, and Metaphysics • Fair Play, Sportsmanship, and Cheating • Drugs and Sport • Gender Issues and Sport • The Morality of Hunting and Animal Liberation • Sport, Aesthetics, and Art

Scott Kretchmar published an undergraduate textbook in 1994, *Practical Philosophy of Sport*, that moved to new heights of engaging readers in "doing philosophy." His goal was to make philosophy of physical activity "come alive" and be useful in people's personal and professional lives. The book leads readers to apply central knowledge in the subdiscipline to (1) examine overall values that define "the good life," and the contributions that physical activity makes toward achieving this sort of life; and (2) examine ways that physical activity professionals can help us move toward "the good life."

Philosophy of physical activity is a small subdiscipline in comparison with others in kinesiology. With only a handful of scholars, it's difficult to identify specific trends in their research. As we just saw, however, there has been an overall expansion of the topics they study. Three book-length research monographs are illustrative of the high level of excellence achieved since the 1970s by top scholars in this area. Bernard Suits's *The Grasshopper: Games, Life and Utopia* (1978) is a delightful investigation into the nature of games. Suits takes his readers on a fascinating and enjoyable excursion into absurdity to demonstrate, and by this means define, the essential characteristics of games. His definition (referred to later in this chapter on page 170) is one of the most frequently cited by other scholars.

Warren Fraleigh's *Right Actions in Sport: Ethics for Contestants* (1984) presents carefully reasoned guidelines for morally right actions in athletic contests. He examines the nature of a good sport contest, lays out practical moral guides for enhancing the possibility of achieving a good sport contest, and offers pointers on how to use these guides most effectively.

William Morgan's *Leftist Theories of Sport: A Critique and Reconstruction* (1994) is an insightful and sophisticated critique of leftist scholarly thinking about commercialized sport, focusing on leftist concerns about the worklike qualities and social injustices of sport. He also suggests ways of moving beyond leftist reasoning toward the goal of making elite-level competition in sport more playlike.

Since the 1970s scholarship in the subdiscipline has grown more sophisticated, and it has also expanded to a wider variety of topics

Research Methods in Philosophy of Physical Activity

Now that you know about the goals of philosophy of physical activity and a bit of its history, let's look at how scholars produce knowledge in the subdiscipline. Systematic reflection about puzzling questions is the central feature. One expert says that philosophy "is done just by asking questions, arguing, trying out ideas and thinking of possible arguments against them, and wondering how our concepts really work" (Nagel, 1987, p. 4). You don't need to be able to do scientific experiments or mathematical proofs. You do need to be able to think carefully and precisely, and you can improve this skill with practice, just as you can improve writing skills or athletic skills by working on them. For some of us, reflection may be a new experience; in our fast-paced, rapidly changing world it's sometimes difficult to find time for contemplation. In chapter 4 we noted how reflection on our past experiences in physical activity can make these experiences more meaningful to our everyday lives. Philosophers may be considered the "reflective specialists."

Clear and systematic thinking—logic—is the major tool of philosophers. Logical thought is important, of course, in all scholarship, not just in philosophy. While logic is indispensable to the research of exercise physiologists, sport and exercise psychologists, sport historians, and scholars in all the other academic subdisciplines in kinesiology, it is the major research tool used by philosophers of physical activity. For this reason, they devote considerable attention to sharpening their logic skills, just as a novelist would hone writing skills, a biomechanist would hone laboratory skills, and a professional athlete would hone movement skills.

Four types of reasoning are central to philosophical research (see figure 5.2) (Kretchmar, 1994, 1996):

- Inductive
- Deductive
- Descriptive and speculative
- Critical and poetic

Inductive Reasoning

Inductive reasoning starts by comparing specific cases in order to develop broad, general principles. For example, how would you go about determining the general nature of exercise? The inductive route would involve looking at numerous physical activities (e.g., rhythmic aerobics classes, strength training to achieve better performance in football, weightlifting to develop muscles for a bodybuilding contest, mowing the lawn, walking to work because you don't own a car, taking a brisk walk at lunch each day to improve your health), deciding whether all of them really belong together in one category, and then identifying their common characteristics.

Deductive Reasoning

Deductive reasoning starts with a broad, general principle in order to examine specific facts that follow from it. A philosopher (or anyone, for that matter) might use deductive reasoning to determine whether a particular activity is a sport. If a necessary characteristic of sport involves using physical skills to achieve a goal, then we may deduce that a man who gets sick and designates a friend to take his place in a golf foursome doesn't engage in a sport even if he keeps in touch with the group by cell phone on every hole. Here's another example of deductive reasoning: If footraces require you to run on a particular course to a finish line, and if you get to the finish line of a particular race by driving there in a car without doing the required running, then we may deduce that you didn't take part in a footrace.

Descriptive and Speculative Reasoning

Descriptive and speculative reasoning involves looking at one example of an event and describing its essential qualities. For example, you might imagine slightly altered forms of basketball and then through a process of descriptive reasoning determine whether these are still the same game. What do you think: Would the following altered versions still be basketball? (1) changing the goal of the game to achieve a tied score at the end, rather than a higher score; (2) eliminating all restrictions on the means of scoring a basket, thus making it legal to use a ladder under the basket or stand on a teammate's shoulders; or (3) playing a computer version of the game to eliminate moving around on the court.

One important research technique in which descriptive reasoning is often used is phenomenology. The aim of phenomenology is to explore subjective experiences (Pearson, 1990). Peak mo-

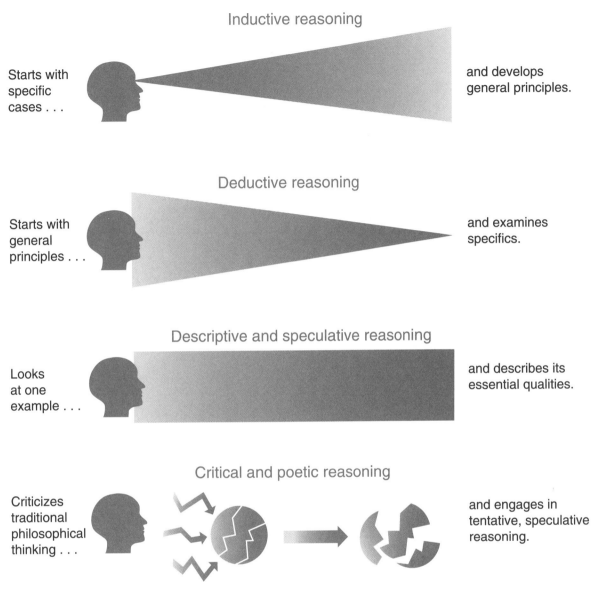

Inductive reasoning

Starts with specific cases . . .

and develops general principles.

Deductive reasoning

Starts with general principles . . .

and examines specifics.

Descriptive and speculative reasoning

Looks at one example . . .

and describes its essential qualities.

Critical and poetic reasoning

Criticizes traditional philosophical thinking . . .

and engages in tentative, speculative reasoning.

Figure 5.2 Four types of philosophical reasoning.

ments in competitive sport—the perfect soccer play, the ski race in which everything came together just right—have been studied quite often using phenomenological techniques. Sometimes researchers examine their own experiences, and at other times they seek to understand the experiences of others. To study others' experiences, they often conduct in-depth interviews, or ask people to write out their impressions. Even nonverbal renderings (e.g., body movements, art, music) of experiences sometimes constitute valuable data. Some investigators believe that descriptions of subjective experiences should not be analyzed further. In their opinion, more analyses only

serve to distance us from the experiences as they were lived. Others, however, do analyses that typically involve looking for common themes among the descriptions.

There are probably as many varieties of phenomenological research techniques as there are scholars using them. In general, however, phenomenological investigators take seriously people's subjective accounts of their experiences, and they consider these to be legitimate data. These scholars also make conscious efforts to be perceptually open to fine nuances in subjective experiences in order to capture as much of their richness and complexity as possible.

Think of an example illustrating your thinking about the nature of exercise using inductive reasoning, deductive reasoning, and descriptive reasoning. For example, you would be doing inductive reasoning if you examine several specific examples of exercise (e.g., jogging five miles per day, doing calisthenics with an exercise class, warming up to play tennis, stretching your hamstring muscles) and then use your detailed knowledge of these examples to make general statements about the nature of exercise.

Phenomenologists argue that scientists who shy away from examining subjective experiences are likely to end up with unnecessarily limited truths about human beings.

Critical and Poetic Reasoning

Critical and poetic reasoning involves skeptical criticism of traditional philosophical thinking. Scholars who take this approach believe that reality isn't as tidy and organized as most philosophical analyses make it out to be. They attempt to show that all philosophical arguments contain biases and reasoning errors, and therefore that traditional philosophical research is a futile activity. For example, some critics have highlighted gender, social class, and racial and ethnic biases in philosophical investigations of sport; they complain that traditional philosophers haven't taken social inequalities into account in their research (Kretchmar, 1996). As you may have guessed, it's hard to do this type of reasoning unless you have extensive knowledge about traditional philosophical research on physical activity. Those involved in critical reasoning often don't want to engage in traditional philosophical thinking themselves, choosing instead to produce more tentative, suggestive, and speculative—perhaps poetic—investigations of things.

Inductive reasoning begins with comparisons among specific cases in order to develop broad, general principles; deductive reasoning begins with a general principle and examines specifics that follow from it; descrip-

tive reasoning begins with one example of an event and examines its essential qualities; and critical and poetic reasoning couples skeptical criticism with nontraditional philosophical reasoning.

Overview of Knowledge in Philosophy of Physical Activity

Now let's take a brief look at several important topics in philosophy of physical activity. While scholars have produced a complex, detailed body of knowledge, we'll only be able to explore a few examples of the fascinating information that makes up this subdiscipline. Specifically, we'll examine

- the nature of the human mind–body relationship,
- the nature of sport and its relationships to work and play,
- values promoted by physical activity, and
- ethical values and sport.

The Nature of the Human Mind–Body Relationship

Have you ever thought about the situations that make you most aware of your body? If you get injured or sick, your pain may call attention to it. If you cut your finger while slicing an apple, for example, the pain during recovery would probably remind you of how central your fingers are in your day-to-day functioning. We are also more aware of our bodies when we move. In most academic tasks such as studying for a chemistry test or reading a novel, we have only a dim awareness of our own bodies and those of others. Playing golf, lifting weights, running marathons, and playing soccer bring them to the foreground. Our bodies play a more prominent role in such activities, and we are therefore more likely to notice them. Most people are aware that thinking is important in human functioning. When they become more aware of the importance of bodies as well, it leads to questions about the re-

Your View of the Mind–Body Relationship

For each item below, mark an × on the continuum in the place that best reflects your opinion.

Physical education classes are more important than academic classes in school.	All classes are equally important.	Academic classes are more important than physical education classes in school.

I can move my body, therefore I know I exist.	I am alive, therefore I know I exist.	I think, therefore I am.

A body is a terrible thing to waste.	A human being is a terrible thing to waste.	A mind is a terrible thing to waste.

Bodybuilding contests are more important than research studies about bodybuilding contests.	My human capabilities make it possible for me to engage in bodybuilding as well as to do research about bodybuilding; both involve my whole being, and both are equally important.	Research studies about bodybuilding contests are more important than bodybuilding contests.

- If your ×s land mostly on the right side, you have a dualistic view and see the mind as superior to the body.
- If your ×s are mostly on the left side, you have a dualistic view and see the body as superior to the mind.
- If your ×s are mostly in the center, you consider mind and body to be fused together in a unified whole, and you see all parts of this lived body as equally important.

lationship between mind and body. Learning about the nature of the mind–body relationship is important for people in all areas of the field of physical activity.

The relationship between mind and body has been a controversial subject in Western thought, dating back at least as far as ancient Greece. Some people consider the mind and body to be separate, while others view them as a fused unity. These two conceptions usually lead to different views about the importance of physical activity. They influence such matters as the status or value of physical activity occupations, the level of budgetary support for physical activity programs, and the importance of research on physical activity. Before we describe the two positions in more detail, complete the questionnaire on your view of the mind–body relationship.

Mind and Body as Separate

The ancient Greek philosopher Plato (427–347 B.C.E.) had a great influence on later thinking about the mind–body relationship. He considered mind and body to be separate from one another and emphasized that the mind is superior to the body. He believed that the body should be kept healthy so that intellectual pursuits can be carried out. In Plato's view, soldiers should have fit bodies to provide adequate protection of the citizenry. But overemphasizing bodily training, such as practicing and getting in shape for sports, lowered a person's status because it would prevent athletes from pursuing more important intellectual matters.

Plato's attitudes became the cornerstone of a philosophical position termed idealism, which holds that reality is centered in consciousness or reason (Thomas, 1983, pp. 25–26). Since idealists believe that the essential, core nature of reality is reason or thought, it is not surprising to find that they consider the mind more important than the body. This belief in the separateness of mind and body, termed **dualism**, continued to be influential for many centuries, first in Europe and eventually in North America. It is still a strong current in American culture today (Kretchmar, 1994, pp. 31–65).

Many centuries after Plato, French philosopher and mathematician René Descartes (1596–1650) took an even more extreme dualistic position on the mind–body relationship. His famous statement "I think, therefore I am" underscores the importance he placed on the mind. Descartes saw the body as an unthinking, material, visible sub-

stance. He believed that the mind—though invisible and immaterial—is the source of our humanity because it is capable of thinking. Since our humanness is rooted in our mind, the mind is more important than the body (Osterhoudt, 1991, pp. 237–238). Although Descartes saw the mind and body as separate, he did acknowledge their interaction.

The dualistic position emphasizing the separateness of mind and body, and usually also the superiority of the mind over the body, has been very influential on attitudes toward physical activity in American society (see figure 5.3). On the positive side, it has encouraged keeping the body healthy and physically fit in order that the mind may go about its intellectual activities as effectively as possible. Those with Christian religious orientations often add that the body should be

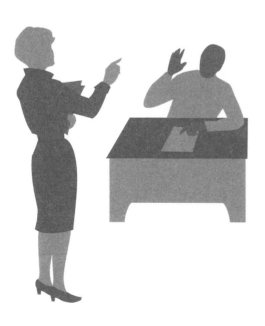

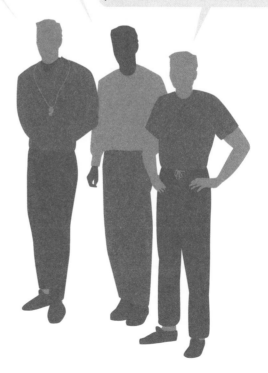

Figure 5.3   Dualistic "mind over body" thinking.

kept fit as a matter of spiritual obligation. An important justification for physical education classes in American schools has been, and continues to be, the improvement of bodily fitness so that students will be able to get the most out of their other courses. More negatively, however, assumptions about the inferiority of the body contribute to cutbacks in physical education courses when school budgets are limited.

Although interscholastic and intercollegiate athletics are considered important, educational administrators often expect these sport programs to be partially or wholly paid for by money from sources other than regular educational budgets. This stems from the fact that varsity sports—along with various campus clubs and other student activities—are not considered to be part of the formal educational curriculum. This is sometimes based on the belief that such programs are less educationally valuable than academic courses. In the case of athletics, this belief is partially supported by assumptions about the inferiority of the body in relation to the mind.

The dualistic view of the mind–body relationship emphasizes the separateness of mind and body, and usually also the superiority of the mind over the body.

Mind–body dualism contributes to the notion that the body is a machine-like object or "thing." Such thinking contributes to scientists' views that physical activity can best be understood by carrying out objective analyses of human bodies engaged in movement, and leaving out the subjective experiences we talked about in chapter 4. With this mind-set, specialists in biomechanics, exercise physiology, exercise and sport psychology, and motor behavior often design research intended to improve motor performance—for example, in elite sport, in physical education classes, and in rehabilitative exercise. While this is, of course, an important goal, it negates the importance of the mind–body relationship. As Meier (1979) states, "The body perceived totally as an object is . . . drained of its humanity; it is a dead body devoid of its vivifying, expressive and intentional abilities and qualities" (p. 197).

A technological, mechanistic view of the human body can pose risks to the health and welfare of athletes in situations in which winning is of utmost importance (Hoberman, 1992; Sage, 1998, p. 149). If an athlete's body or body parts are considered to be merely things, then trainers, sport scientists, coaches, and athletes themselves are free to adjust them (much like a carburetor on a car) to get the best performance possible. Little thought needs to be given to the dangers posed for the people whose bodies undergo such adjustments. The use of medications that eliminate pain so that players can compete while injured and the use of performance-enhancing drugs with serious side effects are examples of two practices that have dangerous implications for athletes' well-being.

There are numerous arguments against the concepts of mind–body dualism and the mind's superiority to the body (Kretchmar, 1994, pp. 31–65)—so many, in fact, that it's amazing that this concept is still prominent and influential in our society! Consider the fact that thinking never takes place independent of a body. Descriptions of bodies as machines, and minds as logic systems, do not produce accurate, full renderings of human beings. Motor performance is often better when we can stop thinking consciously about what we're doing. Thoughts aren't usually necessary to direct skilled performance—instead, they actually seem to get in the way. Gestures (for example, the thumbs-up signal meaning "okay") can often be used in place of verbal language. Also, body movements often express feelings and meanings for which we don't have appropriate words. Thinking (mind) is not necessarily more accurate or truthful than sensing (body); in fact, thoughts are sometimes based on faulty assumptions or faulty logic, and sensations often give us immediate, clear knowledge. For example, if you conclude (think) that a stove burner is hot because it is the right time of day for the stove to be used, you may be wrong because of inaccuracies in your assumption about regular use at a particular time. On the other hand, if you see (sense) a bright-orange stove burner, you immediately know it's hot.

Human Beings as Embodied, Whole People

In modern times, philosophers with holistic conceptions of the mind–body relationship have been influential in Europe and North America. Their viewpoints are referred to as existentialism and phenomenology. A few of the important philosophers who contributed to developing these ideas are Maurice Merleau-Ponty (1908–1961), Gabriel Marcel (1889–1973), and Jean-Paul Sartre (1905–1980). Existentialism and phenomenology are closely intertwined, and there are many variations. Both are oriented toward broadening understanding of subjective human experience, self-awareness, and consciousness. Congruent with this, as you already know, phenomenological research methods are designed to study subjective experience.

Existentialists and phenomenologists shun the idea of the separation of mind and body. Instead, they hold that human consciousness is embodied—body and mind are fused into a unity (Kretchmar, 1994; Meier, 1979). The fusion of the two is referred to as *embodiment*, and the term lived body refers to the dynamic, ongoing life of this unity. Existentialists and phenomenologists believe that by becoming more sensitive to the subjective experiences of our own lived bodies, we can learn much about the nature of human beings in general.

The lived body is somewhat beyond the reach of scientists. To examine it we have to tap our own private, individualistic, subjective experiences, which are not available in their original form to anyone else. We can tell others about them, but no one else can access them in their initial, immediate fullness.

The holistic view of the mind–body relationship emphasizes embodiment—the fused unity of mind and body, and the lived body—the dynamic, ongoing life of unified, whole people.

This way of thinking clashes with traditional scientific ways of seeking knowledge. Scientists favor the use of impartial, objective assessment techniques; they consider subjective experiences of the lived body to be beyond the limits of acceptable knowledge. On the other hand, existentialists and phenomenologists argue that objective, scientific studies have limited potential to give us insight into the full range of lived body experiences that constitute human existence.

When the mind and body are considered a single unity, it is difficult to treat the human body as a machine that can be tuned for maximal performance with little regard for the rest of the person. Those who believe in the importance of embodiment and lived body experiences view athletes as whole human beings; they are more likely to attend to athletes' overall health and welfare than to focus only on improving their sport performance.

From this standpoint of the unified lived body, the mind is not the master of the body. Since body and mind are a blended unity, one cannot be subservient to the other. Physical activity, therefore, is not different from, or inferior to, intellectual activity (see figure 5.4). Both are equally important for learning about ourselves and the world around us, and for expressing ourselves. In short, physical activity involves the dynamic interweaving of cognitions, emotions, nerves, muscles, bones, blood, and all the rest that comprises the lived body. Exercise, sport, dance, and other forms of movement are valued equally with all other sorts of human experience. Physical activity courses are considered as educationally important as the rest of the courses in the curriculum. Extracurricular activities, including competitive sports, are valued because they provide a rich variety of lived body experiences.

The Nature of Sport and Its Relationships to Work and Play

Sport has been conceptualized as serious work, as ecstatically frivolous play, and as a combination of the two (Osterhoudt, 1991, pp. 33–61). Here we will look at its worklike and playlike qualities. Since there is evidence that both qualities exist, it seems reasonable to conclude that sport is indeed a combination of work and play, and that it varies from being more worklike in some cases to being more playlike in others.

Work Elements in Sport

Elite sporting events such as Major League Baseball games, top-level college basketball games, and the Olympic Games are important entertainment commodities—the games are economically valuable. Spectators spend a lot of money to watch them, television companies pay huge sums to broadcast them, star professional athletes are paid millions to play, and professional team owners make untold sums in profits. Labor negotiations between players and team owners are intense and sophisticated, and owners frequently haggle with city leaders over the level of fund-

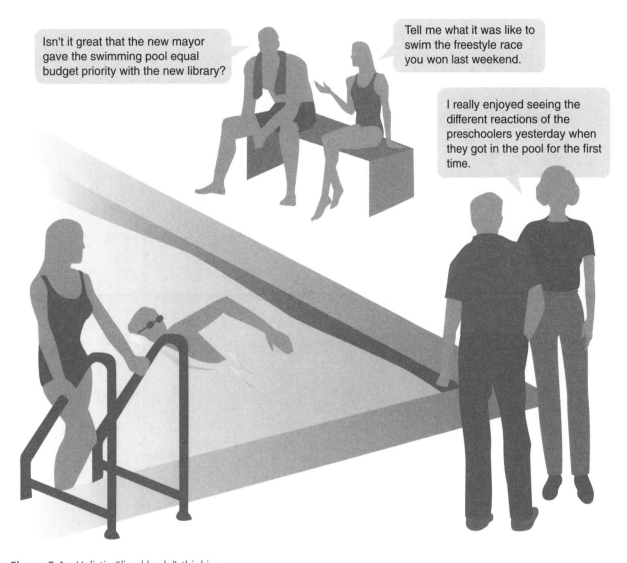

Figure 5.4 Holistic "lived body" thinking.

ing a city will earmark for building new stadiums and arenas.

These examples illustrate work elements in sport (see figure 5.5). **Work** involves purposeful, utilitarian activity to make or do something. It often culminates in products that are sold for profit. In sport, the products are the games themselves. The central goals of worklike sport are extrinsic rewards—most notably status and money (Osterhoudt, 1991). They are extrinsic (external); they come from the outside—primarily from spectators, the mass media, and corporate sponsors. Status is conferred on athletes and coaches by television broadcasters, newspaper reporters, radio commentators, and the general public. Money comes from television and radio

companies, spectators who attend games, and corporations that pay to be associated with popular athletes and teams. Knowledgeable coaching, sophisticated equipment, and high-tech training are necessary to field teams that are entertaining and interesting for spectators.

Work elements in sport are geared toward producing something for consumers to buy—entertaining sports events; the focus is on external rewards, primarily money and status.

Work elements are prominent in professional sports, but you can find them in amateur sports as well. Organized youth sports illustrate an

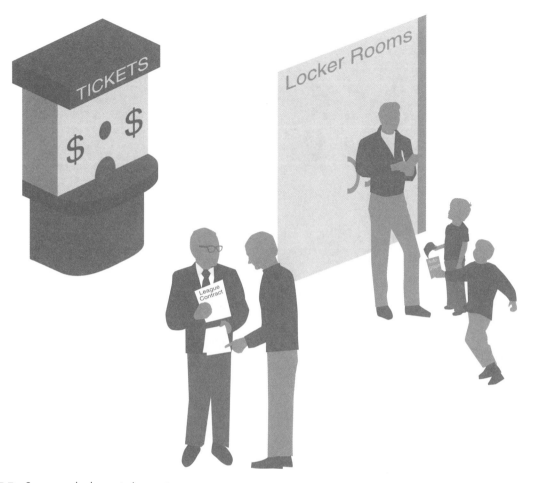

Figure 5.5 Some work elements in sport.

amateur activity in which high priority is sometimes placed on status and other external rewards. Events such as all-star games, radio broadcasts of games, and newspaper coverage encourage an external focus. High school varsity athletes also sometimes get swept up by the notoriety they receive from the mass media in their local cities or towns. Some have their sights set on getting an athletic scholarship to play for an elite college team. Top-level college programs where fame and money are emphasized are other examples of amateur sports in which work elements are prominent.

Play Elements in Sport

In spite of the seriousness of worklike sport, it is often viewed as trivial, absurd, and inconsequential in relation to the larger scheme of things, even though it is utterly absorbing for the athletes (Osterhoudt, 1991). If you asked your friends to compare the importance of sport to education,

religion, family, business, or government, most would probably rank sport close to the bottom. Dualistic thinking about the mind–body relationship is probably partially responsible for swaying them toward this view. As you have just learned, "body activities" are still thought by many to be less important than "mind activities," and the body is prominent in sport. In addition, however, sport's playfulness should probably receive part of the blame.

In play you have more freedom than in ordinary life (including work) to behave as you wish, to begin and end activities when you want, to change goals in midstream, to change your level of commitment to goals, and to fantasize and act out your fantasies (Caillois, 1958/1961; Huizinga, 1944/1950; Osterhoudt, 1991; Thomas, 1983). You don't have to produce anything in particular when you play. Intrinsic (internal) rewards are central; the freedom you have to alter what you do in play is usually experienced as pleasurable.

Although extrinsic goals and rewards are sometimes important in play, they often recede into the background. Instead, players get primary rewards from "just playing"; the process is what counts.

🔑 Play elements in sport frame the activity as different from ordinary life, and as trivial; this gives people more freedom to behave as they wish. The focus is on intrinsic rewards—the pleasures of doing the activity.

Playlike elements are probably more common in pickup games and lower levels of formally organized amateur sports (e.g., NCAA Division III intercollegiate athletics, city recreational leagues, youth sports), but you can also find them in elite professional sports. For example, professional athletes often report that the sheer joy of competition—the "high" they get from a good performance along with the close camaraderie

they develop with teammates—is so satisfying that they continue to compete long after they have achieved fame and financial security, and even while coping with severe chronic injuries such as knee and back problems. These pros are clearly drawn to the process of *doing* the activity, an internal focus. Because most societies place a high value on utilitarian outcomes, however, "just playing" is often regarded as inconsequential.

Laughing, smiling, and subtle body movements tell people "play is going on here." In play, ordinary events often take on different meanings, and they can also be changed in ways that would be inappropriate outside of play (Bateson, 1955). For example, when you play with a dog by getting it to tug on an old sock, the dog often gets so caught up in the activity that it starts to growl. Ordinarily, a growling dog would be something to avoid because you know that growling usually accompanies attacks. In the context of play, however, you are usually not afraid because the dog often has its front legs on the ground with its hind end raised, and its tail is wagging. Growling in play does not mean the same thing as it does in ordinary life. Your fears may mount if you suspect that play has ended, of course, because then the dog's growls mean something much more threatening.

Another example is children's pretend or fantasy play. Here youngsters often alter various events they routinely experience in ordinary life. When they "play house," they may introduce modifications in regular family life, such as babies who die and then come back to life, or a father whose main characteristics are exaggerations of certain qualities of the father of one of the players.

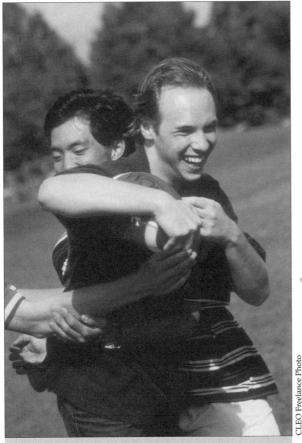

Some play elements in sport.

CLEO Freelance Photo

What are some examples of the sorts of things you might do if you were to engage in play while taking part in sport? What makes these things play? Can you play in ways that would not be disruptive to the sport you are doing? If yes, think of some examples. If no, why not?

While most play theorists emphasize its positive, liberating aspects, play sometimes includes mean-spirited or intimidating actions. Instances of children's cruel and coercive actions toward one another on the playground are evidence that not all play is fun for everyone (Fine, 1988; Schechner, 1988; Sutton-Smith, 1983; Sutton-Smith & Kelly-Byrne, 1984).

Because it has definite rules that are supposed to be followed, sport is clearly not as free as play. If sport were entirely play, participants would be free to change the rules, disregard the rules, or move on to a completely different activity in the middle of a contest. Can you imagine a college basketball game being interrupted by a player who wanted to change the rules so he could take five steps without dribbling? In order to understand why this doesn't happen, we need to look briefly at the nature of games.

Games are activities in which rules specify a goal to be achieved and also limit the means that can be used to reach the goal. These rules exist for the sole purpose of creating the game; they would be absurd in ordinary life (Suits, 1978). Let's consider sport in light of this definition.

A **sport** is a game or contest in which motor skills are necessary. In American football, for example, the goal is to get the ball over the end line enough times to score more points than the other team. This requires a variety of skills including passing, running, kicking, blocking, and tackling. Furthermore, there are certain prohibited actions that might otherwise increase a team's ability to accomplish the goal. To illustrate, offensive linemen are limited in the ways they can block opponents; only certain players are eligible to receive forward passes; clipping is prohibited because it is a frequent source of injury; a player who is advancing the ball must stay within the boundaries of the field; each team may have only 11 players on the field at one time; teams may not use mounted horsemen to outrun their opponents; and players may not use brass knuckles or clubs to beat their opponents into submission.

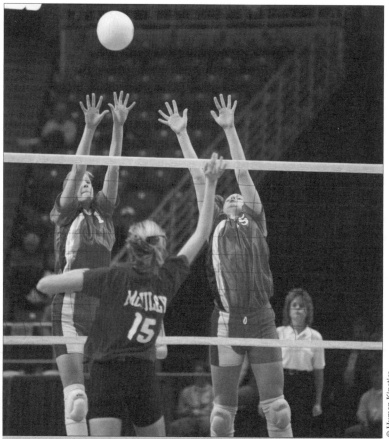

© Human Kinetics

What limitations do the rules require for getting the ball over the net? What is the role of these limitations?

The built-in inefficiencies structured by the rules of games are different from many other realms of life—for example, education, politics, and business—where limits on efficiency come mainly from ethical constraints. For example, we are not permitted to copy someone else's writing and call it our own—this is plagiarism, and it is such a strong breach of ethics that it is illegal. Game rules, however, handicap us in absurd ways that have nothing to do with ethics. Think about the ordinary activity of reading a book. This could be turned into a game if several people agreed to read only every other page with the goal of learning as much as possible about the content. The winner would be declared by scores on a test immediately following the reading. This is not the most efficient way to learn the book's content, but it does turn book-reading into a game.

Rules can be thought of as formal types of play cues. They tell us to give different meanings to the events in a game than we would give these events in ordinary life. For example, in ordinary life it is not particularly important whether we can get a basketball through a hoop consistently while imposing handicaps such as not using a ladder, or whether we can pitch a baseball over home plate consistently while imposing handicaps such as standing a certain distance away. It is only within the rules of the game of basketball or baseball that these activities make sense and take on value. Because of this, when viewed from the perspective of ordinary life, sport has a frivolous quality, and this gives it an element of freedom. Engaging in acts that would be inconsequential in ordinary life liberates us a bit, making it possible to explore and change things more easily. For example, we might make temporary rule changes in an effort to equalize teams with unequal numbers of players, or perhaps just for the fun of experimenting with playing the game using somewhat different rules.

Sport is a game that depends on physical skills; it has rules that specify a goal and limit the means that can be used to reach the goal. These rules exist solely for the purpose of creating the game and give sport a built-in inconsequentiality, contributing to its playfulness.

Values Connected With Physical Activity

Did you ever wonder whether you should notify an official when you violate a rule while competing in a sport; is it okay just to keep quiet about it? What do you think about the merits of focusing more on the aesthetic qualities of team sports such as soccer or American football by giving extra points for the artistic merit of a team's offensive plays (similar to the way figure skating, gymnastics, and ski jumping are judged)? Should cities stop building publicly funded gyms and outdoor fields for sports in wealthy areas where there are lots of private recreational facilities such as country clubs and fancy health clubs, and concentrate instead on low-income neighborhoods? In order to answer these questions, you have to examine your values (see figure 5.6).

All of us use values—our conceptions about the importance of things—to make decisions. In this section we will look at several central values that are promoted by the field of physical activity. Then we'll examine ethical values and sport—a fascinating topic that has attracted a considerable amount of philosophical study. Two other sorts of values have been studied by philosophers of physical activity, and although there isn't space to discuss them here, you may want to look up additional information about them on your own:

- Aesthetic values and sport—an examination of beauty, grace, sensuality, balance, harmony, and expressiveness
- Political values and sport—an examination of the extent to which, and ways in which, sport contributes to the common good of all people

Values Promoted by the Field of Physical Activity

You already know that values are things people consider to be desirable. Your values help you define the good life and steer a course toward achieving it (Kretchmar, 1994, p. 111). Are there values that are especially central in physical activity, and if so, what are they? In his analysis of major values promoted by physical activity programs, Kretchmar (1994, pp. 109–176) identifies four:

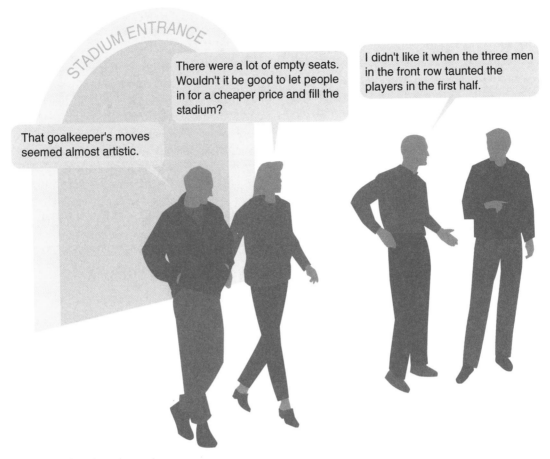

Figure 5.6   Questions based on values.

- Health-related physical *fitness*
- *Knowledge* about the human body, physical activity, and health practices
- Motor *skill*
- *Pleasure*

Each of these values emphasizes a different approach to developing physical activity programs. Valuing physical fitness, for example, relates well with people's interests in health and appearance. From this perspective, physical activity professionals would be primarily concerned about such things as assessment of fitness, measuring fitness changes resulting from physical activity, and promoting physically active lifestyles.

Valuing knowledge connects well with people's desires to obtain more information about such things as how to stay healthy, look good, and perform physical skills better. Taking this view, more research in scholarly subdisciplines

of kinesiology would be encouraged. Physical activity professionals would become well grounded in these with the assumption that having more of this knowledge would make them better practitioners.

Valuing motor skill relates well to the attention our society gives to physical activities. Some might rank this goal highest because of the possibility that becoming more highly skilled could encourage people to stay physically active and thus improve fitness. Being more skilled also might make some physical activities more fun. From this standpoint, physical activity professionals would concentrate on teaching appropriate movement techniques—for example, in school and college physical activity classes—focusing on particular sports such as golf or softball.

Valuing pleasure resonates well with people's conceptions of the good life—fun is important for just about everyone. Enjoyment is heightened when a situation is complex enough to present stimulating challenges, but simple enough so as not to overwhelm people's capabilities (Csikszentmihalyi, 1990b). We get bored if things are too easy, and anxious if the situation is too difficult. To promote fun in sports, the games may need to be simpler for beginners and more complex for advanced players. For example, T-ball is a simplified version of baseball that is better suited to the motor skill levels of young children. The regular rules of baseball seem adequate for producing a complex game that gives advanced players enjoyment. Intense competition notches up complexity even further, and it probably also increases fun as long as players aren't overwhelmed by the challenge. Another way of varying the complexity is to make sure opponents are evenly matched. The higher skills of more talented players would lead to a more complex game, while the skills of beginners would keep the game simpler.

🔑 Each of the four values promoted by physical activity programs—fitness, knowledge, skill, and pleasure—would lead to a different sort of program if used as the central guide to planning.

Before reading further, rank Kretchmar's (1994) four values—health-related physical fitness; knowledge about the human body, physical activity, and health practices; motor skill; and pleasure—according to your opinion about their relative importance. Why did you rank them the way you did? How might these rankings influence your choice of favorite physical activities, your central interests in studying physical activity, and your physical activity career choices?

Of course, these four values don't exist in isolation from one another—all are important in physical activity (Kretchmar, 1994, pp. 126–133). The main task we face is to weigh their relative merits and rank them. Once this is done, we can use them as guides for involvement in physical activity—for experiencing it as performers and spectators, for studying it, and for engaging in professional practice centered in it. To illustrate the latter, professionals might use their value rankings to prioritize the topics they cover in discussions with people who control purse strings (e.g., city government officials, school boards, representatives of private foundations that donate to worthy causes) in an effort to encourage more spending for physical activity programs.

Kretchmar's own ranking of these four values (highest to lowest) are: pleasure, motor skill, physical fitness, and knowledge (1994, pp. 135–176). His thoughts about the intrinsic and extrinsic values associated with each value are important in his rationale for his rankings. He uses three criteria in his rationale:

• Intrinsic values are better than extrinsic values because intrinsic values have immediate, direct worth, while extrinsic values lead only indirectly to an intrinsic value.

• Among intrinsic values, those involving broader satisfaction and contentment are better than those involving more limited pleasure.

• Among intrinsic values involving broader satisfaction, those involving longer-term meaning and coherence in our lives are better than those involving more immediate pleasure.

Ethical Values and Sport

Studies of right and wrong actions in sport deal with topics such as cheating, intentional fouling, participating with a determination to win, using performance-enhancing drugs, promoting justice and equality, and promoting the safety and welfare of athletes. Studies of fair play usually focus on several of these simultaneously.

Moral issues are often magnified at elite levels by the large amounts of money involved. When athletes and coaches have their eyes on valuable prizes, it's sometimes tempting to give less attention to questions of morality. Under such conditions, ethics are severely tested.

Three sources of ethical reasoning exist in sport (see figure 5.7) (Fraleigh, 1984). First, we use our society's customs and conventions such as written laws, religious beliefs, and other common understandings about right and wrong. Deciding to follow game rules simply because they are

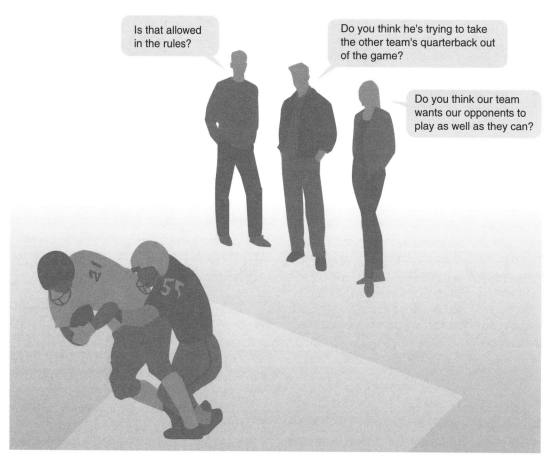

Figure 5.7 Questions of ethical values.

the rules is an example. Second, we sometimes make ethical decisions based on self-interest—we do what is best for ourselves. A lineman in American football uses this sort of reasoning when he decides to help his team by hitting a quarterback extra hard in the hope of causing an injury serious enough to send the quarterback to the sidelines for the rest of the game. Third, we sometimes take the moral high road, focusing on producing the best possible world for everyone. Enabling your opponents to perform at the highest level possible in order to give added worth to your own victory is an illustration of this.

Moral decisions made on the basis of self-interest lead to "chaos, distrust, fear, and rampant disregard of one participant for other participants" (Fraleigh, 1984, p. 12). Deciding to adhere to societal customs and laws is also problematic; they are not necessarily always morally right. For example, during World War II soldiers in Nazi concentration camps followed rules that resulted in the slaughter of millions of people.

Although it is a long way from ethical decisions in concentration camps to ethical decisions in sport, if the rules of particular sports allow you to act in ways that seriously injure others, then perhaps they aren't the best guides to moral action. Decisions about right and wrong actions often require careful thought about what would lead to the greatest good for the most people.

Sources of ethical reasoning in sport include laws, religious beliefs, and other societal understandings about right and wrong; a person's own self-interest; and the goal of producing the best possible world for everyone.

Using the criterion of the greatest good for the most people, and emphasizing sport's playlike qualities, the following are examples of morally right situations that produce a good contest (Fraleigh, 1984):

Although performance-enhancing drugs have been used by athletes for a long time, they became more prevalent in the late 1950s when anabolic steroids came on the scene, and they have been on the rise ever since (Todd, 1987). Although precise figures are difficult to find, data from the U.S. National Football League show that drug suspensions were much higher in 1995 and 1996 than in the previous decade (Boeck & Staimer, 1996). In this section we'll look at the use of performance enhancers—drugs as well as other things—from ethical perspectives (Osterhoudt, 1991, pp. 122–126; Simon, 1991, pp. 71–92).

The main ethical problem, of course, is that performance enhancers give athletes an unfair advantage over opponents. You might ask, then, what improves performance unfairly, and what improves it fairly? Your first answer might be that natural substances (e.g., food, testosterone) are fair, while unnatural substances (e.g., steroids, amphetamines) are not. However, the natural–unnatural distinction is problematic. Technological breakthroughs in facilities and equipment—long-body tennis rackets, artificial track surfaces, sophisticated basketball shoes, and better-engineered racing bicycles—are unnatural. Performance enhancers such as these would generally be considered fair, even though limits are sometimes placed on technology (e.g., golf balls and baseballs could be engineered to travel farther, but there are limits placed on this). On the other hand, testosterone is a natural substance, yet it is usually considered to be unfair when taken in large doses beyond what a person might produce in his or her own body (Brown, 1980).

One solution is just to equalize everyone by giving all competitors access to whatever performance-enhancing aids they want. This sounds pretty good initially, but it's problematic because performance enhancers can drastically change a game, making it

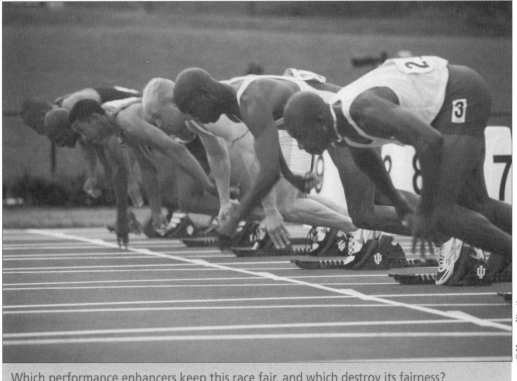

Which performance enhancers keep this race fair, and which destroy its fairness?

© Human Kinetics

into something totally different. For example, if all baseball teams could use ball machines to deliver pitches, then the teams would certainly be equal, but they wouldn't be playing the traditional version of the game. The contest would shift to one focused on which team's engineers could build the best pitching machine.

Another possibility is to distinguish between performance enhancers that actually increase a body's capabilities and those that just make it possible to use more effectively whatever capabilities the body already has (Perry, 1983). From this perspective, things such as carbohydrate loading and high altitude training would be fair because they make the body's performance capabilities more effective. Steroids and amphetamines alter the body's capabilities and would therefore be unfair. However, the distinction between these two is very blurry—it seems to be more a matter of difference in degree of performance enhancement rather than a difference among the techniques used (Osterhoudt, 1991).

Another view is that performance enhancers are unfair if they put the health of an athlete or others at risk. Here we have a second ethical issue in addition to the main one of inequality among players. Since most performance-enhancing drugs have side effects that are risky to health, they could be considered unfair from this standpoint. The rationale is that using such substances violates the playfulness of sport in several ways. It demonstrates lack of respect for oneself and one's opponents as worthy competitors by making it necessary to take risky drugs to stay competitive. As you already know, coercion and cruelty can occur in play, and also in games and sport, but such behavior is ethically inappropriate.

Additionally, youngsters may copy risky drug-taking habits of stars in high-profile, elite sports, and this is clearly problematic from a moral perspective. It goes against the generally held belief that risky performance-enhancing drugs should be kept away from children because youngsters haven't developed the intellect to make adequate judgments about the consequences of using them (Brown, 1984).

Finally, there is the matter of the self-determination and freedom of athletes. When is drug testing acceptable, and when is it an ethically unwarranted intrusion on an athlete's freedom as a human being? If we test athletes for recreational drugs that don't enhance performance, or for illegal drugs that don't enhance performance, some would argue that we are invading their privacy in unacceptable ways (Thompson, 1982).

Clearly, difficult ethical issues are connected with athletes' use of performance enhancers. Uncertainties remain concerning which aids are morally unacceptable, although performance enhancers that present health risks to athletes seem to be viewed as less acceptable than others. Additional investigations are needed to examine the ethics connected with using aids to enhance sport performance.

- Competition between opponents who are close in ability, and who compete with personal resolve to win without slacking off during the event

- Opponents who strive to bring out the best performance in one another, and who compete with mutual respect for each other's athletic talents and general well-being, while moving toward the goal of determining a winner and loser

- Opponents who follow the letter and spirit of the rules of the game, avoiding such things as cheating and intentional fouls

In the golf tournament scenario at the beginning of the chapter, you saw that a lackluster performance by the loser cast doubts on the excellence of the winner. If opponents are evenly matched, then a competitor who doesn't go all out to win, or who doesn't strive to bring out excellence in his or her adversary, is not acting for the good of everyone. In the scenario, of course, the lackluster performance wasn't the fault of the athlete—an illness was the culprit. There was no intent to subvert the contest.

On the other hand, players who try so hard to win that they are willing to injure opponents, cheat, or cause an intentional foul to gain an advantage are also not acting for the good of everyone. Intentionally injuring opponents clearly shows disregard for their welfare, and this diminishes a victory over them. Cheating—intentional, hidden disobeying of the rules—makes the outcome of the contest meaningless because the cheater has a secret advantage not enjoyed by others. Intentionally fouling to gain an advantage may not always be against the rules, but it does subvert the spirit of the rules. Fouls are designed to keep players from breaking the rules, not to provide opportunities for intentional rule-breaking in order to slow down the game, or to prevent an opponent from scoring. When intentional fouling becomes common, a change in the rules to take away the advantage gained by such fouls might help to decrease them.

Wrap-Up

Philosophy offers fascinating new insights by helping to sharpen your thinking about various forms of physical activity as well as the mind–body relationship. It focuses on the general nature of such things rather than on specific instances—broad insights are the ultimate goal. Philosophy of physical activity also includes explorations of knowledge that can be derived through involvement with physical activities and values connected with physical activities. The subdiscipline also points you toward using your philosophical insights to make positive changes in people's lives. For example, you might bring your knowledge of ethics to bear on important decisions you have to make concerning the use of performance-enhancing drugs in a league where you serve as the executive director.

If you find the knowledge in this subdiscipline to be interesting, take time to leaf through some of the philosophy of physical activity texts, as well as the *Philosophy of Sport Journal*. You might also enjoy an introductory course on the topic. You'll learn to think more carefully and precisely about things, and this will help you be a better performer, scholar, and professional.

Study Questions

1. Describe the goals of philosophical study of physical activity, and the three major areas of study.

2. Why were early 20th century philosophical studies of physical activity tied to education? Why did this change by the 1970s, and what was the focus of studies from this point to the present?

3. Describe the four reasoning processes that are central research tools in philosophical studies of physical activity.

4. Discuss the concept of separateness of mind and body, its implications for school physical activity programs, its implications for research on physical activity, and its implications for the well-being of competitive athletes.

5. Discuss the concept of blended unity of mind and body, its implications for school physical activity programs, its implications for research on physical activity, and its implications for the well-being of competitive athletes.

6. Discuss playful elements in sport, play as a source sport's inconsequentiality, and the implications of this for what sport means to people.

7. Discuss the four values promoted by the field of physical activity and the implications of these for designing physical activity programs.

8. Discuss the three sources of ethical reasoning in sport and the relative value of each.

9. Discuss the ethical issues involved with using performance-enhancers in sport.

10. Discuss some examples of sport contests in which opponents strive to bring about the greatest good for the most people involved. In your examples point out what you view as the greatest good.

6

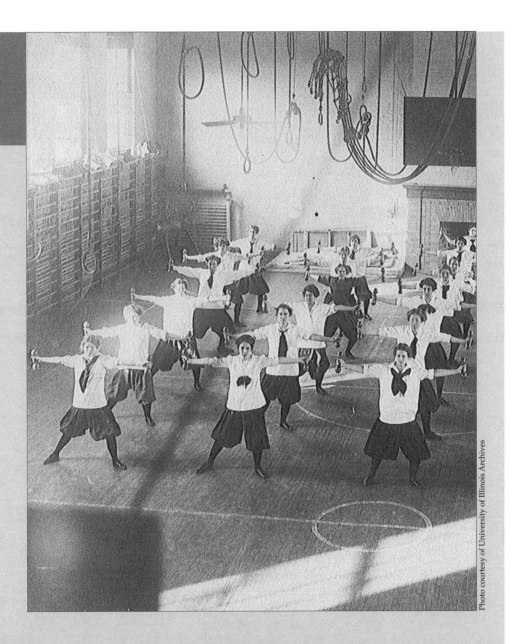

Photo courtesy of University of Illinois Archives

History of Physical Activity

Janet C. Harris

In this chapter . . .

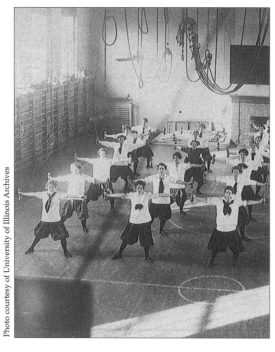

Photo courtesy of University of Illinois Archives

You find a collection of old photos showing life in American colleges and universities. They aren't dated, but from people's hairstyles and clothing you think they must have been taken about 1900. Several snapshots show football players, and one shows people posed with tennis rackets. Other photos are of students in orderly formations doing calisthenics and other exercises with equipment such as dumbbells, long wooden rods, and weights. In one photo, men are working out with larger apparatus such as parallel bars, vaulting horses, and hanging rings. You wonder whether students of the time also participated in other forms of physical activity. Did they do aerobic exercise? What about basketball? Did they do any dancing? You think about the excitement and color surrounding college football today, and you wonder whether students in 1900 experienced that, too. Many other intriguing questions come to mind: Do the exercise photos show college physical education classes, or were the students working out in a campus recreation program? Did men and women engage in similar types of activities? What benefits did students expect from sports and exercise? Were they active in campus intramural sports? How did physical activities fit into overall college life?

Why History of Physical Activity?

Consider what life would be like if you didn't have a memory. You wouldn't be able to recall past experiences such as the 10 years you spent training with a swim team; the pickup basketball games you played at your local neighborhood courts; the time you broke your leg falling off your bike and went to an exercise rehab program for several months; or the details about the fortunes of your favorite professional football team. Memories give you insights about how things came to be the way they are. No one has a perfect memory, and no one can predict the future with total accuracy, but our recollections help us act intelligently and develop reasonable plans for the future.

History offers broad and detailed insights that go far beyond our own memory. It gives us the opportunity to develop a more extensive "memory" than we could ever acquire independently. It consists of a vast collection of information—mostly events that occurred before we were born, often in geographic regions and societies different from our own. The ancient Greek Olympic Games, 18th-century peasant ball games in Great Britain and Europe, and 20th-century American basketball all influenced the physical activities we take part in today. Studying history gives us windows to the past and magnifying lenses to look closely at things that we find especially interesting. It helps us understand how and why our current physical activities are structured the way they are; it allows us to compare them with physical activities from earlier periods; and it gives us the tools to look toward the future from new vantage points.

A kinesiologist who is knowledgeable about history of physical activity would probably interpret such things as the current fitness craze or the popularity of spectator sports in colleges and universities quite differently from someone who lacks this information. A person who has studied history of physical activity would look at the snapshots in our opening scenario and have answers for the questions we asked. For example, the historian would know that gymnastic exercise was especially important at that time; basketball had only been in existence since 1891; and college football had become a "big deal" on quite

a few campuses and was attracting lots of spectators.

American society's current interest in exercise, health, and fitness is a phenomenon that's hard to miss. Exercise studios and health clubs dot the landscape; exercise videos, books, and magazines are available in almost every neighborhood shopping center. However, if you asked teenagers or "twenty-somethings" about the origins of this, most would probably draw a blank.

Kinesiologists would know that interest in exercise picked up in the 1950s due to a variety of influences such as Cold War fears, President Eisenhower's heart attacks, and evidence suggesting that American children were less physically fit than their European counterparts. They would also know about an earlier period in American history when exercise was also very prominent—the late 19th century (Park, 1987b).

Kinesiologists would be able to point out that American fascination with exercise has fluctuated over the years. This is important information: Is the current, relatively high level of interest in exercise likely to decrease in the future, in line with the fluctuating pattern we've seen in the past? If so, this will have serious negative implications for the health of many Americans. Is there anything we can do to prevent this possible downward cycle? Or do we now have such strong scientific evidence confirming the health benefits of exercise that the roller-coaster pattern of the past will be broken? These are questions that could not even be raised without an understanding of history of physical activity.

 History of physical activity teaches us about changes as well as stability in the past, and this helps us understand the present as well as make reasonable decisions for the future.

CHAPTER OBJECTIVES

In this chapter you will learn about these topics:

▪ What background knowledge you already have about history of physical activity

▪ What a historian of physical activity does

▪ The goals of history of physical activity

■ How the subdiscipline of history of physical activity developed

■ How research is conducted in history of physical activity

■ What research tells us about physical activity in American society from the industrial revolution to the present

Think about film coverage you have seen showing people playing a sport a long time ago. Compare this with the way this sport is today.

What Background Knowledge Do I Already Have?

Your previous physical activity experiences, academic studies, and even observations of professional practice have already given you some insights into history of physical activity. From *experience*, you may have participated in competitive team sports such as basketball, volleyball, and soccer and noticed that they are incredibly popular in Western societies. If you have ever wondered how this came to be, you have been on the verge of historical inquiry. Or perhaps you have noticed gender inequities in physical activity and wondered what historical events led to this. Maybe as a man you have at some time feared being teased for your lack of athletic ability or if you are a male athlete you may have noticed uneasily how much more financial support you received to develop your athletic talents in relation to your female counterparts. If you are a woman, perhaps at times you have felt strangely out of place in a competitive environment, or maybe there has not been as much financial support to help you improve your athletic skills. In either case, if you have ever wondered why such situations exist, you were on the verge of delving into history.

From previous *scholarly study*, you are probably familiar with a lot of historical information that will help you understand the history of physical activity. Most of the historical research on physical activity deals with ancient Greece and Rome, Europe and Great Britain, and North America. Knowing something about the overall history of these societies will make history of physical activity easier to learn and remember. For example, if you know that nationalism and national patriotism swept through Europe in the 19th century, then it's not surprising to learn that in countries such as Germany and Sweden people thought that special gymnastics systems could help build a healthy, strong citizenry that could keep their nation strong. Making this connection helps you remember when, and at least one reason why, these gymnastics systems came into being.

Finally, from watching *physical activity professionals* in action, you may have observed some history in the making. Perhaps you know people who work as athletic trainers, sport marketers, personal trainers, and sports physical therapists. These professionals are part of an important historical trend! Not long ago, career opportunities for people in the physical activity field were limited to professors, physical education teachers, and coaches. But in recent years, professional opportunities have greatly expanded, and this is a historical phenomenon.

As your knowledge of history of physical activity broadens, you will see that it is related to both philosophy of physical activity and sociology of physical activity. As you can see in figure 6.1, all three are part of the sociocultural sphere of scholarly study—that is, the sphere of research that focuses on the social and cultural aspects of physical activity.

What Does a Historian of Physical Activity Do?

Historians who study physical activity are usually college or university faculty members, but a handful are librarians, consultants for book publishing companies, archivists in charge of special collections of documents, or museum curators. We will focus on the faculty members. They engage in typical activities consisting of teaching, research, and professional service. They often teach broad survey courses on history of physical activity, and some of their classes are more

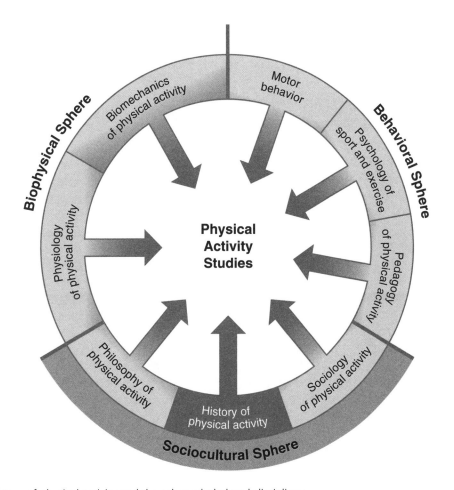

Figure 6.1 History of physical activity and the other scholarly subdisciplines.

narrowly focused on topics such as the ancient Olympic Games, physical activity in colonial America, or sport and ethnic relations in the United States. Examples of professional service include giving a community presentation about the history of a region's minor-league baseball team, participating on an educational TV panel to discuss the history of gender relations in American sport, or helping a city's nonprofit historical society put together a museum display about the history of rehabilitative exercise.

Libraries are perhaps the most important research tools for historians. If you want to study the physical activities of African American slaves prior to the Civil War in the U.S., for example, you could locate library sources such as records of interviews with former slaves who were asked to recall their experiences under slavery, published accounts from white slaveholders written during the time of slavery, and accounts from Northern whites who visited plantations where

slaves worked (Wiggins, 1980). Most historians take great care to develop solid working relationships with librarians. Sometimes library staff act almost as gatekeepers—deciding how much access you should have to rare and valuable materials.

Historians of physical activity sometimes apply for research money from their own college or university, as well as from outside organizations that specialize in supporting historical research. They often use the money to travel to libraries in distant cities, or to pay a research assistant to help collect information. When asking for research money, their proposals must be clearly written and persuasive. They are usually required to describe such things as the topic they want to investigate, why it is important, the sort of information they will collect, the sources where they'll find this information, what makes them competent to conduct the study, how much money they'll need, and what they'll buy with it.

Goals of History of Physical Activity

There are two main goals of history of physical activity. The first is *to identify and describe patterns of change and stability in physical activity in particular societies or cultures during specific time periods.* Whether the focus is on the 1890s "bicycle craze" in the United States, the shrinking attention to physical activity in the education of young boys in the ancient Roman Empire, or the U.S. middle-class notion in the late 19th century that exercise could improve young men's morality, there is a central concern with identifying shifts and continuities. These are always examined in relation to the broader societies in which physical activities took place, and over specific periods of time. Historians provide an enormous number of factual details to give readers a thick, robust description of such things as what it was like to be involved in the particular physical activities being studied, the values and attitudes people had about those activities, people's broader lives, general societal values and attitudes that were prevalent at the time, how people's physical activities fitted into their overall lives, and how they changed their physical activities. Because written historical descriptions require many pages, we can't include examples here.

Sometimes changes occur slowly, giving us the impression that things have stayed the same. For example, the rules, strategies, styles of play, and equipment in many of our sports changed a lot during the 20th century. Because these shifts occurred relatively slowly, however, the games remained recognizable. At other times, changes take place much more rapidly and dramatically. For example, improvements in bicycle design in the United States more than a hundred years ago contributed to a rapid rise in bicycling—the "bicycle craze" in the 1890s (Hardy, 1982).

The other main goal of history of physical activity is *to analyze patterns of change and stability in physical activity in particular societies or cultures during specific time periods.* Most historians go beyond description to demonstrate relationships and influences in an effort to explain why things occurred. They look for individuals, groups, events, and ideas that helped bring about changes or contributed to maintaining stability. For example, Hardy's *How Boston Played: Sport, Recreation, and Community 1865–1915* (1982) focuses on the city-building process that took place in Boston over several decades after the Civil War. During that time the city's population mushroomed as European immigrants and people from the American countryside arrived to take jobs created by the industrial revolution. This led to major problems such as overcrowded tenements, poor health, neighborhood destruction, crime, ethnic conflict, and political and moral disorder—all serious threats to traditional ways of life. Hardy believed that Bostonians were looking for ways to revitalize their sense of connectedness to one another, and sports and recreation played an important part.

Based on what happened in Boston during this period, Hardy created three categories of ways Bostonians responded to the problems in their city: escape from the city and its problems, reform of the city and its problems, and accommodation to new forms of city life by developing a renewed sense of group identity (pp. 197–201). Hardy used these categories to examine the complex ways in which people sought community through building new playgrounds and parks, expanding sport and exercise programs in schools and universities, joining community-based sport clubs, riding bicycles, and conferring hero status on top athletes.

Most physical activity historians are college and university faculty members; through their research, teaching, and service, they pursue the two main goals of the subdiscipline.

Goals of History of Physical Activity

1. To identify and describe patterns of change and stability in physical activity in particular societies or cultures during specific time periods

2. To analyze patterns of change and stability in physical activity in particular societies or cultures during specific time periods

History of the Subdiscipline

A handful of American scholars studied history of physical activity in the early 20th century, and even in the late 19th century at least one physical educator viewed this to be important. In spite of this, it wasn't until the 1960s that the subdiscipline began to develop a recognizable identity in North America.

One of the earliest American reports to emphasize history of physical activity was Edward Hartwell's "On Physical Training" (1899), which included information about ancient Greece, Europe and Great Britain, and the United States (Gerber, 1971). Hartwell believed that professionals who would be charting a course for the future should know about the past, and as early as 1893 he pointed to the need for a textbook on history of physical education. It would be several more decades, however, before such texts would begin to appear.

Historian Frederic Paxson wrote a classic article in 1917 titled "The Rise of Sport." Based on the well-known "frontier thesis" developed by his graduate school mentor Frederick Jackson Turner, Paxson argued that the disappearance of the American western frontier spurred sport to become more popular because it served some of the same escape or release functions as the frontier (Pope, 1997, pp. 1–2; Struna, 1997, pp. 148–149). This "safety valve" function, along with Paxson's belief in the gradual, inevitable social evolution of sport, were central ideas in the research of many sport history scholars for decades to come.

In the 1920s and 1930s physical educators published several textbooks on the history of physical education, as well as articles in professional journals on the development of physical education programs in schools and colleges. Their focus was on instructional programs; they gave much less attention to the wide array of sports and recreational activities beyond school settings (Struna, 1997). In spite of this limitation, these books and articles probably helped open the door in college and university physical education departments to a recognition of the importance of history of physical activity.

Historical Time Line

1886–1940	Beginnings of U.S. historical analyses of sport and physical education.
1923–1942	Physical educators write early textbooks on history of physical education.
1937	Seward Staley writes "The History of Sport: A New Course in the Professional Training Curriculum," calling for an increased focus on the history of sport in physical education curriculums.
1952–1963	Historical analyses treating sport as "active" and "passive" were produced that continued to influence scholars in later decades.
1962	A section for sport history is established in the College Physical Education Association.
1971	Eugen Weber publishes "Gymnastics and Sports in Fin-de-Siecle France: Opium of the Classes?" giving sport history more visibility among scholars in the discipline of history.
1972	The North American Society for Sport History is established.
1974	The *Journal of Sport History* begins publication.
1976	Researchers in sport history begin using modernization theory, and this is still in use today.
1980	Researchers in sport history begin using human agency theory, and this is still in use today.
1980	Researchers begin studying history of exercise and fitness, and this work continues to the present.

Seward Staley (1937), a professor of physical education at the University of Illinois, opened the door wider when he suggested that courses on the history of physical education should be expanded to focus on the history of sport. Staley continued to emphasize this in the years following World War II, and graduate students began studying sport history at the University of Illinois under his direction (Struna, 1997).

In 1940, during the early years of World War II, historian Foster Rhea Dulles wrote his widely read *America Learns to Play: A History of Popular Recreation.* Dulles went beyond Paxson's safety valve and evolutionary perspectives to point out more positively that popular 20th-century American recreational pursuits—including sports—were well liked because they were satisfying to the American public (Struna, 1997). Furthermore,

a broad range of people had access to them, indicating to Dulles that American democracy had come of age (Pope, 1997).

After World War II, historian John Betts completed an important doctoral dissertation titled "Organized Sport in Industrial America" (1952). He stressed that sport played an active role in society by helping bind people closer together, and he also highlighted the ways in which late-19th-century entrepreneurs harnessed a variety of new manufacturing processes, new forms of transportation, and new forms of communication to shape sports into profitable commercial enterprises (Pope, 1997; Struna, 1997). In sharp contrast to Betts's active model, a decade later journalist Robert Boyle's *Sport—Mirror of American Life* (1963) offered a passive model of sport. Boyle viewed sport as a mirror that merely reflected

In Profile

© Burns Library, Boston College

John Rickards Betts

A faculty member in the history department at Boston College for the last 17 years of his career, John Betts conducted important studies about the rise of modern organized American sport. He followed this path at a time when few other historians were interested in sports. Moving beyond mere descriptions of the growth of sport, Betts provided detailed examples of central influences such as urbanization, industrialization, and new technologies such as railroads and telegraph systems. He believed that sport had an active role in shaping social life, primarily serving as a rallying point that encouraged people to be unified and supportive of one another. This approach to sport history was a model that many others used in the years that followed (Lewis, 1972; Metcalfe, 1974; Struna, 1997).

World War II interrupted Betts's education, and during military service he received the Bronze Star for bravery at Leipzig. After completing his influential doctoral dissertation "Organized Sport in Industrial America" at Columbia University in 1951, he continued to study and write about sport and other aspects of American culture. In the late 1960s and early 1970s he developed a new interest in health, exercise, and recreational activities prior to the Civil War.

Betts had many other interests beyond sport history. He was several times the director of the American Studies Institute at Boston College, and also president of the New England American Studies Association. He was active in organizing a chapter of the American Association of University Professors at Boston College, and he was involved in numerous political and religious organizations in the Boston area (Daly, 1972). He passed away suddenly in 1971, a few months after his wife died of cancer (Loy, 1974).

society. Both Betts's and Boyle's works had considerable influence on the subsequent work of sport historians.

Identifying the Subdiscipline

The ranks of sport historians began to grow in the 1960s, but there was still no scholarly association to help the subdiscipline advance. The first attempt to remedy this took place in 1962 when Marvin Eyler, Seward Staley, and Earle Zeigler worked to develop a section for sport history in the College Physical Education Association (soon renamed the National College Physical Education Association for Men), a professional organization for college and university physical education faculty members and administrators. Because this was the only formal organization for sport historians at the time, the NCPEAM *Proceedings* became an important published record of their work (Berryman, 1973; Struna, 1997).

Scholars in the discipline of history became more interested in studying sport when Eugen Weber, a prominent historian, presented "Gymnastics and Sports in Fin-de-Siecle France: Opium of the Classes?" at the 1970 meeting of the American Historical Association and published it the following year in the *American Historical Review* (Berryman, 1973). The program of the 1971 AHA meeting included a whole section on sport history.

The North American Society for Sport History was established in 1972, and it was soon recognized as the main scholarly association for sport historians in the United States and Canada. NASSH was designed to attract a broader scholarly membership including women, Canadians, international scholars beyond North America, and sport historians from disciplines beyond physical education (Struna, 1997). It began publishing the *Journal of Sport History* in 1974, and a report issued in 1985 showed this publication to be the seventh most frequently cited history journal among hundreds in existence (Struna, 1997).

Expanding the Subdiscipline

Research in sport history expanded in several directions during the 1970s and 1980s (Pope, 1997; Struna, 1997). Scholars began using two new **analytical frameworks**, or sets of general concepts or ideas, to make sense of the historical information they collected. The first framework, **modernization theory**, emphasized that the rise of modern sport occurred during the industrial revolution as American society shifted away from being agricultural and locally oriented and developed city-based industries rooted in science and technology. Sports changed from relatively unspecialized games to highly organized contests involving lots of rules and many specialized playing positions. Allen Guttmann pioneered the use of modernization theory in his book *From Ritual to Record: The Nature of Modern Sports* (1978).

The second conceptual framework emphasized **human agency,** suggesting that people were actively involved in developing or "constructing" their own sports. Research focused on the details of how this occurred (Pope, 1997; Struna, 1997). One of the earliest works to use this approach was Stephen Hardy's *How Boston Played: Sport, Recreation, and Community 1865–1915* (1982). Hardy pointed to many local struggles among middle-class and working-class groups—often tinged with ethnic distinctions—that occurred as Bostonians went about structuring their sports and recreational activities.

Other scholars expanded the focus on human agency to look at gender differences. For example, in *Cheap Amusements: Working Women and Leisure in Turn-of-the-Century New York,* Kathy Peiss (1986) examined working women's culture between 1880 and 1920, emphasizing their newfound recreational activities outside the home in dance halls, nickelodeons, social clubs, and amusement parks.

An important research direction inaugurated in the 1980s dealt with exercise and health (Struna, 1997). This was sparked by the American public's growing interest in exercise and physical fitness in the late 20th century and by the expansion of advanced course work on exercise in college and university kinesiology and physical education programs. One of the earliest studies was James Whorton's *Crusaders for Fitness: The History of American Health Reformers* (1982). Whorton showed the role of exercise among the many practices advocated in 19th- and early-20th-century reform movements aimed at improving the health of the American public.

In the 1990s, physical activity scholars continued to use the approaches to historical research that were pioneered in the 1970s and 1980s. In addition, they increasingly linked their work to research in other social science disciplines, especially anthropology, economics, and sociology (Struna, 1997).

🔑 Building on a small base of scholarly knowledge gathered earlier in the century, the history of physical activity subdiscipline grew in size, sophistication, and scope from the 1960s onward. Scholars initially focused on sport, but beginning in the 1980s exercise and physical fitness received greater attention.

Research Methods in History of Physical Activity

Remembering what you've learned about the goals of history of physical activity, as well as the chronology of the development of the subdiscipline, let's look at how scholars produce this knowledge. How do they find out what happened, who was involved, when and where things took place, and why? The process has similarities to what detectives and attorneys do when they hunt for evidence that helps reconstruct important details of a crime (see figure 6.2). It involves locating evidence; critiquing and examining evidence; and piecing it together in a coherent, insightful framework that explains how and why things occurred. We can divide this process into three stages: finding sources of evidence; critiquing the sources; and examining, analyzing, and synthesizing the evidence.

Finding Sources of Evidence

Think about the many different physical activities that currently exist in our society. If historians two hundred years in the future wanted to study these, what sorts of items would be useful? All kinds of things come to mind: aerobic workout videos; popular books, articles, and magazines about exercise and physical fitness; business records of professional sport franchises; videos of televised sporting events; school physical education curriculum guides; videos of dance concerts; policy statements from the National Collegiate Athletic Association; and the 1996 United States government report *Physical Activ-*

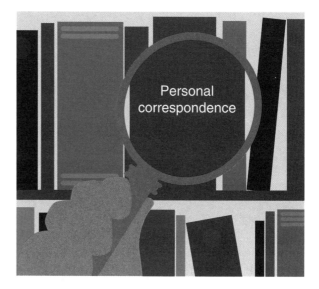

Figure 6.2 Historians have to search carefully for important evidence.

ity and Health: A Report of the Surgeon General. The list could go on and on.

These items are all **primary sources** of information, meaning they were produced in the society and time period being studied. But where would scholars find them? It's hard to say where these things might be stored in the future, but we know where historians look today—libraries, archives (storage facilities for documents from important people and organizations), and private collections (Struna, 1996a). Sometimes they also interview people to tap their memories of life in earlier times.

Materials are scattered throughout the country. For example, the Avery Brundage Collection (Brundage was president of the International Olympic Committee 1952–1972) is at the University of Illinois. It contains items such as letters to and from Brundage, books, pamphlets, scrapbooks, Brundage's notes on various topics, speeches given by Brundage, and policies from the IOC and other sport governing bodies (Guttmann, 1984). Copies of the *Boston Medical and Surgical Journal* from the 19th century are located at the National Library of Medicine in Bethesda, Maryland, as well as a library at the University of Chicago (Struna, 1996a). Local historical societies are often rich sources of information, along with archives located in the library at your own college or university.

Historical reports written by people in later time periods—**secondary sources**—are also useful for finding primary sources. Examples of secondary sources include a journal article written in the 1980s about African Americans who participated in intercollegiate athletics in the 1930s and 1940s, or a book-length report produced in the 1990s on physical activity in the American colonies. Authors include detailed notes pointing to the nature and location of specific information (primary sources and other secondary sources) used in their investigation. Most libraries have electronic databases to help you locate sources, and some of these are accessible via the Internet.

Critiquing the Sources

Once you locate primary sources, it's important to scrutinize them carefully for authenticity and credibility. Sources that are authentic and credible make your historical research believable. Let's concentrate on written documents such as newspaper articles, books, and letters. Determining **authenticity** involves such matters as who authored the piece and the date it was written. You might learn, for example, that a document was actually written many years after the events it describes took place or that the author listed on the document was not the actual person who wrote it. For example, if a letter dated in the 17th century uses the phrase "didn't get to first base," you can be quite sure that the piece was written much later because this term comes from American baseball and the game didn't exist in the 17th century (Shafer, 1980, p. 131). If ink used to publish a report wasn't manufactured until several years after the date listed, then you know that the piece was written later. (Such a determination would require a technical specialist.)

Determining the **credibility** of written documents helps you interpret them. First, the "rule of context" encourages you to make sense of a document's language in relation to what the words meant to people in the society in which it was produced. Second, the "rule of perspective" requires you to examine an author's relationship to the events he or she describes, and how the author obtained the information. Finally, the "rule of omission or free editing" reminds you that you always have partial records of events—not the complete events themselves; it is thus important

to locate multiple sources to add more details to your evidence (Struna, 1996a).

If you want to study the television coverage of the 1984 Los Angeles Olympic Games, where would you look for primary sources? What kinds of data might you find?

Examining, Analyzing, and Synthesizing the Evidence

Once you've located authentic and credible sources, it's time to examine the evidence to find information that addresses the tentative hypotheses or research questions you established at the beginning of your investigation. The goal is to describe events in detail, and then analyze them to learn how and why things took place. Historians accomplish this by placing events in an analytical framework that uses (1) trends and relationships in the events themselves and/or (2) theoretical models from the social sciences. You have already seen examples of analytical frameworks—the "revitalizing a sense of connectedness" framework, the "modernization" framework, and the "human agency" framework. There are probably as many approaches to analysis and synthesis as there are researchers. The main goal is to piece together the evidence to gain a detailed understanding of what happened, as well as how and why (Shafer, 1980; Struna, 1996a).

Historical research involves finding sources containing evidence about past events, critiquing the sources for authenticity and credibility, and analyzing the data contained in the sources to learn how and why things happened.

Overview of Knowledge in History of Physical Activity

Now that you know what historians of physical activity do, let's take a brief look at some of the fascinating information they've discovered. The body of knowledge is large and complex; it deals with many societies worldwide, and it covers many different time periods. Here we will touch on a few of the interesting highlights.

If you were a boy living in ancient Greece during the 6th century B.C.E. in the city-state of Sparta, for example, you would have received more extensive and harsher physical activity training than in the city-state of Athens, where you would have gotten a more balanced physical and intellectual education. In both places, however, your physical activity instruction would have been aimed toward preparing you for warfare. And even though the ancient Greeks considered the Olympic Games to be similar to the competitiveness of warfare, this prestigious event for fullfledged citizens was distinct from the brutal gladiators' contests—mostly among slaves and convicts—staged several hundred years later in the Roman Empire. And the Roman contests were very different from the informal, rough team ball games played by European peasants in the Middle Ages, and also distinct from high-profile women's gymnastics in the Olympics of the late 20th century. And we haven't even mentioned other forms of physical activity such as dance and exercise. Understanding the ways in which physical activities have fitted into societies around the world since the beginning of history is indeed a monumental task.

In North America we know a lot about the history of physical activity in Western civilizations—especially ancient Greece and Rome, Europe, Great Britain, Canada, and the United States. It's important to recognize, however, that rich physical activity traditions were developed by people in Africa, Asia, Australia and New Zealand, the Indian subcontinent, Central and South America, the Caribbean region, and the Pacific Islands. These include a variety of martial arts in Asian societies, Sumo wrestling in Japan, ball sports such as lacrosse in native North American tribal societies, ball games played in high-walled courts in native Central American civilizations, an African martial art brought to the Atlantic and Caribbean coasts of South America, and a sport in Afghanistan involving hundreds of mounted horsemen who simultaneously try to gain possession of a dead goat or calf carcass. Historical information exists about all of these. In this text,

however, we will focus on the history of physical activity in the United States.

British and European colonists began arriving in North America in greater numbers beginning in the early 1600s, swelling an earlier trickle. Initially, people worked hard to establish themselves in unfamiliar and often harsh environments. This, coupled with strict religious prohibitions against idleness and amusements in some areas of the colonies, meant that participation in sports and games was rather limited. Nevertheless, people sometimes engaged in their own versions of traditional British and European sport and recreational activities. Participation grew as the colonists became more established and religious sanctions were lifted. Activities included horse racing, fishing, hunting, sailing, boat racing, golf, bowls, team ball games, sleigh races, skating, foot racing, boxing, wrestling, animal baiting (in which a wild animal such as a bear was tied by a chain and attacked, often by dogs or rats), cockfighting, and billiards. Some of these were commercialized and yielded profits for promoters; gambling was also common (Baker, 1988; Lucas & Smith, 1978; Struna, 1996b).

We'll look more closely at physical activity in the United States during three periods of time:

1840–1900 American society was characterized by industrialization, growth of science and technology, immigration, urbanization, democratization, and westward expansion; the Civil War occurred.

1900–1950 American society was characterized by the growth of consumerism, immigration, and democratization; a major economic depression and two world wars occurred.

1950–2000 American society was characterized by the growth of electronic communication, the growth of global trade, immigration, and democratization; the Cold War, Korean War, and Vietnam War occurred.

For each of these periods, we'll examine

- participation in physical activity,
- physical activity professions, and
- scholarly knowledge about physical activity.

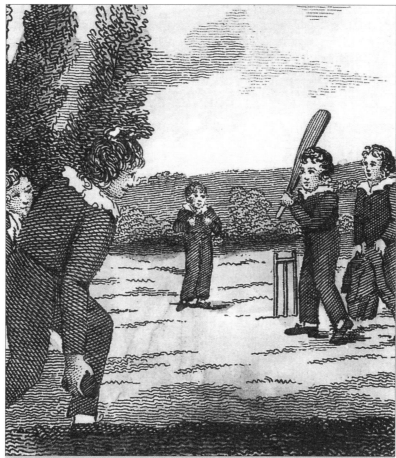

Cricket, a sport that came from England.

From P.D. Welch, *History of American physical education and sport*, 2d edition, 1996. Courtesy of Charles C. Thomas, Publisher, Ltd., Springfield, Illinois.

Physical Activity in the United States: 1840–1900

From the mid-1800s to 1900 the United States economy, population, and geography all expanded. New developments in science and technology fueled the growth of business and industry. City populations mushroomed, producing major sanitation problems that threatened everyone's health. The advent of more leisure time sparked an interest in building city parks and playgrounds, as well as in developing more commercial entertainment and amusements. Many new schools and colleges opened. The citizenry started buying more products in response to newspapers, magazines, and eventually movies that offered glimpses of "the good life." Westward expansion continued, highlighted by the completion of the transcontinental railroad. Massive numbers of European and British immigrants arrived, along with Asians on the West Coast. The Civil War (1861–1865) exacted a terrible toll of death, destruction, and disruption, but it led to legal affirmation of the ideal of racial equality, an important goal in American society ever since.

Participation in Physical Activity: 1840–1900

Liberal religious and philosophical currents had begun to flow together in the early decades of the 19th century, emphasizing that a human being's body, mind, and soul were an integrated whole. From this perspective, it was considered important to keep one's body healthy in order to achieve peak mental functioning as well as the highest possible level of moral reasoning. Some believed that good health practices indicated a morally righteous person in the eyes of God. This thinking, combined with squalid conditions in overcrowded cities and a nationalistic desire to make the United States self-sufficient, led to widespread efforts throughout most of the 19th century to improve people's health. Proper diet and exercise were among the recommended practices (Berryman, 1989; Whorton, 1982).

Physicians, writers, and teachers, addressing primarily the middle class and social elites, called for more vigorous physical activity—especially for boys and men. They coupled their notions of the importance of health reform with ideas from England about the value of sport for developing moral character and manliness. As the century progressed, physical activity grew increasingly attractive and popular.

Many professionals also recommended moderate exercises for improving the health of girls and women. However, straining too hard in exercise or competitive sports was usually considered unladylike and dangerous for women's physical well-being and future childbearing capabilities (Vertinsky, 1990). By the end of the 19th century, some girls and women were involved in more vigorous physical pursuits.

European systems of gymnastics, especially those from Germany and Sweden, gained an important American foothold during this time. German cultural societies called Turnvereins eventually offered well-equipped gymnastics facilities in many American cities. There were 148 of these by 1867 serving 10,200 members (Swanson &

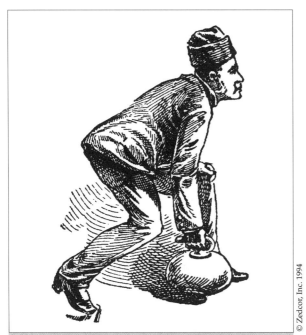

Curling stones gliding on ice, a favorite Scottish winter sport.

© Zedcor, Inc. 1994

Spears, 1995, p. 128). The centerpiece was exercise on heavy equipment such as parallel bars, vaulting horses, and hanging rings. By contrast, the Swedish system involved calisthenics and exercises with lighter equipment such as dumbbells, long wooden rods, and weights. Elements from both systems, as well as other exercise programs developed by Americans, grew increasingly popular in YMCAs, YWCAs, and city parks and playgrounds.

Sports were popular with many of the new immigrants who arrived in the United States from 1840 onward. They played American baseball, and when American football came on the scene later in the century, they played that too. Youngsters often learned American sports and games at local playgrounds, and many civic leaders hoped this would speed their assimilation into American society. However, immigrants also sought to keep the cultures of their homelands alive through participation in physical activities. Many belonged to special clubs where sports, exercise, and other recreations were often prominent. Examples in the city of Boston included the Boston Turnverein, featuring gymnastics and catering to German immigrants; the Caledonian Club, devoted to Scottish culture and including an array of sports and games such as caber toss, races, and pole vault; the Irish Athletic Club, the Irish-American Athletic Club, the Ancient Order of Hibernians, the Boston Hurling Club, and the Shamrock Hurling Club—all focusing on Irish sports and games, including oarsmen's regattas, stone throwing, and hurling; and cricket clubs formed by West Indian immigrants (Hardy, 1982, pp. 136–138).

Other immigrants took part in sports and amusements which, at the time, were considered less than respectable by members of the mainstream society. These included prize fighting, billiards, bowling, cycling, and wrestling. Prize fighting was dominated by the Irish for several decades, and later in the century boxing gyms could also be found in African American neighborhoods (Gorn, 1986; Hardy, 1982; Rader, 1990). After the Civil War, African Americans found their way into mainstream sports—professional baseball and horse racing, for example—but by 1890 racial prejudice forced most of them out.

In school and college physical activity classes, gymnastic exercise was preeminent. The Swedish and German systems were common, as well as other exercise programs developed by Americans that focused on calisthenics and lightweight equipment. Sports were not usually included in classes, but instead existed as extracurricular activities. Originally low-key intramural activities, they were a rich supplement to often stodgy exercise classes (Rudolph, 1962; Smith, 1988). Student-run intercollegiate competition appeared about mid-century and gathered steam in the 1870s. The most common intercollegiate sports were American football, crew, baseball, and track and field.

In the late 19th century, physical education programs focused on calisthenics; sports were not usually included in physical education classes. What types of activities have your physical education classes in high school and college included? What do you think caused the change between what was offered in the 1890s and what is offered today?

College and university administrators believed that intercollegiate sports could be helpful for recruiting new students, attracting alumni contributions, and promoting a sense of community among an increasingly diverse student body. According to thinking that arrived on American shores from England, sports could also develop leadership, vigorous manliness, and upstanding moral character, all qualities considered desirable for college men. For all of these reasons, athletics were believed to be too important to be left in the hands of students. Control was gradually taken over by campus administrators, faculty, and coaches.

During this era fewer sports opportunities were available for college women—occasional intercollegiate competition and somewhat more frequent intramural competition. Women who wanted to compete faced societal concerns about overly strenuous and highly competitive physical activities for women and girls. Sports in which injuries were more likely (football, for example) were avoided. Basketball, tennis, golf, and baseball were popular. Women's sports usually took place in secluded places with only a few specta-

tors present. A delicate balance had to be struck between making competition available to college women and keeping the activities acceptable to faculty and campus administrators (Park, 1987c).

Beyond schools and colleges, by the 1860s many amateur baseball teams were on their way to becoming professionalized; common practices by that time included charging admission and paying players. Baseball had an avid following, and newspapers gave it the most coverage of any sport (Adelman, 1986, p. 174). In the 1880s the most popular sports were horse racing, baseball, and prize fighting (Oriard, 1993, p. 60).

American athletes also competed in a new amateur event developed by Europeans and first held in Athens, Greece, in 1896—the modern Olympic Games. The United States fielded a team of 10 male track and field competitors—all collegians or ex-collegians—who participated in the fledgling Games; they chalked up 9 victories in 12 events, along with 5 second-place finishes (Smith, 1988, pp. 115–116).

American interest in physical activity—for example, gymnastic exercises, baseball, football, crew, track and field, horse racing, boxing, bicycling, and less-well-known sports tied closely to people's ethnic origins—grew throughout the 19th century.

Physical Activity Professions: 1840–1900

An identifiable physical activity profession didn't appear in the United States until late in the 19th century. Nevertheless, a variety of practitioners in earlier decades focused at least some of their work on physical activity. These included physicians, successful athletes, journalists, educators, ministers, health reform advocates, business entrepreneurs, and a handful of European gymnastics specialists who immigrated to the United States. Some of them wrote about the physical, intellectual, and moral benefits of exercise and sport. Some developed exercise programs in schools and colleges. Others worked to establish various European gymnastics systems on American soil. Some wrote popular self-help manuals on achieving healthy lifestyles that included "how-to" information on exercise routines. A few became professional athletes in sports such as horse racing, pedestrianism (long-distance walking), boxing, and baseball. Some tried to sort out the best training techniques for athletic success. Some became coaches. And some bankrolled professional sports (Adelman, 1986; Berryman, 1989; Gorn, 1986; Park, 1992; Whorton, 1982).

By the 1880s a climate of intense interest in exercise and sport that had been building throughout much of the century existed in the United States. In addition, numerous professions were beginning to organize in response to the growing need for people with specialized knowledge and skills in technologically based businesses and industries. There were efforts to develop more stringent educational standards for new practitioners.

In this atmosphere, the physical education teaching profession took root (Park, 1987b), the first recognizable physical activity profession in the United States. In 1885 the American Association for the Advancement of Physical Education was formed by about 60 people who wanted to have an organization that would promote the new profession (Park, 1981; Swanson & Spears, 1995, pp. 181–182). After several name changes, it is today known as the American Alliance for Health, Physical Education, Recreation and Dance, an important professional association for practitioners in several fields.

Several physical education teacher training programs were inaugurated, primarily in the Northeast, and they varied in length from a few weeks to about two years. Some of the most famous were the Sanatory Gymnasium (opened near Harvard in 1881 by Dudley Sargent, and in 1894 renamed the Normal School of Physical Training); the Harvard Summer School of Physical Education (opened in 1887 by Dudley Sargent); and the Boston Normal School of Gymnastics (opened in 1889 by Mary Hemenway and Amy Morris Homans)(Gerber, 1971). Around the turn of the century, several four-year bachelor's degree programs were initiated for the preparation of physical education teachers (Rice, Hutchinson, & Lee, 1969).

The earliest identifiable American physical activity profession—teaching physical education—was established in the late 19th century during a period of high interest in physical activity among the general public.

Scholarly Knowledge About Physical Activity: 1840–1900

Scientific discoveries in the 19th century produced a lot of new information about human anatomy and physiology. By the 1840s improved microscopes permitted more detailed studies of phenomena such as oxygen transport in blood, energy transformation in muscles, and the anatomy and functioning of the nervous system (Park, 1987b, p. 144). Later in the century, such information was occasionally used by scholars who wanted a better understanding of the biological effects of physical activity on the human body. Educators also sometimes incorporated this knowledge into physical education teacher training programs.

For example, Edward Hartwell, an associate in physical training and director of the gymnasium at Johns Hopkins University, published an article in 1887 titled "On the Physiology of Exercise" (Gerber, 1971; Park, 1987a, 1987b). George Fitz, an instructor and researcher in physiology and hygiene at Harvard University, established a four-year undergraduate program in "Anatomy, Physiology, and Physical Training" (Park, 1987b). Not far from Harvard, the Boston Normal School of Gymnastics—a two-year physical education teacher training institution that attracted mostly female students—offered a curriculum focused on Swedish gymnastics that also included a variety of basic science courses taught by well-known scholars from major universities around Boston (Gerber, 1971; Park, 1987b). This excursion into the biological sciences by early leaders in physical education is important because it demonstrates the value they placed on developing a scientific base for the emerging physical education teaching profession (Park, 1987b).

Despite this new interest in the sciences, scientific curriculums were outnumbered by professional programs focused on learning physical activities and how to teach them. By the end of the 19th century the emphasis was clearly on the professional programs, as well as on the positive social values that students could learn through participating in play and sports. Investigations into the biological mechanisms underlying physical activity were not completely curtailed, but it was not until the 1960s that scientific information again moved to center stage in college and university physical education curriculums (Park, 1987b).

One of the most interesting fads in American history occurred when people's fascination with bicycling mushroomed in the mid-1890s. This brief craze blossomed between 1893 and 1896. City dwellers used their "silent steeds" to commute to work, have fun on local streets, escape on short jaunts through the countryside, and take longer tours involving overnight stays. Delivery boys rode bicycles; police sometimes used them to patrol; postmen occasionally delivered mail on them; physicians, ministers, and salesmen rode them to call on people; and at least one ambulance service experimented with them (Harmond, 1971–1972; Smith, 1972).

At the peak of the fad in 1896, there were approximately four million cyclists in the United States (Harmond, 1971–1972), about 1 out of every 18 people. At first glance, this figure may not seem very impressive, but the ratio is based on the entire American population— country folks as well as city dwellers. The percentage of riders was much higher in the cities. Estimates of the yearly bicycle production demonstrate the rise and decline of the frenzy (Harmond, 1971–1972; Tobin, 1974):

1890	40,000
1896	1,200,000
1904	225,000

In the six years between 1890 and 1896 a whopping thirtyfold increase in production occurred! Although the number of new bicycles remained steady at about a million each year through the late 1890s, the softening of the American market after 1896 led manufacturers to export more to other countries (Harmond, 1971–1972).

Bicycles had been in the United States as early as 1819, but it was not until the "safety" bicycle was perfected in the late 1880s that people's cycling passions were sparked (Hardy, 1982). Earlier versions were uncomfortable, difficult to balance, and unsafe; they appealed primarily to men with athletic ambitions. Manufacturers brought together a number of technological advances to make bicycles safer: the frame was stronger and made of lighter steel tubing; the chain and sprocket system was well suited for propulsion; the saddle was better balanced between two equal-sized wheels; the ball bearings in the wheel hubs reduced wear; the pneumatic (air-filled) rubber tires reduced vibration; and the coaster break improved the ability to stop (Harmond, 1971–1972; Smith, 1972). The new bicycle was a testament to the mechanical advances that had been occurring since mid-century when the industrial revolution spread to North America.

In addition, the bicycle industry aggressively promoted its new machine. The goal was to inoculate the population with desire—especially a desire for "this year's model." The task was challenging because current models were sometimes no better mechanically than ones from the previous year—the changes were often cosmetic. The industry's promotional campaign featured advertisements in trade journals, major daily newspapers, and upscale magazines. In addition, new bicycles were displayed at annual trade shows in major cities; racing events and successful racers were subsidized; and promotional contests were held for consumers (Harmond, 1971–1972; Smith, 1972). All of this helped the bicycle industry create consumers for its product (Hardy, 1982), a practice that became critical to most industries in the 20th century.

Bicycles also caught on because they resonated well with problems and concerns facing urban residents. Bicycling was thought to be a "tonic for the mental stress of business life in the city," offering exercise, plenty of fresh air, and escape from urban problems (Hardy, 1982, p. 162; Harmond, 1971–1972; Tobin, 1974). Enjoyment of intoxicating freedom while spinning through city streets and parks, or touring for several

→

days in the countryside, added a new dimension to leisure. A large number of cycling clubs brought people together for friendship, recreation, and the promotion of cycling. And most physicians recommended cycling to improve circulation, strengthen lungs, and improve muscle tone (Smith, 1972).

An overarching fascination with speed—and thoughts about greater speed, saving time, and progress—also drew city people to bicycles. Rapid transportation and communication—for example, railroads and telegraph—had proven to be indispensable to the development of the nation. New equipment such as typewriters, high-speed presses, and sewing machines saved time at work. In this context, the speed with which people could travel on bicycles was another sign of progress (Harmond, 1971–1972).

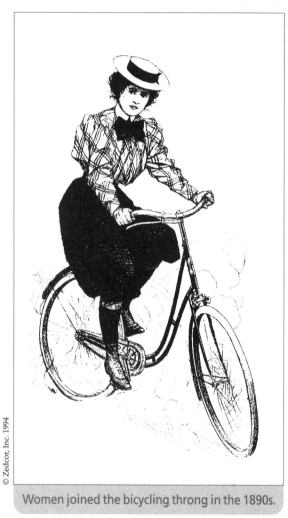

© Zedcor, Inc. 1994

Women joined the bicycling throng in the 1890s.

Attracted to the late-19th-century ideal of an independent and adventuresome New Woman, many middle-class and society women eagerly took up cycling. Although there were special concerns about their health, as well as what they should wear, the flood of women on bicycles presented daily displays of new styles of dress (including split skirts and bloomers) and new levels of independence (Smith, 1972).

In spite of people's massive commercial and emotional investments in cycling, the craze was not long-lived. By the end of the century, a new machine promised even faster and more comfortable transportation—the automobile. Reliable interurban railways also moved people from the suburbs to the central city without the extra demands of cycling—the effort of exercise and the special clothes required (Harmond, 1971–1972; Smith, 1972). Although bicycles were no longer on the cutting edge of progress, the bicycle craze had contributed to the development of consumerism and tourism, and both of these would become important and pervasive in 20th-century American society.

Scholarly knowledge about physical activity—mostly information from the biological and physical sciences—became important in a few professional teaching training curriculums in the late 19th century, but in most programs this took a back seat to learning physical activities and practical knowledge about how to teach them.

Physical Activity in the United States: 1900–1950

In the first half of the 20th century, American industry perfected mass production and churned out a wide variety of consumer goods from automobiles to canned food to refrigerators. With readily available products, entrepreneurs stepped up their advertising to encourage the general public to become enthusiastic consumers. Many new immigrants—especially from Southern Europe—arrived on American shores, adding more ethnic diversity to our already multifaceted population. American society made progress toward the democratic ideal of equal opportunity and social justice: Women got the right to vote, and African Americans were hired in greater numbers for federally funded jobs. However, full achievement of social equity remained distant and elusive. The severe economic depression that began in 1929 left personal, lifelong scars on massive numbers of Americans who suffered through it. And many other horrible and unforgettable disruptions occurred during World War I (1914–1918) and World War II (1939–1945).

Participation in Physical Activity: 1900–1950

Competitive sports were in the limelight during the first half of the 20th century. Professional baseball, professional boxing, horse racing, and American collegiate football—all men's sports—were especially popular with fans. Professional baseball's American League and National League joined forces in 1903 to keep player salaries in check and reduce competition for fan loyalty. American professional football and basketball gained a degree of prominence by the 1930s, although they were still fledgling enterprises. World War II temporarily put a damper on men's professional athletics because most healthy young men were drafted. This spurred Chicago Cubs owner and chewing gum magnate Philip K. Wrigley to organize the All-American Girls' Baseball League that played in the Midwest from 1943 to 1954 (Guttmann, 1991; Lucas & Smith, 1978).

Intercollegiate athletics were dominated by American football during this era. Major college games received widespread news coverage, and they were occasions for lively partying and revelry. By 1903 Harvard had a stadium that could seat 40,000 fans (Smith, 1988, p. 169), and by 1930 seven of the concrete giants on college campuses could hold over 70,000 people (Rader, 1990, p. 182).

Competitive sports for boys were also common in high schools, elementary schools, playgrounds, and youth service agencies such as YMCAs. By the 1930s elementary school competition began to decline when physical education teachers complained about the high stress of competition. Many people still wanted competition for young-

sters, however, and the void was filled by new programs designed by city recreation departments and organizations such as Little League Baseball, Inc. (formed in 1939), and Biddy Basketball (formed in 1950)(Berryman, 1975).

Girls' and women's sports were subdued in comparison to the publicity and hoopla connected with major boys' and men's events. A few women achieved national and international success in sports such as tennis, basketball, golf, long-distance swimming, and track and field. For the most part, they trained and competed outside the educational system in settings such as private country clubs and industry-sponsored leagues. For example, in 1930 Mildred "Babe" Didrikson was offered a job as a stenographer at Employers Casualty Insurance Company in Dallas so that she could play for the company's Golden Cyclones basketball team. The company also sponsored her to compete at the Amateur Athletic Union's national track and field championships in 1932. Her phenomenal success led her to the 1932 Olympics where she won two gold medals and a silver (Guttmann, 1991).

In schools and colleges during the 1920s, women physical educators turned toward intramural sports and low-key "extramural" competition for girls and women. They wanted to avoid the stress of high-level competition and encourage all girls and women to participate. Although a few institutions continued to sponsor elite sports for females, "fun and games" became the goal at most schools and colleges, and this greatly curtailed the development of elite female athletes in educational settings. Things didn't begin to change until the late 1950s.

Public interest in competitive sports was so pronounced in the early decades of the 20th century that sports replaced gymnastic exercises as the centerpiece in most school and college physical education curriculums. A large number of physical education teachers believed that student participation in sports would help develop high moral character and other qualities needed to be a good citizen. And students seemed more interested in physical activities that were sparked with competitive excitement, compared to the tedium of repetitious, traditional gymnastic exercises.

Exercise did not completely disappear from physical education classes, however. Teachers sometimes replaced the old gymnastics systems with expressive movements designed to

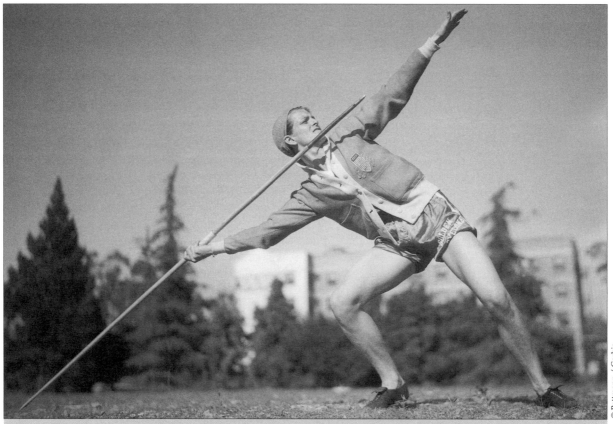

Mildred "Babe" Didrikson, 1932 Olympic champion.

© Bettmann / Corbis

communicate ideas and feelings, or with sport-related exercises such as shooting baskets or batting baseballs (Van Dalen & Bennett, 1971, p. 460). By the 1920s "corrective" physical education classes also offered special exercises to students with posture, fitness, and health challenges (Van Dalen & Bennett, 1971, pp. 461, 468).

The United States military recognized the need for physical training during World War I, when approximately one-third of U.S. draftees were initially declared unfit to serve. Moreover, overseas hospitals were deluged with recruits with musculoskeletal incapacities such as flat feet and backaches. Recreational sports—organized by about 345 military athletic directors—were widespread and popular with the troops (Murphy, 1995; Rice, Hutchinson, & Lee, 1969).

Physical education teachers on the home front added military training such as marching drills and calisthenics to school and college physical education programs. People could also exercise by following an instructor on the radio. Recognition of the poor physical condition of the troops served as a wake-up call after the war, and this

spurred the expansion of school and college physical activity programs (Murphy, 1995; Rice, Hutchinson, & Lee, 1969; Van Dalen & Bennett, 1971; Welch, 1996).

Racial discrimination eliminated most African Americans from the highest levels of competitive sport by 1900. In spite of this, a few were active in boxing (Jack Johnson and Joe Louis were heavyweight champions); a small number participated in intercollegiate athletics at predominantly white schools; a few competed in the National Football League until 1933 when racial barriers were raised; and a handful took part in the Olympic Games (track star Jesse Owens won four gold medals in the 1936 Berlin Games). African American baseball players had no choice but to play for African American teams until Jackie Robinson signed with the Brooklyn Dodgers in 1945 and played on one of their minor-league teams in 1946; he moved up to the Dodgers in 1947.

Cultural heritage also influenced the sport involvement of people in many other racial and ethnic minority groups. For example, baseball, basketball, and boxing served as a "middle ground" for second-generation Jews, providing at the same time a place to celebrate Jewish heritage and a place to assimilate into mainstream American society (Levine, 1992, pp. 3–25, 270–274). First-generation Japanese immigrants who arrived early in the 20th century often used traditional perspectives from their homeland to make sense of American sports, sometimes recalling samurai (historic Japanese knight-warriors) principles of courage and honor (Regalado, 1992).

> Think of as many examples as you can of groups of people with a particular ethnic heritage getting together to: (1) play or watch sports associated with their own cultural heritage and (2) play or watch sports that are widely popular in the United States. Is there any overlap between your two lists? Why do you think there are such overlaps?

World War II renewed people's interest in exercise. After the war, educators expanded many school and college physical activity curriculums in response to weaknesses observed in the fitness of wartime military recruits, and sports were again at center stage (Swanson & Spears, 1995).

> Sports—in elite-level competition, community recreation programs, and school and college physical education classes—were Americans' favorite physical activities in the first half of the 20th century. Americans paid less attention to exercise, although interest picked up during the two world wars in order to improve physical fitness.

Physical Activity Professions: 1900–1950

Bachelor's degree programs in physical education grew in the early 1900s, expanding to about 135 by 1927 (Park, 1980). Master's degrees were available just after the turn of the century, and doctoral programs began in the 1920s. Undergraduate programs focused on training physical education teachers, continuing the trend that had started in the late 19th century. Graduate pro-

grams offered advanced training for teachers, as well as the academic preparation to become a college or university faculty member. The quality of these programs improved as research on physical activity picked up in the late 1920s.

Despite the popularity of sports during the first half of the 20th century, college and university physical education curriculums didn't include much course work to prepare students for the occupations of coach or athletic trainer. Coaches most often came from the ranks of successful athletes. If they worked in a school or college, they were often required to teach physical education classes as well, so they earned the necessary college degrees and professional teacher certifications.

The few athletic trainers on the scene during this period had little formal education in health care. In colleges and universities, they often began as a gymnasium jack-of-all-trades with custodial responsibilities as well as other duties such as repairing equipment and facilities, laundering clothes, driving the team bus, and maintaining outdoor playing fields. They sometimes met their counterparts from other institutions at intercollegiate athletic events and shared training techniques (Smith, 1979). Because elite sports were primarily for boys and men, most coaches and athletic trainers were men.

The Cramer Company, founded in 1922, identified a commercial niche and began selling liniment for sprains as well as other products for athletic training. In 1933 Cramer inaugurated *The First Aider*, which soon became a popular newsletter aimed at helping high school coaches understand training techniques. For many years, Cramer also sponsored educational seminars for athletic trainers. The profession grew, but it wasn't until 1950 that a professional organization was founded—the National Athletic Trainers Association (Smith, 1979).

Interest in physical therapy was sparked by the outbreak of World War I. By the end of the war, United States military reconstruction aides—an entirely female corps of therapists trained to help the war wounded—were receiving training in massage, anatomy, remedial exercise, hydrotherapy, electrotherapy, bandaging, kinesiology, ethics, and the psychological effects of injuries. In 1921 the reconstruction aides formed the American Women's Physical Therapeutic Association, the organization that eventually became the present-day American Physical Therapy Association, the main professional association for physical therapists (Murphy, 1995, pp. 54, 71).

Teaching physical education continued to be the main profession for which students were prepared in college physical education programs during the first half of the 20th century; bachelor's degree programs increased in number, and master's and doctoral programs came on the scene.

Scholarly Knowledge About Physical Activity: 1900–1950

At the turn of the century, a number of scholars were investigating topics such as neuromuscular fatigue, the vascular effects of exercise, kinesiology (today called functional anatomy or biomechanics), body measurements and proportions, the psychological aspects of play, and the history of physical education and sport (Park, 1981). However, it was the late 1920s before research on physical activity gained more visibility. Investigations were conducted by faculty members in physical education as well as other disciplines. The prestigious Harvard Fatigue Laboratory, focused on research in exercise physiology, opened in 1927. The *Research Quarterly*, a scholarly journal devoted to physical activity, began in 1930. One issue in 1934 contained the following topics: "physiology of respiration, reflex/reaction time, measurement of motor ability, effects of temperature on muscular activity, and test construction" (Park, 1980, p. 5). Due to the importance of teacher training in college and university physical education departments, physical educators often did research that could be applied to teaching. For example, studies of techniques for assessing motor skills could be used to help teachers develop ways to evaluate student progress.

A handful of physical educators began doing research on aspects of physical activity not centrally applicable to teaching. For example, Charles McCloy initiated work at the University of Iowa to examine what he thought were the more basic factors underlying physical activity such as "motor ability" and "motor capacity" (Gerber, 1971); T.K. Cureton developed an extensive research program on physical fitness at the

University of Illinois (Buskirk & Tipton, 1997); and Franklin Henry conducted work on metabolic responses to exercise at the University of California, Berkeley (Park, 1981). Research on topics not closely allied with teaching continued to grow in the 1940s and 1950s, but it was not until the 1960s that such research mushroomed.

Research on physical activity started to expand in the late 1920s. Most physical educators studied topics relevant to teaching physical education; a few examined other aspects of physical activity.

Physical Activity in the United States: 1950–2000

In the second half of the 20th century, electronic communication expanded at a breathtaking pace. Television—in its infancy in 1950—became a common fixture in most homes in less than two decades. Digital computers grew from massive, room-sized arrays of vacuum tubes with limited capabilities, to tiny but enormously powerful collections of memory chips and electronic displays. Communications satellites were placed in orbit, greatly simplifying intercontinental communication. Air travel became faster and easier. Global trade expanded, accompanied by greater worldwide political and economic interdependence. New immigrants continued to arrive in the United States—especially from Asia and Latin America. Progress was made toward the American democratic ideal of equal opportunity and social justice—federal civil rights legislation mandated greater equality in education, business, and housing. Nevertheless, complete achievement of this goal remained elusive. The Cold War between communist and capitalist countries was a worldwide reality for over 40 years. The Korean War (1950–1953) and the Vietnam War (1960s–1975) were hot, disruptive episodes in the Cold War. However, communism unraveled after the fall of the Berlin Wall in 1989, leading to vast global changes in political and economic relations.

Participation in Physical Activity: 1950–2000

A dramatic increase in health-related exercise began in the United States in the 1950s and continued for several decades. A number of events contributed to this. The Korean War again underscored the importance of physical fitness for military preparedness. The USSR's 1957 launch of Sputnik—the first earth satellite—graphically displayed the continuing threat of communism. A highly publicized 1953 report showed that over 50% of American children failed a strength and flexibility test, compared to less than 10% from European countries. After President Eisenhower's heart attacks in the mid-1950s, people were well aware that his doctor prescribed exercise for recovery, a radical idea at the time. And in the early 1960s President Kennedy continuously demonstrated an active lifestyle—touch football, tennis, swimming, sailing, horseback riding, badminton, and general exercise (Rader, 1990, p. 242).

By one estimate, commercial health clubs increased from 350 in 1968 to over 7,000 in 1986 (Rader, 1990, p. 243). By another, the number of health clubs and physical fitness centers was about 24,000 in the late 1980s (Eitzen & Sage, 1993, p. 390). Marathon races throughout the United States increased from fewer than 25 in 1970 to over 250 in 1996. Between 1980 and 1996, road races covering shorter distances increased from 4,100 to over 20,000 (Eitzen & Sage, 1997, p. 316). Adult membership in commercial and nonprofit health, racquet, and sports clubs reportedly grew by a whopping 51% between 1987 and 1996, increasing from about 13.8 million to about 20.8 million (Carey & Mullins, 1997).

The proportion of children and adults who said they did something on a daily basis to help keep physically fit rose from 24% in 1961 to 59% in 1984. Conversely, adults who said they had a sedentary lifestyle dropped from 41% in 1971 to 27% in 1985. Activity levels increased by greater amounts for people over the age of 50 than for younger adults, although older Americans were still less active. The trend was also more pronounced among women than men (Blair, Mulder, & Kohl, 1987; Ramlow, Kriska, & LaPorte, 1987; Stephens, 1987). These increases leveled off in the 1990s, and it is hard to predict in what direction things will move in the future (U.S. Department of Health and Human Services, 1996, p. 186).

Americans' well-established fascination with sports grew more widespread—both for participants and spectators—in the latter half of the 20th century. For example, between 1950 and 1996 the number of youngsters competing in Little League

Baseball, Inc., increased by more than 140 times, from 18,300 to 2,571,330. This was staggering in light of the much smaller growth in the population of 10- to 14-year-olds in the United States (from 11,119,000 to 17,060,000 between 1950 and 1990) (U.S. Bureau of the Census, 1961, 1996; Little League Baseball, Inc., personal communication, May 1997). In the last two decades of the century, the number of youngsters playing soccer sponsored by the American Youth Soccer Organization, Soccer Association for Youth, and the United States Youth Soccer Association grew by 3.4 times from 888,705 in 1980 to 2,983,826 in 1995 (Soccer Industry Council of America, personal communication, May 1997).

Elite athletic competition for girls and women reappeared in high schools and colleges beginning in the late 1950s. In 1972 the United States Congress approved Title IX of the 1972 Education Amendments to the 1964 Civil Rights Act, requiring equal opportunity for males and females in educational programs—including athletic programs (Swanson & Spears, 1995). Between 1971 and 1995 participation in athletic competition among high school girls increased 600% from 294,015 to 2,240,461. During the same period, the number of boys in high school athletics actually declined slightly (Eitzen & Sage, 1997, p. 292). Similar dramatic increases occurred in the number of female players in colleges and universities.

In the 1950s African Americans trickled back into elite professional athletics, and by the 1960s this trickle grew to a fast-moving stream. African Americans constituted about 10% of the players in professional baseball, basketball, and football in the late 1950s. These proportions diverged in the 1960s, and by 1994, 77% of the basketball players were African American, along with 65% of the football players, and 18% of those in baseball (Eitzen & Sage, 1997, p. 264; Leonard, 1998, p. 212). In addition, Latinos comprised about 17% of the baseball players in 1993 (Coakley, 1994, p. 251), and by the late 1990s several Japanese players had joined major-league teams.

Enthusiasm for outdoor physical recreation skyrocketed during this period. Between the mid-1960s and the mid-1970s the increase in interest was so rapid that it sometimes outstripped manufacturers' ability to supply people with proper clothes and equipment. Cross-country skiers increased from about 2,000 in 1964 to 500,000 in

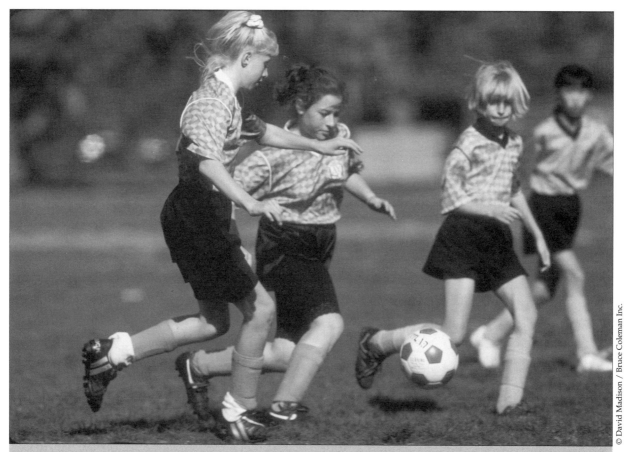

© David Madison / Bruce Coleman Inc.

Organized sports for youngsters mushroomed in the second half of the 20th century.

1974. Backpacking at Kings Canyon and Sequoia National Parks in California increased 100% between 1968 and 1971. Visitors at New Hampshire's White Mountain National Forest zoomed from 234,000 in 1968 to 482,000 in 1972. Bike paths in the United States went from almost none in 1965 to over 24,140 km (15,000 miles) in 1974 (Wilson, 1977).

Americans also increased their spectator involvement. Attendance at Major League Baseball games was four times greater in 1993 than it was in 1950. Professional football attendance mushroomed to 7.4 times its size during the same period. And attendance at professional basketball games in 1993 was a whopping 9.6 times larger than in 1960. These increases far outstripped a more modest U.S. population growth over the same period (U.S. Bureau of the Census, 1966, 1996).

Although soccer is a preeminent spectator sport throughout most of the world, it didn't gain much of a foothold in the United States as an entertainment event until the 1990s. The final rounds of the 1994 World Cup were held on American soil, and in 1996 entrepreneurs developed a relatively stable professional league—Major League Soccer—with teams that held special allure for Latino spectators (Brewington, 1998; O'Connor, 1999).

By the early 1960s Roone Arledge, head of sports programming at ABC, was incorporating the highly innovative and popular instant replay technique into sports broadcasts. He unveiled additional novel production technologies—for example, close-ups of players and fans, multiple cameras, and directional microphones—in 1970 with the inauguration of ABC's *Monday Night Football* (Gorn & Goldstein, 1993, p. 239). These made televised sports much more exciting to watch and drew new spectators. The commercial success of sports on TV—primarily men's team sports—provided vast amounts of money for professional and big-time intercollegiate athletics.

The Internet took off with phenomenal growth in the 1990s. Anyone with a computer attached to phone lines had instantaneous access to worldwide news and discussions about sports through electronic chat rooms and Web sites.

 Americans' enthusiasm—both as direct participants and as spectators—for a widening array of sports and exercise mushroomed in the second half of the 20th century.

Think of all the sports and exercise programs you have (1) participated in directly and (2) watched as a spectator throughout your lifetime. Which list is longer? Why did you do more of the one than of the other?

Physical Activity Professions: 1950–2000

At mid-century, most American college students who majored in physical education—the name used almost universally at the time—became high school teachers, and some also coached. Things began to change in the mid-1960s with the development of kinesiology—the body of knowledge about physical activity that included many different scholarly subdisciplines. It soon became apparent that there were a lot of other careers centered in physical activity. Let's look at a few examples.

With the growing American interest in exercise and physical fitness, it is little wonder that new health clubs, cardiopulmonary rehabilitation programs, worksite health promotion programs, and health maintenance organizations began offering physical activity programs. People with specialized training in exercise began working in a variety of jobs such as cardiopulmonary rehabilitation, personal training, aerobics instruction, and strength training. Some rapidly advanced to management and business ownership roles.

Certification of practitioners is important because it helps ensure professional competence. Two of the most demanding certifying bodies for exercise specialists are the American College of Sports Medicine (founded in 1954) and the Na-

tional Strength and Conditioning Association (founded in 1978 as the National Strength Coaches Association). In 1974 ACSM began certifying practitioners, and by 1995 it had awarded 10,896 certifications (Berryman, 1995, p. 333). The NSCA began its strength and conditioning certification program in 1985, and by the end of 1999 it had awarded 11,570 certified strength and conditioning specialist certifications and 2,990 certified personal trainer certifications.

The National Athletic Trainers Association was founded in 1950 to support the growing number of specialists who worked to prevent and treat athletic injuries. The membership was almost entirely men until 1972 when Title IX (requiring equal opportunity for males and females in educational settings) became law, encouraging women to enter the field in greater numbers. As of 1995 there were about 125 NATA-accredited degree programs—a mixture of master's and bachelor's programs—and about 12,700 NATA-certified athletic trainers (Paul Grace, National Athletic Trainers Association Board of Certification, personal communication, April 5, 1995; National Athletic Trainers Association Board of Certification, personal communication, April 4, 1995).

At mid-century there was little by way of standard educational preparation for most careers in sport management and leadership. As you already know, the sport industry experienced enormous growth during the second half of the 20th century. As a result, there were more jobs, and a wider variety of jobs, in sport settings. Job opportunities were available, for example, with intercollegiate athletic departments, professional athletic teams, city stadiums, and participant-oriented nonprofit organizations such as Boys and Girls Clubs and YMCAs. Some jobs didn't even require a college degree (e.g., ticket sales in minor-league baseball, YMCA program leader), while some required extensive high-level leadership experience and/or advanced degrees (e.g., big-time intercollegiate athletics director, city arena or stadium manager). This unevenness made it difficult to accredit degree programs or certify practitioners.

Nevertheless, in 1987 the National Association for Sport and Physical Education (affiliated with AAHPERD, the American Alliance for Health, Physical Education, Recreation and Dance) and the North American Society for Sport Management jointly published curriculum guidelines for

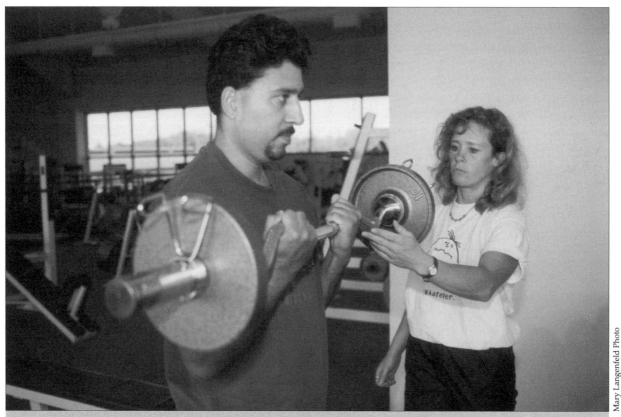

Growing interest in physical fitness has led to an increase in jobs in this area.

Mary Langenfeld Photo

bachelor's and master's degree programs in sport management. These were revised in 1993 and published as voluntary accreditation standards. It is not yet clear whether these will promote higher standards and greater uniformity in the educational preparation of sport managers.

Physical therapy continued to grow as a profession. The number of physical therapy jobs in the United States in 1960 was estimated to be 8,000; this grew over twelvefold by 1994 to 102,000 (Bureau of Labor Statistics, 1961, 1996). In the 1950s students were trained in undergraduate physical therapy degree programs, or in older, hospital-based certificate programs designed for people who had competed a bachelor's degree in another field. By the late 20th century, hospital-based programs were phased out, undergraduate programs were in decline, and master's programs were on the rise. In 1981 accredited physical therapy curriculums included 100 undergraduate degree programs, 7 certificate programs, and 8 master's programs (Bureau of Labor Statistics, 1982, p. 166). In 1995, only 14 years later, there were 65 undergraduate programs and

80 master's programs (Bureau of Labor Statistics, 1996, p. 170).

Most college students majoring in physical education in the middle of the 20th century entered the same profession—physical education teaching; by the end of the century, students had a wide array of physical activity careers to choose from.

Scholarly Knowledge About Physical Activity: 1950–2000

Scholars developed new knowledge about physical activity at a feverish pace during the final 35 years of the 20th century, a trend that is continuing today. You will learn a lot more about this in the chapters of this text on the other scholarly subdisciplines—each has a section on history. Here we'll focus on the big picture.

By the 1950s researchers had already produced a lot of information about physical activity. Problematically, knowledge was scattered throughout many different research journals, and no one had taken the time to make it easily accessible. Warren Johnson, Professor of Health Education and Physical Education at the University of Maryland, attempted in 1960 to remedy this by publishing a book titled *Science and Medicine of Exercise and Sports*. It contained 36 essays summarizing current knowledge. Another early attempt at organizing research knowledge appeared in the May 1960 supplement to the *Research Quarterly*. Edited by several scholars headed by Raymond Weiss of New York University, each paper summarized research concerning a different aspect of physical activity (Karpovich, Morehouse, Scott, & Weiss, 1960).

Calls from politicians and educators in the early 1960s for better quality control in college and university teacher education programs resulted in scrutiny and criticism of physical education curriculums because they were mostly teacher education programs at the time. In response to this, physical education faculty began charting new directions for their discipline. Franklin Henry, a physical education professor at the University of California and top-notch scholar in exercise physiology and motor learning, published a paper outlining his views on the nature of the discipline titled "Physical Education: An Academic Discipline" (1964).

As discussed in chapter 13, Henry envisioned a body of knowledge about physical activity that would draw from "such diverse fields as anatomy, physics and physiology, cultural anthropology, history and sociology, as well as psychology" (p. 32). He also believed that the discipline should be cross-disciplinary. By that he meant it should bond together knowledge from various disciplines to form a distinct, new body of knowledge concerning human movement.

Henry's vision of the discipline spurred rapid changes during the rest of the 1960s and 1970s. A nucleus of physical educators who were already heavily engaged in research began pushing to make scholarship more central in university physical education departments. They continued their own research, and they trained a new cadre of doctoral students who expected to be centrally involved in inquiry throughout their own careers. They communicated frequently with scholars in other disciplines—for example, physiology, medicine, psychology, history—who were also studying physical activity. This led to rapid growth in the size and scope of the body of knowledge.

The knowledge also became more specialized, and this soon led to the formation of subdisciplines. By 1970 the earliest ones were clearly identified, and most of the others were on the drawing boards. You already know the names of the subdisciplines and how they fit together to form the scholarly source of knowledge in the discipline. Throughout the rest of the 20th century, scholars formed many new associations and worked with publishers to inaugurate a host of new research journals to support the growing subdisciplines (see figure 1.13). In the 1980s and 1990s the amount and quality of research continued to increase, and the subdisciplines became stronger and more identifiable (Massengale & Swanson, 1997; Park, 1981, 1989).

Beginning in the 1960s the discipline of kinesiology grew rapidly and branched into numerous scholarly subdisciplines.

Wrap-Up

History extends your "memory" with fascinating, evidence-based stories about how and why physical activities such as exercise and sports came to be shaped the way they are. Knowledge of the past gives you important, broad understandings about the present that you can use to make better-informed personal and professional decisions for the future. Since the 1970s scholars have gone beyond earlier descriptive approaches to put more emphasis on analytical frameworks that help answer questions about why things happened as they did. So far, this subdiscipline has focused mostly on sport, but since the 1980s scholars have given greater attention to exercise.

If you are intrigued by what you have learned here, you might have fun venturing into sport history textbooks, taking an introductory course, looking through the book-length research studies mentioned in this chapter, and leafing through the major journals such as the *Journal of Sport History* and the *International Journal of the History of Sport*. This interesting and provocative subdiscipline will give you a new outlook that will help enrich your understanding of physical activities as you step into the future.

Study Questions

1. List and discuss the goals of history of physical activity.

2. Describe the expanding research directions in history of physical activity from 1970 to the present.

3. List and discuss the three stages in research focused on history of physical activity.

4. Describe participation in physical activity in the United States during the following three periods: 1840–1900, 1900–1950, 1950–2000.

5. What factors led to the bicycle craze of the 1890s? Give some examples of evidence that there was, indeed, a greatly increased interest in bicycling during that time.

6. Describe professional practice centered in physical activity in the United States during the following three periods: 1840–1900, 1900–1950, 1950–2000.

7. Describe scholarly knowledge about physical activity during the following three periods: 1840–1900, 1900–1950, 1950–2000.

7

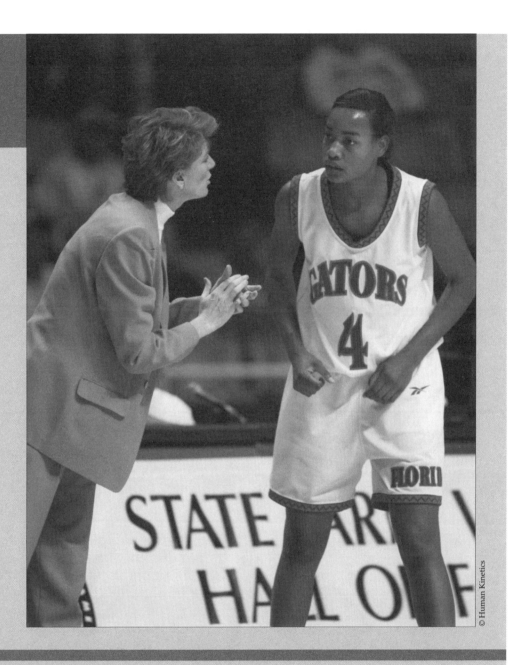

© Human Kinetics

Sociology of Physical Activity

Janet C. Harris

In this chapter . . .

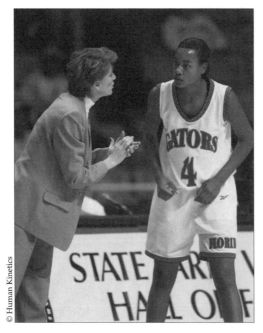

© Human Kinetics

You're the coach of a top-ranked women's college basketball team. Your team gets strong media coverage and enjoys tremendous fan support. You learn from Shanna James (not the player pictured here), a sophomore who is one of your best players, that she's interested in coaching college basketball after she graduates. You have known Shanna since she was a junior in high school and have helped her blossom into a top collegiate player who after another two years might have the skills to play professionally. Over the years you have developed an especially close relationship with Shanna and know her well enough to see that she will strive to excel in whatever career she chooses, but you want her to consider all her options carefully. You realize that before sitting down with her to discuss her future, you have some questions to answer for yourself: What are Shanna's chances of entering college coaching? What should she know about the job market? Are coaching opportunities for women better or worse than they were 5 or 10 years ago? With whom would she be competing for jobs? Should she apply to both women's and men's programs? How would she fare in other occupations such as playing basketball professionally, telecasting games, or officiating? You realize that getting all of these questions answered for Shanna is going to take some time and research.

Why Sociology of Physical Activity?

Many of our physical activities (e.g., circuit training, 10K fun runs, aerobic exercise classes, American football, X-Games, tennis, and clogging) revolve around interaction with other people. Without these opportunities for social interaction, our physical activities would be very different. Most of us would probably engage in basic movements such as walking, running, and jumping, but if we never interacted with others—never watched them, never communicated with them, never played with them—each of us would probably develop our own unique style of moving that would be unfamiliar to anyone else.

In such an absurd, asocial world, sports would be impossible; without communication there would be no way to decide on game rules. People also wouldn't have a mutually shared concept of exercise (i.e., physical activity done to improve human functioning or appearance), and they probably wouldn't be consciously aware that people's health can improve with moderate physical activity on a regular basis. Some individuals would probably do strenuous physical activities such as running fast or lifting heavy loads, and if they did these things often enough their health would probably improve. But other people would never learn about this. Exercise, sport, dance, and many other specific forms of physical activity have been brought into being, and are continuously being modified, through social interaction. Without it, these activities wouldn't exist.

Our **social life** is made up of mutually influential **social practices** (everyday behaviors) and shared beliefs; these are so commonplace that we rarely think about them. Whether we're playing soccer, coaching a basketball team, rehabilitating a leg after a tibia break, cheering for our favorite football team, or working out at a local gym, our social practices as athletes, coaches, exercisers, and spectators are influenced by commonly held beliefs in our society. And in turn, it is through our social practices that we come to have beliefs or understandings that we share with others. Although this is true, few of us spend time analyzing the social arrangements—social practices and shared beliefs—that underlie physical activity. But when we do look more closely, we gain insights about ourselves and our culture. It is the job of sociologists of physical activity to give this a closer look.

Although the subdiscipline of sociology of physical activity is focused primarily on sport, there has been a growing interest in exercise and in the ways in which people in our society conceive of the human body. By exploring how we, as a culture, view our bodies, we can come to a renewed understanding of what it means to be human.

Let's look again at our opening scenario to see how a well-educated kinesiologist with knowledge of sociology of physical activity might arrive at answers to the questions facing the basketball coach that would be different from that of a lay person without such training. For example, a kinesiologist would know that there are many more women coaching basketball now than in earlier decades. However, in spite of an enormous growth in the number of female basketball teams, and in spite of an increase in the absolute number of female basketball coaches since 1972 (when Title IX was passed giving males and females equal opportunity in educational settings), many of the new coaching positions have been occupied by men. In intercollegiate basketball, for example, 79% of the coaches of female teams were women in 1978–1979, but by 1991–1992 this had dropped to 64% (Acosta & Carpenter, 1994). Clearly young women looking for coaching jobs with women's teams face increasing competition from men. And there is almost no opportunity for a woman to coach a male team. Two women's professional basketball leagues are now in existence in the United States, so a few of the top collegiate players can aspire to continue playing beyond college.

Sociology of physical activity focuses on the shared beliefs and social practices that constitute specific forms of physical activity (e.g., sport, exercise); sociological information adds to the breadth of knowledge of a well-educated kinesiologist.

CHAPTER OBJECTIVES

In this chapter you will learn about these key topics:

▌ What background knowledge you already have about sociology of physical activity

▌ What a sociologist of physical activity does

▌ The goals of sociology of physical activity

▌ How sociology of physical activity came into being

▌ How research is conducted in sociology of physical activity

▌ What research tells us about inequitable power relations relevant to physical activity, especially gender relations, ethnic and racial relations, and socioeconomic relations.

What Background Knowledge Do I Already Have?

Through your previous physical activity experiences, scholarly studies, and observations of professional practice, you are already familiar with some aspects of sociology of physical activity. Your *experiences* have probably already exposed you to a number of issues sociologists of physical activity study. Perhaps you played on the girls' basketball team in high school and wondered why the boys' scores showed up on the television news but yours didn't, or why the boys' games were packed to capacity, but bleachers sat empty at your games. Or maybe as a young boy you felt pressured to compete, to show coordination, and to be stronger and play better than your female counterparts. Perhaps you watched sports from around the world on television—soccer, sumo wrestling, cricket—and wondered how

How often have you taken time to reflect on your physical activities? Have you ever wondered how similar other people's experiences are to yours? Spend a few moments thinking about your answers to the following questions.

1. What were your most memorable experiences with formally organized physical activity (e.g., youth soccer team, aerobic exercise class, taekwondo class, jazz dance class, summer basketball camp, hiking club trip, varsity football)? What were your most memorable experiences with informally organized physical activity (e.g., after-school pickup basketball, dancing at a local night spot, neighborhood skateboarding, working out at a local gym)? Do you remember these experiences as being rewarding or disappointing? Which were more rewarding? Why?

2. Considering the activities you thought of in the first question, who participated in these activities with you? Do you think the other participants shared your views of what was rewarding or disappointing? If so, why? If not, why do you think their experiences might have been different from yours?

3. Defining the words *excel* and *fail* however you want, think of one person from your past who excelled and one who failed at performing a physical activity. Reflect on your definitions of *fail* and *excel* and why you think the first person excelled whereas the second failed. Do you think the people in your two examples would have perceived themselves the same way you did? Why or why not?

4. Do you remember someone from your past who did not have the same opportunities as others to participate in physical activities? In your opinion, how and why did this occur? How did you respond? How would you respond to the same situation if it occurred today? Why?

and why those sports developed as they did. Maybe you have noticed how racial and socio-economic issues affect physical activity participation. It is likely you have noticed your ethnic or racial group's dominance or lack thereof in the sports you enjoy the most. All of these issues that you have recognized through experience are topics that sociologists of physical activity investigate.

From your previous classwork or *scholarly studies*, you may be familiar with basic principles from sociology, cultural anthropology, economics, political science, and communications. All of these will help you understand sociology of physical activity. You don't have to know all these disciplines in depth, but the more information you have, the more insightful you will be about the social side of physical activity. For example, if you know a little about the general nature of socialization—the process of learning about your own society and how to get along there—it will be easier for you to understand how young boys become socialized into participating in sports, or how certain people become members of subcultures centered in activities such as surfing, triathlons, mountain climbing, skateboarding, or rugby. If you know a lot more about socialization, however, you will likely notice many more details and fine nuances when you study socialization into physical activity. For example, your advanced knowledge might lead you to ask questions about the extent to which, and the ways in which, youngsters contribute to socializing their parents into participating in physical activity, rather than being content to think that socialization flows in only one direction—from parents to children.

Even your observations of *professional practice* have lent you some insight into sociology of physical activity. Perhaps you have noticed that there are few female athletic trainers for American football teams, that many people cannot afford to belong to a country club, and that it has taken years for African Americans to reach the ranks of college and professional coaching. All of these observations are ripe for sociological study, and many of them have already been documented and analyzed by sociologists of physical activity.

As you can see in figure 7.1, sociology of physical activity joins philosophy and history of physical activity to complete the sociocultural sphere of study. Like philosophers of physical activity and historians of physical activity, sociologists of physical activity use their expertise to study the social life and patterns associated with physical activity. By examining physical activity from yet another standpoint, they bring new insights into our understanding of the human experience of being physically active.

What Does a Sociologist of Physical Activity Do?

Sociologists of physical activity are usually faculty members in colleges or universities. They teach classes, offer professionally related service, and engage in research. They may teach an introductory class on sociology of sport and offer courses on specialized topics such as the Olympic Games; interscholastic and intercollegiate athletics; or the ties between physical activity and phenomena such as gender relations, violence and aggression, or the mass media (e.g., television, magazines, the Internet).

Sometimes sociologists of physical activity combine teaching with professional service by encouraging their students to assist in physical activity programs located in nearby neighborhoods. In so doing, they help local communities and foster a sense of civic responsibility in students. Faculty service activities might also include speaking to a community group about TV coverage of the Olympics, or participating in a panel discussion about gender equalities and inequalities in high school sports.

Sociologists of physical activity don't do their research in a typical laboratory. Even if you could bring a "slice of life" (e.g., fans watching an NFL football game, an aerobic exercise class) into a lab for study, in most cases your analyses wouldn't be very useful. This is because when you move such an event into a lab, you alter the very thing you're trying to study. You would be studying "an aerobic exercise class in a lab" rather than "an aerobic exercise class in ordinary life." Sociologists usually prefer to study their subjects "in the field"—for example, professional golfers on the LPGA tour, a television production crew covering a downhill ski race, the political processes that underlie the preparation of elite Canadian athletes for international competition, or an

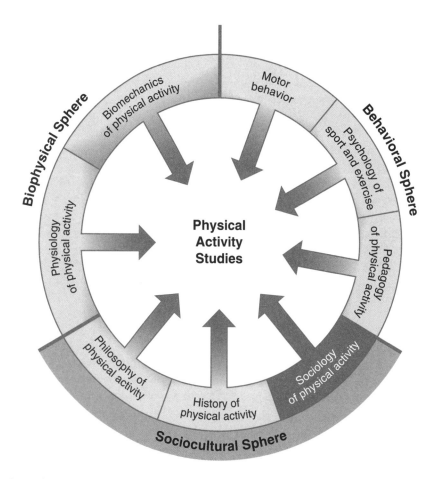

Figure 7.1   Sociology of physical activity and the other scholarly subdisciplines.

American NCAA Division I men's college basketball team.

Investigators usually spend a lot of time making contacts with the people they wish to study and gaining their confidence. A sociologist of physical activity wanting to study an NCAA Division I men's basketball team, for example, would probably need permission from the university, the athletic director, the coach, and the team members themselves. He or she would need to develop especially good rapport with the coach and the team members in order to give them confidence in the worth of the project. The quality of such relationships has an important bearing on the quality of the research.

Sociologists of physical activity usually study ongoing social life as it ordinarily occurs; they don't often bring it into a laboratory.

Sociologists of physical activity often apply for small grants from their own colleges or universities to fund their research. Writing a grant proposal involves stating what the main focus of the research will be, why it is important, the methods they intend to use to gather and analyze data, what makes them qualified to carry out the research, the amount of money they need, and how they plan to spend the money. This has to be stated clearly and concisely so it persuades others that their project is important and that they are competent to carry it out.

Goals of Sociology of Physical Activity

Sociology of physical activity has three main goals. The first is *to look at physical activity with a penetrating gaze that goes beyond our common understanding of social life.* This is a habit that must

Take a few moments to think about the following questions or situations and how you would address them. If you are particularly interested in one of these issues, you may want to get additional information from others on campus, or from the library. If your instructor desires, discuss your solutions with others in class.

• Your football coach constantly says things like "No pain, no gain" and "Play through the pain." Why does he say this? Do you think you will gain anything worthwhile if you play while you have a painful injury? What are the costs and benefits?
• Your 15-year-old sister says she looks fat, and she's planning to diet and exercise more. She doesn't appear overweight to you. You wonder what to say to her.
• Your city's competitive swim program for youths is privately run, charges a participation fee, and operates in public pools for which the city receives rent. What are the implications of such a program? Is the program really available to all the youths in your city?
• You've heard from physical fitness experts that it's up to each individual to adopt a more active lifestyle. Do societal barriers make doing this more difficult for some people than for others?
• On a trip to the Trobriand Islands in the South Pacific, you see a sport that is like the English game of cricket, but the players wear local costumes, more than 60 people play at once for each team, the home team always wins, and the fielders dance for a while each time a batsman from the other team gets put out. You wonder why their rules are so different.

be developed, and acquiring it involves a dash of skepticism about common assumptions. If you remember that the inner workings of social life are usually not readily observable, it will be easier to form the habit of looking more closely. For example, on the surface it appears that sport is a place where a person's wealth makes little difference, but if you look more closely, you'll find that economic inequalities in a particular society are influential in the sports of that society, too. To illustrate, in the United States becoming an Olympic competitor in sports such as figure skating, gymnastics, or speed skating often requires an athlete's parents to make financial sacrifices for many years in order to pay for coaching, living away from home for months at a time in the city where a coach is located, and traveling to competitions. Middle-class parents sometimes decide to make this extreme financial commitment, but working-class parents usually can't even consider it. Youngsters from economically impoverished families must usually turn toward sports that are available at low cost in their own neighborhoods, and where coaching is provided at almost no charge (e.g., public schools, community recreation facilities).

The second goal of the subdiscipline is *to identify and analyze patterns of change and stability in*

physical activity. Once you start looking beneath the surface of social life, then your goal is to identify changes as well as ongoing regularities. Let's look at one change in physical activity that occurred in the middle of the 20th century. Since the late 1960s there has been tremendous growth in the prescription of exercise for the rehabilitation of heart patients. This recommendation is now commonplace, but as recently as the mid-1960s the usual suggestion was bed rest. This dramatic turnaround occurred because of increased societal interest in exercise and physical

Goals of Sociology of Physical Activity

1. To look at physical activity with a penetrating gaze that goes beyond our common understanding of social life

2. To identify and analyze patterns of change and stability in physical activity

3. To critique physical activity programs in order to identify problems and recommend changes leading to the enhancement of equality and human well-being

fitness beginning in the late 1950s, accompanied by greater clinical and scholarly understanding of the medical benefits of exercise.

A third goal of sociology of physical activity is *to critique physical activity programs in order to identify problems and recommend changes leading to the enhancement of equality and human well-being.* As you have probably already guessed, sociologists point to the constant stream of social interaction that goes on in any society (rather than to our individual psyches or genetics) as the most important source of societal problems, although they don't deny that psychological and biological factors have important influences in our lives. They study this social interaction, and more important, they *evaluate* it—pass judgment on its contributions to overall human well-being and equitable social relationships (e.g., relationships among racial and ethnic groups, men and women, or people at different socioeconomic levels).

Consider this example. It has been found that locker-room banter among intercollegiate male athletes sometimes includes uncomplimentary, disparaging comments about women and gay men (Curry, 1991). Although we don't know for sure, many people believe that constant exposure to this sort of environment might serve to reinforce inequalities between men and women and between gays and straights. This locker-room practice is therefore considered to be problematic, and sociologists often suggest working to modify it.

In keeping with the third goal, sociologists of physical activity are not oriented toward supporting or reinforcing status quo physical activities such as present exercise programs and competitive sports. For example, an athletic trainer might work with a basketball player to improve her ankle strength, and therefore her physical toughness in a game, through rehabilitative exercises; a biomechanist might design an exercise machine that meshes with the human body to improve fitness. Both of these are examples of working within the status quo—working to improve performance in activities *as they are currently structured.* But a sociologist might actually advocate *changing the structure* by questioning the desirability of fierce competition in basketball or treating the human body like a piece of machinery that needs to be "meshed" with other pieces of machinery.

Sociologists of physical activity look beneath the surface of social life in order to see things from different angles; they often point out social problems in an effort to encourage people to make changes that would enhance human well-being and promote equitable social relationships.

History of Sociology of Physical Activity

Beginning in the late 19th century and continuing through the first six decades of the 20th century, American research on the social aspects of physical activity was sporadic and diverse (Loy & Kenyon, 1969a; Loy, Kenyon, & McPherson, 1980; Sage, 1997). Research about sport was sometimes embedded in broader studies of play and games, an approach that continued through the 1970s. Exercise received virtually no attention because it fell outside this domain. Scholars described game rules and equipment, studied paths by which games spread to different societies, and examined ways in which play and games teach children about their society (Schwartzman, 1978).

One of the earliest American critiques of sport appeared as a chapter in Thorstein Veblen's *The Theory of the Leisure Class* (1899/1967). Veblen complained that members of the American upper class used sport to show off their wealth. In his opinion, they participated partially to demonstrate that they had enough money to avoid work and enjoy leisure. He also thought that sport distracted the wealthy from more beneficial philanthropic activities that could help improve society.

A few U.S. studies focused specifically on sport. Some of these dealt with the relationship between participation in intercollegiate athletics and academic achievement. Athletic competition mushroomed on college campuses during the last three decades of the 19th century, and this was accompanied by growing faculty concerns about its effects on players' academic work. For example, Paul Phillips's article "Competitive Athletics and Scholarship" appeared in *Science* in 1908. Phillips compared the scholastic standing of athletes on varsity teams at Amherst College in Massachusetts with students at the same institution who were nonathletes during the period from 1886 to 1903. He concluded that athletes had lower grades than nonathletes and that their weaker academic performance was due to their athletic involvement. Based on data accumulated through the 20th century, however, we now know that many factors are related to college grades, and athletic participation by itself is not a very good predictor.

Several prominent American sociologists did excellent research on sport in the 1950s and early 1960s. For example, David Riesman and Reuel Denney (1951) examined early American football; Reuel Denney (1957) wrote about American spectators; E. Digby Baltzell (1958) investigated sporting practices in a broad study of upper-class men in Philadelphia; James Coleman (1961) examined the role of sport in public schools as part of a larger study of American education; and Gregory Stone (1969) studied the content of urban adults' conversations about sport. These researchers demonstrated that sociological investigations of sport had the potential to be informative and useful.

Early sociological studies of physical activity were often part of larger studies on games and play; occasional investigations focused directly on sport.

Identifying the Subdiscipline

Europeans took the lead in developing the first scholarly association in sport sociology and the first research journal, but several North Americans were also involved. The International Committee of Sport Sociology was founded in 1964, and in 1966 it inaugurated a scholarly journal— the *International Review of Sport Sociology*—still in publication today. Over the years, the ICSS (later called the International Committee for Sociology of Sport, and presently named the International

Historical Time Line

1895–1910	Beginnings of U.S. sociological analyses of sport.
1951–1961	Several well-known sociologists do sport research that demonstrates the value of such investigations.
1964	The International Committee of Sport Sociology is established.
1965	Gerald Kenyon and John Loy write "Toward a Sociology of Sport," an important statement envisioning a scholarly subdiscipline focused on the social aspects of sport.
1966	The *International Review of Sport Sociology* begins publication.
1970	Socioeconomic inequalities and class relations in sport begin to grow in importance as research topics, and they continue to be major research topics through the 1980s.
1977	The *Journal of Sport and Social Issues* begins publication.
1980	North American Society for the Sociology of Sport is established.
1980	Gender relations in sport begins to grow in importance as a research topic, and it continues to be a major research topic at present.
1984	The *Sociology of Sport Journal* begins publication.
1985	Exercise and societal conceptions of human bodies begin to grow in importance as research topics, and they continue to be major research topics at present.
1990	Racial and ethnic inequities begin to grow in importance as research topics, and they continue to be major research topics at present.
1990	Sport in the context of global, national, and local relations begins to grow in importance as a research topic, and it is still a central topic today.

Sociology of Sport Association) has conducted numerous seminars, workshops, and annual conferences throughout the world (Sage, 1997).

The subdiscipline began to take shape in North America in the mid-1960s. One notable influence was English physical educator Peter McIntosh's 1963 book *Sport in Society,* dealing broadly with the social significance of sport. His analysis encouraged several North American scholars to channel their careers toward this emerging area (Sage, 1997).

Canadian physical educator Gerald Kenyon, a faculty member in physical education at the University of Wisconsin, was also very influential. Beginning in 1965 he and his colleagues brought the subdiscipline to the attention of North American scholars through numerous papers, books, and conference presentations.

Kenyon supervised the doctoral education of several early leaders in the growing subdiscipline. One of them, John Loy, went on to become one of the most prominent and creative scholars in sport sociology, and he mentored a large number of doctoral students who subsequently became well-known researchers in their own right. Taken together, their scholarship spans a wide variety of topics across the subdiscipline.

The social upheavals in the United States in the late 1960s spurred several people to write critiques of sport, often from personal experiences as athletes. Examples include Dave Meggyesy's *Out of Their League* (1971) and Paul Hoch's *Rip Off the Big Game* (1972); both are about football. These authors pointed to what they considered to be dehumanizing aspects of the game, such as the use of performance-enhancing drugs, au-

In Profile

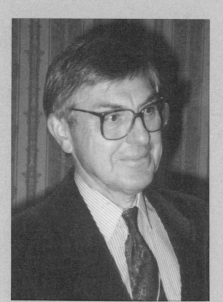

Gerald Kenyon

As a professor at the University of Wisconsin from 1961 to 1970, Canadian Gerald Kenyon was key in the establishment of sport sociology as an academic specialization in North America. This influential scholar was educated in Canada (BPE, University of British Columbia, 1954) and the United States (MS, Indiana University, 1957; PhD, New York University, 1960). He was a prime mover who developed contacts with European and English sport sociologists, wrote articles and spoke at numerous conferences and symposia on the social importance of sport and the framework he envisioned for the new subdiscipline, and guided some of the first North American doctoral students in this specialization.

His 1965 article "Toward a Sociology of Sport," coauthored with his doctoral student John Loy and published in the *Journal of Health, Physical Education and Recreation,* was a benchmark statement that charted a path for the new area. This paper helped to place the sole focus of the subdiscipline squarely on sport, an emphasis that continued until the mid-1980s. In 1969 Loy and Kenyon edited an early anthology of scholarly articles in the specialization, *Sport, Culture, and Society.* Kenyon continued to pursue numerous other academic interests including sociology of the arts and culture, sociology of leisure, comparative sociology, and sociology of information technology. He returned to Canada in 1970 to take a dean's post at the University of Waterloo in the province of Ontario. In 1982 he became a vice president at the University of Lethbridge in the province of Alberta. He returned to a faculty post in sociology at the University of Lethbridge in 1987 and retired in 1995. His active retirement has included teaching an annual course at the university.

thoritarian coaches, and bone-crunching violence. The general atmosphere of social criticism in American society during the late 1960s and early 1970s, along with specific indictments of sport by some of the players, led to greater scholarly recognition of the fruitfulness of studying sport from social perspectives.

Several other early investigators also helped define the growing academic specialty in North America. Gunther Luschen, a sociologist from West Germany, had been involved with the International Committee of Sport Sociology in its formative years in Europe. When he moved to the University of Illinois to be a faculty member in physical education and sociology beginning in the late 1960s, he had the opportunity to contribute directly to the development of the subdiscipline in the United States and Canada. His contacts with European scholars were useful to North Americans.

Eleanor Metheny, a physical educator at the University of Southern California, used philosophical, historical, and social concepts in her analyses of sport. Her well-known work on the symbolic meanings of movement, *Connotations of Movement in Sport and Dance* (1965), was applauded as exciting, cutting-edge thinking in the mid-1960s. Her examination of the feminine image in sport, and its role in censuring females in athletics, has often been referred to by sport sociologists. Many of Metheny's doctoral students specialized in philosophy or history of physical activity. One of her students who went on to influence the sociological subdiscipline was Marie Hart, who wrote and spoke on the topic of women's involvement in sport, taking the position that outmoded, stereotypical gender role expectations in athletics tend to stigmatize female athletes.

Through the late 1960s and 1970s sessions on sociology of sport were held at major conferences in physical education and sociology throughout North America. Several universities sponsored sport sociology symposiums. The *Journal of Sport and Social Issues* began publication in 1977 and is still in operation today. Two of the most prominent textbooks in the subdiscipline—currently still in publication after several editions—first appeared in 1978: *Sociology of American Sport* by sociologist Stanley Eitzen and physical educator George Sage, and *Sport in Society: Issues and Controversies* by sociologist Jay Coakley.

Perhaps because the early leaders in North American sport sociology had strong ties with scholars in Europe and England, an academic organization in North America was slow to develop. Such a group finally formed in 1978—the North American Society for the Sociology of Sport—under the leadership of physical educators Susan Greendorfer and Andrew Yiannakis. The society held its first annual conference in 1980 and began publishing an academic journal in 1984—the *Sociology of Sport Journal*. Both the society and the journal are still going strong.

During the 1960s, 1970s, and early 1980s sociology of physical activity became increasingly identifiable as a subdiscipline: more scholars were attracted to this area, special academic meetings were held, scholarly associations were formed, research journals appeared, and introductory textbooks were published.

Expanding the Subdiscipline

Since the mid-1970s the number of scholars in sociology of physical activity has increased, and they have used a wide array of theories and research methods. The hottest topics have focused on social inequities—especially those connected with gender, race, ethnicity, wealth, sexual orientation, and different cultures around the world. In the 1970s and early 1980s socioeconomic inequalities (tied to differences in such things as wealth, education, and occupational prestige) were of central importance. Richard Gruneau's *Class, Sports, and Social Development* (1983) was a classic, and it continues to be so widely read that it was reprinted in 1999.

In the 1980s more scholars began to study gender inequities, and this continued through the 1990s. Paul Willis's seminal article "Women in Sport in Ideology" (1982) is still widely read, and by 1988 there had been enough investigations for Susan Birrell to write a review of research titled "Discourses on the Gender-Sport Relationship: From Women in Sport to Gender Relations." A listing of a few titles from the 1990s will give you a sense of the wide range of interests: *Power at Play: Sports and the Problem of Masculinity*

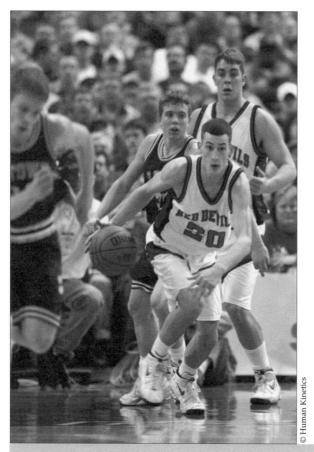 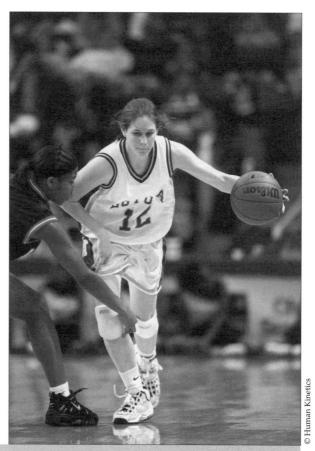

Studies of gender inequities constitute a major line of research in sociology of physical activity.

(Messner, 1992); *Unbearable Weight: Feminism, Western Culture, and the Body* (Bordo, 1993); "Gender Stereotyping in Televised Sports" (Duncan, Messner, Williams, & Jensen, 1994); "The Status of Women in Intercollegiate Athletics" (Acosta & Carpenter, 1994); *Outsiders in the Clubhouse: The World of Women's Professional Golf* (Crosset, 1995); and *The Swimsuit Issue and Sport: Hegemonic Masculinity in Sports Illustrated* (Davis, 1997).

In the 1990s the focus widened even further as scholars gave greater attention to racial and ethnic inequities, especially those faced by African Americans. Investigators also attempted to look more often at intersections among race, ethnicity, social class, and gender, rather than addressing only one of these at a time. The explosion of important works dealing with racial and ethnic inequalities included "Deconstructing Michael Jordan: Reconstructing Postindustrial America" (Andrews, 1996); *In Black and White: Race and Sports in America* (Shropshire, 1996); *Muhammad Ali: The People's Champ* (Gorn, 1995); *Darwin's*

Athletes: How Sport Has Damaged Black America and Preserved the Myth of Race (Hoberman, 1997); *Birth of a Nation 'Hood: Gaze, Script, and Spectacle in the O.J. Simpson Case* (Morrison & Lacour, 1997); "Reading Nancy Lopez: Decoding Representations of Race, Class, and Sexuality" (Jamieson, 1998).

Another topic that has moved to center stage in the subdiscipline is global sport relations. The focus here is on inequities in the dissemination of national and regional cultures throughout the world. Sports are clearly part of this. For example, American culture—and American sports (especially basketball, football, and baseball)—are spreading rapidly via television and other mass communication media. In some cases, they are perceived as threats to other national or regional cultures. For example, baseball fans in Japan have learned about doing "the wave" in stadiums, probably from watching American spectators do it on TV. This runs counter to the decorum expected among Japanese baseball fans, so in at least one stadium there are now signs saying "No Wave" (Sugimoto, 1996). Clearly, there is a struggle going on over what constitutes appropriate spectator behavior—a struggle probably brought on by mass media portrayals of other fans (especially American fans) behaving differently.

Rooted in global politics and economics as well as in the rapid expansion of new communication technologies, worldwide cultural exchanges (of such things as movies, videos, sports, fashions, customs, and political and economic processes) are expanding at a dizzying pace. The following titles show you some of the topics being studied: *Games and Empires: Modern Sports and Cultural Imperialism* (Guttmann, 1994); "Sport, Identity Politics, and Globalization: Diminishing Contrasts and Increasing Varieties" (Maguire, 1994); and *Baseball on the Border: A Tale of Two Laredos* (Klein, 1997).

Beginning in the 1980s and continuing through the 1990s, sport sociologists also extended their studies beyond sport to examine exercise and societal conceptions of the human body. Many of the works on sport mentioned in the preceding paragraphs include a focus on people's conceptions of gendered bodies or racialized bodies. Concerns about bodies have also filtered into studies of exercise, as demonstrated in the following titles: "Participant Perceptions of Exercise Programs for Overweight Women" (Bain, Wilson, & Chaikind, 1989); "Firm but Shapely, Fit but Sexy, Strong but Thin: The Postmodern Aerobicizing Female Bodies" (Markula, 1995); and "The Composite Body: Hip-Hop Aerobics and the Multicultural Nation" (Martin, 1997). Perhaps signaling the strength of this new focus on the human body and exercise, in 1997 kinesiologists James Bryant and Mary McElroy published a textbook titled *Sociological Dynamics of Sport and Exercise.*

In the 1970s, 1980s, and 1990s sociology of physical activity expanded as scholars explored a wider variety of topics, especially those concerning sport and societal inequities related to socioeconomic, gender, racial and ethnic inequalities; globalization, and regional and national differences; and exercise and societal conceptions of the human body.

Research Methods in Sociology of Physical Activity

Now that you know something about the subdiscipline and its historical roots, you may be wondering how sociologists of physical activity produce their knowledge. What methods do researchers use to answer important questions about the social side of physical activity? They gather both quantifiable data (things you can count or measure) and qualitative data (e.g., interviews, direct observations of social life, written documents, artifacts). We'll look at six different methods: survey research, interviewing, thematic analysis, ethnography, societal analysis, and historical research. Of course, sometimes two or more of these are used in the same study.

Survey Research

Doing **survey research** involves using questionnaires that are completed directly by respondents or filled out by a researcher during highly structured, brief interviews. Questionnaires allow data to be collected from a large sample of people. The largest survey project in the country is the U.S. census conducted every 10 years. Political polls about voting preferences are also surveys. Surveys dealing with physical activity have been conducted on numerous topics including youngsters' opinions about what led them to become involved in sport, former collegiate athletes' thoughts about leaving competition at the end of their four years of eligibility, and college athletic directors' opinions about the characteristics of successful coaches.

Interviewing

Researchers use interviews when they want broader and deeper information than they can get through a questionnaire, or when they want information about activities that would be difficult or impossible to observe themselves. Because **interviewing** is time-consuming, studies often focus on a small number of people. Typically, interviews are tape-recorded and later transcribed. Researchers often ask relatively open-ended questions and then probe to get details. One investigator asked top high school, college, and

Following is an example of a questionnaire used in survey research about sport. It was designed to gather information about young athletes' general television viewing habits and their televised sport viewing habits. It was part of a larger 1976 Canadian study of prosocial and antisocial behavior of boys and girls participating in three sports—ice hockey, baseball, and lacrosse (Hrycaiko, McCabe, & Moriarty, n.d., p. 28). Take a few minutes to complete the items for yourself. Compare your answers with others.

Player Questionnaire

1. Age _____   2. Sex: M ___ F ___   3. Sport _____   4. Team name _____

5. What do you like most about your sport? Circle your choices.

Rewards	Game itself	Winning
Action	Fun and enjoyment	Fitness
Skills	Aggression	Achievement

6. What do you like least about your sport? Circle your choices.

Aggression	Losing	Equipment
Injuries	Nothing	Referees
Drills and practices	Not playing	Coaching

7. Number of hours/week that you watch television during the summer: _____

8. Time of day when you watch the most television during the summer:

Morning ___   Afternoon ___   Evening ___

9. Number of hours/week that you watch television during the winter: _____

10. Time of day when you watch the most television during the winter:

Morning ___   Afternoon ___   Evening ___

11. What type of show do you like best? Rank 1–6.

Mystery __	Adventure __	Cartoons __
Comedy __	Drama __	Sports __

12. Of these sports programs shown regularly on television, which do you watch the most? Rank 1–9.

Hockey __	Wrestling __	Golf __
Basketball __	Bowling __	Football __
Car-racing __	Baseball __	Tennis __

13. Of these sports programs shown occasionally on television, which do you watch the most? Rank 1–9.

Gymnastics __	Horse-racing __	Swimming __
Track and field __	Volleyball __	Skiing __
Boxing __	Soccer __	Synchronized swimming __

professional athletes to discuss their initial involvement in sport, their participation over the years, and their disengagement from sport. Another asked young people about the characteristics of their athletic heroes.

Thematic Analysis

Thematic analysis, sometimes called content analysis, is used to investigate cultural material such as magazine and newspaper articles, photos, the verbal and visual content of television programs, and interview data. The procedure involves examining the material and then categorizing the content in various ways. For example, magazine photos of female and male Olympic athletes were analyzed using the categories of physical appearance, poses, position of the body, emotional displays, camera angles, and groupings of people. A researcher often ends up with several main categories or themes along with a set of subthemes within each. Sometimes investigators count the number of times each theme and subtheme occurs. In other cases they are more interested in qualitative data, such as describing the richness and complexity of the themes. The themes help to organize a large mass of data into a manageable number of categories that can be analyzed further in relation to theories of interest to the researcher.

🔑 Research methods used in sociology of physical activity include survey research, interviewing, thematic analysis, ethnography, societal analysis, and historical analysis.

Ethnography

Researchers using this method spend many months and even years observing in a particular social setting. They "hang around" while ordinary day-to-day events take place, often taking part themselves, talking with people about what's happening, and keeping careful field notes to remember details. While observation is their primary source of information, they may also look at local documents or use interviews and questionnaires. Most of the data they collect are analyzed using thematic analyses. Ethnography has been used to study a wide variety of sport set-

tings including minor-league ice hockey, baseball in the Dominican Republic, women's softball, the Olympic Games, women's professional golf, rodeo, and boys' Little League baseball.

Societal Analysis

In societal analysis the researcher's goal is to examine the sweep of social life usually from the perspective of a broad social theory. This method, of course, isn't the only one tied to theory—all good social research is theoretically based. However, the theories used in societal analysis are extremely broad—they attempt to explain the most fundamental ways in which societies operate. Examples of these include Marxism (and its many derivatives), modernization, structural-functionalism, figuration theory, various strands of feminism, various cultural studies frameworks, and various forms of postmodernism. These theories are extremely complex; for each there are massive collections of scholarly papers and books aimed at supporting, refuting, or expanding them. Illustrations of societal analysis in sociology of physical activity include a study of modernization that focuses on sport in preindustrial and postindustrial societies (Guttmann, 1978), and an investigation—focused on social class—of societal constraints and human freedoms in sport (Gruneau, 1983).

Historical Analysis

Social scientists interested in large-scale social change frequently incorporate historical research into their work. Historical analyses often are part of a larger study involving theoretical explorations of the kind just noted. Examples of historical research by sociologists of physical activity include an examination of the ways in which development of sport in Canada was related to socioeconomic inequities (Gruneau, 1983), and a study of unruliness among soccer spectators in England from the 1890s to the 1980s (Dunning, Murphy, & Williams, 1988).

🔑 Research in sociology of physical activity involves collecting quantitative and qualitative data using a variety of different methodologies.

Methods of Research

Of the six research methods highlighted—survey research, interviewing, thematic analysis, ethnography, societal analysis, and historical analysis—which do you think would yield the most useful and interesting data on violence among fans at high school football games? Why? How would you use the method(s) to collect data? In what ways are the methods you chose connected with what you wanted to learn about violence among fans? If your instructor desires, compare your answers with other students in class.

Overview of Knowledge in Sociology of Physical Activity

Now it's time for a brief overview of topics in sociology of physical activity—a snapshot that shows you some of the information produced by scholars in the subdiscipline. Remember, though, that this short excursion into the subdiscipline cannot do justice to the richness and variety of the knowledge that scholars have produced. The body of knowledge is far-reaching. It is especially complex because it concerns many different societies throughout the world, and social life is not the same everywhere. It is also important to remember that knowledge about any particular form of physical activity—for example, sport or exercise—gives us only a partial understanding of ourselves and others. Abstract theoretical generalizations are useful to a point, but they must be grounded in specific examples in order for us to make use of them.

We will focus primarily on American society, and because sport remains the central focus of the subdiscipline, it will be mentioned most frequently. We'll look primarily at links between physical activity and inequitable power relations based on gender, ethnicity and race, and socioeconomic status. Power inequalities such as these are central to a large portion of the research currently being conducted in the subdiscipline.

Before going on, it's important to note other topics that have been especially interesting to sociologists of physical activity:

- Children, socialization, and youth sports
- Interscholastic and intercollegiate athletics
- Physical violence, performance-enhancing drugs, delinquency, and sports
- Aggression and sports
- Commercialization, transnational corporations, and sports
- Sports in relation to local, national, international, and transnational politics
- Mass media (e.g., television, newspapers, magazines, the Internet) and sports: production, content, and audiences
- Relationships between sports and religion

Investigators often look at these other areas from the standpoint of the power relationships we're going to consider in the next section. Once you learn a bit about these power relationships, you may begin to see them almost everywhere. And you'll be able to look more carefully—with a more penetrating gaze—at the other fascinating social aspects of physical activity just listed above.

For the purposes of this chapter, though, we will focus on inequitable power relationships and physical activity. Although our democratic system promises equal opportunities for all, inequalities still exist. Some of the most vexing are tied to differences in gender, ethnicity, race, and socioeconomic status. Wealthy, white, non-Latino men are most likely to gain positions of power; poor women of color, and women from ethnic minorities, are least likely. The U.S. Congress, for example, is heavily lopsided toward white men. There is also a preponderance of men in top corporate executive positions. Among Fortune 500 companies in 1996, women made up 46% of the workforce, but only 10% of the corporate officers. Only 2% of the top 2,500 earners in these companies were women (Neuborne, 1996). At the other end of the continuum, there are much higher proportions of Latinos/Latinas and African Americans living in poverty than non-Latino/Latina whites, or Americans who trace their heritage to Asian countries or to the Pacific Islands. And families headed by single women are much more likely to be in poverty than those

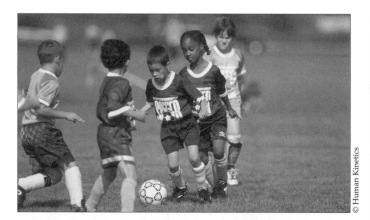

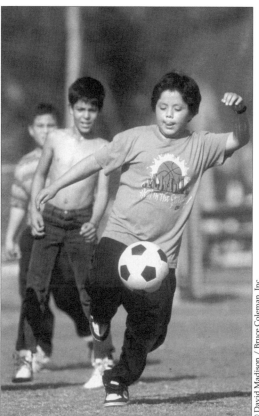

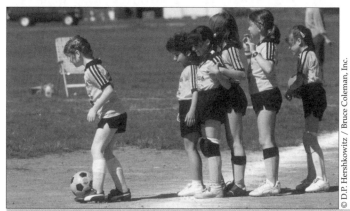

Overall quality of life and opportunities for future advancement may depend on gender, ethnicity, and socioeconomic status.

headed by married couples or single men (U.S. Department of Commerce, 1993).

Power is the ability to do what you want without being stopped by others. Money, prestige, body size and strength, information, and weapons are major sources of power, and hence major sources of inequity. Powerful people usually have more opportunities to move toward their personal and professional goals. The quality of your life as well as your future chances for advancement can be severely limited if you don't have much power.

Looking specifically at physical activity, power inequities sometimes affect our participation as performers as well as our opportunities for involvement in influential leadership roles such as health club owner, coach, athletic director, or cardiac rehabilitation program director. People with more power can usually get involved more easily. Those with less power often face social barriers that make involvement more difficult. For example, African American players in the NFL have a more difficult time being hired for coach-

ing and administrative positions in the league than whites.

Furthermore, current power differences in American society are frequently displayed—and thus reinforced—in movies, television, music, and physical activities. Whether we participate directly in activities such as sport, dance, and exercise, or whether we watch others performing, a lot of subtle information is expressed that tends to support and reinforce status quo power differences. For example, telecasts that highlight the physical appearance of female athletes—with special focus on their clothes and hairstyles—contribute to undermining, and thus trivializing, their athletic accomplishments.

Power relations underlie social inequalities; they affect people's quality of life and their chances for a better life in the future.

Our examination of power relations will lead us to look at gender relations, ethnic and racial relations, and socioeconomic relations. We'll focus on three areas: participation, leadership, and expression. Where appropriate, we'll also look at societal conceptions of the human body, a topic that received increasing attention from sociologists beginning in the late 1980s.

Gender Relations

Gender is different from sex. A **gender** is a set of norms or expectations about how we should behave, and these are linked to societal understandings of sexuality and procreation. At birth, babies are assigned to a sex category based on the appearance of the genitalia (Lorber, 1994). This assignment process, and the subsequent differential treatment of youngsters based on different sex categories, constitutes the gendering process. Genders are not natural, biological categories—they are socially defined. You can't inherit a gender—you have to be assigned to it and learn it.

In American society, men are typically more powerful than women. The situation has improved greatly during the 20th century, but many inequalities remain. In the field of physical activity, inequalities prevail as a result of beliefs about the appropriateness of certain forms of physical activity for each gender.

Participation

It's common today to see many girls playing in organized youth sports and many of their older sisters playing on high school and college teams. We also see females of all ages engaging in other physical activities such as aerobic dance, lap swimming, jogging, mountain biking, yoga, dance, and weight training. Nevertheless, overall we still find a lot more males participating in sports (Coakley, 1998, pp. 222–224). While men and women engage in moderate levels of activity with equal frequency and for about the same length of time, men make up a much higher proportion of high-energy exercisers (Stephens & Caspersen, 1994).

In our society, sports are considered important avenues for exploring and confirming masculinity. They are thought to sharpen a number of qualities traditionally considered appropriate for men and boys, such as toughness, aggressiveness, roughness, working well under pressure, and competitiveness. You probably know girls and women with some of these qualities, which shows

the indistinct boundaries between these two genders. Nevertheless, in our society these qualities are still typically conceptualized as masculine.

Although many sports attract large numbers of both males and females, some are more gender-specific. For example, girls and women rarely engage in boxing, football, wrestling, or weightlifting contests. American boys and men almost never play field hockey, even though it's a sport for men in international competition. If a woman or girl you know started training to be a boxer, what would you think? Many Americans would judge this negatively. But what makes it inappropriate? Although there are now many females developing muscular strength and endurance through weight training, few take part in sports requiring great strength, physical domination of an opponent through bodily contact, or the manipulation of heavy objects. Furthermore, it is only in recent decades that women have taken up competition in strenuous, long-distance runs,

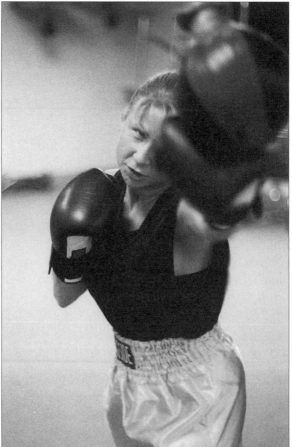

What is your immediate reaction to this boxer?

including marathons. In an early, cutting-edge analysis, the sports we judge to be more appropriate for females, such as gymnastics or tennis, were observed to entail little body contact, the manipulation of light objects, and aesthetically pleasing movements (Metheny, 1965).

The continued emphasis on masculinity in sport, and the preponderance of male participants, often results in downplaying women's competition. Examples include fewer resources for female sports (e.g., less travel money, lower coaching salaries, fewer publicity funds, less media exposure, fewer corporate sponsorships), and sometimes team nicknames that reflect physical ineptitude, such as the Teddy Bears, Blue Chicks, Cotton Blossoms, or Wild Kittens (Coakley, 1998, pp. 221–222).

Although much larger numbers of girls and women are participating in physical activities today compared with several decades ago, there are still far fewer females than males, and they tend to be more attracted to sports involving less body contact, prominent aesthetic dimensions, and less extreme strength development.

Leadership

We know that opportunities for women in coaching, sports telecasting, and officiating are growing but are still more limited than they are for men (Acosta & Carpenter, 1994; Eitzen & Sage, 1997, pp. 238–239). Moreover, from the 1970s into the 1990s there were sharp decreases in the percentage of female coaches of female high school and intercollegiate teams, and the proportion of female administrators heading women's intercollegiate programs. For example, in 1977–1978, 79% of the coaches of female basketball teams were women; by 1991–1992 that number had dropped to 64% (Acosta & Carpenter, 1994). The percentage of female administrators heading women's intercollegiate programs went from 90% in 1972 to only 21% in 1994. It's unlikely that these percentages have changed significantly in recent years.

Why are more men now coaching and administering women's teams and programs? Researchers have postulated a number of reasons. To be-

gin with, the larger number of male players constitutes a larger pool of qualified candidates. Also, the fact that women's coaching salaries still lag behind those of men may cause some of the top female players to seek careers outside of athletics. One estimate of the gender ratio among applicants for coaching jobs in women's collegiate basketball was five or six men to one woman (Marcy Weston, personal communication, September 1996). Also, men occupy most of the influential athletic leadership positions (e.g., collegiate athletic directors, leaders in the Olympic movement). When they make decisions about hiring coaches or appointing people to important committees, it is likely that they use their network of connections with other men in athletics—usually referred to as the "old boys" network—to find candidates. Finally, it's possible that men favor applicants with stereotypical masculine qualities (e.g., aggressive, dominating, physically tough), and this puts many well-qualified women at a disadvantage (Knoppers, 1987).

Women occupy a relatively small proportion of coaching and leadership positions in sport.

Expression

Knowing that gender inequalities exist in American society, and that all physical activities have expressive dimensions, it's not surprising that our physical activities frequently demonstrate such inequities. For example, in some forms of dancing (e.g., the waltz, many country-western dances) men usually move forward and "lead" women who usually move backward. There is a subtle message communicated here about men's superiority.

Our most popular sports—the ones we see constantly on TV—are celebrations of heterosexual manhood centered around aggressiveness, roughness, and the ability to dominate physically. Girls and women have most often been relegated to marginal positions as spectators of boys' and men's competition, or to playing their own less popular versions of these and other sports. One of the messages communicated by this is that females don't matter much in "real sports." Coaches sometimes criticize weak or ineffective plays by boys and men by calling them "a bunch of girls" or "sissies" (Coakley, 1998, p. 236).

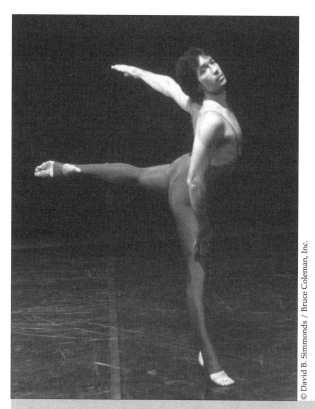

© David B. Simmonds / Bruce Coleman, Inc.

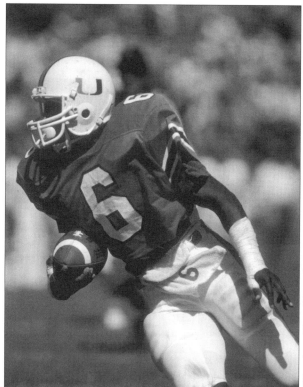

© Tony Aruza / Bruce Coleman Inc.

What are your initial thoughts about the ballet dancer and the football player?

Intended to spur better performance, such comments send a message that females are inferior. A similar message is communicated when coaches tell players they "throw like a girl." These are examples of ways in which sports tend to reinforce ideas about the acceptability of heterosexual male dominance.

Girls and women are not the only ones shortchanged by the macho attitudes that prevail around sports. Our society often questions boys and young men who aren't interested in athletics or lack ability. They are called "sissies," and their sexual orientation may be challenged with taunts of "gay," "fag," or "queer" (Coakley, 1998, p. 236). In high school, boys' popularity is closely connected with being good in athletics. A group of white college graduates who had not played varsity sports in either high school or college said that as boys they experienced social ostracism and name-calling because of their poor athletic ability. One said, "I identified sports as a major aspect of what I was supposed to be like as a male, which oppressed me because I could not do it,

no matter how hard I tried" (Stein & Hoffman, 1978, p. 148).

Have you ever really thought about the degree of coverage of men's and women's sports in the media (e.g., television, newspapers, magazines)? About 5% of sport on television focuses on women's athletics, while men's competition constitutes 92%. In newspapers, the space devoted to women's athletics is about 15% of the total for all sports (Eitzen & Sage, 1997, p. 284). This disparity trivializes women's athletic accomplishments and sends an underlying message that women's events aren't worth much.

Beyond the amount of coverage, there are differences in the way men's and women's athletics are presented. Male athletes tend to be portrayed as strong, competent, highly skilled competitors who confidently pursue victory. Female athletes, on the other hand, are depicted more ambivalently. For example, in a comparison of television coverage of men's and women's basketball games in the NCAA tournament, Duncan and Hasbrook (1988) noticed that coverage of the women's contests focused more on the artistic qualities of players' movements and less on skills and strategic knowledge.

Winning at elite levels in the sports our society likes best requires bodies that are big and strong, qualities almost always associated with male bodies. This situation is often highlighted in the mass media. For example, when men's and women's winning times are compared in Olympic swimming, skiing, or track events, men always prevail. Comparative times for events such as the New York City Marathon or the Boston Marathon show the male winners far ahead of the female winners. If top male and female tennis players, basketball teams, or soccer teams ever played each other, the men would have an easy win. And it is laughable to think of women competing against men in football! Because men are superior to women in these sports, this is thought to be an important symbolic statement about male superiority in general (Messner, 1988; Willis, 1982).

Although this may strike you at first as a bit outlandish, it is an important matter. We use symbols to communicate things, and sports are a major symbol system. For example, athletic teams often represent schools, cities, or nations. When a team wins, it not only demonstrates the superiority of the players and coaching staff, but also suggests symbolically the superiority of the group it represents. When your high school or university team wins and you chant "We're number 1," you're doing more than telling others that your team is tops. You're expressing something about the superiority of your school or university—and perhaps yourself—as well. In Olympic competition, American victories are wrapped up in the virtues of our national way of life. Similarly, the superiority of men in popular, highly visible sports supports and reinforces men's more superior position throughout our society. No one knows for sure how much this influences our thinking, but it is not likely to encourage thoughts of gender equity.

🔑 Many sports serve as vehicles for exploring, celebrating, and giving privilege to masculinity, and because of this they express ideas that are problematic for girls and women as well as for boys and men who are not athletically inclined.

The outward appearance of bodies is important in most societies, and by exercising and dieting we can achieve a more slender, muscled look—the current ideal in American culture. A quick glance through fashion and fitness magazines will show you that this look is "in" for both males and females. However, it's important to realize that Americans are especially attentive to the bodies of girls and women because appearance is a major definer of female sexual attractiveness (Bain, Wilson, & Chaikind, 1989; Bordo, 1993, p. 166).

Anorexia and bulimia are two of women's extreme responses to today's societal dictates to be slender (Bordo, 1993). These have filtered into women's sports such as figure skating and gymnastics where societal ideals for attractive bodies and graceful movements are important. At the other end of the weight continuum, heavy women find themselves in a predicament because they compare unfavorably to current American standards of female beauty. For example, among a group of 18 women weighing an average of 200 pounds, most of them thought other people disapproved of their body size and consequently also disapproved of them as people (Bain, Wilson, & Chaikind, 1989).

Bodybuilders are well known for using steroids to achieve a muscular appearance. In addition, football players and athletes in other strength-dependent sports often report using steroids to increase their performance. Because steroid use is commonly reported by the media, and because our society favors the heavily muscled look for men, many teenage boys use steroids to improve their appearance. While many consider such use an extreme response to societal pressure by insecure teenagers, it is so widespread that you probably know someone who has tried it.

Evidence suggests that children's physical attractiveness influences physical education teachers' expectations for physical performance. Teachers expect less from students who appear less attractive (Martinek, 1991, p. 63). Given what we already know about the importance of physical attractiveness for girls and women, it would not be surprising to find this operating more often among girls. Similar expectations might be found to operate in exercise classes in community recreation centers or health clubs, or in physical training programs for occupations such as police or military work.

Ideals for good-looking bodies in the 1990s—lean and taut for both genders, with accentuated muscles for men—have led to extreme responses from both males and females who find these ideals hard to reach.

Think about situations you have encountered in physical activities in which questions occurred about a male's masculinity or a female's femininity. What do these examples show us about our shared beliefs concerning appropriate activities for boys and men, and girls and women? What do they show us about gender inequalities in these activities? What do they show us about our society's definitions of masculinity and femininity?

Ethnic and Racial Relations

A race is a group of people defined by society as different from others based on genetically inherited traits such as skin color, eye shape, or hair type. It is important to keep in mind that race is socially defined on the basis of the characteristics we select; it is not a natural, biological category.

Ethnicity refers to cultural heritage. People who share important and distinct cultural traditions—often developed over many generations—are classified as an ethnic group. Ethnic markers include such things as language, dialect, religion, music, art, dance, games and sports, and style of dress. Latinos/Latinas, Jews, Eskimos, Amish, and Cajuns are examples of ethnic groups in the United States. Sometimes race and ethnicity overlap. For example, African Americans are defined as a racial group, yet they also have distinct cultural traditions. In addition, there is enormous ethnic diversity within the African American population itself (e.g., distinctly different African tribal cultures, heritages from the various African nation-states, influences from different Caribbean cultures, and a variety of European colonial influences).

In the United States, members of racial and ethnic minorities have typically held less power

than the white majority. While they have become more equal during the 20th century, many difficulties still remain. Physical activity, of course, is not immune to such problems. Our focus will be mostly on sport, and we'll highlight comparisons between African American and white males because they have been at the center of the research.

Participation

In elite team sports and in track and field, African American male athletes are overrepresented in relation to their proportion in the general population. For example, in 1994 about 12% of the U.S. population was African American, while in major-league professional sports their numbers were much higher: 77% in basketball, 65% in football, and 18% in baseball. These high participation rates are probably tied to African American cultural traditions as well as to American social structure (Eitzen & Sage, 1997, pp. 254–269). Whether they are local playground heroes or major-league players, African American male athletes receive much public applause by African American men and women alike. Some of the most visible and popular African American role models are top male athletes, and this may give young African American boys the incentive to spend long hours practicing their sport skills.

But this doesn't account for their high participation rates in a few sports and their low involvement in most of the others. Opportunities—and lack of opportunities—probably influence this (Eitzen & Sage, 1997). African Americans tend to be more visible in sports with easy access to facilities and coaching—primarily in school and community recreation programs. Sports requiring private coaching, expensive equipment, empty land for playing fields, or facilities at private clubs—for example, tennis, golf, swimming, soccer, or gymnastics—are less popular. The extent to which these various factors are influential on African American athletic involvement remains unclear. It will be interesting to see how much influence golf phenomenon Tiger Woods will have on increasing golf participation among young people of color in the years ahead.

Recreational physical activities in which competition is not essential, as well as exercise programs geared toward improving health and appearance, are probably subject to some of these same factors. For example, surfing, backpacking, exercising at a health club, swimming, and skiing require various combinations of expensive equipment, facilities, lessons, and travel. Because a disproportionately higher percentage of African Americans live at the poverty level (26.1%) than non-Hispanic whites (8.2%), it is little wonder that we observe relatively few African Americans taking part in such activities (U.S. Department of Commerce, Bureau of the Census, September 30, 1999).

🔑 Large numbers of African American athletes play major team sports and participate in track and field, but few are involved in other sports in our society.

Leadership

If our society had complete racial equality, then in sports with high proportions of African American players—football, basketball, and baseball—we would expect to find rather high proportions of African American coaches. However, this is not the case. In 1994 African Americans numbered only 4 out of 28 Major League Baseball managers, 2 out of 28 NFL head coaches, and 5 out of 27 NBA head coaches. Among NCAA Division I-A intercollegiate programs in 1995, African Americans were head coaches of less than 6% of the football teams, 13% of the basketball teams, and none of the baseball teams (Eitzen & Sage, 1997, p. 274).

In addition, very few minorities officiate games; they made up only 28% of NBA basketball officials in 1993 (14 African Americans and 1 Latino). This is a very poor showing when we remember that in 1994 a whopping 77% of the players were African Americans (Eitzen & Sage, 1997, p. 274).

There are two major explanations for these leadership inequities. First, racist stereotypes featuring erroneous conceptions of inferior intellectual capabilities of African Americans are probably operating to keep them from attaining athletic leadership roles in which thinking and working well under pressure are viewed as crucial. When people doing the hiring have racist views, African Americans are likely to get short-changed (Shropshire, 1996). Ricky Stokes, an African American assistant basketball coach at Wake Forest University, put it this way: "As an African American assistant coach, sometimes you can be

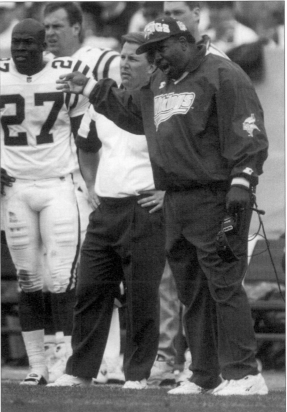

© Ron Vesely

Dennis Green of the Minnesota Vikings became a head coach in spite of unfavorable odds.

labeled as a recruiter. A lot of times people think that's all you're supposed to do. Sometimes people don't think you can do the job on the floor—coaching, teaching the fundamentals and, taking another step, speaking to booster clubs." Although Stokes expressed optimism about the likelihood that he would land a head coaching job, he realized that people might perceive hiring him as "taking a chance" (Ross, 1996, pp. C1–C2).

A second reason for leadership inequities is that white athletic administrators in charge of hiring people for entry-level coaching or management positions are likely to learn about candidates from their professional friends in other athletic programs, most of whom are also white and may think in similar ways. Because ethnic and racial minorities are not usually involved in these "old boys" networks, they are easily overlooked. There are also relatively few people from ethnic and racial minority groups in leadership positions in programs featuring expensive sports and exercise regimens (Coakley, 1998; Eitzen &

Sage, 1997; Shropshire, 1996). A quick tour of facilities such as health clubs, soccer fields, skating rinks, ski areas, gymnastics schools, and tennis courts would probably reveal only a handful of minority coaches and administrators.

 Few African Americans reach important sport leadership positions, even in team sports that boast many African American players.

Think about the local physical activity programs with which you're familiar in schools and community recreation centers (e.g., physical education classes, high school and college varsity athletic teams, rhythmic aerobics classes at a local YMCA, pickup basketball games on inner-city courts, gymnastics instruction at a private center, youth sport leagues formed by groups such as the American Youth Soccer Organization or Little League Baseball, Inc.). From your observations, what ethnic and racial minorities are represented among the people in leadership roles in these programs (e.g., supervisors, directors, coaches, officials)? How do the proportions of different ethnic and racial minorities in these positions compare with the proportions of ethnic and racial minorities among the players? What are possible reasons for the similarities or differences?

Expression

For many African Americans, sports give high visibility to commonly understood expressions of masculine creativity, strength, and pride. At the same time, however, stereotypical views of minorities are sometimes communicated through sports, and these reinforce racial and ethnic inequities.

Expressive behavior by African American athletes may be one way of dealing with barriers to achieving manhood that are faced by many African American males in our society (Majors, 1990). Because their access to education, jobs, and power is restricted, African American males often work on proving their masculinity in other ways. One of these is constructing an expressive "cool pose" consisting of "styles of demeanor, speech, gesture, clothing, hairstyle, walk, stance, and handshake" (Majors, 1990, p. 111). Cool pose sends a message that the person has a potent, interesting lifestyle that deserves respect. Sports are a ready-made arena for cool pose. Examples include football end-zone dances and spikes; Tommy Smith's and John Carlos' raised, black-gloved fists on the victory stand at the 1968 Olympics; Muhammad Ali's boasting, poetry, and dancing in the ring; and Julius Erving's gravity-defying moves to the basket that often began at the foul line (Majors, 1990). Many current African American athletic stars continue to create images rooted in the traditions of cool pose. In addition, cool pose is threaded through a variety of stylish gestures and "walks" that are embedded in the ordinary activities of African Americans, and also in distinctive dances such as hip-hop.

Young African American boys and men develop their own renditions of cool pose at playgrounds and school athletic facilities. Their style is a crucial part of their sports—especially basketball (Carlston, 1983; Kochman, 1981; Majors, 1990; Wilson & Sparks, 1996). They challenge each other with their creative, flashy moves, assertively daring other players to top them. Their goal is to heighten their reputation by combining effective game skills with a spectacular "look"—a look that can even been seen in TV sneaker commercials.

Unfortunately, sport also communicates ideas that help maintain racial and ethnic inequities. For example, the fact that many top athletes are African American seems to send an upbeat message to African American boys and young men telling them that they can make it to the pros if they work hard enough. However, this is misleadingly positive. While 43% of African American high school varsity basketball and football players think they have a chance of playing in the pros, a minuscule number actually make it. And since their constant athletic practice usually gets in the way of acquiring other job skills, they have little to offer employers when they fail to make it in athletics (Coakley, 1998, pp. 312–316). White youths in higher socioeconomic brackets who dream of playing professional sports also often end up short of their goal; however they don't face racial discrimination and are from higher-income families that have more contacts with potential employers and thus are usually in a better position to pursue other job opportunities.

Racist stereotypes are sometimes used in television portrayals of white and African American athletes (see figure 7.2). In two articles published in 1989 and 1996, Derrick Jackson studied the comments of TV sportscasters about African American and white athletes. He noticed that sportscasters tended to recognize white basketball and football players for their brains: intelligence, thoughtfulness, and strategy. African Americans, on the other hand, were noted more

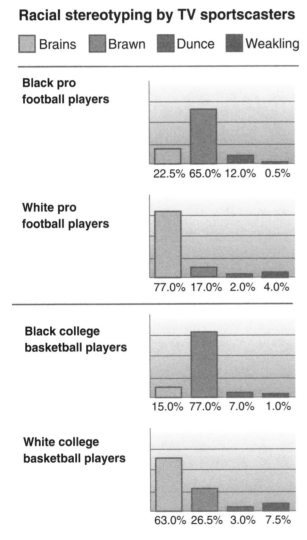

Racial stereotyping by TV sportscasters

☐ Brains ☐ Brawn ■ Dunce ■ Weakling

Black pro football players
22.5% 65.0% 12.0% 0.5%

White pro football players
77.0% 17.0% 2.0% 4.0%

Black college basketball players
15.0% 77.0% 7.0% 1.0%

White college basketball players
63.0% 26.5% 3.0% 7.5%

Figure 7.2   Racial stereotyping by TV sportscasters.
Data from analysis of seven NFL Playoffs games and five NCAA basketball games during 1988–1989.
Data from D.Z. Jackson, 1989, "Calling the plays in black and white," *Boston Globe*, (January 22): A30, A33.

for their brawn: physical skills, moves, and muscular strength. Such behavior reinforces a prominent racist stereotype. It is heartening to learn, however, that although brains were still mentioned more often in 1996 television portrayals of white athletes, this tendency was not as strong as in 1989. Unfortunately, however, over the same period the "brawn gap" between African Americans and whites doubled. African Americans were twice as likely to be praised on television for their physicality in 1996.

In addition, the media sometimes portrays African Americans in a way that strips away some of their "blackness" in order to make them more appealing to white Americans. A collection of articles devoted exclusively to Michael Jordan, probably the most visible athlete in the world in the 1990s, demonstrate the ways in which he was constructed as a media icon that transcends race (Andrews, 1996). Part of this involved stripping away some of his "blackness"—his racial identity. Media portrayals of Jordan give us a collage of meanings, some lending positive support to a distinctive African American culture, and others reinforcing old ideas that help to maintain racial inequalities. It's not easy to sort out which are which.

🔑 African American athletes who engage in "cool pose" express creativity, strength, and pride associated with masculinity; however, mass media professionals (e.g., journalists, broadcasters, advertisers) sometimes use racial stereotypes to characterize African American athletes, and sometimes they also characterize them in ways that strip away some of their racial identity.

Socioeconomic Relations

Wealth, education, and occupational prestige are all ingredients of socioeconomic status. People with larger amounts of money, more education, and greater occupational prestige have higher socioeconomic status and usually more power. To illustrate, it's not hard to think of the many advantages of being a corporate chief executive compared to being a custodian at the corporate headquarters. The chief executive can afford a

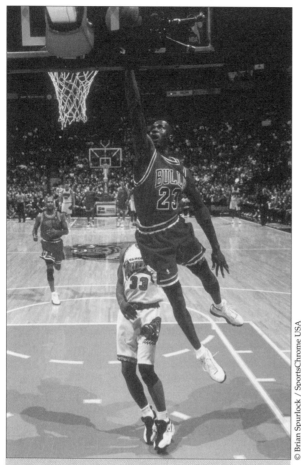

Michael Jordan: were his athletic performances an expression of "cool pose"?

© Brian Spurlock / SportsChrome USA

That's more than a sixfold increase in 21 years! By contrast, in 1995 German chief executives earned only about $14 for every worker's dollar (Hout & Lucas, 1996).

This vast and growing income disparity in the United States has important implications for many aspects of American life including education, recreation, health care, and physical activity. For example, among industrialized nations, citizens of countries with wider income gaps generally are less healthy (Siedentop, 1996). Much evidence also indicates that poor people are more likely to suffer from health problems. Yet, in the United States we have seen an enormous growth in private health and exercise clubs that charge membership fees and cater to the upper middle class and the wealthy. There has also been a decline in publicly funded programs in schools and recreation departments that are more accessible to middle- and working-class people (Wankel, 1988). For example, it is increasingly common for students to pay user fees to participate in varsity athletics in the public schools, and for families to pay user fees for youngsters to compete in community youth sport programs (Coakley, 1998). Most U.S. citizens could benefit from physical activity, and yet barriers are in place that make programs less accessible to low-income people.

Participation

As we saw in chapter 2, people's level of education is clearly tied to participation in physical activity. Highly educated groups were found to be 1.5 to 3.1 times more likely to be active than least educated groups (Stephens & Caspersen, 1994). Salaried professionals are much more likely to participate in corporate fitness programs than hourly workers (Eitzen & Sage, 1997).

Income is also linked to the types of sports and recreational activities in which people take part. Wealthy adults tend to participate in individual activities such as tennis, golf, and skiing, while those with lower incomes tend to bowl and play team sports such as football, basketball, and baseball (see table 7.1). There are at least two explanations for this. Equipment and facility costs are so high in some sports that they don't attract people with low incomes. In addition, the working hours of higher-income professionals often fluctuate, making it more difficult to schedule regular competition with a team. Blue-collar workers tend to have standard working hours,

luxurious lifestyle, while the custodian might have to scrimp to make ends meet. The chief executive can send his children to the most expensive universities, while the children of the custodian might have to work to put themselves through college. The chief executive can make major decisions affecting future directions of the company, while the custodian might only be able to make recommendations to his boss about better ways to do clean-up work.

Abundant evidence indicates that the income gap between rich and poor is widening in the United States. For example, after taking inflation into account, between 1968 and 1994 the average income among the top 20% of households grew by 44%, while among the bottom 20% it only grew by 7% (Income gap, 1996). In 1974 chief executive officers of U.S. corporations made about $35 for every dollar earned by workers, and by 1995 this had grown to $224 for every worker's dollar.

and this makes it easier to schedule regular team sport competition (Eitzen & Sage, 1997, pp. 244–245). Many expensive physical activities can be scheduled flexibly, and this may appeal more to higher-income people. Examples include skiing, scuba diving, mountain climbing, hang gliding, and white-water kayaking.

We can point to many athletes who grew up in poverty and eventually acquired enormous wealth and fame as professional players. This leads a lot of people to think that talented athletes have a sure path to upward social mobility. However, this route is only traveled successfully by a tiny minority of mostly male athletes. In 1992, for example, the 2,490 major-league professional players in football, basketball, and baseball represented only 0.14% (less than 1%) of the 1,900,000 high school boys playing these sports. About 15,000 players from colleges and universities are eligible to be drafted as rookies in the National Football League each year, but only about 160 actually end up on the final team rosters (Eitzen & Sage, 1997, pp. 254–255).

Socioeconomic status influences the types of physical activities to which people have access; physical activities requiring expensive equipment, facilities, and coaching are mostly beyond the reach of people at lower income levels.

Leadership

It comes as little surprise to learn that the people who control elite sports are generally quite wealthy. At the top are the owners of professional team sport franchises, sports media moguls, and an occasional corporate executive. In 1993 the individual net worth of U.S. pro team owners was estimated to range from a high of $3.2 billion (Paul Allen, sole owner of the Portland Trailblazers) to a mere $3 million (George W. Bush, owner of 5% of the Texas Rangers). Most were sole or partial owners of several other businesses, and many were (or had been) corporate chief executives (Steinbreder, 1993). In 1996 the three most

TABLE 7.1
Participation in Selected Sports Activities by Household Income

Sport	% total participants in the activity by household income	
	< $15,000	≤ $75,000
Baseball	14.6	8.3
Basketball	13.5	10.1
Bowling	15.7	8.1
Football	16.5	8.7
Softball	13.0	7.4
Hunting (with firearms)	13.5	6.9
Fishing (fresh water)	17.5	7.2
Tennis	10.3	18.6
Skiing	6.5	25.1
Skiing (cross country)	8.8	17.2
Exercising with equipment	12.4	13.2

Data from 1992 census; for persons 7 years of age or older, based on a sampling of 10,000 households.

Adapted from *Statistical Abstract of the United States: 1994* (Washington, DC: U.S. Census Bureau), 258.

Remember the opening scenario that focused on an outstanding women's collegiate basketball team—a team that had lots of media coverage and wonderful fan support? The hype and excitement surrounding the team's success, coupled with extra income from tickets, special promotions, and donors, might lead the players to feel some of the same pressures experienced by their male counterparts in "big-time" men's intercollegiate sports. Nevertheless, the much larger amounts of money involved in top men's football and basketball make these activities different from the other men's, and all women's, intercollegiate sports.

One of the most controversial socioeconomic issues in "big-time" men's intercollegiate athletics concerns conflicts between professionalism and amateurism. While some of the big money that comes in as a result of a team's enormous popularity goes to coaches and athletic directors (in the form of salaries) and to television companies (in the form of profits), athletes receive comparatively meager financial rewards for their efforts.

Players on major intercollegiate men's football and basketball teams often experience large conflicts between their athletic and academic roles. They are expected to be major contenders for national athletic supremacy while performing well enough in classes to progress toward a degree and eventually graduate. Of course, many other college athletes also have difficulty juggling their athletic and academic roles, but they are not under pressure to produce high-quality entertainment that pleases paying spectators, donors, and the mass media.

On one NCAA Division I men's basketball team, many of the players came to college as freshmen expecting to be able to achieve in the classroom as well as on the basketball court. However, during their four years of athletic eligibility, most readjusted their sights. Basketball became so all-consuming that athletes who originally enrolled in difficult majors switched to easier ones. Those who started in easier ones gave up the hope of graduating and just tried to do well enough in the classroom to remain eligible to play (Adler & Adler, 1991).

As freshmen, the players were awestruck by the university. They thought it was giving them a lot and asking very little in return. By the time they were seniors, however, most viewed themselves as exploited. They felt their athletic scholarships were not adequate compensation for four years of helping the university generate large sums of money through basketball. And those who were on track to graduate felt that their college degree wouldn't be enough additional reward.

What leads to a situation in which talented basketball players believe they are vastly underpaid, and at the same time a university's promise to give them an education gets undermined by the enormous athletic commitments it expects them to make? What are the roots of this predicament? The problem develops because of tensions between amateurism and professionalism. Let's look more closely.

Under the amateur model, student-athletes are considered to be in school primarily to acquire an education; their athletic involvement is thought to be secondary. Efforts are made to prevent athletic excesses that might sway players away from education. For example, the NCAA requires a specified grade-point average and demonstration of progress toward graduation to be eligible to play. It strictly limits the formal length of playing seasons, and it avoids scheduling championships when most campuses have final exams. It limits the size of an athletic scholarship as well as expenses that can be reimbursed during recruiting. Student-athletes who transfer to another institution lose part of their eligibility because it is thought that unrestrained movement might lead to continuous recruiting by rival coaches, and this could interfere with academic work.

→

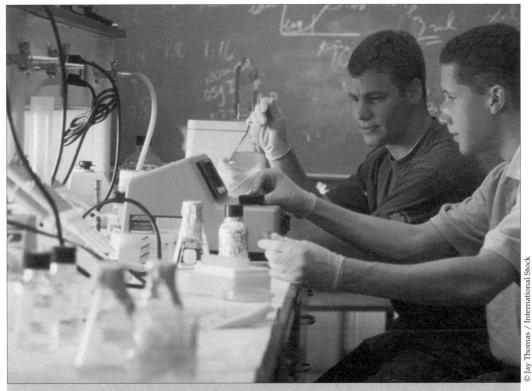

How compatible are academic studies and university sports?

Under the professional model, student-athletes are considered valuable resources. Their elite playing skills contribute to exciting games that often receive national attention. Victories in this electrifying public arena are thought to bring prestige, notoriety, and a sense of community to the university, along with money to the athletic program. Student-athletes are pressured to spend more time, not less, on athletics. The goal is to develop elite players who are entertaining to watch. Recruiting top high school players and then working closely with them as collegians through long hours of intense training and practice are the typical ways in which this goal is achieved.

In "big-time" men's intercollegiate basketball and football, the high level of professionalism is at cross-purposes with amateurism (Eitzen & Sage, 1997; Sage, 1998). Here the professional model has been whole-heartedly accepted for everyone except student-athletes. For example, major intercollegiate athletic departments have multimillion-dollar annual budgets. Coaches, athletic directors, and other staff members are paid what their talents are worth on the open employment market. The construction of new arenas and stadiums requires major outlays of money, and subsequent team performances are expected to justify this. Men's college football and basketball programs are expensive to operate; they often must keep all the revenue they generate just to stay afloat. Their games are also profitable beyond campus borders—for the mass media, commercial advertisers, and corporate sponsors.

In the midst of this, student-athletes are expected to maintain simultaneous allegiance to both professionalism and amateurism. They are required to spend major portions of each week practicing to be elite athletes, traveling to games, competing, and recovering from competition (the professional model). Without them, there would be no games to attract paying spectators. In return, however, athletes receive only modest financial rewards in the form of their official athletic scholarships and are supposed to do well academically (the amateur model).

→

These expectations of conformity to both models lead to exploitation from both directions. From the perspective of professionalism, student-athletes get the short end of the stick when they don't receive the level of financial compensation that their outstanding athletic talents would bring in an open employment market. From the standpoint of amateurism, they are abused when they aren't able to acquire the education that was promised upon enrollment.

There are no easy solutions. The most obvious would be to align expectations for student-athletes in men's football and basketball more fully with one of the two approaches. This would mean either treating student-athletes more like professionals, or adjusting athletic programs more toward amateurism. To illustrate the former, student-athletes could be exempted from attending classes and instead could be given four years of free education once their playing days are over. They could also be allowed to receive money for endorsing commercial products during their collegiate competitive years. At the extreme, the monetary value of athletic scholarships could be permitted to vary in relation to players' athletic talents.

Moving more toward the amateur orientation might mean eliminating scholarships and recruiting altogether and focusing on encouraging athletes to put their highest priorities on getting an education. In the extreme, if a football player has a special chemistry review session scheduled during a football practice, he would be expected to attend the review session. The amateur orientation is more prominent at NCAA Division III schools. If this model became common in all colleges and universities, professional football and basketball leagues might have to start minor leagues to train future major-league professionals.

powerful people in sports identified by the editors of *Sporting News* were Dick Ebersol (president of NBC Sports), Philip Knight (chairman and CEO of Nike), and Steve Bornstein (president and CEO of ESPN and president of ABC Sports) (Coakley, 1998, p. 294).

Increasingly, corporate heads are being hired as athletic directors in NCAA Division I college and university programs, and their salaries and other financial compensation have to be high enough to lure them away from private business. Top coaches are also well paid. In 1997 NCAA Division I-A football coaches averaged about $140,000 in base salary plus another $208,000 for shoe and clothing endorsements, radio and television shows, and public appearances. About two dozen coaches had total income packages worth over $500,000. The top two were University of Florida's Steve Spurrier (over $2 million) and Bobby Bowden of Florida State University (over $1 million). In some cases, a coach's salary is about three times that of his university's president (Dodd & Pearson, 1997). These incomes are justified in the minds of some people because many top college coaches are in contention for jobs with professional teams that can offer huge sums of money.

There are few opportunities for the less affluent to occupy important leadership roles. In the commercial enterprises of our most popular spectator sports, the goal is to make money—either for profit (e.g., professional sports franchises, media companies) or to improve the program (e.g., nonprofit, "big-time" intercollegiate sports). People who are particularly adept at doing this (e.g., winning coaches; astute collegiate athletic directors; efficient professional franchise managers, television executives, and production personnel; forward-looking team owners) usually get rewarded with higher incomes or more profits. Less affluent people have few opportunities to occupy important leadership roles in this high-stakes business.

Chances are much better for people with average incomes to assume leadership roles in lower-level collegiate programs, high school athletics, and community recreational programs such as organized youth sports and adult athletic leagues. The competitive structure of these programs often mimics elite athletics, of course. For example, youth sport teams are often named after major professional squads. Procedures involving cutting players from teams, having play-offs, and naming all-star teams are derived from elite

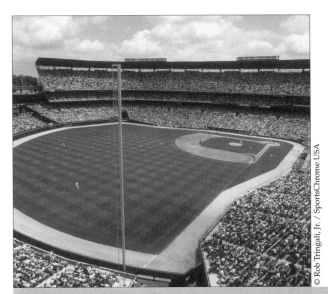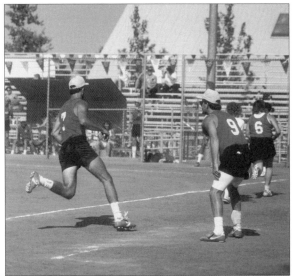

What differences would you expect to find between the personal wealth of leaders in major professional sports and the personal wealth of leaders in grassroots community recreational sports?

college and professional sports. People at the lowest income levels don't participate in sports as frequently, and because of this they are not likely to advance to positions of leadership even in lower-level programs and leagues.

Leaders in other types of physical activity programs—for example, noncompetitive recreational activities, instructional programs, and health-related exercise programs—also range from people who are extremely wealthy to those with modest incomes. For example, owners of health club chains, ski resorts, and golf courses are probably among the most affluent. Since these are private businesses, specific financial information is difficult to obtain. Like any industry, there is undoubtedly wide variation in profitability. People who manage or teach in such facilities are probably from the middle and upper-middle classes. Most individuals at the low end of the socioeconomic continuum probably don't participate enough to make it into the leadership ranks in these types of programs.

Influential leadership positions in our popular spectator sports, as well as in selected recreational physical activities, are occupied by wealthy people, while people of average means are often found in leadership roles in lower-level competitive sports and many grassroots recreational programs. People at the lowest levels of the socioeconomic continuum rarely find themselves in positions of leadership.

Expression

Sports such as golf and sailing, as well as physical activities that are not essentially competitive such as skiing and scuba diving, are sometimes used to mark economic affluence. Belonging to private country clubs or indulging in vacations at fancy sport and recreational resorts lets others know that you have enough time and money to enjoy luxurious physical activities.

In similar fashion, well-exercised, lean, taut bodies serve as status symbols. They adorn magazine and television advertisements, model the latest designer clothes, and appear in popular movies and television shows. A thin, well-contoured "hard body" accentuated by spandex tells others that you have the time, money, and self-discipline to shape yourself according to today's difficult-to-attain standards. These ideals are readily observable in almost any magazine or movie. Having a personal trainer sets you off as even more affluent. Most people can't afford all the bodywork—exercising, dieting, beauty treatments, plastic surgery, and other procedures—needed to achieve this look. The "look" thus be-

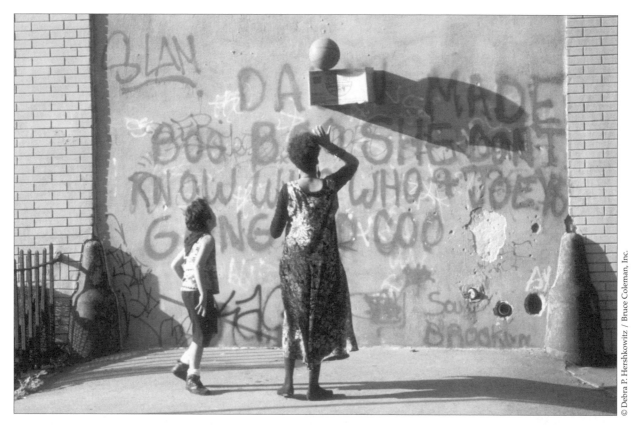

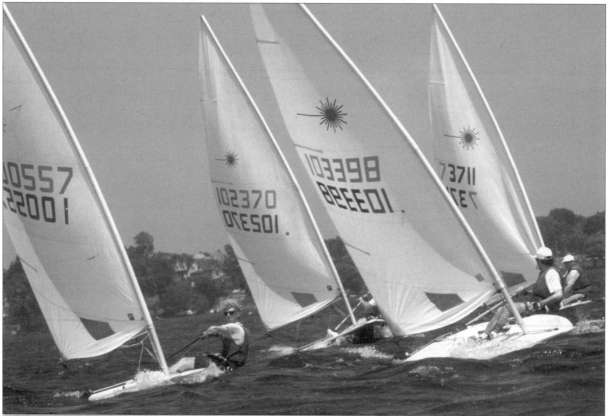

Physical activity sometimes reflects socioeconomic inequalities.

© Debra P. Hershkowitz / Bruce Coleman, Inc.

Mary Langenfeld Photo

comes a scarce commodity—something that marks you as wealthy and stylish.

Beyond highlighting socioeconomic differences, sport sends other messages that support socioeconomic inequities. For example, winning is the most prevalent organizing theme in newspaper stories and telecasts of sporting events (Kinkema & Harris, 1998). Winning is usually attributed to self-discipline, talent, and hard work. If an athlete or team doesn't win, then it is assumed that they were lazy or lacked talent and so didn't deserve to win. Such beliefs underscore the American conception of merit—we often link hard work and talent to financial success. The flip side is that if someone fails financially, it must be because she or he isn't very talented or didn't work very hard. This reasoning allows us to hold the belief that the rich and poor both deserve whatever money they have. The point here is not that merit is a bad idea. The problem is that this logic often leads us to overlook the societal barriers (e.g., poor nutrition, neighborhood gang violence, poor access to libraries and computers, dysfunctional families, lack of child care) that prevent poor people from developing themselves to the fullest and becoming valuable members of society (Coakley, 1998, p. 292).

Think about the things coaches typically tell players when a team loses a game. You can recall your own direct experiences or talk to other people about theirs. How often did coaches tell players that they didn't work hard enough and if they'd practiced harder or given more in the game, victory would have been theirs? How often did coaches tell players that they obviously tried hard but lost to a team that was just more talented? What other reasons did coaches offer for why the team lost? Did any of these (or all) make the players feel that they really didn't deserve to win?

Finally, our popular team sports also send messages about the importance of obedience and teamwork. These are valuable qualities for most workers. While some employers may need employees who can break out of traditional molds and be creative, most simply need people who can work well with others and follow directions. Because sport tends to reinforce obedience and teamwork, it helps maintain our current economic system.

A well-sculpted, lean body and participation in expensive sports are often markers that a person is wealthy. In addition, sports express other ideas that reinforce the socioeconomic status quo, such as the notion that winners and losers deserve what they get, and the value of obedience and teamwork.

Wrap-Up

Sociology of physical activity takes us beyond common, everyday understandings of sport and exercise. It illuminates patterns of change and stability, identifies social problems, and urges modifications aimed at enhancing equality and human well-being. This subdiscipline has so far emphasized sport, but there is increasing interest in exercise and societal conceptions of the human body. While researchers have analyzed relationships and trends in social life, for the most part they have not completely nailed down causal factors underlying these trends and relationships. This is not unusual in the **social sciences** because it is difficult to bring a "slice of social life" under the strict laboratory controls needed to demonstrate causation.

If you are interested in what you have learned here, you might enjoy looking through some of the sport sociology textbooks, taking an introductory course, and exploring major journals such as the *Sociology of Sport Journal*, the *Journal of Sport and Social Issues*, and the *International Review for the Sociology of Sport*.

Sociology of physical activity provides information that we can use to increase our understanding of our own experiences as participants, spectators, and professionals, as well as the experiences of others. It also helps us think more clearly about the changes we would like to make in these physical activity programs, as well as the things we would like to keep the same.

Study Questions

1. List and discuss the goals of sociological study of physical activity.

2. Give an analysis of the expanding research directions in sociology of physical activity from 1970 to the present.

3. List and discuss the six research methods commonly used in sociology of physical activity.

4. Describe the ties between participation in physical activity and power relationships based on gender, race and ethnicity, and socioeconomic status.

5. Describe the ties between leadership in physical activity programs and power relationships based on gender, race and ethnicity, and socioeconomic status.

6. Describe the ties between physical activity expressiveness and power relationships based on gender, race and ethnicity, and socioeconomic status.

7. Discuss the amateur and professional models of intercollegiate athletics. Point out how student athletes can be exploited in each.

PART II

BEHAVIORAL SPHERE

In this part . . .

8

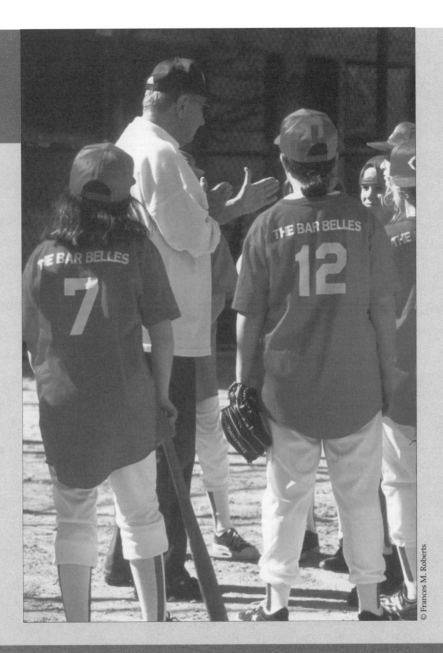

© Frances M. Roberts

Motor Behavior

Jerry R. Thomas and Katherine Thomas Thomas

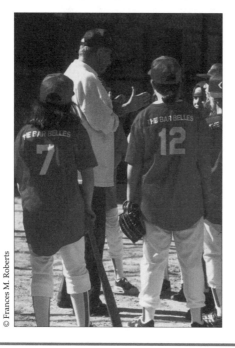

© Frances M. Roberts

You are the coach of a Little League baseball team. Jenny, a 12-year-old, is the shortstop on your team. She has played baseball for four years and is a very good fielder, but her hitting is weak. Prior to the season, Jenny's dad has been helping her with her hitting. They have developed a practice routine with a baseball fastened to a 6-meter (19.69-foot) length of string. Jenny's dad swings the ball around in a circle. Jenny stands at the circle's edge holding a bat. Jenny tries to hit the ball each time it comes around. As Jenny's coach, you wonder if this is a good practice technique. Even if Jenny becomes more skilled at hitting the ball during this practice routine, will her increased skill transfer to improved hitting in baseball?

Why Motor Behavior?

You are probably very good at certain physical activities. Perhaps you pitch a great fastball, run a quick 5K, have a killer volleyball spike or a terrific backhand in tennis. Maybe on the weekends you like to mountain bike, hike, rock climb, or kayak. Have you ever wondered how your body executes these activities?

Take dribbling a basketball for example. How did you learn to dribble? What types of practice experiences worked best for you? How did you learn to coordinate the movements of your feet, your hands, and the ball? Remember those early years when you dribbled slowly, couldn't turn very quickly, could only dribble with one hand, and sometimes lost control of the ball? In what ways did your brain and nervous system develop and adjust in order for you to improve your control and coordination? It is one thing to be able to perform an activity; it is quite another to understand how you learned it and how the motor skill is controlled. This is the content of the study of motor behavior.

We have seen in chapter 3 that practice is a specific form of experience that leads to increases in performance called learning. Parents urge children to practice playing the piano, athletes ask coaches for help practicing a sport skill, and students are given practice exercises to learn keyboard typing. Clearly, however, some forms of practice are superior to others. *What*, *how*, and *how much* are important questions about the rituals of practice. Further, we must consider what we expect as a result of practice—what can we change with practice? Is the expert better because of practice, or was she born with special talent? While the maxim that practice makes perfect persists, many factors influence the effectiveness of practice.

Think back to the Little League scenario described earlier—is 12-year-old Jenny using good practice technique? The answer is probably no—Jenny's practice routine will not improve her batting during a baseball game. Jenny may improve her batting stroke, but this routine will not be useful to improve the timing of her swing, in conjunction with the pitcher's movement that is critical to hitting a pitched ball. Athletes use many special practice drills hoping to improve their playing performance. However, only practice conditions that are very similar to actual game performance will benefit future game performance. This principle, called specificity of practice, is one of the most solid principles in motor behavior. In addition, other factors such as talent, confidence, and growth fit into the equation determining the skill Jenny will demonstrate at bat. More will be said about specificity of practice and other principles and theories within the subdiscipline of motor behavior in this chapter.

While teachers and coaches should be experts on practice, we all might encounter situations, such as the following, that call for knowledge about practice and skill acquisition:

- Your golf partner asks you to watch her swing and advise her on how to avoid slicing her drive.

- You're on the board of directors for a youth league football program. The topic of discussion is how best to group kids for fair competition.

- You regularly lose to your tennis opponent and you're afraid he's getting bored. How can you plan a practice schedule to improve your game?

- You volunteer time at a local home for the elderly. You're asked to help improve the residents' control of self-sufficient ADLs such as reaching, grasping, and picking up small objects.

- You and your dad are watching an NBA basketball game, both of you marveling at the graceful moves and expert skills of the players. How would you explain some players' attaining such a high level of expertise?

You have probably faced situations similar to these examples, and if you're like most people, you weren't entirely sure what to do or what to say. While most of us can talk at a superficial level about motor skill performance—"Did you see how long he was off the ground? He floated through space to dunk that ball!"—few people really understand how motor skill is controlled, learned, and developed over time. When practice is working—that is, performance is improving—we believe we understand skill acquisition. However, when practice doesn't work, we may feel frustrated and may begin to question the routines of practice. An understanding of motor skill acquisition is the essence of the science of motor behavior.

 CHAPTER OBJECTIVES

In this chapter we will focus on these key topics:

- What background knowledge you already have about motor behavior

- What a motor behavior researcher does

- The goals of motor behavior, including motor learning, motor control, and motor development

- The evolution of motor behavior within the field of physical activity

- The research process used by scholars in motor behavior

▪ Principles of motor learning—rules about practice, feedback, transfer, and individual differences

▪ Principles of motor control—coordination, motor equivalency, serial order, and perceptual integration

▪ Principles of developmental motor learning and motor control (motor development)—growth and motor performance, fundamental movements, and learning and control of motor skills

This chapter will serve as an introduction to the subdiscipline of motor behavior and will establish the relationship of motor behavior with other scholarly subdisciplines in the discipline of kinesiology. You'll begin to understand why motor behavior is of interest to performers who want to improve movement *experience*, scientists who contribute to *scholarly study*, and practitioners in *professional practice* who seek to assist others in developing motor skills.

What Background Knowledge Do I Already Have?

You already have a good deal of knowledge about motor behavior. Think back for a few minutes about your physical activity *experiences*. You can probably remember practicing new skills that were hard to learn, such as softball batting or throwing a football with a good spiral. And you can probably recall gaining better control of the bat or the football through the years. Finally, you can see how much more developed your movements are now than when you were a small child. Perhaps you have also witnessed the other end of the age spectrum and noticed the decline of motor skill in older people. All of these experiences have given you insights into the subdiscipline of motor behavior.

Through previous *scholarly study* you have accumulated a large body of knowledge from which to draw as you learn about motor behavior. You will recognize some of the theories and research methods used in motor behavior from your introductory, developmental, or experimental psy-

chology course. Motor behavior is a derivative of psychology that has application to movement or physical activity and focuses less on feelings and emotions than do other areas of psychology. Information from biology or zoology is incorporated into the subdiscipline of motor behavior as heredity, aging, and growth impact physical activity. In addition, researchers in the subdiscipline apply principles and laws from physics to their study of humans in motion.

Finally, from watching *physical activity professionals* in action, you may have already witnessed some results of motor behavior research. You probably remember your physical education teachers or coaches having you repeatedly practice bumping a volleyball or swinging a golf club or dribbling a soccer ball. They likely gave you feedback about your practice: "Bend a little more at the knees," "Follow through with a smooth stroke," "Keep the ball as close to your feet as possible." They were implementing the motor behavior principles that correct practice and appropriate feedback improve performance.

The subdiscipline of **motor behavior** is part of the behavioral sphere within the study of physical activity, along with psychology of sport and exercise, and pedagogy of physical activity (see figure 8.1). As people practice physical activity, they *experience* the essence of motor behavior as they try to control and learn movements. Scholars of motor behavior *study* how motor skills are learned, controlled, and developed to assist people as they practice and experience physical activity. Some of the knowledge from motor behavior research is used in *professional practice* by professionals who try to improve individuals' physical skills. Physical education teachers and coaches are two of the many types of professionals who base their practice on motor behavior knowledge. Other examples include the gerontologist who wants to improve the motor skills of the elderly, the physical therapist who rehabilitates the movements of injured patients, and the athletic trainer who attempts to prevent injuries and rehabilitate injured players.

Motor behavior is related to sport psychology and biomechanics as well as the pedagogical areas of physical education and physical education for individuals with disabilities (adapted physical education). Sport psychology research and motor behavior research often use the same performance measures (some aspect of skill); however, motor behavior research examines the control and learning of these skills, while sport psychology addresses other cognitive and emotional characteristics (e.g., motivation and arousal) that moderate the skills. Motor behavior also differs from sport psychology in that sport psychology typically studies elite athletes in competitive settings, while motor behavior studies people of all skill levels.

Motor behavior and biomechanics both study movement control and how motor control changes with age and experience. The difference between the two lies in the nature of the research questions. Motor behavior researchers may ask how this control is achieved. For example, how do the brain and nervous system coordinate all the movements involved when you're swimming the butterfly stroke? Biomechanic researchers may ask instead how effective the movement is—

for example, what is an efficient butterfly stroke?

Finally, the pedagogical areas of physical education and adapted physical education may use motor behavior knowledge to design instructional programs and evaluate motor skill. For example, a physical education teacher may use motor behavior information to plan a series of instructional classes for sixth-graders to improve soccer dribbling techniques.

Motor behavior is part of the behavioral sphere of kinesiology. It is linked to the other behavioral subdisciplines—psychology of sport and exercise and pedagogy of physical activity. Motor behavior is also closely associated with biomechanics from the biophysical sphere of study.

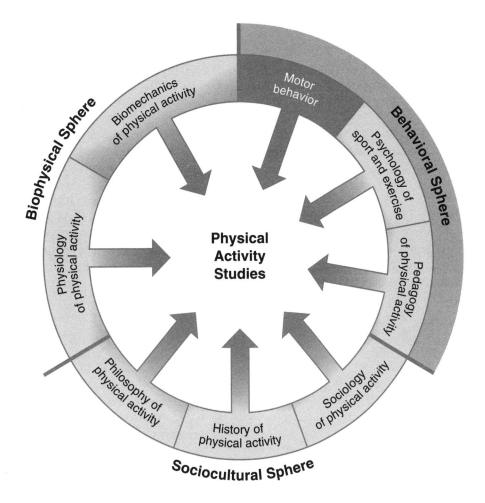

Figure 8.1 Motor behavior of physical activity and the other scholarly subdisciplines.

What Does a Motor Behavior Researcher Do?

Scholars who study motor behavior are often employed at universities where they teach and do research and service; however, some work in research facilities not associated with universities. Motor behavior research can be conducted in a university laboratory, in a clinical setting (e.g., a hospital), or in an industrial/military setting.

Motor learning and motor control research has industrial and military applications. Researchers might study, for example, how night vision glasses influence pilots controlling helicopters, or what the optimal method is for training workers to assemble a product. In addition to conducting research, industrial and military researchers also do grant writing and perform professional services, such as reviewing manuscripts for scholarly journals.

Medical and educational researchers often study motor learning, motor control, and motor development. They might study how the nervous system changes across age in the control of movement, what the best methods are for teaching rehabilitation protocols to patients in physical therapy, how the game performance of youth soccer players can be improved, or what the causes are of movement deterioration with Parkinson's disease.

The duties of a motor behavior scholar at a university typically include research in the area of learning, control, or development; teaching; and service. Scholars may write grants to support research or programs related to practice. Teaching duties could include courses in motor behavior (learning, control, and development) or related courses such as biomechanics or sport psychology, research methods, measurement and evaluation, or pedagogy and youth sport. Service for a university faculty member might include evaluating motor disorders or managing a program for individuals with motor disorders and doing workshops or clinics about motor disorders.

Goals of Motor Behavior

The subdiscipline of motor behavior produces knowledge of how motor skills are achieved across the human life span and involves three areas: motor learning, motor control, and motor development (a developmental view of motor learning and motor control). One goal of motor behavior is *to understand how motor skills are learned*. The second goal is *to understand how motor skills are controlled*. Motor learning research deals with "the acquisition of skilled movements as a result of practice," whereas work in motor control seeks to understand "the neural, physical, and behavioral aspects of movement" (Schmidt, 1988, p. 17); both are often evaluated across the life span, resulting in a developmental view. This brings us to the third goal of motor behavior, which is *to understand how the learning and control of motor skills change across the life span.*

Remember when you were learning to drive a car? Name one task that was difficult for you to master (e.g., using the clutch, slowing down to turn without stopping completely while signaling, parallel parking). Now think about the last time you drove somewhere familiar, for example, driving to school today. Sometimes we cannot remember anything about a familiar drive. First, you can see how your skill has changed as a result of learning to drive and then continuing to practice. Second, you can identify skills that are so well learned that you don't think about the skill at all during or after the performance. In other words, driving your car on a familiar route is well learned and automatic. Can you think of a situation when you have to think about a well-learned skill? For example, when there is a lot of traffic or during a storm, you are forced to pay more attention to driving.

Motor learning and motor control are not distinctly different areas, but they tend to ask slightly different questions. The goals of motor learning can be summarized as understanding the influence of feedback, practice, and individual differences, especially as they relate to the retention and transfer of motor skill. The goals of motor control are to understand how the muscles and joints are coordinated during movement, how a sequence of movements is controlled, and how to use environmental information to plan and adjust movements. In addition, motor development scholars are often interested in exploring how motor learning and motor control vary with different age groups from children to senior citizens.

Goals of Motor Behavior
1. To understand how motor skills are learned
2. To understand how motor skills are controlled
3. To understand how the learning and control of motor skills changes across the life span

When you think of motor behavior, you may think of sport skills. But consider the many other types of movements people use in their daily activities:

- Babies learning to use a fork and spoon
- Dentists learning to control the drill while looking in a mirror
- Surgeons controlling a scalpel; microsurgeons using a laser while viewing a magnified TV picture of the brain
- Children learning to ride a bicycle or roller skate
- Students learning to use a computer keyboard
- Teenagers learning to drive
- Dancers as they perform carefully choreographed movements
- Pilots learning to control an airplane
- Young children learning to control a pencil when writing

All of these activities and many others involve motor behavior and are of interest to researchers and practitioners in this area. Thus, the goals of motor behavior are important not only in sport but in the total field of physical activity. As we saw in section 1, understanding the learning, control, and development of movements plays an essential role in our culture and society. For example, the first clue parents may have that their

baby is developing normally may be when they observe a reflex or motor milestone, such as reaching. Individuals have probably been asking questions about motor behavior since the beginning of time; scientists have been seeking the answers to those questions for over a hundred years.

History of Motor Behavior

Long before the subdiscipline of motor behavior was recognized, researchers in the field of psychology began studying motor skills (Adams, 1987; Thomas, 1997). While motor behavior and its components of motor learning and motor control were not recognized until recently, some of the motor skills research from the end of the 1800s until the modern period falls within the purview of the area we now call motor behavior research. Therefore, we will begin our study of the history of motor behavior by looking at the early work in motor skills, then review the middle period, and finally examine the modern period in which researchers explored the subjects of motor learning and motor control. Motor development will be discussed in the next section.

Early Work in Motor Skills

In the late 1800s and early 1900s researchers investigated vision and hand movements (Bowditch & Southard, 1882), force reproducibility (Fullerton & Cattell, 1892), telegraphy (Bryan & Harter, 1897, 1899), transfer of learning in dart throwing (Judd, 1908), and limb positioning accuracy (Leuba, 1909). However, these researchers were primarily interested in using motor skills as a means to understand the mind; motor skills were a tool to examine cognition (Abernethy & Sparrow, 1992).

Woodworth's (1899) attempt to identify rapid arm and hand movement principles was the first research devoted to understanding motor skills in their own right. Adams (1987) identified five themes from this early work that have persisted through the years: "knowledge of results, distribution of practice, transfer of training, retention, and individual differences."

Thorndike's (1927, 1932) Law of Effect indicated that rewarded responses became stronger and were selected more often, thus "learned."

Historical Time Line—Motor Learning and Control*

1846–1892	Beginnings of motor control research—springlike quality of muscles, relation between brain electrical activity and muscle.
1897–1920	Beginnings of motor skill research.
1927, 1932	Thorndike develops Law of Effect, which influenced learning research and knowledge-of-results research.
1910–1935	Development of five themes of motor skill research—knowledge of results, distribution of practice, transfer of training, retention, and individual differences.
1940s	Influence of World War II on motor skill research, particularly pilot training.
1948–1954	Craik develops the idea of the human brain as a computer; Fleishman works on abilities and motor learning; Fitts develops Fitts's Law—the relation between movement speed and accuracy.
1960	Henry and Rogers publish the "memory drum theory," the first real theory of motor behavior.
1968	Singer publishes first textbook on motor learning and performance.
1969	Establishment of the *Journal of Motor Behavior (JMB)*.
1971	Adams publishes the "closed-loop theory" in *JMB*.
1975	Schmidt publishes the "schema theory" in *Psychological Review*.
1975–1977	Stelmach organizes two conferences and subsequently edits a books on motor control and learning.
1995	Kelso proposes the dynamical systems model, challenging information processing as the dominant motor behavior theory.

*Summarized from Thomas (1997).

Thorndike's work influenced motor behavior research and practice for 40 years and was an early example of research on feedback (called "knowledge of results" by Adams).

Early research from the field of physical education was related to motor behavior; examples include McCloy's (1934, 1937) research on measurement in sport and athletic performance, and Griffith's (1930) research on learning plateaus in motor skills, reaction time, decisions in sport, and muscular tension and skill. McCloy's research was more influential in the measurement of physical performance capacity, while Griffith's was more influential in sport psychology.

Five themes have persisted over the years in motor behavior research: knowledge of results (more generally called feedback), distribution of practice, transfer of training, retention, and individual differences.

Motor control research can be traced to research in the late 1800s on the "springlike" qualities of muscle (Blix 1892–1895) and the relation between brain electrical activity and movement control (Beevor & Horsely 1887, 1890). Sherrington's (1906) seminal work on neural control is still useful in explaining how the nervous system controls muscles during movement and resulted in terms that are still in use, such as *reciprocal innervation, final common path, muscle tension and length*, and *proprioception*.

These scholars studying motor control were in the field of neurophysiology. Unfortunately, there was virtually no contact between motor skills researchers and neurophysiology researchers (Schmidt, 1988). The only place where the two areas were integrated was in Russia with Berstein's studies of coordination in the 1930s and 1940s, but his research was not known in the United States until its translation into English in 1967.

The middle period covers the time from 1940 to 1970. The World War II era, from 1941 to 1945, was one of great interest in motor behavior research (Thomas, 1997). Because the military needed to select and train pilots, attention was focused on applied work (Adams, 1987). Transfer of training was important to assist instruction of pilots who had to learn to fly one aircraft, then transfer to another plane that might be of a different size and have different controls. Errors occurred when going to the second plane, particularly when the planes had different cockpit setups. When the pilots returned to the original training aircraft, there was evidence of a new set of errors. Did learning the setup of the second airplane interfere with the capability to fly the first plane (negative transfer)? The most famous work of this period was by Fleishman (1953, 1956). He found that different motor abilities affect motor performance early and late in learning.

World War II was an important time for applied research in motor learning and motor control because the military needed to select and train pilots.

Motor Behavior as a Subdiscipline of Physical Activity—the Modern Period

Beginning in the 1960s and increasing in the early 1970s, motor behavior evolved as a scholarly subdiscipline of kinesiology. Scholars doing motor behavior research were no longer primarily neurophysiologists or psychologists; they were specialists in kinesiology. Franklin Henry's (Henry & Rogers, 1960) memory drum theory was the first major theoretical paper from the discipline of kinesiology (at the time called "physical education"). Henry's theory stated that reaction time was slower for more complex movements because these movements took more planning time. For example, movements with several segments—involving moving from one position to a second position and then to a third position—required a longer reaction time than did single-segment movements. This is because the brain requires more time to specify the needed information for the more complex movement. The

current work on motor programs (central representations in the brain of the plan for movements) evolved from Henry's memory drum theory.

During this time, scientists were being trained by Franklin Henry (referred to as the father of motor behavior, see profile on page 252) at the University of California at Berkeley, Fritz Hubbard (and psychologist Jack Adams) at the University of Illinois, and Arthur Slater-Hammell at Indiana University. Often called the three H's of motor behavior, they prepared many scholars in the newly emerging motor behavior subdiscipline within the study of physical activity. John Lawther from Pennsylvania State University was also one who influenced the study of motor control and learning by preparing doctoral students.

Two of these scholars were Richard Schmidt and George Stelmach. Schmidt's work on motor programs using schema theory (Schmidt, 1975) is probably the most frequently cited paper in motor behavior (Thomas, 1997). Stelmach's organization of a motor control conference and his subsequent book (1976) set the tone and direction for research in motor behavior from the late 1970s well into the 1980s. Both Schmidt and Stelmach continue their research and function today as scholars in the subdiscipline of motor behavior.

Robert N. Singer of the University of Florida wrote the first book to organize the subdiscipline of motor behavior—*Motor Learning and Human Performance* (1968). His work and the work of doctoral students he mentored have had a significant impact on the subdiscipline. His former student Richard Magill's research at Louisiana State University on the influence of practice in skilled learning (Lee & Magill, 1983; Magill & Hall, 1990), as well as Magill's motor learning textbook (1989) have moved the field of motor learning forward.

Since 1970 these scholars and numerous others have led motor behavior to a prominent place in both theory and practice. In the early periods of research, motor behavior tended to select theories from psychology and apply them to motor skills. However, beginning with Henry and Roger's (1960) memory drum theory and continuing with Adams's (1971) closed-loop theory and Schmidt's (1975) schema theory, motor behavior has evolved to study and explain movement with its own theories and models. This is a common and essential evolutionary process for disciplines

In Profile

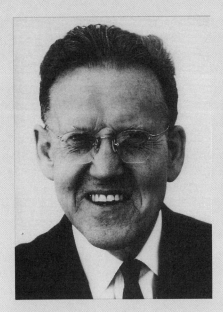

Franklin "Doc" Henry

Franklin "Doc" Henry is often called the father of motor behavior. This designation is appropriate as he developed the first theory about the control of movement, the memory drum theory (Henry & Rogers, 1960), suggesting that as movements become more complex, reaction time increases because greater detail about the movement must be specified in memory. This paper is likely the most frequently cited paper from *Research Quarterly for Exercise and Sport*. In addition, Henry's famous paper on physical education as an academic discipline charted a course for the developing discipline and led to the development and consolidation of the subdisciplines discussed in this book.

Henry was born on April 4, 1904, and died on September 13, 1993, at the age of 89. He spent his academic career at the University of California at Berkeley. His scholarly work spanned the subdisciplines of exercise physiology and motor learning and control and included 121 scholarly papers, among them 45 papers published in *Research Quarterly for Exercise and Sport*—the first in 1938 and the last in 1976. Henry also published papers in the most prestigious journals in the scientific field, including five or more papers in *Science, Psychological Bulletin,* and the *Journal of Applied Physiology.*

This academic record was established by a boy who dropped out of high school at 15 to join the navy by convincing his mother to say he was 17. He talked his way into the University of California without a high school diploma, earned a BA degree *summa cum laude* in 1935, an MA in 1936, and a PhD in 1938, all in psychology. He was hired as an instructor of physical education at UC Berkeley in 1938, progressed through the academic ranks to professor, and retired in 1971. He was a Fellow in the American Academy of Kinesiology and Physical Education and received its Hetherington Award in 1972. He was also honored as the first Distinguished Scholar of the North American Society for Psychology of Sport and Physical Activity.

and subdisciplines. In fact, the subdiscipline, while retaining its connections to psychology and neurophysiology, is now recognized as a subdicipline of kinesiology.

A model called **dynamical systems** has recently challenged the information processing view of movement (e.g., motor programs) embraced by earlier researchers. This view of movement control and learning promoted by Scott Kelso (1995) at the Center for Complex Systems (Florida Atlantic University) suggests that certain, or possibly most, movement patterns are the natural and stable choice of the neuromuscular system; a central controller, such as a motor program, does not play as prominent a role. According to Kelso, the neuromuscular system is set to choose this natural action pattern unless something else interferes.

 An information processing view of motor behavior (motor programs or schema), based on the role of cognition and a central processing mechanism, has dominated the research in motor behavior for over 30 years. However, the dynamical systems view (movements organized by environmental constraints) has provided an alternative explanation and challenged information processing as the dominant theory in recent years.

Another debate within motor behavior is the issue of basic versus applied research. In laboratory (basic) research, gaining and maintaining control over subjects, treatments, and measurements is easier than in real-world (applied) settings. However, results from laboratory research sometimes don't apply very well to the real world (e.g., how skills are learned and controlled in sports). This issue has led to discussion about whether motor behavior research should focus on basic or applied issues. Christina (1989) has provided a good summary of this debate and potential solutions. One outcome of this debate is that principles are being tested in a variety of settings from the controlled laboratory to the field in order to ensure the validity of the principles in application.

Can you think of an example of applied research and another example of basic research that you have read or heard about? The TV news and newspapers often present research findings. Watch the news tonight or read the paper and see if there is an example. Do you think the general public is more interested in basic or applied research? Have you ever thought about doing research or perhaps being a subject in an experiment?

The subdiscipline continues to evolve as a result of research, technology, and differing theoretical models. Motor learning and motor control are distinct but linked by a common goal—to understand physical activity.

Developmental View of Motor Behavior

The areas of motor learning and motor control tended to evolve from experimental psychology with connections to neurophysiology; however, a developmental approach to motor learning and motor control (also known as motor development) originated in developmental psychology and child development. Motor development grew from the "baby biographies"—many done before 1900—which were descriptions of the changes in reflexes and movements of infants.

The early work used twins to establish the role of environment and heredity in shaping behavior (Galton, 1876). Early research during the 1920s and 1930s by Gesell (1928), McGraw (1935, 1939), and Dennis (1938; Dennis & Dennis, 1940) provided careful descriptions of the sequences and unfolding of reflexes and movements in infant twins and young twins exposed to different circumstances. Bayley's (1935) motor development scales for evaluating infant development are still widely used today (in modified form) for screening young children's motor development. Finally, Wild's (1937, 1938) careful description of the stages of development in overhand throwing established a model that is still in use. She described the systematic age-related changes in the fundamental skill of the overhand throw.

In the 1940s and 1950s developmental psychologists lost interest in the developmental aspects of motor learning and motor control and focused their attention on cognitive and emotional development. Research in the developmental aspects of motor learning and motor control might have died out altogether if not for the work of three people: Ruth Glassow and Larry Rarick (see profile on page 254) at the University of Wisconsin and Anna Espenschade at the University of California at Berkeley. The emphasis of their work was different from the developmental psychologists' in that it focused on how children acquire skills—for example, how fundamental movement patterns are formed and how growth affects motor performance. These three maintained the developmental nature of motor learning and motor control in their research through the 1950s and 1960s.

Just as research in motor learning and motor control increased around 1970, developmental research addressing the questions of motor learning and motor control also became popular during that period (Clark & Whitall, 1989; Thomas & Thomas, 1989). Motor development was considered part of the subdiscipline of motor behavior because the same topics were studied developmentally.

Two research themes in motor development continued from the years prior to 1970—the influence of growth and maturation on motor performance and the developmental patterns of fundamental movements. While these topics may seem less connected to motor behavior, motor patterns can be considered to be an applied view

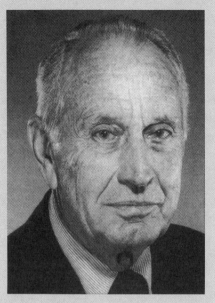

G. Lawrence Rarick

Larry Rarick received two BAs (1933) and an MS (1935) from Fort Hays State College (Kansas). He taught in a junior–senior high school and then went to the University of Iowa where he earned a PhD in 1937 while working with the famous measurement scholar, C.H. McCloy. After teaching at the University of Wichita and Boston University, he moved to the University of Wisconsin where he taught from 1940 to 1968. He then moved to the University of California at Berkeley until his retirement in 1979. He maintained an active doctoral program in both institutions. G. Lawrence Rarick died on December 15, 1995.

A mainstay in motor development research from 1950 well into the 1980s, Rarick was a leader in establishing motor development as a scholarly subdiscipline in the field of physical activity. His research focused on the influence of maturation, age, and sex on motor performance as well as on motor development in disabled children. He published work in *RQES*, the *Journal of Mental Deficiency Research, Human Biology,* and many other journals of physical activity, human biology, and special education. His edited book *Physical Activity: Human Growth and Development* (1973) defined the broad nature of motor development.

Rarick was honored (along with Franklin Henry) as one of the first two Distinguished Scholars of the North American Society for Psychology of Sport and Physical Activity. He is Alliance Scholar for the American Alliance of Health, Physical Education, Recreation and Dance, and an elected Fellow in the American Academy of Kinesiology and Physical Education.

Historical Time Line—Developmental Motor Learning and Control*

1797–1906	Baby biographies—descriptions of day-to-day changes in young infants—are published.
1928	Gesell publishes *Infancy and Human Growth*.
1935	Biographies of Jimmy and Johnny, development of the California Infant Scale of Motor Development.
1937	Wild publishes her dissertation on overhand throwing.
1956–1962	Studies on growth, strength, and motor performance are conducted.
1967–1973	Four books on motor development are published, including Connolly's *Mechanism of Motor Skill Development*.
1975	Malina publishes a book on growth and development.
1980	Thomas reviews cognitive factors in motor skill development in *Research Quarterly for Exercise and Sport*.
1982	Kelso and Clark edit a book on applying dynamical systems theories to children.
1985	Thomas and French publish a paper in the *Psychological Bulletin* on the development of gender differences.

→

1989	A series of papers appear in *Quest* on "What is motor development?"
1991	Thelen and Ulrich write a monograph on dynamical systems applied to motor development.
1993	Thomas, Thomas, and Gallagher review developmental factors in children's skill acquisition.

*Summarized from Thomas (1997).

of motor programs. Because consistent patterns are observed within and between individuals, these fit the criteria for motor programs. Growth clearly influences the performance of motor skills, and some of the studies on growth relate growth to performance. Since all of the improvement in motor performance during childhood cannot be explained by growth, developmental scientists have turned to motor control, motor learning, and biomechanics for more information.

The areas of growth and maturation and motor performance were a major part of Larry Rarick's work (e.g., 1973) and continue to be explored by one of his doctoral students, Robert Malina at Michigan State University (Malina, 1975; Malina & Bouchard, 1991). Following the model established by Wild (1937), Ralph Wickstrom (1970), Lolas Halverson of the Uni-

versity of Wisconsin, Mary Ann Roberton (e.g., 1982) from Bowling Green State University, and Vern Seefeldt and John Haubenstricker (1982) of Michigan State University continued the work on fundamental skill development.

Motor Expertise

Motor expertise, an area of research that has gained prominence in recent years, can be considered related to motor development since researchers in this area often use age as a variable. Research on motor expertise often compares novices and experts to determine how they differ within various sports. Bruce Abernethy from the University of Queensland (Brisbane, Australia) uses an action–perception model to understand expertise in sport. He believes that the major

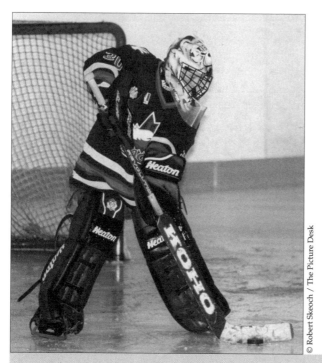

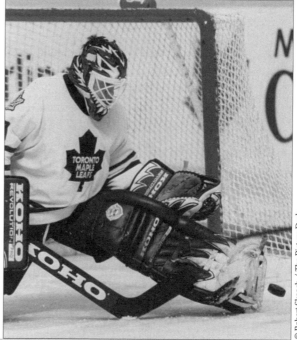

© Robert Skeoch / The Picture Desk

Research on motor expertise compares novices and experts. What differences do you see?

factor distinguishing experts from novices is the use of perceptual information. Jerry Thomas and his former students, Karen French from the University of South Carolina and Sue McPherson from Western Carolina University, suggest that faster and more accurate decision making gives the expert an advantage. Janet Starkes (1993) of McMaster University has examined the relationships among experience, age, and expertise.

Research Methods in Motor Behavior

While methodological approaches to the study of motor behavior must match the questions being asked, motor behavior researchers have concentrated on the use of techniques to measure movement speed and accuracy. Motor control and motor learning researchers use technology similar to that used by researchers in biomechanics. The major change over the past 30 years has been the use of increasingly sophisticated technology (e.g., computers, high-speed video, electromyography [EMG]) to control the testing situation as well as to record and analyze the movements. Technology has allowed the use of "real-world" movements.

Types of Studies

Three experimental designs/techniques are used frequently in motor behavior research. The "between-group" design gives two or more groups different treatments but tests them using the same task. In the second design, "within-group," all subjects are exposed to two or more different treatments and are tested on the same task.

Suppose you want to study whether a subject's reaction time—how quickly the movement begins after a signal—varies as a function of the size of the target. You could design an experiment in which, upon a verbal signal, the subject must move a stylus (like a pencil) as rapidly as possible to a target 30 centimeters (11.8 in.) away. The target is a circle either 2 or 4 centimeters (.79 or 1.57 in.) in diameter (see figure 8.2). Does the time between hearing the signal and beginning the movement (reaction time) change depending on the target size? Using a between-group design, one group could move to the 2-centimeter target

and the second to the 4-centimeter target. Using a single group (within-group design), half of the subjects could move to the 2-centimeter target first and then to the 4-centimeter target, and the other half could move to the 4-centimeter target first, then to the 2-centimeter target. In deciding which design to use, an investigator should consider whether changing target sizes interferes with subjects' performances. If so, then a between-group design is preferred; if not, a within-group design is often used for economy.

The third type of experimental design used in motor behavior research is descriptive research in which subjects are measured or observed performing a task. Sometimes the same subjects are observed several times to trace changes, for example, measuring reaction time at four, six, and eight years of age. Other times, the performances of different groups are compared, for example, four-, six-, and eight-year-old children are tested for reaction time. This technique is often used to describe age differences or differences between experts and novices. Descriptive research is different from the first two techniques because the subjects are given no treatment.

Studying the Early Stages of Learning

In the past, motor learning has used individuals in the early stages of the learning process as subjects (e.g., beginners or novices). In order to be certain that no subject had tried the task, investigators used novel learning tasks, tasks that were created for use in experiments. Figure 8.3 shows

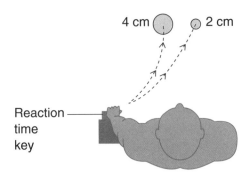

Figure 8.2 A reaction time study measures how fast a movement occurs after a signal and whether the size of the target object affects the movement.

an example, a linear positioning task with a handle that can be moved on a track with very little friction. The goal of this task is to move the handle to a location (target) previously presented to the subject. Usually subjects are blindfolded so they are not able to see the location when it is presented to them or while they are moving. Responses are scored in terms of distance from the target location. The subject's score is the measure of motor learning and is called the dependent variable. Subjects are unlikely to have ever done this task before (it is novel), particularly while blindfolded.

Many have questioned whether the results of novel learning experiments can be applied to real-world, complex movement situations. Because of the nature of the design, only the early stages of learning can be evaluated, not to mention that performers are seldom blindfolded in real-world situations. In order to allow more experimental control, the tasks tend to be simple so that improvement occurs during the testing time. In addition, the outcome of the movement rather than the nature of the movement itself is studied (Christina, 1989). Novel learning experiments also may not be helpful for researchers interested in physical activity or sport tasks in which performers have had thousands of trials (e.g., keyboard typing or baseball batting).

Studying Expert Performers

Having realized the limitations of studying novices, some scholars began to study expertise, asking the question, what do expert performers do during practice and competition? Some created descriptive studies that compared expert performers to novice performers to evaluate how they differ on perceptual knowledge—particularly decision making, skill, and game performance variables. In such studies, expertise is established by criteria such as national team membership or ranking in the sport.

Sport has been an especially interesting area to study because knowledge and skills are often unique to individual sports (Thomas & Thomas, 1994). For instance, videotapes of badminton players have been used to determine how age and expertise influence shot prediction ability. By altering the video (for example, erasing the head, arm, or racket, or zeroing in on certain motions), investigators are able to examine one of several time periods from just after the swing was initiated to just after contact with the birdie. As predicted, expert players could make better, faster predictions, with less information, about where the birdie would land than novices. Experts also looked at different body parts than novices and therefore based their decisions on different sources of information than did novices. The novices looked at less helpful body parts such as the head; experts gained task-relevant information from the racquet and arm. The advantage seemed to be a result of experience rather than age. Similar techniques have also been used to examine expertise in other physical activities such as tennis, ballet, basketball, keyboard typing, and microsurgery.

Before the early 1980s motor behavior research tended to use novel tasks that resulted in the study of early skill learning; more recently, scholars have begun to focus on expert performers in physical activity. While this has the advantage of being valid and applying to the real world, the real world is complex, and so experiments can be difficult to conduct.

Measuring Movements

The tasks used in motor behavior research provide a number of ways to measure movement and their outcomes. For example, suppose senior citizens perform a movement that involves

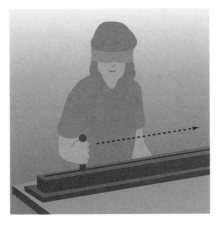

Figure 8.3 Using a linear positioning task to study early stages of learning through novel learning tasks.

Suppose you wanted to research a women's softball team. You have available standard data that are kept on the players—batting averages, RBIs, home runs, and fielding percentages. But you think these data don't always reflect the contributions players make to the team. You have videotapes of five games the women have played, which were taken using a wide-angle camera that shows the complete field. What kind of data can you get from the videotapes to help you answer the following questions:

- How many times did each player hit the ball hard while at bat?
- How many times did each player make a special effort that doesn't show up in the score book (e.g., backed up a throw, saved a bad throw, moved up a runner)?

reaching 30 centimeters (11.8 in.), then grasping and lifting containers of different sizes and weights. A high-speed video of the movement can be taken with two cameras to evaluate how this movement differs for 55-, 65-, and 75-year-old subjects. From such videos, researchers can measure kinematics (location, velocity, acceleration—see chapter 11 on biomechanics), muscle activity (EMG) of the arm and hand during the movement, and the pinching force between the forefinger and thumb during the grasp. In addition, dependent variables from the tasks may measure error in the movement, speed of the movement, reaction time before the movement begins, or accuracy of the movement. Since it is impractical to measure all variables during a movement, motor behavior scientists must use care in selecting the appropriate measurements.

Characteristics of Movement Tasks

Motor behavior scientists must consider the characteristics of the movements they study (Gentile, 1972). For example, some movements are continuous, such as a gymnastics routine, and some are discrete, having a beginning and an end, such as striking a ball with a bat. Some movements are more open in nature, whereas others are more closed. An example of an open movement is hitting a thrown ball—the environmental characteristics change from trial to trial as the batter must respond to the speed and location of the oncoming ball. A closed movement is undertaken in a more consistent environment, in which the performer tries to do the same thing each time (e.g., in archery or bowling). By choosing skills from certain categories, researchers can obtain results that apply to similar skills.

Measuring Learning and Transfer

At the end of the semester, how much do you remember when taking a comprehensive final exam? Motor behavior researchers, particularly those studying motor learning, often examine how much of what is learned is retained over time. Because of the importance of such information, nearly all studies of learning evaluate retention after a period without practice. In addition, researchers often evaluate subjects' ability to transfer to a slightly modified type of performance after a period of no practice, for example, from a football practice to a football game.

In order to study motor skill acquisition, researchers must also study how well skills are retained and how they transfer to similar situations.

Overview of Knowledge in Motor Behavior

Now let's take a look at what motor behavior researchers have learned from years of study. This section is organized according to the goals of motor behavior presented previously. While this section provides a general overview of topics and research in the subdiscipline of motor behavior, only selected topics will be covered. See table 8.1 for the main topics that have been studied as well as a selected reading for each topic.

Motor behavior is often considered within a framework called information processing. This view was adopted to help scientists conceptual-

TABLE 8.1
Topical Readings for Motor Learning and Control

Topic and subtopics	Reading
Motor Learning (overview)	Schmidt 1991 (pp. 1–12)
Feedback	Salmoni, Schmidt, & Walter 1984
Practice	Chamberlin & Bjork 1991
Retention and transfer	Christina & Bjork 1991
Individual characteristics	Keele & Hawkins 1982
Motor Control (overview)	Rosenbaum 1991 (pp. 3–28)
Coordinating movements	Stelmach & Nahom 1992
Sequencing movements	Magill 1989 (pp. 30–32)
Planning/adjusting movements (motor programs)	Schmidt 1975
Developmental Motor Learning and Control (overview)	Thomas, Thomas, & Gallagher 1993
Growth and motor performance	Malina & Bouchard 1991
Fundamental movements	Seefeldt & Haubenstricker 1982
Developmental cognitive views of movement aging	Spirduso & MacRae 1990
Expertise (overview)	Abernethy, Thomas, & Thomas 1993
Dynamical Systems (overview)	Kelso 1995
Developmental issues	Clark & Phillips 1991
History of Motor Behavior	Thomas 1997
Motor skills	Adams 1987

ize the brain as the master controller in planning, organizing, selecting, and controlling movements. General commands are sent from the brain through the spinal cord—which probably reduces the complexity of the information into relatively simple commands—to the muscles or muscle groups. From this perspective, the goal of motor behavior is to explain response selection (how the skill to be used is selected) and response execution (how the skill that is selected is performed). The following concepts are tested in research:

- Motor learning asks how processes such as practice and feedback improve the efficiency and effectiveness of response selection and response execution.
- Motor control analyzes how the mechanisms within response selection and response execution control the body's movements.
- Developmental motor learning and control tests how the response selection and re-

sponse execution processes change over the life span—generally improving across childhood and adolescence, and then deteriorating with aging.

Motor Learning

Motor learning usually focuses on the average performer, usually someone who has little or no experience with the task. The reason for this is to separate the influence of previous practice and experience from learning. Research studies in motor learning try to observe the behavior during the acquisition or learning process and typically try to eliminate all but one possible explanation for the observable behaviors. Unfortunately, learning is an internal process that cannot be observed and measured directly; it must be inferred from performance. Therefore, motor learning has often relied on the study of laboratory tasks that are quite simple and novel (such as the one displayed earlier in figure 8.3, p. 257).

Because the process of acquiring real-life motor skills takes so long and is often influenced by many variables at once, research with real-world skills is difficult to carry out. As technology has improved, however, more skills used in real-world activities are being used in research.

Motor learning is an internal state that is relatively permanent; it requires practice to occur and is difficult to observe and measure.

Based on the results of many individual experiments, the skill acquisition process can be described as an orderly progression. The learner begins by making many large errors while trying to understand the task. Early in learning, the cognitive demands are great; in fact, the task may be more cognitive than motor (Adams, 1987; Fitts & Posner, 1967; Gentile, 1972). With practice the errors become more consistent—rather than making a different error on each trial, performers make the same errors over and over. At this point the demands are less cognitive and more motor, and the errors are smaller and less frequent—response execution is improving. When the learner can execute the skill with fewer and smaller errors and doesn't have to think about the skill while performing it, the skill is considered learned or automatic. Now the performer can think about the opponent or strategy when deciding which response to select and execute, instead of what each body part is doing (response execution).

Motor learning studies try to explain and predict conditions that will make skill acquisition easier or faster as well as make learning relatively more permanent. Such conditions include individual differences in the learner such as speed of movement and coordination. Task differences are also important conditions in skill acquisition, since tasks may be more open, such as batting, or closed, such as bowling. Environmental conditions that may affect learning include practice, extrinsic feedback, and transfer.

Before undertaking a more in-depth discussion of the factors that may enhance or reduce learning, a distinction between learning and performance is necessary. While learning reflects the successful acquisition of a skill, performance reflects the degree to which someone can demonstrate that skill at any given time. Performance is the current observable behavior—in other words, what the learner is doing right now. Sometimes performance reflects learning, such as when a player is able to demonstrate successfully his or her newly acquired skill, but at other times it does not. For instance, most of us have taken an exam and after turning in the paper were able to remember an answer we knew but could not put on the paper. We argue that we had learned the material, but just could not produce it for the exam! In this case we are saying that performance does not represent learning.

One way to distinguish between performance and learning variables is to remember that performance variables have a temporary effect while learning variables have a relatively permanent effect. You may have trouble typing a term paper after you have been working and typing late into the night and are tired. Yet, the next day—after some rest—you may type rapidly with few errors. Your performance was depressed by fatigue, but you had learned the keyboard as a result of practice and could demonstrate it at a later time when you were not tired.

The distinction between learning and performance can also be illustrated by the occasional poor performance of a great athlete, or the marked improvement of a student from the end of one class to the beginning of the next (with no practice between). Examples of performance variables are fatigue and arousal. Fatigue or other short-term variables often explain poor performance; skill has not been lost—it is simply masked temporarily. When the fatigue is gone, performance improves and is a better indicator of learning.

Because performance does not always reflect learning, researchers prefer to measure learning with retention and transfer tests (Christina, 1992; Magill & Hall, 1990). Comprehensive final exams are an example of retention tests for which you must retain information for a long period of time (often with little or no practice over that time). In sport, retention means how much of a skill a performer can demonstrate after a period of no practice. Examples of retention include being able to swim at the beginning of the summer after learning the previous summer, or typing after a vacation without typing. Transfer tests require that you use the information in a slightly different way. Using a principle from physics to solve a biomechanical problem would be an example. Transfer is used in several ways—for example, transferring skills learned in practice to a game, or using your experience throwing a baseball when throwing a javelin for the first time.

🔑 Since motor performance can be influenced by variables such as fatigue, motor learning is best measured by tests of retention and transfer.

As mentioned earlier, one of the goals of motor learning is to explain, predict, and ultimately improve the skill acquisition process. In order to do this, researchers have developed principles that generalize to many situations. While these principles apply to most people under similar circumstances, they cannot explain every person and all situations! Certain individuals respond differently, and that in itself is one of the topics studied in motor learning. However, while all individuals are unique and are comprised of varying combinations of strengths and weaknesses, most of us are more alike than we are different.

Practice

After considering many practice variables, motor behavior scholars have arrived at two general conclusions, or principles. First, more practice is usually associated with better performance and is a requirement for learning. Second, practice should be organized differently depending on whether the objective is performance (short term) or learning (long term). Before the learner even tries the task, several important practice concepts can facilitate learning.

Before Practice: Goal Setting, Instructions, and Demonstrations. Goal setting—in general, setting specific and moderately difficult goals—has been shown to improve performance. Having a target goal of, say, 5 hits out of 10 pitches produces better gains in performance than simply being told to "do your best" (Locke & Latham, 1985).

In addition to setting goals, instructors of physical activity can facilitate learning by limiting instructions to one or two important points with very few details. Because forgetting occurs

quickly in our information processing system, simple instruction can help learners remember.

In addition, observational learning—or modeling—is a good way to provide learners with the general idea (McCullagh, 1993). After some practice, instructors should then model again since learners seem to have a better idea of what to look for in the demonstration after a bit of practice. It's critical, of course, that the instructor model correct form.

Other helpful techniques include verbal and mental rehearsal. Researchers have found that it is often beneficial to learners to have them verbally repeat cues or steps, along with or just after the model (Weiss & Klint, 1987). This is especially helpful in tasks with several components that must be reproduced in order. Mental rehearsal, in which the learner thinks about the task as if he or she were actually doing it, is another helpful practice strategy (see figure 8.4). Mental practice is best when accompanied by physical practice. Both verbal rehearsal and mental practice have been found to work better with certain tasks than with others.

It should come as no surprise that different tasks benefit from different practice strategies. For example, tasks with relatively independent parts, such as dance steps or parts in a gymnastics routine, benefit from practicing the individual parts before joining the parts into the sequence since the parts are relatively independent of each other. A common example of this is to learn the round-off before learning the round-off–back-hand-spring combination. Another skill, such as spring-board diving, may be more difficult to break into parts since it would be impossible to practice a dive without also doing the water entry.

🔑 Practice conditions—goal setting, modeling, verbal and mental rehearsal, separating tasks into parts, and random and variable practice—require the performer to think about and attend to the skill in order to increase retention and the transfer of skills.

Scheduling Practice. The type of task and the goal (performance or learning) of practice determine how practice should be scheduled. Periods of rest and work should both be considered when scheduling practice. The length of time the

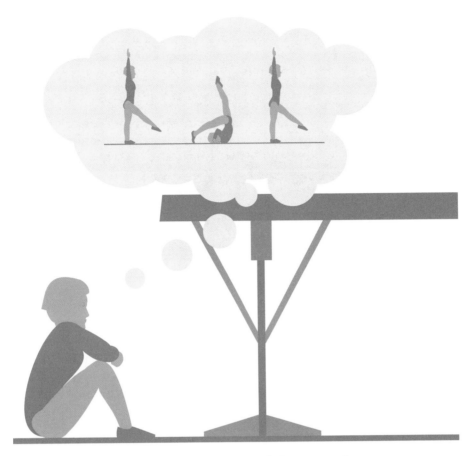

Figure 8.4   Mental rehearsal combined with physical practice usually improves performance.

performer can maintain attention to the practice and task—before fatigue sets in—should be considered. If learners are too tired, injury is possible. Sometimes, however, practicing while fatigued does not hurt and may help! For example, if players must sometimes perform during a game when fatigued, some practice when tired may help them to prepare. In other instances, practicing while fatigued may result in poorer performance. In any case, adequate gains in learning are often found when measured after a rest/retention interval. The object is to balance rest and practice to make the most of the available time for practice without risking injury or learning decrement.

Context of Practice. A final practice consideration is the context of practice (Chamberlin & Lee, 1993). The easiest practice procedures tend to produce the fastest gains in skill acquisition. An example is doing a simple skill over and over, with as little error as possible and perhaps lots of feedback. This is called constant practice. Most motor skills are not simple, however, and often require unique responses (particularly for open skills).

Difficult practice conditions will produce better results for most skills, especially complex or real-world skills. This is another rule or principle of practice. Even though the rate of acquisition will be slower, the long-term gains will be greater. Examples of various practice conditions are trial-and-error learning, variable practice, and contextual interference. In trial-and-error learning the learner must discover solutions by making errors. In variable practice each trial has different conditions. For example, in basketball shooting, players practice the jump shot from a different distance and location on each shot rather than taking many shots from one spot, then switching to another spot. Contextual interference occurs when different skills are practiced in a random condition. For example, the clear, smash, and drop shots are different skills used in badminton depending on the situation. Practicing all smash shots, then all drop shots—blocked practice—is not as valuable to learning as practicing them in a random order that produces a certain amount of interference.

Each of these forms of more difficult practice enhances learning because each demands the full concentration and involvement of the learner. When practice trials are blocked, the performance becomes automatic very quickly, and the learner can "tune out" the process. Both variable and random practice—more difficult practice organizations—seem to be more valuable when the goal is to develop motor programs (and learning), while blocked practice gives a false sense of learning (Schmidt, 1991).

Think about learning to type. As you practiced a phrase, your speed increased and errors decreased. Unfortunately, when you switched to a new paragraph or phrase, your speed usually decreased and errors increased. The final goal of typing is to be able to type new information rapidly and accurately; typing the practice phrases is of little value outside of a typing class. As you use typing to type assignments or play computer games, skill increases. The way we use typing is the ultimate form of random practice—and the results are continued improvement and long-term retention.

You want to practice to improve your golf game. You have available a practice range with target distances marked (91.44 meters [100 yards], 137.16 meters [150 yards], etc.), a practice putting green with several holes, and a sand trap. You also know about blocked and random practice from the theory of contextual interference. Using the principles you have learned, how would you plan your practice sessions to best improve your golf game?

Feedback—Knowledge of Results and Performance

Feedback is an integral part of the practice regime. Learning a skill correctly cannot occur without feedback. Feedback serves to guide the learner toward performing the task correctly as well as reinforcing correct performance. Feedback can be intrinsic or extrinsic (also called augmented). **Intrinsic feedback** is information about performance that you obtain for yourself as a result of the movement. **Extrinsic feedback** is information provided by an outside source such as a teacher or a videotape.

In addition to distinguishing between intrinsic and extrinsic feedback, motor behaviorists also categorize extrinsic feedback as **knowledge of results (KR)** and **knowledge of performance (KP)** (see figure 8.5). KR is information about the result (you missed the target); it helps advanced performers more than beginners because advanced performers understand how to make corrections based on KR. That is, they are more likely to understand how to change the movement to influence the outcome. A good typist who is told he keyed in *Hybe* instead of *June* would know that the right hand was one key away from home. Because he is an advanced typist, he is able to use KR feedback. A beginner typist, however, might need a cue ("check your home position") to correct the error. This typist is said to be using KP feedback. The goal of feedback is ultimately to help performers detect and correct their own errors. The study of feedback has focused on KP and KR with regard to frequency, precision, modality, and processing time. Feedback may also be reinforcing ("that was a good effort") or negative ("you didn't try very hard"). However, KR and KP are the forms of feedback discussed here.

How Often Do We Need Feedback? Frequency of feedback refers to the percentage of the practice trials on which feedback is given (e.g., 50% or every other trial versus 100% or all trials). On the surface, more would seem better. However, the performer can become dependent when feedback is too frequent. If the goal is to detect and correct your own errors, the detection and correction processes are not learned when feedback is given all the time. KP (or KR) should be given more often at the beginning of learning, and then gradually reduced (Salmoni, Schmidt, & Walter, 1984), often referred to as fading the feedback.

Knowledge of performance is given by an instructor who provides feedback about the nature or process of the movement. Knowledge of results is information about the

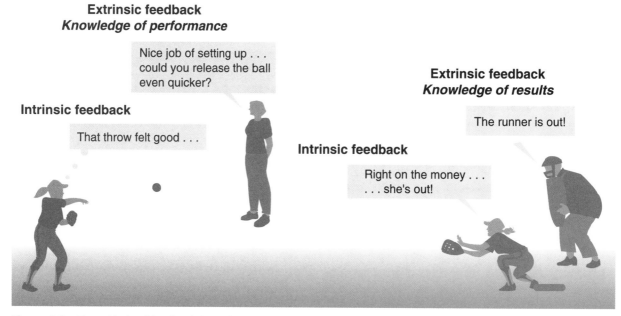

Figure 8.5   Three kinds of feedback for a shortstop.

outcome of the movements. It may be supplied by a teacher, coach, or trainer.

Precision. Precision of feedback refers to the type of information, from general ("good performance") to specific ("your error was 45 milliseconds"). A performer's ability to use feedback is dependent on two things, the usefulness of the information and the performer's skill level. As we become more skilled, we can use more precise information. Beginners usually improve with information such as "your hand was too high," while more advanced performers may need more specific information such as "you took a three-quarter swing, not a half swing; keep your wrists straight and your hands below your waist."

Modality. Feedback can be provided through numerous modalities, for example, verbal, visual, or physical manipulation. The modality through which the information is presented may change as skill increases. For example, manually guiding a beginner through the correct movement is often helpful. This is typically not helpful to a skilled player, however, because the sensory feedback for passive movements (someone else's) and active movements (his or her own) are different. Alternatively, beginners might not be able to detect their errors from a videotape, whereas advanced performers might.

Processing Time. The amount of time between when KR is given about the movement and the beginning of the next movement is called the post-KR interval. This is the time when KR can be used to adjust the next movement. The post-KR interval must be longer in children and beginners, and sometimes must be increased as the complexity (or precision) of the KR or KP increases. In any case the time must be sufficient for the learner to think about the feedback and produce a corrected plan for the next movement based on the feedback. If the time is too short, the feedback will not help.

Learning requires both practice and feedback. Extrinsic feedback (e.g., KR or KP) must be information the learner could not obtain alone, should be corrective, should be provided on about half the trials, and must be followed by sufficient time to make corrections before the next attempt.

Transfer

Transfer refers to the influence of previous practice on a related but new skill. The general rule is that the more similar the two skills are, the more successful the transfer will be. At times, transfer can be negative; sometimes previous experience may hurt future performance. For example, there may be negative transfer between badminton and tennis. Early in play there is an advantage since the order of play and rules are similar. The motor skills, however, have critical and essential differences. In tennis the wrist is firm, while in badminton shots are made by using the wrist. In this case there is both positive (game play) and negative (wrist versus no wrist) transfer.

Transfer is a major concern in planning practice and learning situations (Lee & Weeks, 1987). Coaches and teachers who use drills must be certain that these will transfer to (i.e., benefit) performance in the game situation. The more similar the activities the better, except in some rare circumstances in which there is more to be gained than lost. Recall the springboard diving example presented earlier. One major challenge in diving is confronting the fear associated with injury. Guidance belts, trampolines, and diving pits have all been used to reduce the risk of injury and the fear associated with attempting difficult dives. While the transfer may not be perfect, practice under these circumstances has great benefits. The benefits of transfer in practice usually are less as learning progresses. This means drills, simulators, and lead-up activities are more helpful to beginners, whereas practicing the actual activity under performance conditions is of more benefit to the more skilled performer.

In motor learning, skill acquisition is studied by isolating the individual elements of the study

You may be interested in physical activity because of sport, but consider other types of motor skills from everyday life, such as driving a car. As in our earlier example, recall learning how to drive. How did you practice? Did you learn to drive a standard transmission? If so, did you learn with an automatic first and then a standard, or vice versa? (What is the term in motor behavior used to describe learning on one and switching to the other?) How difficult was learning to use the clutch when shifting a standard transmission? How did you practice that? How difficult was learning to control the car when parallel parking? How did you practice that?

(characteristics such as ability and motivation) or environmental elements (external variables such as practice opportunities). We had previously been discussing environmental characteristics such as practice and tasks that influence skill acquisition. Next we will discuss some individual differences that influence motor behavior.

Individual Differences

As we saw in chapter 4, our individual differences are a result of both inherited talents and environmental influences. These differences can be studied in relation to motor learning, motor control, and motor development. Experience can be gained by practicing, observing, and in sport, competing. Experience usually changes our knowledge of a skill; in fact, experts typically structure their knowledge about a skill in rather unique ways. Knowledge has been used to study and explain expertise in motor learning and developmental research.

A player must know what to do on two levels. First, to make a movement he needs to know how to execute the movement, for example, the order of events in a movement or the location of a body part. As we learn movements, we first know, then do. When movements are well learned, we know a great deal about the movement, such as how to alter the movement slightly so the outcome will match unique conditions. Second, in sport, a player must know what to do. In baseball, for example, when the batter hits the ball, he must know to run to first base. The fielder must know where to throw the ball; experts know when to throw to first and when to throw to second. However, just because somebody knows how a movement should be done or which movement to do does not mean he can actually do the movement correctly. This is where practice and inherited talents enter the picture.

The inherited characteristics that contribute to individual differences are things such as speed and coordination of movements; such characteristics are studied in motor control research. The following three types of individual differences influence performance (Keele, Pokorny, Corcos, & Ivry, 1985):

- Timing—the ability to coordinate body parts during skilled movements; for example, shooting a jump shot

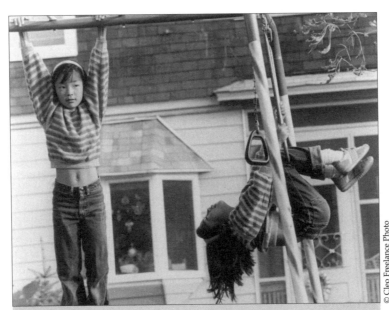

Some individual differences are inherited.

- Maximum rate of repetitive movements—the ability to move the limbs rapidly for a period of time; for example, running a sprint
- Force control—the ability to produce the same force repeatedly in the same limb or across different limbs; for example, rowing

Knowledge/experience and inherited characteristics are found in varying levels and combinations. As the level of performance changes from beginner to expert, the role of knowledge may vary in its value to performance.

A novice baseball player who knows what to do has an advantage over other novices, even if he or she may not be able to execute the proper task each time. For example, imagine a team of five-year-olds playing T-ball. The ball is hit to the second baseman, who knows the ball needs to get to first base. The second baseman also knows that the first baseman is not likely to catch the ball, so the second baseman runs the ball to first base. By eight years of age all the players know the ball must go to first base, and the skills associated with accurate catching and throwing are performed better. An eight-year-old second baseman in the same situation as the five-year-old may simply throw the ball to first base.

Professional baseball players vary in their individual skills—a pitcher is not expected to be a good hitter; fielders are expected to be good hitters, but some hit only left- or right-handed while some are switch-hitters. Knowledge—or knowing what to do—becomes important in the highest levels of baseball because it may narrow the number of choices and therefore help a player respond more accurately and quickly. For example, knowing when a batter is likely to bunt is an advantage to the fielding team. If there is no chance a batter will bunt, the fielders have narrowed their choices of what may happen. We see a similar use of strategies in other physical activities. A typist may slow down when using an old typewriter because the cost of an error is greater than when using a word processor where error correction is either easy or even automatic. An experienced driver is more attentive in heavy traffic or inclement weather than when the road is vacant and the sky is clear. We apply strategies and use our experience to make good decisions about our motor skills. In these examples the skills of throwing and catching, typing, and driving didn't change, but the consequences of actions were taken into account in our decisions.

The characteristics of the sport may determine how important a specific ability will be. In running the 100-meter dash, knowledge is relatively unimportant, while speed is critical. For a football quarterback, speed is important but is of limited value without the knowledge of plays as well as knowing when to throw or run. A quarterback must evaluate what the defense is expecting when making his decisions.

Sport is unique in part because many sports demand that performance be completed quickly (in the briefest possible time). Further, the movements in sport often must start, stop, or be coordinated with something outside of the athlete. The two characteristics of timing—speed and external factors—taken together are the timing demands of the task. Some tasks have less timing demand (e.g., golf, bowling), because both speed and external demands are low. Other tasks have other timing demands; for example running the 100 meters requires the runner to start on signal and move as quickly as possible. Finally, movements like the option play by a quarterback in football include both speed and external demands. Sports that have offensive and defensive components like football also bring another dimension to timing. The quarterback must make decisions quickly and accurately. Complex decisions, or decisions where information evolves over time (e.g., the defense changes), present a situation where having more time before deciding is an advantage. However, if we take more time to decide, we must compensate by making the movement after the choice more quickly.

In baseball the batter watches the pitcher for critical information that may give a clue about the pitch; the batter ignores the crowd yelling and gathers only related advance information about the pitch and where to hit it. Figure 8.6 provides an example of how long the batter has to make decisions about swinging the bat once the pitcher releases the ball. The figure demonstrates how a batter has more decision time (150 milliseconds versus 130 milliseconds) if the batter waits longer and speeds up the swing (140 milliseconds versus 160 milliseconds). The example also demonstrates how critical advance information is to successful performance. Thus, it becomes obvious why batters want to know in advance whether a pitcher is likely to throw a curve or a fastball

$\longrightarrow$

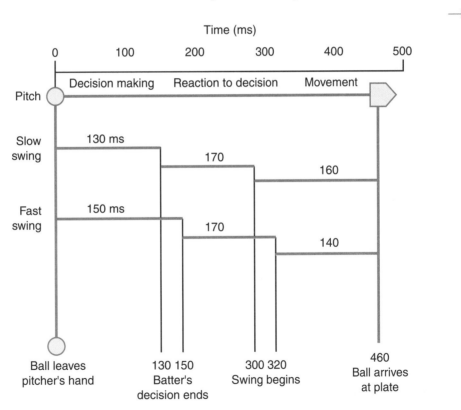

Figure 8.6 Time line showing the critical events in hitting a pitched baseball. The movement time is 160 milliseconds for the slow swing, 140 milliseconds for the fast swing.
Reprinted, by permission, from R.A. Schmidt, 1991, *Motor learning and performance: From principles to practice* (Champaign, IL: Human Kinetics), 122.

as well as the potential location of the pitch. You may hear a baseball commentator say, "The count is three balls and one strike; the batter will be looking for a fastball high and inside" (a certain pitch in a specific location). The batter is trying to reduce the potential decisions to a "go or no-go" situation—I'll swing if the pitch is what I expect—rather than all possible options. This is because the batter can decide not to swing in this situation even if the pitch is a strike. If the count were three balls and two strikes, the batter would be less likely to look for a specific pitch.

The ability to select critical cues changes with age and experience. Young children tend to focus on only one aspect of the visual and auditory array, older children are distracted by many (often irrelevant) aspects of the array, and adults are usually able to select the important information. This selection process and vigilance are important; they enable performers to focus on the key elements of the situation.

One of the tasks of the baseball coach is to help players learn how to hit. Practice situations and cues from the coach about what to look for during the pitch are essential in improving batting. Acquiring batting and anticipation skills (learning cues) begins with young children as they practice and play baseball, but improvements in skill continue even into professional baseball.

Motor performance is the result of a complex relationship among various individual differences, which vary greatly from person to person, and cognitive/neurological systems, which may respond quite consistently from individual to individual. Both improve with experience, which produces learning.

At what physical activity are you most expert? Think about how much you have practiced this sport or activity over the years to attain your level of expertise. Then, answer the following questions:

• How many years have you been playing and practicing the skills of this sport or activity?

• Who helped you develop your skills the most? What did he or she encourage you to do that improved your skills?

• Think back over the last several years that you have been involved with this physical activity. Did you practice all year? How many hours per week did you practice? What were the drills and practice routines you used the most? After reading the material in this chapter, do you think you had some poor practice routines? Is so, which ones, and why were they not a good way to practice?

Motor Control

Motor programs (Schmidt, 1975) are the theoretical explanation for our ability to successfully produce and control movements. A motor program can be compared to a computer program that does math problems. First, you select the program to use—this is response selection. The program has the ability to add, subtract, multiply, and divide. If you put in the numbers and indicate what math operations to perform, the program outputs the answer—response execution. A motor program is like that; you select the program (response selection) and indicate what it should do (operations). Then the program specifies how to do it and sends signals through the spinal cord to the muscles that perform the movement (response execution). Schmidt (1991) indicates that motor programs, at a minimum, must do the following five things:

• Specify the muscles involved in the action
• Select the order of muscle involvement
• Determine the forces of muscle contraction
• Specify the relative timing and sequences of contractions
• Determine the duration of contractions

If we had to remember every single movement we have made, our memory would be overloaded. Motor programs explain why we do not have a storage problem. Instead of storing each movement we have ever done in memory, we store groups of movements with similar characteristics. These are called "schema" and are the foundation of motor program theory (Schmidt, 1975).

🔑 Motor programs are a proposed memory mechanism that allow movements to be controlled. As motor programs are developed, they become more automatic, allowing the performer to concentrate on the use of the movement in performance situations.

As explained earlier in the chapter, some motor behavior experts contested the motor program theory, arguing that it overemphasized the role of the brain in performing complex movements. They proposed another theory called dynamical systems (Haken, Kelso, & Bunz, 1985; Kelso, 1995), which suggested a more direct and less cognitive link between information the perceptual system picks up and the motor action that occurs. This direct link is called a coordinated structure.

You may be wondering which theory—motor program or dynamical systems—more accurately represents the process of motor control. An acid test for theories of motor control is how well they explain motor learning and the development of motor expertise (Abernethy, Thomas, & Thomas, 1993). The fact is that neither the motor program theory nor the dynamical systems theory has provided clear explanations for these important aspects of motor behavior. Nevertheless, these are two of the most important theories in motor behavior today.

🔑 Future research that contrasts predictions and key elements from a dynamical systems view of motor behavior or motor program view is likely to be both exciting and controversial.

The study of motor control addresses five areas:

1. Degrees of freedom—coordination (Rosenbaum, 1991)
2. Motor equivalency

3. Serial order of movements—coarticulation (Rosenbaum, 1991)
4. Perceptual integration during movement (Rosenbaum, 1991)
5. Skill acquisition (Rosenbaum, 1991)

The brain initiates the planning of movements, then the nervous system sends signals through the spinal cord to the muscles, which in turn make the movements. What is not known is how the brain represents the information to be sent to the muscles. Motor control tries to explain what the brain, nervous system, and muscles are doing to direct movements. While skill acquisition—the notions of learning and improvement—is the focus of motor learning, it is critical in motor control as well. One reason skill acquisition is interesting in motor control research is that learning is difficult to explain in some theoretical models, for example, dynamical systems. Another is that skill acquisition accentuates the relationship between motor learning and motor control.

The previous section discussed skill acquisition (learning) issues, so those will not be repeated here. Further, the amount of information covered in this section is less for two reasons. First, some topics that apply across the subdiscipline of motor behavior (e.g., individual differences, motor expertise) were covered in the section on motor learning. Second, the area of motor control has developed more recently than that of motor learning and so information is more limited.

Coordination of Movement

The issue of coordinating the degrees of freedom in a movement is best understood using a robot analogy. Robots have been designed to be very simple, with fewer joints and limited movement in each joint, because their programs cannot handle the complexity of humanlike movements. A robot can be programmed to make certain movements with very few variations. In addition, robots usually move more slowly than humans, especially in more precise movements. The robot can move only in patterns that are programmed or that respond to feedback. When the robot uses feedback to control a movement, the adjustments are slow because the robot has to process a huge amount of feedback to make the adjustments. The amount of programming for each movement is extensive, so the number of available programs is limited.

Humans perform a nearly unlimited variety of movements—often rapidly—so the human brain must be dealing more effectively than the robot's computer with all of the ways a movement can be done. The task a human faces in coordinating all the muscles and joints to produce a movement is called the degrees-of-freedom problem. A joint such as the elbow, which can flex and extend, has one degree of freedom. Many joints have more than one degree of freedom (e.g., the ankle), and most movements involve many joints. Thus, the human system must have some way to limit the degrees of freedom of a movement while maintaining the flexibility to respond to a variety of possible alternatives (Stelmach & Nahom, 1992). One explanation for the human's ability to create coordinated movements with so many degrees of freedom is that we program groups of muscles rather than individual muscles. The issue is complex, and how the neuromuscular system functions is not well understood.

> The human motor system manages to control complex movements. One explanation is that the system reduces the number of degrees of freedom, or items that need to be controlled, so movements are rapid, accurate, and coordinated.

Motor Equivalency

The robot analogy alluded to the fact that humans can solve the same motor task in many ways. An example is turning a doorknob. One way is to reach, extend your arm at the elbow, then rotate your shoulder and wrist. What happens if you have a cup of coffee in one hand and a book under your other arm? You lean toward the knob without reaching and, while gripping the book, you rotate your wrist carefully so as not to move your elbow or shoulder. With a broken wrist and coffee in the other hand, you could still open the door by tilting your entire body while holding your wrist immobile. The point is that each movement task has many solutions—often unique ones that have not been used before.

The fact that we can adapt rapidly, and often without giving new solutions a thought, is fascinating. How does that happen? Further, when

individuals have trouble adapting to changing or new movement demands, we may be able to learn more about how the motor system works. This is because when a specific part of the motor system does not work, the impact of that part on the movement is removed. The resulting adaptation can be observed in a movement. The evidence for motor equivalency (more than one motor response to the same motor task) and the research on motor equivalency may impact our ideas about how motor programs work.

Serial Order of Movements

Another motor control issue is that of serial order of movements (Magill, 1989). The human motor system prepares for a movement, such as lifting the arms while standing, by first contracting the muscles of the legs. Why would the legs be involved when the movement is in the arms? The system is preparing for the loss of stability created by moving the arms—the order of these events is critical. Figure 8.7 shows the order and when muscle contractions begin (as defined by EMG recordings) for the movement of lifting the arm in response to a signal. Note that after the "stimulus onset" (step 1 in figure 8.7), the ipsilateral biceps femoris (step 2, BFi) located in the legs is the first muscle to show EMG activity. How the system makes these compensations is unknown.

Perceptual Integration During Movement

Perceptual integration is the use of visual and other sensory information in the control of movement. Clearly the human has more efficient control than the robot. How does the system include information from the environment in planning and adjusting movements? This question becomes even more complex when you consider that during movements that require a longer time period, the environment is influenced by the movement, requiring subsequent adjustments. For example, as a tennis player, you use information about the shot and location of an opponent in planning the upcoming shot. When you hit your shot, the environment changes as the opponent is now in a different location, which influences your court movements. Motor programs (Schmidt, 1975) are one explanation of how all this complex cognitive and motor action is learned and controlled.

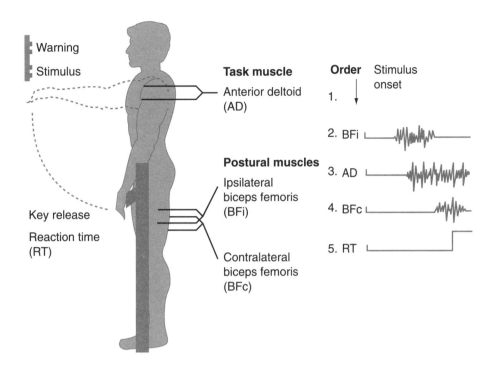

Figure 8.7 Using EMG recordings to measure a movement response. Shown are the reaction-time apparatus, where each electrode was placed to record the EMG for each muscle group of interest, the reaction-time interval for the response, and the EMG recordings for each of the three muscle groups.

Reprinted, by permission, from R.A. Magill, 1998, *Motor learning: Concepts and applications*, 5th ed. (Madison, WI: WCB: McGraw-Hill).

Developmental Motor Learning and Control

After watching a baby and a child perform a motor task, you see there are clear differences and similarities related to age. Infants demonstrate more random movements, have a smaller repertoire of movements, and tend to do the same movement over and over. Children have a larger repertoire of motor skills, do more voluntary skills, and exhibit greater skill than infants (Seefeldt & Haubenstricker, 1982) but less than adults. Children are not miniature adults—their movements are not simply scaled-down versions of adult movements. One explanation for the relative inefficiency of children's movements may be their lack of practice. Also, adults probably select and plan movements better than children do, which is a cognitive process.

Virtually all of the questions in motor learning and motor control can be studied as part of motor development—by examining the same questions across age. In addition, there are some unique problems related to studying infants, children, and the elderly. Children differ from adults

in several ways: physical growth, information processing, experience, and neurological development (Thomas, Thomas, & Gallagher, 1993). This section will cover the topics that were not covered in the sections on motor learning and motor control. Again, you can see some overlaps among development, learning, and control.

The mechanics of movements are different at different ages partly due to different sizes and proportions of the body executing the skill. For example, a baby's head is one-quarter of its height, while an adult's head is only one-eighth. The legs also change dramatically during childhood. At birth the legs are typically less than 30% of the body length; adult leg length is often over half of the body length. Obviously, balance and locomotion will be influenced by these physical characteristics.

Growth is also a factor in motor behavior; children are growing until around 13 to 14 years of age for females and around 18 to 20 years of age for males, whereas growth is not a factor in adult motor learning studies. Children grow in three physical dimensions: overall size, proportions (e.g., leg length, shoulder breadth, chest depth), and body composition (e.g., increases in muscle). Growth influences motor performance, in part, because children must deal with changes in their bodies, which is not an issue for adults. Further, the adult–child differences can be factors explaining child to child differences. For example, there is a positive relationship between size and strength: larger children are stronger. As children grow, the increase in size produces increases in strength; however, strength also increases due to neuromuscular efficiency. Since growth is not under our control, we must understand how growth influences performance in order to accommodate the challenges of physical growth.

 If you are planning to study physical activity, you must understand the physiology, biomechanics, and motor behavior underlying the development of movement in order to address problems such as how children gain control of movement skills, how expertise is achieved, and how these skills deteriorate as people age.

Imagine that you are coaching a 6- and 7-year-old girls' basketball team. Last year you coached a 10- and 11-year-old boys' basketball team. You want to plan your practice to improve skill and game performance. What changes should you make this year because the children you are coaching are younger?

• Will the younger children use feedback (KP and KR), benefit from practice, and learn the same way as the older children?

• How will four years less experience influence the performance of these children?

• Should you expect girls to be different from boys?

In addition to studying the effects of growth on motor performance, developmental motor learning and control also examines the effects of aging on motor performance; thus, it is sometimes referred to as *life span development* (Spirduso & MacRae, 1990; Stelmach & Nahom, 1992). Changes in strength and motor coordination are most rapid at the extremes of the age continuum. Growth is less important after adolescence, because the changes in physical parameters are less dramatic in adults and the elderly than in infants and young children.

Cognitive processes also change during childhood due to the developing nervous system and experience. Children use fewer cognitive processes and use them less effectively than adults. For example, when asked to remember a movement, a 5-year-old child might "put on his thinking cap"—not a very effective strategy for remembering. A 7-year-old might do the movement over and over, while a 12-year-old could repeat the movement in a series composed of several movements. Adults and older children know they must do something to learn and remember, while younger children may not recognize the importance of deliberate practice, or they may select an ineffective practice regime. Some researchers refer to such cognitive issues as software issues (analogous to a computer program for word processing or statistics) that develop over childhood in the information processing system (Thomas, Thomas, & Gallagher, 1993).

Processing time, discussed in the section on motor learning, is an important issue developmentally. Children process more slowly than adults and therefore need more time or less information to be successful in solving motor problems. One of the reasons for the increasing interest in cognitive processing during motor skill acquisition in children is that the strategies used by adults can be given to children to actually improve performance. In other words, this is an area where research enhances teaching!

Experience was presented as a factor in children's performance. Experience can help the elderly and can be a negative factor for children. In a situation where experience is a benefit, the elderly have an advantage and children have a disadvantage because children lack experience and the elderly have more experience. Clearly, we can enhance experiences for children in two ways—quality and quantity. Research shows that children with experience can outperform adults with less experience—which means practice and experience help. This has clear implications for pedagogy and curriculum development. In other words, curriculum and instruction need to provide experience to enhance sport performance in children. Further, we know that the quality of the experience can be improved too, for example, by using what we know about information processing to help children get more out of the practice. So, by providing children adult learning strategies, children will benefit more from the same amount of experience. The key is that children need practice; and that to be effective, practice must help children retain information, skill, and decision making, which would normally be lost in children. To do this, we teach children adult learning strategies.

The hardware (analogous to the computer itself and its disk drives and monitor), or neurology, is also different in children than it is in adults. Infants have fewer synapses (connections between neurons in the nervous system) and less myelin (the covering of nerve cells with a fatty sheath that aids nerve impulse transmission). In addition, babies at birth have fewer neurons than adults. The hardware is nearly complete as children are beginning school, but it may not be functioning as well as in older children and adults.

Performance may be negatively impacted by the deteriorating nervous system in the elderly. As people age, they lose neurons in the brain and motor neurons in muscles. This results in slowness and variability in movement control. However, older people benefit from experience and use experience to compensate for the loss of speed, strength, and control. Understanding the changes in the central nervous system is important, since we have little opportunity to accelerate or decelerate these changes.

Motor control issues are important in understanding adult motor behavior, and they are important in developmental learning and control. Critical issues are similar to those listed in the previous section on motor control (for a review, see Clark & Phillips, 1991). However, one additional point is important—how does growth become integrated into the motor control system? As previously mentioned, children may change very rapidly, particularly at puberty (Malina, 1984; Malina & Bouchard, 1991). How are these changes in size, proportion, and mass accounted for in the motor control system? Consider a boy who played baseball from March until July at 12 years of age. By the next March he is 13 years of age, he has grown 4 inches in height, his arms

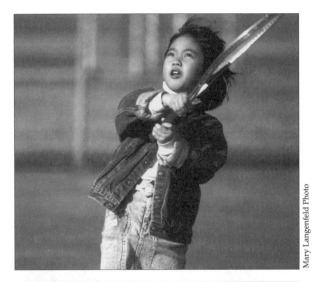

Mary Langenfeld Photo

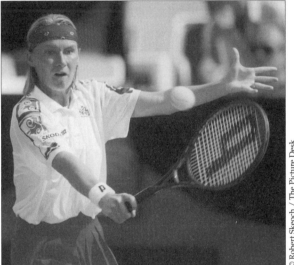

© Robert Skeoch / The Picture Desk

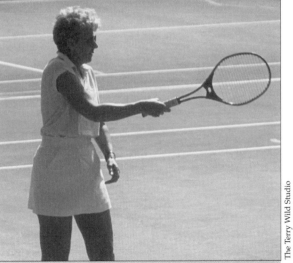

The Terry Wild Studio

As we grow and develop across the life span, our ability to perform movements changes.

We have all seen examples of people of different ages and genders showing markedly different physical abilities. But can these differences be documented? And what are the reasons for them? Here we will take a look at what researchers have learned about overhand throwing. First we need to examine physical growth and development. See tables 8.2 and 8.3 for a summary of growth in terms of stature and weight. Then we will see how this affects overhand throwing skills.

Physical growth is rapid during infancy, constant during childhood, and rapid during the growth spurt associated with puberty (Malina, 1984; Malina & Bouchard, 1991).

TABLE 8.2
Important Growth Changes in Body Length and Stature

Age	Selected growth information
Conception	0.14 mm in diameter
Birth (median length)	Boys: 20 in. (50.8 cm) Girls: 19.75 in. (50.2 cm)
6 months (median length)	Boys: 26.75 in. (67.9 cm) Girls: 26 in. (66 cm)
Year 1 (median length)	Boys: 30 in. (76.2 cm) Girls: 29.25 in. (74.3 cm) Length increases approximately 50% during the first year.
Year 2	Length increases about 4.75 in. (12.1 cm).
Year 3–5	Decelerated growth rate to about 2.75 in./yr (7 cm/yr).
Year 6–adolescence	Decelerated growth rate to about 2.25 in./yr (5.7 cm/yr).
Adolescence	20% of adult stature is attained during this 2 1/2 to 3 yr period. Approximately 4 in./yr (10.2 cm/yr) growth for males and 3 in./yr (7.6 cm/yr) for females.
16 1/2 years	Females attain 98% of adult stature.
18 years	Males attain 98% of adult stature. Average adult stature of 69 in. (175.3 cm) is roughly 3.5 times larger than that of the newborn. Females attain final 2% growth in stature.
20 years	Males attain final 2% growth in stature.
20–30 years	Growth of vertebral column may add another 1/2 in. (1.3 cm) to stature.
30–45 years	Stature is stable.
Above 45 years	Possible decrease in stature from disk degeneration.

From *Human Motor Development: A Lifespan Approach, Fourth Edition* by V. Gregory Payne and Larry D. Isaacs. Copyright © 1999 by Mayfield Publishing Company. Reprinted by permission of the publisher.

→

TABLE 8.3
Important Growth Changes in Body Weight

Age	Selected growth information
Conception	Ovum weighs roughly 0.005 mg.
19th week of gestation	14 oz (400 g)
34th week of gestation	Fetus is 20 times heavier than at 14 weeks (5.5 lb).
Birth (median weight)	Boys: 7.5 lb (3.4 kg) Girls: 7 lb (3.1 kg) Small mothers tend to have small babies. Later-borns are heavier than firstborns (6.8 oz). Twins are approximately 1.5 lb lighter than singletons.
1–3 days	Weight loss upwards of 10% of birth weight.
10 days	Weight is equal to birth weight or slightly heavier.
First 6 months	Gains about 2/3 oz (20 g)/day. Birth weight generally doubles at 5 months.
Last 6 months of year 1	Gains decelerate to about 1/2 oz (15 g)/day.
Year 1	Median weight of boys: 22.5 lb (10.15 kg) Median weight of girls: 21 lb (9.53 kg) Birth weight triples during first year.
Year 2	Gains about 5.5 lb (2.5 kg)
Years 3–5	Gains about 4.5 lb (2 kg)/yr
Year 6–adolescence	Slight increase in rate of weight gain to 6.5 lb (3 kg)/yr
Adolescence	Males add about 45 lb of body weight and females about 35 lb of body weight during this 2 1/2- to 3-yr period.
Year 18 (median weight)	Males: 151 lb (68.49 kg) Females: 27 lb (12.25 kg) lighter (124 lb [56.25 kg]) Mature body weight is approximately 20 times greater than birth weight.
Above 19 years	Weight becomes a matter of nutritional and exercise status. Some weight gains during pregnancy appear permanent.

From *Human Motor Development: A Lifespan Approach, Fourth Edition* by V. Gregory Payne and Larry D. Isaacs. Copyright © 1999 by Mayfield Publishing Company. Reprinted by permission of the publisher.

Children's limbs grow more rapidly than their torso or head. The increase in proportion of total height attributed to leg length explains some of the improvement in running and jumping performance during childhood. The shoulders and hips also become wider, with males' shoulders becoming much broader on the average than females' shoulders, giving them an advantage in activities in which shoulder power is helpful, such as throwing. Growth is orderly, with length then breadth and circumferences increasing. Children in upper elementary school grades often look awkward—their legs

$\longrightarrow$

and arms appear to be long and skinny. Figure 8.8 provides an example of the variation in physical growth among upper elementary children. After most of the length of a limb has been attained, the limb gains thickness. The bone circumference and muscles (and fat!) increase to make the body look more proportional: the children "fill out." In fact, men's shoulders and chests usually grow (bones and muscle) until about 30 years of age, while most women have stopped growing by their late teens.

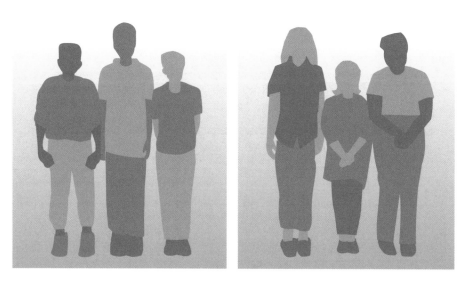

Figure 8.8 Three boys and three girls of the same chronological age but of different biological ages.

The changes in physical growth present three challenges: mechanical, adaptive, and absolute. The mechanics of movement change due to different body proportions; the individual must adapt to a rapidly changing body. These changes are especially problematic in seasonal sports. Consider the wrestler who experienced a rapid growth spurt from the end of one season to the beginning of the next. The center of gravity has changed, which may influence balance and the location of optimal points for exerting maximal force. Finally, the absolute changes in size may influence performance. Females gain fat at puberty, which adversely influences performance in most physical activities, but males gain muscle, which has a positive influence on performance. During childhood, physical growth interacts with all of the other factors that are developing (e.g., motor programs) and therefore must be considered for instruction and research.

A good way to examine structural and functional change and its influence on skill across childhood and adolescence is to consider overhand throwing. Figure 8.9 shows the changes in throwing for distance and velocity for girls and boys that occur across childhood and adolescence. Figure 8.10 shows stick figures (developed from high-speed cameras) of an expert male and female throwing and a young boy and girl (about five years of age) throwing. Note that the expert male is considerably different even from the expert female (e.g., longer step, more complete body rotation). The young boy has a much more mature (more like the adult male pattern) throwing pattern (e.g., longer step, greater lag of arm behind shoulder, more body rotation) than the young girl even though both are only five years old. Table 8.4 shows the developmental nature of the overhand throw across childhood and early adolescence. This description is separated into various body actions during the throw (e.g., arm, trunk, foot). Figure 8.11 provides a look at a very immature pattern (*a*), a moderately mature pattern (*b*), and a very mature pattern (*c*) for overhand throwing.

→

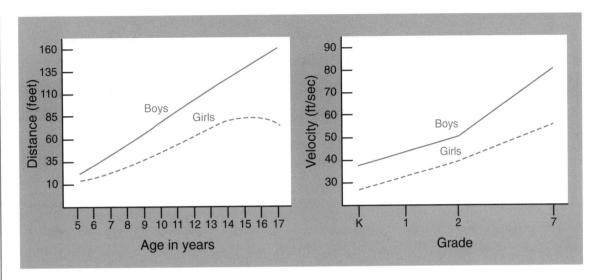

Figure 8.9 Age differences in boys and girls for throwing for (*a*) distance and (*b*) velocity.

Data for distance are from "Motor Development" by A. Espenschade, 1960, in W.R. Johnson (Ed.), *Science and Medicine of Exercise and Sports* (p. 439), New York: Harper and Row. Copyright 1960 by W.R. Johnson and E.R. Buskerk. Reprinted by permission. Data for velocity are from "Development of the Overarm Throw: Movement and Ball Velocity Changes by Seventh Grade" by L. Halverson, M.A. Roberton, and S. Langendorfer, 1982, *Research Quarterly for Exercise and Sport, 53,* pp. 198–205. Copyright 1982 by AAHPERD. Reprinted by permission of the American Alliance for Health, Physical Education, Recreation and Dance, 1900 Association Drive, Reston, VA 22901.

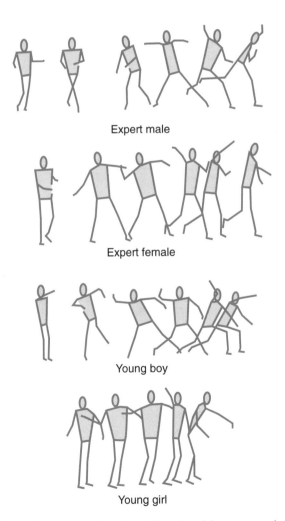

Expert male

Expert female

Young boy

Young girl

Figure 8.10 Stick figures of throwing patterns of male and female adult experts and male and female five-year-olds.

TABLE 8.4
Development of Body Actions During Throwing

Level	Body actions
Preparatory arm backswing	
Level 1	Child's hand moves directly forward to release from where the ball is first grasped.
Level 2	The forearm is moved backward beside the head and then forward in ball release.
Level 3	The ball is moved backward with a circular and upward backswing with elbow flexion.
Level 4	The ball is moved backward with a downward swing below the waist and then up behind the head with elbow flexion.
Arm action	
Level 1	The upper arm moves backward and forward at an angle to the body. The forearm is linked to the upper arm movement and does not lag behind it.
Level 2	The upper arm is aligned with the shoulder and moves with it until near release, when the upper arm leads the shoulder. The forearm lags behind the upper arm (i.e., appears to stay at the same point after the shoulder and upper arm have started forward).
Level 3	The upper arm lags behind the shoulder as the forward movement of the arm begins. The forearm lags even farther behind the upper arm and shoulder, reaching its final point of lag as the body is front facing.
Trunk action	
Level 1	Little or no trunk action; the throw is accomplished by just the forward and backward action of the arm.
Level 2	The trunk rotation is in one block; the spine and hips move together in one rotating action.
Level 3	The hips lead in forward rotation followed by the spine (differentiated rotation).
Foot action	
Level 1	Feet do not move during throwing action.
Level 2	Step occurs but with the foot on the same side as the throwing hand.
Level 3	Step occurs but with the foot on the opposite side of the throwing hand.
Level 4	Same as Level 3 except the step is longer (about one-half of standing height).

Reprinted from M.A. Roberton, 1984, Changing motor patterns during childhood. In *Motor development during childhood and adolescence*, edited by J.R. Thomas (Minneapolis: Burgess), 73-74. Used with permission.

Given that prepubescent boys and girls are very similar structurally, differences as large as those observed in throwing are quite unusual. In fact, Thomas and French (1985) noted that the gender differences in throwing at five years of age were three times the size of any of the 20 tasks they reviewed. While it seems likely that practice, encouragement, and opportunities account for a large part of these differences, throwing may be one of the very few motor skills in which biological factors play a signifi-

→

cant role in gender performance differences before puberty. Findings such as these pose some of the most interesting and provocative questions in the developmental aspects of motor learning and motor control.

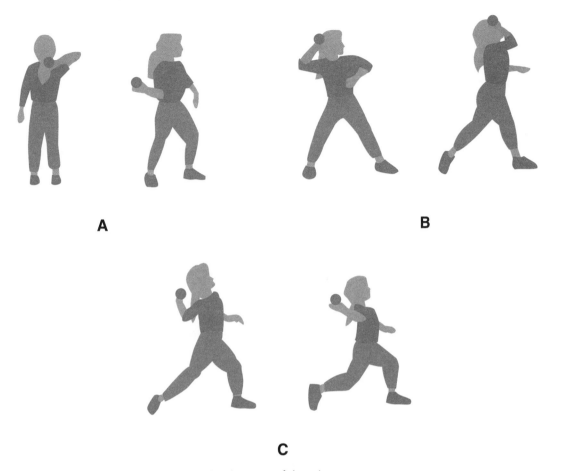

Figure 8.11 Important changes in the development of throwing.

Reprinted from M.A. Roberton, 1984, Changing motor patterns during childhood. In *Motor development during childhood and adolescence*, edited by J.R. Thomas (Minneapolis: Burgess), 75. Used with permission.

have grown in length, and he weighs more. He has not practiced batting or throwing very much since the last summer, yet he can still bat and throw successfully. How does the nervous system compensate for these changes, yet still produce coordinated movements?

At the other end of the age continuum are the elderly. How are loss in cognitive function, body mass, flexibility, and strength accounted for in a system of motor control that has functioned for years using different parameters? No good explanation has been found for these important issues from the developmental aspects of motor learning and control, although some progress is being made (for reviews, see Thelen, Ulrich, & Jensen, 1990; Thomas, Thomas, & Gallagher, 1993).

While some topics are unique to developmental motor learning and control, there is considerable overlap with the previous two goals of motor behavior—motor learning and motor control. So, while this section is shorter, this does not mean it is less important, nor that less research has been conducted.

One of the most intriguing developmental questions in motor behavior is, how does the brain and nervous system adjust its control in response to increases in cognitive function, body size, and strength across childhood and to decreases in these same variables as people age?

Wrap-Up

While motor behavior has produced important knowledge for human behavior since the late 1800s, it began to evolve as a significant subdiscipline in the field of physical activity in the 1960s. A particularly important part of that evolution was Franklin Henry's classic paper on memory drum theory, which led to the development of other theories within the field of motor behavior and a shift away from relying on the application of theories from psychology. Schmidt's schema theory is the best known and most influential of these.

Knowledge developed through motor behavior has become increasingly important in all aspects of society. While we often think of learning and control of sport skills as being the main issue, in fact our society depends on human movement in many ways: babies learning to use a fork, surgeons using a scalpel, pilots learning to control airplanes, children learning to control a pencil in writing, and dentists using a drill are some examples. Understanding the development, learning, and control of these and other motor skills so that they may be more effectively used in our culture and society is the goal of motor behavior.

Knowledge of motor behavior is essential for several professions, including physical or occupational therapy, physical education, coaching, or working with children in community organizations such as the YMCA or YWCA or boys' or girls' clubs. If you want to know more about this subdiscipline, you might want to read some of the journals that regularly publish research in motor behavior, such as the *Journal of Motor Behavior* or *Research Quarterly for Exercise and Sport*. Your school probably offers at least one undergraduate course in motor learning, motor control, and motor development.

Study Questions

1. How does motor behavior differ from the psychology of sport?

2. Within motor behavior, explain the differences between motor learning and motor control.

3. Why is the change in motor learning and motor control across the life span of interest?

4. Why are characteristics of practice important as they influence motor performance, retention, and transfer?

5. How can you judge if practice sessions influence the learning of a skill? What characteristics of practice might disguise whether or not skills are being learned?

6. Think about the practice issues that were discussed, such as feedback, retention, transfer, goal setting, and scheduling. Pick a sport you are familiar with as well as a specific age group or performance level and discuss how the practice characteristics would influence your planning if you were a coach.

7. How does the motor program theory explain the motor control issues of coordination of movements (degrees of freedom), serial order of movements, and integration of information about the movement?

8. Think about children's performance in a seasonal sport such as baseball, basketball, or football. How might changes in size and muscle–fat ratio from one season to the next influence performance for a 12- to 13-year-old girl or boy?

9. Can you think of an example in which more difficult practice conditions result in better retention and transfer? Why does that happen? Can you plan practices to promote this? How?

10. Discuss when it might be best to provide either knowledge of performance or knowledge of results to a person learning a motor skill.

11. The opening example in this chapter was about how a certain practice routine (trying to hit a baseball at the end of a string) was not useful for learning to bat in a game. Can you think of other practice routines you have seen that are probably not useful? What are they? Why don't they help?

12. Figure 8.8 shows boys and girls of the same age but of varying sizes. Discuss why size and skill level might be important to consider for participants in a specific children's sport.

9

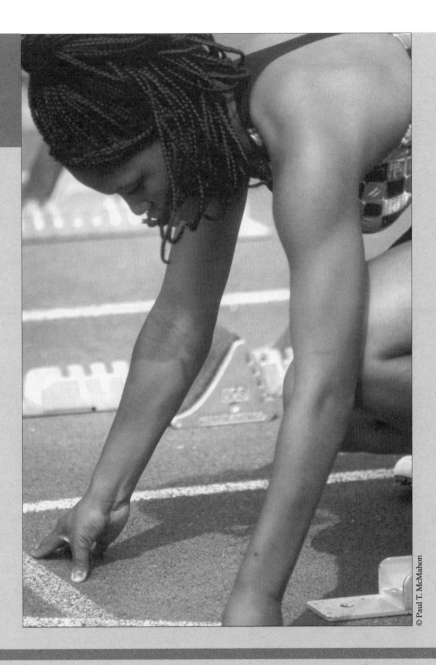

© Paul T. McMahon

Psychology of Sport and Exercise

Robin S. Vealey

In this chapter . . .

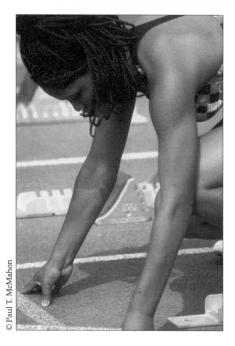

You are crouched in the starting blocks for the final race of the 100-meter dash at the Olympic Games. The athletes in the other lanes are top sprinters in the world who, like you, have trained for years—all in preparation for this moment. Your muscles are coiled as tightly as springs waiting to explode at the sound of the starter's pistol. What are you thinking? Should you even *be* thinking? Where is your attention focused? Do you have negative thoughts and fears about not performing well, or do you feel a confident excitement that you are ready to meet the challenge? Do you feel a relaxed inner calmness or a feverish emotional intensity?

Why Psychology of Sport and Exercise?

The psychologist William James wrote that "the greatest discovery . . . is that human beings, by changing the inner attitudes of their minds, can change the outer aspects of their lives." How true

that is! All types of physical activity involve a mental or psychological component as well as the more obvious physical component. This psychological component of physical activity is the focus of study in psychology of sport and exercise. Specifically, sport and exercise psychology focuses on the mental and behavioral processes of humans as they engage in physical activity.

Recall the opening scenario in which you were crouched in the starting blocks at the Olympic Games. The following questions were asked, What are you thinking? Should you even *be* thinking? Do you feel relaxed? and so on. Sport and exercise psychology research has enabled us to understand how and to what extent your psychological state—as reflected in your answers to these questions—affects your performance. Obviously, the physical skill and fitness of you and your competitors will be major factors in the race, but each of your psychological skills, your mental mind-set, will also be crucial to your sport performance.

Research shows that athletes perform best when they are in their optimal performance zone, which includes the disciplined practice of what is called a competition focus plan. As an Olympic athlete, you have such a plan, and it directs your attention to productive, energizing thoughts instead of worries and distractions. It involved preprogramming your mind and body to respond optimally without any thoughts of the pressure to win or the stress of performing in front of an international television audience. You have planned and mastered the mental focus and physical readiness that you will need for your best performance, and now your body and mind are one, waiting to explode from the blocks for the performance of your life!

Most of us will not have the opportunity to compete in elite sport competition such as the Olympic Games. However, we can engage in many types of physical activity that provide us with tremendous personal satisfaction and fulfillment. Let's consider some more true-to-life scenarios that you may encounter:

- You take up mountain biking and are amazed at how your self-esteem and confidence are enhanced along with your physical health.
- You begin an exercise program to enhance your personal fitness, but you lack the motivation to persist in your program.
- You really enjoy your weekly bowling league, but you get so nervous about bowling poorly and letting your team down that it interferes with your performance and enjoyment of the game.
- Your grandfather's physician recommends that he begin a progressive aerobic exercise

program, and your grandfather asks you to help him establish a physical activity routine that he will enjoy.

All of these examples illustrate the critical and fascinating link between mind and body that is inherent in physical activity.

 Physical activity always involves the mind as well as the body. The mental aspect of physical activity is the realm of sport and exercise psychologists.

You may have noticed that we have used a different name for this subdiscipline than for most of the others in this book. That is, we have used *psychology of sport and exercise* instead of *psychology of physical activity*. Why is that? Both motor behavior and sport and exercise psychology grew out of the discipline of psychology. As you will soon learn, the subdiscipline that this chapter covers is rapidly evolving into two distinct areas—that of sport psychology and that of exercise psychology, both with two separate and distinct focuses. Therefore, we have chosen to title this chapter "Psychology of Sport and Exercise," and you will see frequent references to sport and exercise psychology.

CHAPTER OBJECTIVES

In this chapter you will learn about these key topics:

- What background knowledge you already have about sport and exercise psychology
- What sport and exercise psychologists do
- The goals of sport and exercise psychology
- How sport and exercise psychology evolved within the field of physical activity
- How professionals in sport and exercise psychology engage in research and practice
- What research tells us about personality, motivation, and group processes in sport and exercise settings
- How intervention techniques are used to enhance participation in sport and exercise

▌ How your personal thoughts, feelings, and behaviors influence and are influenced by your participation in sport and exercise

If you succeed in learning the material in this chapter, you will have gained information about experience, scholarly study, and professional practice connected with physical activity. First, you will gain insight about the psychological aspects of experience in sport and exercise, which should hopefully enhance your physical activity participation. Second, you will gain understanding about the scholarly study or research conducted in sport and exercise psychology. Third, you will learn how professionals engage in the practice of sport and exercise psychology to enhance people's experiences in physical activity. Also, the information in this chapter should help you understand the mental processes involved in the scenarios presented at the beginning of the chapter. Check your understanding at the end of the chapter by again imagining yourself in the starting blocks at the Olympic Games and putting your newfound knowledge about sport and exercise psychology to work!

What Background Knowledge Do I Already Have?

You already know a lot about sport and exercise psychology. Without knowing it, you have gained knowledge prior to reading this chapter through your physical activity experiences, prior study in related areas, and your observations of people in professional practice.

Knowledge Based on Experience

Much of your knowledge about the psychological aspects of sport and exercise is experiential. For example, if you have a lot of experience in competitive sport, you probably have learned that certain precompetitive rituals help you gain the most optimal mental mind-set for performance. If you are an experienced exerciser, you've probably learned that you have particular preferences for exercise behavior, such as lifting

weights with a partner or listening to music when you run. As you saw in section 1, experiential knowledge is rich and insightful and provides a basis for the more systematic study of sport and exercise psychology.

Knowledge Based on Prior Learning in Related Areas of Study

You also may have acquired some background knowledge of sport and exercise psychology from related scholarly areas of study. Throughout this chapter you will see that sport and exercise psychology, although a subdiscipline of kinesiology, has close ties to the discipline of psychology. Psychology is the science that deals with human thoughts, feelings, and behavior, so sport and exercise psychology is the study of these same phenomena within the unique environments of sport and exercise. For this reason, sport and exercise psychology naturally incorporates many of the theoretical models and approaches from psychology. For example, researchers attempting to understand why people begin or discontinue participation in fitness programs often apply motivational theories that have been developed in the discipline of psychology.

🔑 Sport and exercise psychology incorporates many models and approaches from the discipline of psychology.

You have also gained background knowledge related to sport and exercise psychology from reading previous chapters in this book. In chapter 4 the idea of subjective experience in physical activity introduced you to the significance of thoughts and feelings of individuals as they participate in physical activity. Much of what is studied in sport and exercise psychology relies on the subjective experiences of individuals.

The scholarly study of sport and exercise psychology is also closely tied to the philosophy, history, and sociology of physical activity, which you have read about in chapters 5 through 7. Because sport and exercise occur within a sociocultural context, an understanding of human behavior requires some background knowledge of social and historical structures in physical activity. For example, understanding gender differences in confidence and assertiveness in sport requires a historical and cultural understanding of the different social support given to female as compared to male athletes in our society. Likewise, understanding the relationship between body image and the exercise behavior of females requires a clear understanding of the deep sociocultural pressure that equates the worth of women to their physical attractiveness. Recently, you have acquired some background knowledge by reading chapter 8 on motor behavior, a subdiscipline that, as you shall see, is closely aligned with sport and exercise psychology.

Knowledge Based on Observing Professional Practice

Finally, through your observations of and experiences with professional practitioners in physi-

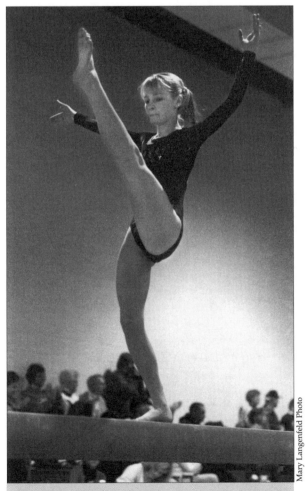

Gymnasts and figure skaters know that judges evaluate their bodies as well as their performances.

cal activity, you have probably gained interesting insights into sport and exercise psychology. If you have ever taken an aerobic dance class, you have observed the ability of the teacher to motivate participants and help them to feel more confident about their physical abilities. If you've ever participated in competitive sport, you have observed the leadership and communication styles of a coach. You may also recall past teachers whom you have had in physical education and consider the ways they used modeling, feedback, and verbal reinforcement to help students gain physical competence in various movement skills. We can all learn much about sport and exercise psychology by observing skilled professional practitioners in the field of physical activity.

The subdiscipline of sport and exercise psychology involves the systematic, scholarly study of human thought, emotion, and behavior in physical activity. Such study offers an appreciation of the fascinating mind–body link by providing information about the psychological aspects of physical activity participation. You can see from figure 9.1 that psychology of sport and exercise is considered a subdiscipline of the behavioral sphere, along with motor behavior and pedagogy, in the study of physical activity.

Psychology of sport and exercise, as a subdiscipline of kinesiology, is the systematic scholarly study of human thought, emotion, and behavior in sport and exercise contexts.

Although in this chapter the collective term *psychology of sport and exercise* is used to encompass the two main aspects of physical activity studied in this subdiscipline, sport psychology and exercise psychology have grown into distinct areas of study. Exercise psychology emerged in the 1980s from the more established study of sport psychology and today is a highly important area devoted to the study of the psychological aspects of fitness, exercise, health, and wellness. Conversely, sport psychology focuses more on the psychological aspects of competitive sport participation. However, since the two areas are closely related and share a great deal of theoretical content, they are both covered in this chapter.

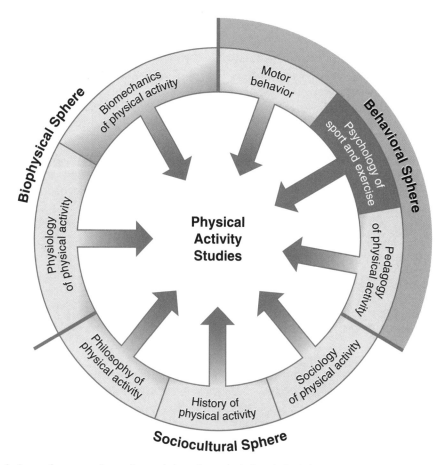

Figure 9.1   Psychology of sport and exercise and the other scholarly subdisciplines.

Consider the following questions:

1. Recalling that we've defined physical activity as intentional and purposeful movement (chapter 1), think of several forms of physical activity in which you participate. What do you think your motivation is for performing each of these activities?

2. Do you think participation in physical activity has influenced your character? If so, what was the activity and how do you think it affected you? If not, why do you think participation has not influenced your character?

3. Have you ever been involved in or watched any form of violence in sport? If so, what happened and why? What do you think caused the violence to occur?

4. Why do you think so few Americans participate in habitual exercise when it has been clearly shown to enhance health and longevity?

In summary, keep in mind that you probably have quite a bit of background knowledge about sport and exercise psychology that you have gained from your own experiences in physical activity, from your prior study of related areas, and from observing skilled professional practitioners in sport and exercise. This chapter offers you a closer look at how our thoughts, feelings, and behaviors influence and are influenced by our participation in sport and exercise.

What Does a Sport or Exercise Psychologist Do?

To really understand what sport and exercise psychology is all about, it's helpful for you to learn about what professionals in sport and exercise psychology actually do. As in any subdiscipline of physical activity, sport and exercise psychology professionals work in many career areas.

Professors of sport and exercise psychology at universities fulfill the multiple roles of researcher, teacher, and service provider. That is, a college professor may develop theory and conduct research on the psychological benefits of aerobic exercise, teach courses in exercise psychology, develop a health promotion program within the university, and conduct workshops for the community on motivation and stress management.

Some sport and exercise psychology professionals focus more exclusively on practitioner or service provider roles. For example, a sport psychology specialist may work on performance enhancement, personal development, and lifestyle management issues of athletes within a university athletic department or professional sports team. Likewise, an exercise psychology specialist may focus on worksite health promotion for a large corporation. Sometimes sport and exercise psychology professionals become consultants for sports medicine or physical therapy clinics to help injured people through the psychological aspects of injury rehabilitation.

It is important to differentiate between an exercise or sport psychologist trained as a physical activity specialist and one trained as a clinical or counseling psychologist. Clinical or counseling psychologists are licensed to provide psychotherapy and consultation for individuals with clinical conditions such as depression, phobias, or anorexia nervosa. The focus of practitioners of sport and exercise psychology within the physical activity field is on education or the teaching of skills to enhance the performance or personal fulfillment of individuals involved in sport or exercise. Although some clinical and counseling psychologists provide services for athletes and exercisers, the main focus of their practice is quite different from that of sport and exercise psychology as a subdiscipline of the physical activity field.

 Career opportunities in sport and exercise psychology include positions as university professors, athletic counselors, corporate health promotion specialists, and sports medicine consultants.

Have you ever considered a career in sport and exercise psychology? If so, what positions most interest you? What are the specific reasons for your interest?

Goals of Psychology of Sport and Exercise

The first goal of sport and exercise psychology is *to understand the social–psychological factors that influence participation in physical activity*. For example, why are some individuals motivated to exercise and others are not? Why do some athletes "choke" in pressure situations in competition? Why do children drop out of youth sport programs? Is it better to exercise alone or with others?

The second goal is *to understand the psychological effects derived from participation in physical activity*. For example, does youth sport participation build character? Can weightlifting enhance self-esteem and decrease stress? Do ice hockey players learn to be violent and aggressive? Does running reduce depression?

The third goal of the subdiscipline is *to enhance the sport and exercise experience for those who participate in physical activity*. This third goal logically follows the first two as sport and exercise psychology professionals attempt to "plug in" knowledge gained through research to implement sound practices. Examples might include using behavior management techniques to increase adherence in exercise programs, modifying children's sport for greater enjoyment and development of self-worth, and helping athletes engage in effective mental training to perform better.

As discussed previously, sport and exercise psychology overlaps with other kinesiology subdisciplines. What makes each of these subdisciplines distinct are the goals within each area of study. Although sport and exercise psychology overlaps significantly with sociology of physical activity, the goals of the two subdisciplines are different. Sport and exercise psychology focuses on factors within the individual, whereas sociology of physical activity focuses more on understanding broader cultural structures and processes. Thus, a sport psychologist would focus on how a large crowd might affect the aggression levels of ice hockey players, whereas a sport sociologist would be more focused on the cultural glorification of fighting and aggression in hockey as a societal phenomenon.

The subdiscipline of motor behavior (chapter 8) is closely aligned with sport and exercise psychology due to its focus on cognition (thought) and perception. However, the study of motor behavior is more oriented toward basic movement and motor skill development as compared to sport and exercise psychology, which focuses specifically on the broader, more social contexts of physical activity. Whereas motor behavior specialists concentrate on understanding the neurophysiological bases of learning and performing skills so that applications can be made to instructional and clinical settings, sport and exercise psychologists tend to be more interested in the motivations and other psychological dispositions that bear on performance. Specifically, the goal of sport and exercise psychology is to understand social behavior such as achievement or exercise adherence and people's thoughts and feelings associated with this behavior, such as anxiety, self-esteem, and motivation.

> Sport and exercise psychology specifically studies social behavior such as achievement or exercise adherence and the thoughts, feelings, and experiences associated with this behavior, such as anxiety, self-esteem, and motivation.

Goals of Psychology of Sport and Exercise

1. To understand the social–psychological factors that influence participation in physical activity

2. To understand the psychological effects derived from participation in physical activity

3. To enhance the sport and exercise experience for those who participate in physical activity

As mentioned earlier, the goals of sport and exercise psychology are pursued by professionals in educational, scientific, and clinical settings. Although sport and exercise psychology shares the parent discipline of psychology, their respective goals differ slightly based on their distinctive contexts. The goal of exercise psychology is to understand and enhance thoughts, feelings, and behaviors related to planned and repetitive bodily movement used to improve performance, health, and/or bodily appearance. The goal of sport psychology is to understand and enhance thoughts, feelings, and behaviors associated with participation in the unique context of competitive sport. Keep in mind, however, a great deal of overlap exists between sport and exercise psychology. For example, early participation in youth sports may help children appreciate the importance of physical activity—both sport and exercise—in maintaining physical and mental health throughout their lives.

History of Psychology of Sport and Exercise

Sport and exercise psychology is often called the youngest of the sport sciences, and the history of the subdiscipline is marked by significant periods as opposed to a smooth, continual progression. The historical perspective presented here focuses on the development of sport psychology in North America, although other sources have documented the development of the subdiscipline around the world (Cratty, 1989; Williams & Straub, 1998).

Around the turn of the 20th century, early physical educators began to write about the psychological benefits of physical activity. Motor behavior research was being conducted in such areas as reaction time, skill transfer, and the use of mental practice in learning motor skills. Also at this time, researchers began assessing the social influences of the presence of others on motor performance, a research area that later became known as social facilitation. The first person to examine these social influences was Norman Triplett, who in 1898 studied the effects of the presence of other people on cycling performance as well as on a fishing reel winding task.

However, the true beginning of sport psychology dawned with the work of Coleman Griffith, who, as a professor at the University of Illinois, engaged in the first systematic examination of the psychological aspects of sport between 1919 and 1938 (see profile). Unfortunately, Griffith may be thought of as a "prophet without disciples" as his significant work was not continued. Although sporadic publications about psychological aspects of sport and exercise appeared after Griffith's time, the subdiscipline largely lay dormant until a reawakening in the 1960s.

Coleman Griffith began systematic research in sport psychology in the 1920s, but because his early work was not extended, the area was not recognized as an academic subdiscipline of physical activity until the 1970s.

In the 1960s motor behavior research served as an antecedent to an upsurge of interest in personality and social–psychological factors associated with physical activity. The research of this period focused primarily on personality traits related to sport participation and social facilitation or audience effects on motor performance. Bruce Ogilvie, a clinical psychologist at San Jose State University, began early work examining personality in athletes and also began applied psychological interventions with athletes. Dorothy Harris at Pennsylvania State University is also considered a pioneer of this period as she began a systematic research focus on women in sport. The first meeting of the International Society of Sport Psychology (ISSP) was held in 1965, and the first North American Society for the Psychology of Sport and Physical Activity (NASPSPA) conference was held in 1967; both served as important forums for the dissemination of knowledge in sport psychology.

In Profile

Coleman Griffith

Photo courtesy University of Illinois Archives

As a professor at the University of Illinois, Coleman Griffith engaged in the first systematic examination of the psychological aspects of sport between 1919 and 1938. Griffith established the Athletic Research Laboratory at Illinois, published numerous research articles, and wrote two classic books—*Psychology of Coaching* in 1926 and *Psychology and Athletics* in 1928.

Interestingly, Griffith also interviewed sport celebrities of that time, such as Red Grange and Knute Rockne, about the mental aspects of their sports and was also hired by Phillip Wrigley in 1938 as a sport psychology consultant for the Chicago Cubs baseball team. During this work, Griffith developed psychological profiles for specific players, such as Dizzy Dean, and researched methods of building confidence and increasing motivation.

Griffith did much of his groundbreaking work in relative isolation, years before the subdiscipline of sport and exercise psychology was recognized as a worthy pursuit. His commitment to his work remains an excellent model for all within the subdiscipline. Griffith is widely recognized as the father of sport and exercise psychology.

The decade of the 1970s is commonly viewed as the point at which sport psychology became recognized as a legitimate scientific subdiscipline within kinesiology. Systematic research programs in the subdiscipline were established at leading universities, graduate study became available in the subdiscipline, and in 1979 the *Journal of Sport Psychology* began publication. Much of the research during this time was experimental research conducted in laboratory settings that involved testing theory from the parent discipline of psychology. During the late 1970s and early 1980s Daniel Landers and colleagues paved the way for research in exercise psychology, emphasizing a psychophysiological approach (Hatfield & Landers, 1983). In this approach, thoughts and emotional responses of individuals are inferred from physiological measures such as heart rate, skin conductance, and brain waves.

It was not until the 1980s that the subdiscipline expanded with a growth in field research and increased interest in applied sport psychology or mental training with athletes. The establishment of two new applied journals, *The Sport Psychologist* in 1987 and the *Journal of Applied Sport Psychology* in 1989, and a new organization, the Association for the Advancement of Applied Sport Psychology (AAASP) in 1986, were indicative of the expansion of the subdiscipline to include applied interests. As with most scientific areas of study, tensions arose during this time and have continued today as to the appropriate relationships among theory, research, and practice in the subdiscipline.

Also during the 1980s, exercise psychology as a hybrid subdiscipline combining exercise science, health promotion, and psychology emerged, addressing increased attention to the psychological aspects of fitness, exercise, health, and/or wellness. Prior to this time, pockets of research investigating the psychological components of exercise existed, but it was during the 1980s that systematic research programs and graduate program offerings in exercise psychology were developed. To reflect this trend, the *Journal of Sport Psychology* became the *Journal of Sport and Exercise Psychology* in 1988. Today, the growing literature base on exercise psychology is derived from exercise science, health education, health psychology, behavioral medicine, and sport psychology, among other diverse sources.

Systematic research in exercise psychology began in the 1980s. It combined knowledge from exercise science, health promotion, and psychology to address a growing interest in the psychological aspects of exercise, fitness, and health.

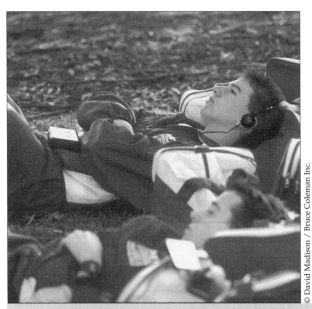
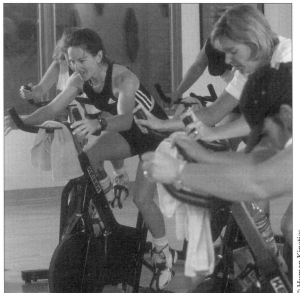

© David Madison / Bruce Coleman Inc.

© Human Kinetics

Not until the 1980s did the subdiscipline expand to systematically examine mental training with athletes as well as the psychological aspects of exercise.

Historical Time Line

1898	Triplett examines the influence of the presence of others on bicycling performance and a fishing reel winding task.
ca. 1900	Physical educators begin to write about the psychological benefits of physical activity.
1919–1938	Coleman Griffith engages in the first systematic examination of the psychological aspects of sport.
1960s	Upsurge of interest in personality and social facilitation effects on physical activity occurs.
1965	The first meeting of the International Society of Sport Psychology (ISSP) is held.
1967	The first meeting of the North American Society for the Psychology of Sport and Physical Activity (NASPSPA) takes place.
1969	The first meeting of the Canadian Society for Psychomotor Learning and Sport Psychology (CSPLSP) is held.
1970s	Sport psychology emerges as a legitimate scientific subdiscipline as systematic research programs are established at several universities.
1979	The *Journal of Sport Psychology* begins publication.
1980s	Interest in applied sport psychology and exercise psychology grows.
1985	The U.S. Olympic Committee hires the first full-time sport psychologist.
1986	The first meeting of the Association for the Advancement of Applied Sport Psychology (AAASP) takes place.
1987	*The Sport Psychologist* begins publication.
1987	The American Psychological Association Division 47 (Sport and Exercise Psychology) is established.
1988	The *Journal of Sport Psychology* becomes the *Journal of Sport and Exercise Psychology*.
1989	The *Journal of Applied Sport Psychology* begins publication.

Research Methods in Psychology of Sport and Exercise

By now you should understand the goals and historical development of sport and exercise psychology as a scientific area of study. But how is science conducted in this subdiscipline? What methods do researchers use to ask important questions about the psychological aspects of physical activity participation?

Researchers use six methods to systematically assess thoughts, feelings, and behaviors in sport and exercise psychology. The first method, the *questionnaire*, is widely used in the subdiscipline. Questionnaires may be survey instruments that

assess demographic variables such as age, sex, or socioeconomic status as well as general information such as the type, frequency, and duration of exercise engaged in during the past week. Most questionnaires used, however, are psychological inventories, which are standardized or objective measures of specific samples of behavior (Anastasi, 1988). For example, inventories are used in the subdiscipline to measure the amount of anxiety, motivation, and confidence an individual feels about exercising or competing in sport.

Consider for a moment how difficult it is to accurately measure the thoughts, feelings, and behavior of people. Assessing individuals' levels of self-esteem is much different from measuring the amount of oxygen they expend during a fitness test or how much weight they lose in the preseason (figure 9.2). For this reason, psychological inventories must meet rigorous standards of uniformity of procedures in developing, administering, and scoring the inventories so that researchers can gain a valid and reliable assessment of behavior. Therefore, psychological inventories used by researchers are not simply a list of questions thrown together, but rather carefully constructed and tested assessment tools that have met specific standards set by experts in the subdiscipline.

Because most of the inventories developed in sport and exercise psychology have been validated for research purposes only, it is inappropriate and unethical to use these test results in sport settings for the purposes of team selection or diagnosis of "problems." That is, it would be inappropriate for coaches to use a test to decide which athletes will make their teams. As you will learn later, no one personality type is destined for success in physical activity more than others, so no test is available to predict who will be successful. Appropriate and ethical use of psychological inventories means that inventories should be used only in situations in which they are valid or supposed to be used.

The second method used in sport and exercise psychology research, the *interview*, is useful when the research question being pursued requires an in-depth understanding of individuals' beliefs, experiences, or values. For example, interviews may be useful in attempting to understand why children drop out of youth sport programs because they allow children to explain things in their own words as opposed to responding to questionnaires. However, interviews, like

Test your anxiety level! Complete the following questionnaire by marking a response for each item.

	Hardly ever	Sometimes	Often
1. Before I compete, I feel uneasy.			
2. Before I compete, I worry about not performing well.			
3. When I compete, I worry about making mistakes.			
4. Before I compete, I am calm.			
5. Before I compete, I get a funny feeling in my stomach.			
6. Just before competing, I notice my heart beats faster than usual.			
7. Before I compete, I feel relaxed.			
8. Before I compete, I am nervous.			
9. I get nervous waiting to start the competition.			
10. Before I compete, I usually get uptight.			

Score your responses this way: For items 4 and 7, Often = 1, Sometimes = 2, and Hardly ever = 3. For all other items, Hardly ever = 1, Sometimes = 2, and Often = 3. Add the scores for all responses to get a total score.

Your total score represents your level of trait anxiety, or how anxious you tend to feel in competitive sport situations (Martens, Vealey, & Burton 1990). Your score can range from an extreme low of 10 (extremely calm in competition) to an extreme high of 30 (extremely anxious in competition). An average score for college athletes is 20. How anxious are you in competitive situations? Do you think this questionnaire accurately measures how you feel prior to competition?

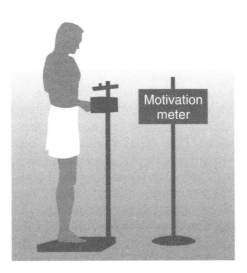

Figure 9.2 Assessing individuals' thoughts and feelings is a bit more difficult than assessing their body weight!

any other scientific method, must be structured to be systematic, and researchers must be appropriately trained in the use of interviews for them to be effective and valid.

The third method used in the subdiscipline is *observation* of behavior. For example, researchers often observe the behavior of coaches during practice or competition to assess the frequency of various types of feedback and communication they provide to athletes. Research examining the motivation of children to engage in physical activity or vigorous play activities would benefit from using behavioral observation. Typically, observation studies employ some type of behavior checklist or timing or coding system to ensure that the behavior is being observed within a particular set of parameters. Also, two observers are typically used to code behavior, and their results are checked against each other to ensure a consistent, reliable assessment.

Physiological measures of physical, mental, and emotional responses are the fourth method used in sport and exercise psychology research. These are sometimes referred to as biofeedback. For example, measures of blood pressure and heart rate may be used to quantify the effects of psychological stressors. Exercise psychologists use measures such as these to study the effects of exercise on stress reactivity and existing anxiety levels. Sport psychologists might measure the amount of tension in muscles to assess how well athletes can learn to relax physically through

mental training. Brain waves can even be measured to assess levels of attention or relaxation.

A fifth research method, *biochemical measures*, is used less frequently in sport and exercise psychology but should be mentioned here briefly. This type of assessment involves drawing and analyzing blood or urine for chemicals from the body that represent responses to stressors or emotions. Examples would be epinephrine and cortisol, which are released by the adrenal gland in response to certain types of stressors.

Finally, a sixth method used in sport and exercise psychology research is *content analysis*. This procedure is used to systematically analyze written material from various sources such as government documents, newspapers or magazines, or even television programming. For example, a researcher could analyze several popular television shows to assess the levels of physical activity being modeled by the media to viewers. Written or dictated physical activity logs are useful to exercise researchers as they provide a detailed accounting of all or selected types of physical activity performed within a given time period.

Thus, researchers in sport and exercise psychology have various methods available to them. Often, two or more methods are used within a single research study. For example, a study examining exercise adherence in an adult fitness program could use observation to assess participation rates, intensity of exercise, and instructor behavior; questionnaires to measure participants' self-confidence and perceived benefits about exercising; and physiological measures of participants' resting heart rate and lung volume. But remember, all methods are designed to be used in a systematic manner to ensure that accurate and consistent measures are obtained. This systematic approach is the mark of science—and it is very different from the casual observations we all make in everyday social interactions.

It is important to remember that all scientific methods in sport and exercise psychology have limitations. Questionnaires typically provide a systematic measure of some phenomenon, but they lack the depth and richness of interviews. On the other hand, it is more difficult to establish consistency and a systematic approach when using interviews as compared to questionnaires. Think back to the anxiety questionnaire. If you were interviewed about your competitive anxiety, how would the interview results differ from your questionnaire results? Of course they would be very different! Scientists in sport and exercise psychology look at the "menu" of research methods available to them and then select the method that best fits the "recipe" of their particular research study. This menu also has other choices for researchers such as whether the study should be conducted in a laboratory or field setting and what type of participants should be used in the research.

Research methods in sport and exercise psychology include questionnaires, interviews, observation, physiological measures, biochemical measures, and content analysis.

Overview of Knowledge in Psychology of Sport and Exercise

This section provides a brief overview of sport and exercise psychology topics to give you a glimpse of the knowledge that has been produced by researchers and practitioners. The topics in this section are divided into five main areas: personality, motivational processes, interpersonal and group processes, developmental concerns, and intervention techniques for physical activity enhancement.

Personality

One of the most popular issues in sport and exercise psychology concerns the relationship between personality and physical activity participation (Vealey, 1992). Personality is typically thought of as the unique blend of the psychological characteristics and behavioral tendencies that make individuals different from and similar to each other. Our personalities determine our thoughts, feelings, and behaviors in response to our environment.

Personality Types in Sport

Most of the early research in personality and sport attempted to (1) find a "personality type" that differentiates athletes from nonathletes, (2) find a "personality type" that differentiates successful athletes from less successful athletes, and (3)

demonstrate that athletes in certain sports have different personalities than athletes in other sports. Interestingly, the popular notion that distinct personality types exist in sport has not been supported by research. No distinguishable "athletic personality" has been shown to exist. That is, there are no consistent research findings showing that athletes possess a general personality type distinct from the personality of nonathletes. Also, no consistent personality differences between athletic subgroups (e.g., team vs. individual sport athletes, contact vs. noncontact sport athletes) have been shown to exist. Although personality differences between certain groups have been identified in some studies, the findings are inconsistent overall.

The early personality research showed that no unique set of personality traits, or relatively enduring and consistent internal attributes, exists in athletes, certain types of athletes, or more successful athletes. However, research since that time has adopted an interactional approach to studying personality in which behavior is viewed as being codetermined by internal characteristics (traits) as well as environmental or situational factors. Many studies now examine personality states, which are manifestations of personality that occur at one specific moment and result from the interaction of traits and situational factors. Anxiety is an example of a personality characteristic that can be traitlike (how you typically respond across situations) or statelike (how you feel during one crucial point in time).

Using the state approach, Morgan (1985) proposed a "mental health model" in which the presence of positive mood states in athletes is associated with higher performance levels as compared to the performance levels of athletes possessing less positive mood states. The pattern of mood states associated with positive mental health was termed the "iceberg profile" by Morgan (because the profile resembles an iceberg) and is characterized by scores above the population norm on vigor and below the population norm on tension, depression, anger, fatigue, and confusion (see figure 9.3).

Morgan's mental health model was an important contribution to the study of personality and sport because it spawned a significant line of research examining the relationship between state personality characteristics and physical activity performance. However, the accumulation of research over time has shown that the iceberg profile contributes little to the prediction of physical activity performance. Substantial individual differences occur in mood functioning, and many individuals perform well despite having theoretically "negative" profiles (Terry, 1995). Mood state profiling is effective, however, when looking at intra-individual fluctuations of mood over time to better understand such factors as staleness, overtraining, and burnout, as well as to assess optimal and dysfunctional patterns of emotions preferred by specific athletes (Hanin, 1997).

Also, as a result of an emphasis on the interactional approach to studying personality, cognitive psychology emerged based on the idea that humans continuously process information from the environment and then respond behaviorally based on their appraisal and interpretation of the situation. Cognition means thought; thus, the cognitive approach focuses on how people's individual thoughts about themselves and the world around them influence their behavior. That is, the athlete or exerciser first interprets, then reacts to the environment. Prior to this, sport and exercise psychologists focused on the underlying traits or drives that supposedly drove people's behavior without their consciously thinking about why they were behaving this way.

While researchers have not been able to find any significant differences between successful and less successful athletes in personality traits, researchers using a cognitive approach have found that successful athletes (compared to less successful athletes) are

- more self-confident;
- able to use more effective cognitive strategies and coping mechanisms to retain optimal competitive focus in the face of obstacles and distractions;
- able to self-regulate activation efficiently;
- positively preoccupied with sport, in terms of thoughts, images, and feelings; and
- highly determined and committed to excellence in their sport.

No set of traits exists for an "athletic personality," but successful athletes possess more positive self-perceptions and use more productive cognitive coping strategies as compared to less successful athletes.

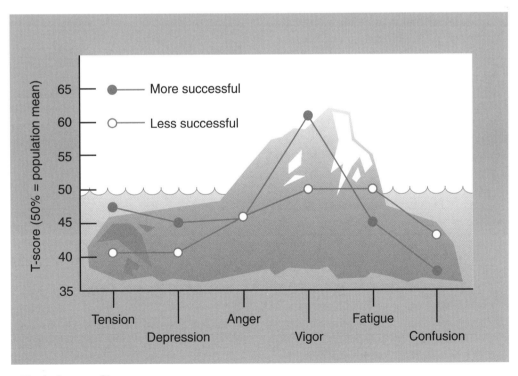

Figure 9.3 The iceberg profile.

Personality Types in Exercise

As in sport, researchers have found no "exercise personality" or set of personality characteristics that predict exercise adherence. Exercisers cannot be differentiated from nonexercisers based on personality type. Instead, exercise adherence is the result of several cognitive, social, and environmental factors.

However, research has identified various personality types that relate to health and exercise concerns. Researchers studying the type A behavior pattern (Friedman & Rosenman, 1974) of time-urgency, competitive drive, and hostility in relation to cardiovascular disease have been able to link only the hostility component to decreased physical health. The type B pattern is simply defined as the absence of type A behavior. Type A behavior patterns, which seem to reflect a society that values achievement and success, offer an interesting insight into the mind–body link as it relates to health and fitness. Despite some disagreement on the exact reasons, it is generally assumed that individuals with a type A behavioral pattern have an increased risk of coronary heart disease. Interventions tailored to type A individuals are needed to enhance exercise adherence for these individuals.

The personality style of "hardiness" enables individuals to cope effectively with stress and life obstacles (Kobasa, 1979). This personality type is characterized by a sense of control, feelings of commitment and purpose in daily life, and flexibility and adaptation skills. This personality type has been shown to be less susceptible to illness, and individuals high in both hardiness and exercise participation remained healthier than individuals who either only exercised or scored high in hardiness alone. Thus, this personality type coupled with exercise participation has been shown to be a very strong predictor of health.

A personality type termed "obligatory exercisers" has been used to describe individuals who participate in exercise at excessive and even harmful levels (Coen & Ogles, 1993). For these individuals, exercise becomes the central focus of life and their behavior becomes pathological in terms of their need to control themselves and their environment. Clinical evidence demonstrates a similar link between anorexia nervosa, a psychopathological eating disorder, and compulsive exercise. Specialists in exercise psychol-

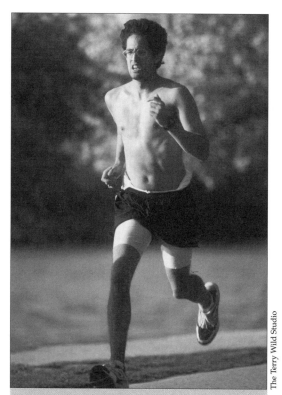

The benefits of exercise are numerous, yet exercise can be harmful when used excessively or when it becomes "obligatory."

The Terry Wild Studio

ogy attempt to help individuals plan and engage in exercise behavior that is healthy and noncontrolling to enhance total well-being.

Effects of Sport on Personality

Although most sport personality research has focused on the influence of personality on sport behavior, some researchers have examined the effects of sport participation on personality development and change. A notion commonly held in American society is that "sport builds character," or that socially valued personality attributes may be developed through sport participation. However, research shows that competition serves to reduce prosocial behaviors such as helping and sharing, and this effect is magnified by losing. Sport participation has been shown to increase rivalrous, antisocial behavior and aggression, and sport participation has also been linked to lower levels of moral reasoning.

Nevertheless, there is a positive side to the sport story. Research in a variety of field settings has demonstrated that children's moral development and prosocial behaviors (cooperation, acceptance, sharing) can be enhanced in sport settings when adult leaders structure situations to foster these positive behaviors (Shields & Bredemeier, 1995). Interventions with children were successful in building character when naturally occurring conflicts arose and were discussed with the children as "teachable moments" to enhance their reasoning and values about sport and life events. The moral of the story is: sport doesn't build character, people do!

Effects of Exercise on Personality

Echoing the idea that sport builds character, exercise or fitness training has also popularly been associated with positive personality change. The various psychosocial outcomes related to exercise participation are shown in figure 9.4.

The personality characteristic that researchers have most frequently examined in this area is self-concept or self-esteem. Research has generally confirmed that fitness training improves self-concept in children, adolescents, and adults (Biddle, 1995). Interestingly, the research indicates that these changes in self-concept may result from perceived, as opposed to actual, changes in physical fitness. The assertion that mere involvement may not lead directly to enhanced self-esteem has important implications for fitness training pro-

grams. Research has also shown that exercise positively influences perceptions of physical capabilities (self-efficacy). This is an especially important finding because self-efficacy is directly linked to the achievement behaviors of approaching challenging situations, exerting effort, and persisting in the face of obstacles (Bandura, 1986).

Many people also associate exercise with changes in mood and state anxiety. Most individuals admit they "feel better" or "feel good" after vigorous exercise, which emphasizes the important link between physical activity and psychological well-being (Morgan & Goldston, 1987). Also, research documents that state anxiety and tension is reduced following acute physical activity. This effect of exercise on anxiety begins within five minutes after acute exercise and continues for at least two hours. Reductions in state and trait anxiety are associated with activities involving continuous, rhythmic (aerobic) exercise rather than resisted, intermittent exercise. The greatest reductions in trait anxiety occur in exercise programs that continue for more than 15 weeks. Much research has been conducted to determine whether exercise or fitness reduces people's susceptibility to stress, with the generally accepted conclusion being that aerobically

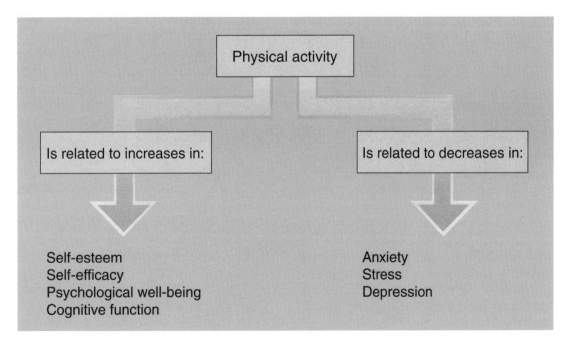

Figure 9.4 Psychosocial outcomes related to physical activity.
Adapted, by permission, from E. McAuley, 1994, Physical activity and psychosocial outcomes. In *Physical activity, fitness, and health: International proceedings and consensus statement,* edited by C. Bouchard, R.J. Shephard, and T. Stephens (Champaign, IL: Human Kinetics) 551–569.

fit individuals demonstrate a reduced psychosocial stress response (Crews & Landers, 1987). A tentative explanation for this finding is that exercise acts either as a coping strategy that reduces the physiological response to stress, or it serves as an "inoculator" to foster a more effective response to psychosocial stress (Willis & Campbell, 1992).

Prolonged physical activity is also associated with decreases in depression and a lessening of depressive symptoms in individuals who are clinically depressed at the outset of the exercise treatment. Explanation for these changes range from the "distraction hypothesis," which maintains that exercise distracts attention from stress, to other hypotheses that focus on the physiological and biochemical changes in the body after exercise. Also, many aspects of intellectual performance have been related to physical activity, suggesting that cognitive functions respond positively to increased levels of physical activity.

While exercise has not been successful in reducing type A behavior, overall, physical activity in the form of exercise has been shown to enhance certain aspects of personality that are important for mental health (McAuley, 1994).

 Sport has not been found to build socially valued attributes, or "character," but exercise has shown several benefits including enhanced self-concept and psychological well-being and decreased anxiety and depression.

Motivational Processes

Although personality was the first major research area in sport psychology, motivation is by far the biggest area of inquiry in the subdiscipline today. Think of motivation as a complex process that influences individuals to begin an activity and pursue it with vigor and persistence. That is, we assume people are motivated when they make choices to join a fitness program, work intensely during the program, and continue to adhere to their training program when their lives get busy. Motivation directs and energizes our behavior in sport and exercise. Consider how you would answer the following two popular questions about motivation: (1) What is the best way to motivate people? and (2) What makes some people motivated and others not?

What is your favorite physical activity? What motivates you to participate in this activity? Is your motivation more internal or external? Explain your answer.

The first question assumes that motivation is something that you give to others—like a cup of water. You might recall from chapter 4 that this type of motivation is termed extrinsic motivation, which means that people engage in a certain behavior to gain some external reward from that participation such as trophies in sport or losing weight in exercise. Reinforcement techniques such as rewards and punishment are often used as incentives to motivate individuals to exercise or exert effort in sport. The fact that people's behavior is modified through reinforcement shows that these techniques clearly work. Gaining popularity in school or eliciting parental approval from sport achievement clearly motivates children to continue this behavior. Adolescent boys gain motivation to lift weights when their bodies become muscular and admired by others.

However, extrinsic motivation and rewards only serve to enhance motivation in the short term and do not fuel the long-term commitment to achievement in sport or fitness training. Thus, although extrinsic motivators are always present in society and offer powerful incentives, this type of motivation is short-lived. Enduring motivation that is necessary for achievement and success is not something that you can give to another individual. Rather, enduring motivation comes from within.

Thus, the second question—why are some people motivated and others not—is more interesting to sport and exercise psychologists. This motivation from within—called intrinsic motivation—involves engaging in behavior because you enjoy the process and gain pleasure and satisfaction from that participation. Athletes who are intrinsically motivated perform because they love the sport. People who exercise regularly do so because they enjoy physical activity. Intrinsic motivation serves as a long-term fueling process for commitment and achievement of important goals in sport and fitness training. Thus, it is important to understand how intrinsic motivation is developed and enhanced, rather than focusing on the "quick fix" use of rewards and gimmicks to extrinsically motivate individuals.

The answers to the two motivation questions, then, are (1) the best way to motivate people is to help them develop or increase their intrinsic motivation, and (2) people that are more motivated than others typically have higher intrinsic motivation to achieve in a certain activity. But that brings up another question—how is intrinsic motivation developed?

🔑 Intrinsic motivation is self-fueling over the long term because it is based on controllable feelings of enjoyment and competence as compared to extrinsic motivation that relies on external reinforcers from the social environment.

Developing Intrinsic Motivation

Current theory views motivation as a cognitive process in which our behavior is a direct result of how we think and process information about ourselves and the world. Although there are numerous theories about motivation, one common thread they all share is that people are motivated to feel competent, worthy, and self-determining.

From the time we are born, we all attempt to be competent in our environment—even toddlers are motivated to gain independence by learning to crawl and walk. As our lives continue, our need to be competent is channeled in various areas through socialization. Some people are motivated to achieve in sport or through fitness training, others in music, others in a career.

🔑 The key to understanding motivation is realizing that all humans, regardless of their individual goals, are motivated to feel competent, worthy, and self-determining.

While we are all intrinsically motivated to be competent and self-determining, competence and self-determination mean different things to different people. Research in sport and exercise psychology has shown that individuals have different goals for achievement in sport and exercise. Therefore, to truly understand motivation we must understand how each person defines success or competence for him- or herself. Because

people engage in exercise programs for diverse reasons, including social affiliation, personal mastery and fitness, or competitive bodybuilding, exercise programs must assess the goals of participants to fuel individual motivation.

Researchers have found that young children participating in physical activity are motivated to have fun, affiliate with their friends and meet new friends, and develop skills. Although adults often think otherwise, children are more motivated by these goals than by the goal of winning! For this reason, it is important for physical activity programs to provide opportunities for children and youth to attain these goals. Practices and competitions should be structured to be challenging and enjoyable for all children so that they develop their skills, learn important cooperative and social skills, and experience the fun and enjoyment of physical activity. It's really a simple formula. If we like something, we do it more. If we do it more, we get better at it. When we get better at it, we like it more. Think of this as the positive cycle of motivation (see figure 9.5).

Another important factor that influences motivation is what psychologists call perceptions of control. Humans are motivated to be self-determining, which means that we want to be in control of our own actions and behavior. Individuals with more internal perceptions of control are more motivated than individuals who feel

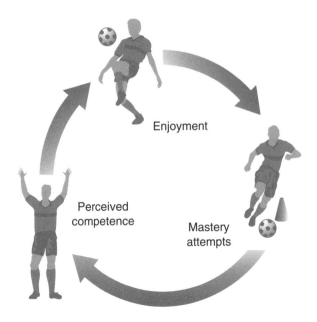

Figure 9.5 Positive cycle of motivation.

others control them or that they are in the hands of fate. Think about a recent success you have achieved. Why were you successful in this endeavor? Identify the reason or reasons for your success in this situation. Are these reasons internal, or controllable by you, such as your ability, hard work, or preparation? Or are your reasons external or uncontrollable, such as luck or the relative ease of the task?

These reasons—called attributions—that individuals use to explain why they succeed or fail influence motivation greatly. The key to motivation is to help people make attributions that fuel their motivation by making them feel proud, satisfied, and expectant of future success. Individuals who begin exercise programs need to internalize feelings of personal accomplishment based on their personal choice to enhance their fitness and health. Athletes need to feel that their successes reflect their competence, mastery, preparation, and hard work. Such beliefs fuel motivation because athletes feel in control of the situation and certain that success can occur again. When athletes fail, they need to take responsibility for the outcome but believe that they can overcome this failure by working hard, gaining skill, or using other strategies. If they feel they have no control over changing their behavior, they will not be motivated to try.

The same is true for individuals involved in exercise programs. If they see and feel progress, and believe they are gaining competence and control over this progress, they will be more motivated to exercise. Individuals who believe they cannot control their behavior ("Why join an exercise program? I'll never be able to stick to it.") must rely solely on extrinsic motivators and incentives, which fall short in helping them make long-term fitness commitments. Feelings of enjoyment and well-being are much more likely to enhance exercise adherence than concerns about health.

Self-Esteem and Self-Confidence

Two important psychological constructs that affect motivation are self-esteem and self-confidence. **Self-esteem** is our perception of personal worthiness and the emotional feelings associated with that perception. Self-esteem is usually thought of as how much we like ourselves. Many psychologists view self-esteem as the most central core component of our identity, and thus it

has a major influence on our motivation in physical activity. Self-worth or self-esteem is an important need for all individuals and it emanates from feeling competent and in control of our behavior in an achievement area that is important to us. The literature emphasizes that self-esteem is the direct result of social interactions, so social support and positive reinforcement for individual mastery attempts are crucial to the development of self-esteem.

Self-confidence is also a critical factor in motivation and is similar to perceived competence as it involves individuals' perceptions that they can successfully perform a specific task. Remember our motivational cycle—if we like something, we do it more; if we do it more, we become better at it; if we become better at it, we like it more. Self-confidence drives motivation because it is the "doing it better" part of the cycle. Athletes who feel more competent and self-confident are motivated to work harder and improve in their sport. Exercisers who gain competence and self-confidence about their fitness level are fueled with additional motivation to continue. If we lack confidence in our ability, then elaborate extrinsic incentives are needed to motivate us. Research supports the notion that people who develop strong confidence in their physical abilities based on early success in exercise programs persist longer than people who fail to develop confidence in their physical abilities.

Self-esteem is based on feelings of personal worthiness, whereas self-confidence involves perceptions of one's ability to be successful in particular achievement areas.

Arousal, Anxiety, and Stress

Remember that motivation involves intensity of behavior and the urge to be competent and successful. It is easy to see, then, that for some people this motivation that was once positive and enjoyable can turn into anxiety and become stressful. Consider the following two examples of how motivation works positively in one situation and negatively in the other.

Jill, a high school tennis player, is very motivated to excel in her sport. She plays a match in which she is "out of her head" or "in the zone" and performs exceptionally. Brad, a college high jumper, is very motivated to excel in his sport. However, at the conference championship meet, he "chokes" and fails to perform near his personal best in his event. What is the difference between these two athletes? They are both motivated, yet their psychological mind-sets for competition are very different.

These athletes differ in their levels of **arousal**, which is defined as physical and psychological readiness to perform. Think of arousal as a specific state of motivation in a particular situation. This state runs on a continuum from deep sleep in which our bodies and minds are at their lowest levels of arousal to extreme activation such as a situation in which we fear for our lives. A popular misconception is that you can never be too motivated or highly aroused, but research has shown that high levels of arousal can hurt performance.

Optimal arousal, in which our muscles work without tension and in congruence with each other, is very personal—every individual has a unique optimal arousal zone. Some athletes perform better when their arousal levels are high and they feel extremely "psyched" about competition. Other athletes perform better when they control their arousal at lower levels so they feel more relaxed yet intense. Exercise behavior is also influenced by arousal; individuals should attempt to be in their optimal arousal zone during exercise bouts. This usually has occurred when people remark, "I was really in the zone today. I felt like I could run for hours without getting tired."

Another consideration in arousal is the type of task the person is performing. Tasks involving high levels of precision such as putting in golf, surgery, or foul shooting in basketball will require lower levels of arousal for successful performance. Would you like your dentist to fill a cavity when he was really "psyched up"? Probably not. On the other hand, tasks involving application of high levels of force in less precise ways such as power lifting, defending the line in football, or shot putting will require higher levels of arousal for successful performance. In the examples pictured below the optimal level of arousal for the archer is likely to be lower than the optimal level of arousal for the wrestlers.

All people have their own unique optimal arousal zone for performance that is influenced by the type of activity they are doing.

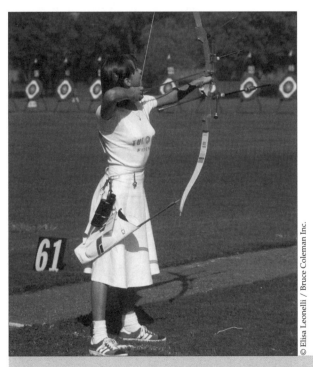
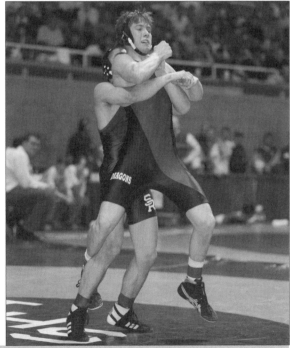

Why will the archer function best at a lower level of arousal than the wrestlers?

When arousal goes past the optimal zone, it usually is perceived negatively and becomes anxiety. Anxiety, then, is simply a negative response to a stressful situation in which individuals feel apprehension and threat to their self-esteem. Thus, while arousal is a generic state of activation (neither good nor bad), anxiety is a state typified by high levels of arousal interpreted as negative. Research has demonstrated that social physique anxiety, or apprehension about one's body and appearance, is predictive of exercise behavior (Crawford & Eklund, 1994). For instance, the less apprehensive people feel about their appearance, the more likely they'll be to participate in activities that require them to reveal more of their bodies (e.g., gymnastics or swimming).

Think about your physical activity participation. How would you describe your optimal level of arousal? What is the optimal level for the type of activity in which you participate? Explain your reasoning.

Stress is a term often used synonymously with anxiety, such as when we hear people say they are "stressed out." However, stress should be thought of as a process rather than a response or state such as anxiety. Stress begins with a situation that places a demand on individuals. If the individuals perceive that the situational demand is greater than their response capabilities, they perceive threat or stress. This perceived threat or stress then leads to certain types of responses such as anxiety. Finally, the individuals' behaviors are influence by their responses to the perceived stressor.

If a diver perceives that she lacks the ability to perform a required dive successfully in competition, she will be threatened by that perception and respond with anxiety. If a retired older adult perceives that he lacks the skills to learn a physical activity such as tennis, he will not take up the game. If an adolescent perceives that she will be laughed at because of her obesity, she will drop out of her swimming class. This is the stress process. However, the key to understanding the concept of stress is the word *perception*. Although we don't always believe it, we have the ability to control our stress because it is a perception. This is why a popular saying is that "pressure is something you put on yourself." A great deal of intervention in sport and exercise psychology focuses on reducing individuals' perceptions of stress in physical activity situations. Similarly, exercise is often prescribed to help individuals cope with stress, as the physical activity serves to distract them from thinking about the stressor to enhance their mood and induce relaxation.

Research has shown that most of the stress associated with physical activity participation is based on fear of failure and fear of evaluation. Both of these fears result from threat to our self-worth. Although some high-risk physical activities involve some fear of physical harm, most participants in these sports indicate that their skill level and mental toughness help them to combat this fear or perception. Stress associated with fear of evaluation can also occur in exercise settings where beginning participants are unfamiliar with equipment such as weight machines or are embarrassed by their lack of experience in such activities as aerobic dance classes.

A popular question is whether sports competition is too stressful for children. Interestingly,

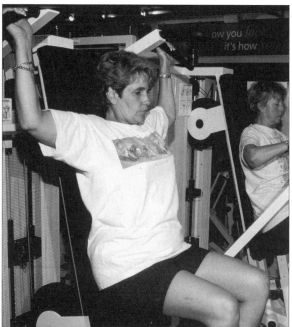

Beginning physical activity is stressful for many individuals who lack experience with technical fitness training.

© Marijo Erzinger

research has shown that sport per se is not stressful, but rather the social evaluation inherent in any competition produces the stress. Thus, sport can be stressful for some children, but it is no more stressful than any other achievement activity that involves social evaluation.

Research Profile

How many parents worry about sport being too stressful for their children? In a research study, Simon and Martens (1979) measured the anxiety levels of children performing in various activities (e.g., academic exams, different sports, band, physical education classes). They found that the highest anxiety was experienced by children performing band solos followed by children participating in wrestling and gymnastics. The researchers concluded that sport is no more stressful than any other evaluative activity in which children engage. The key is to make evaluation in physical activity settings as nonthreatening as possible so children learn to enjoy the challenge of achievement situations.

Stress in physical activity is the perception of threat to self-worth brought on by fear of failure and evaluation.

Burnout is a term often associated with stress and anxiety. **Burnout** is an extreme state of mental, emotional, and physical exhaustion that occurs due to chronic stress. Burnout also involves a loss of interest in a formerly enjoyable activity because the rewards associated with this activity have lost personal meaning. Recent research has indicated that burnout is a complex occurrence related to perfectionism and the controlling nature of high-performance sport (Coakley, 1992; Gould, Udry, Tuffey, & Loehr, 1996). As in the case of obligatory exercisers discussed previously, exercise burnout can result from emotional and physical exhaustion coupled with the stress and pressure of feeling an overwhelming need to exercise. Burnout in fitness training is likely to occur when motivation is focused solely on extrinsic outcomes as opposed to enjoyment.

Interpersonal and Group Processes

Our overview of knowledge has examined the two broad areas of personality and motivation as they relate to sport and exercise behavior. In this section, our focus is on interpersonal or group processes that influence individuals' behaviors in different ways; these include the presence of others, group membership, and leadership. Also, the areas of aggression and gender socialization are explained briefly as behaviors or characteristics that result from interpersonal social processes.

Presence of Others

How is your behavior different when you are alone as opposed to when you are with other people? Why do some people prefer to exercise at home while others like to exercise with others in a public gym? Why do some athletes perform better in front of a big crowd? Does the "home advantage" really exist? Since the turn of the 20th century, researchers have been fascinated with the effects of an audience on human performance, or **social facilitation**. In applying social facilitation to sport, research has shown that the presence of other people increases our arousal, which then may hurt or help our performance. Generally, spectators have a negative effect on someone who is learning a skill and a positive effect on someone who is very skilled (Zajonc, 1965). Think about a beginning golfer who is learning the game and has to tee off in front of a large group on the first hole. The presence of spectators increases his arousal, and because his skills are not well learned, this arousal causes him to hit a bad shot. But consider a professional tennis player who makes the finals at Wimbledon for the first time and whose performance is inspired and elevated by the huge crowd at center court.

Although this sounds like a simple explanation, the social facilitation process is much more complex than it seems. For example, research has shown that it is not the mere presence of others that causes this effect, but rather peoples' perceptions that they are being evaluated by others (Cottrell, 1968). Thus, from a cognitive perspective, we would need to know how different individuals perceive evaluation to really understand how spectators affect them. Also, we know from the previous section that every individual has a different optimal arousal zone, so the presence of others could influence performance differently based on individual responses to changes in arousal. One thing we do know from research in this area, however, is that people should avoid situations of excessive evaluation or analysis when learning sport skills; this pressure can hurt the learning process by adversely affecting beginners' arousal levels and quality of attention.

Generally, the presence of spectators impairs the learning process of sport skills for novices by affecting their arousal and attentional processes.

Researchers have also documented the "home advantage," which shows that teams playing at home sites win a greater percentage of the time as compared to those playing at away sites. The reasons for this home advantage, however, are less clear and could even be attributed to expectancy or the fact that athletes expect to play better at home because they believe in this popular notion.

Although a "home advantage" in sport has been documented, the reasons for this advantage are unclear.

Social facilitation applies a bit differently to exercise, because the people present are usually socially supportive workout partners or simply other individuals concurrently exercising on their own (e.g., while weight training at a public facility). Family social support is a strong predictor of exercise maintenance for women, and individuals who exercise with their spouses have higher rates of exercise adherence than those who exercise alone. Research has demonstrated that physical activity levels of children are related to the modeling of such activity, shared activities, social support, and encouragement within families. Several studies have demonstrated that active children perceived more parental encouragement than inactive children (Taylor, Baranowski, & Sallis, 1994). The social isolation of many elderly people is problematic in that the social incentives to engage in physical activity decrease with age. Community-based programs are needed to ensure the important social support for

habitual physical activity participation for all ages.

The physical activity participation of children is highly predicted by family support and modeling, while elderly people tend to become less physically active due to social isolation.

What sport and exercise activities do you like to engage in with other people present? What sport and exercise activities would you rather perform alone? Try to explain the reasons for your answers.

Group Membership

While social facilitation focuses on the effects of others on individual behavior, the area of group dynamics focuses on how being a part of a group influences behavior as well as how certain psychosocial factors influence collective group behavior. Are people more likely to adhere to exercise programs if they participate in groups versus individually? Why is it that some teams have better "chemistry" than others? And why do teams with better chemistry often perform better than more talented teams with poorer chemistry?

Groups perform better and group members are more satisfied when they are cohesive. **Cohesion** is the tendency for groups to stick together and remain united in pursuing goals (Carron, 1982). Thus, coaches and exercise leaders should strive to develop and nurture cohesion in their teams or groups in several different ways. Cohesion is facilitated by emphasizing uniqueness or a positive identity related to group membership. Nicknames, such as the "Fab Five" or the "The Lunch Bunch," often reflect cohesion and group identification. Athletes sometimes shave their heads or wear team jackets to demonstrate their solidarity and commitment to the group. Cohesion is also facilitated when individual members of teams understand and accept their role within the group. Studies on adherence to exercise programs indicate that most people prefer to exercise with another person or in groups, which enhances enjoyment through affiliation and social support and strengthens commitment to the program. Cohesion and friendship within the group is one of the strongest predictors of exercise adherence.

We also know that success breeds cohesion, so some early successes are crucial in the development of group dynamics. When groups experience success initially, cohesion develops accordingly. However, it is important to realize that cohesion is a dynamic quality that is always changing within a group. For example, conflicts may arise that must be resolved, but this does not mean that the group is not or cannot be cohesive. Also, the quest for cohesion can go too far, resulting in extreme cohesion that involves conformity and elitism. While a strong positive group identity is needed, it is important that diversity within groups is celebrated and respected.

Also of interest in group dynamics is how group membership influences individual performance. **Social loafing** refers to a decrease in individual performance within groups (Latane, Williams, & Harkins, 1979). This occurs because

individuals believe their performance is not identifiable and that other group members will "pick up the slack." It is not a conscious process—people do not decide to socially loaf—rather it is a psychological tendency when performing in a group. However, social loafing is easily reduced by increasing the identifiability of individuals by monitoring their performances. This is typically done in sport via video analysis of individual performance and individual statistics that break out a single athlete's performance from the total performance of the team. Social loafing can be monitored in exercise groups if performance totals (e.g., number of sit-ups, amount of weight lifted, distance run) are recorded so that progress can be checked. Research clearly demonstrates that when individual efforts are identified and monitored, social loafing disappears.

Cohesion and group membership facilitate physical activity performance, but social loafing may occur unless individuals are monitored and their inputs are viewed as important to overall performance.

Leadership and Reinforcement

Obviously, a huge influence on physical activity participation is effective leadership. Although motivation to achieve in sport or fitness largely comes from within a person, effective leadership and appropriate reinforcement can help individuals build feelings of competence and success, which leads to higher motivation. **Leadership** is a behavioral process of influencing individuals and groups toward set goals (Barrow, 1977). Early research in this area attempted to find a set of traits that defined effective leadership. However, think of the many successful leaders you know and how their personalities differ. There is no one set of personality characteristics that make an effective leader.

Leadership is an interactional process that must take into account the situation, the characteristics of the athletes or group members, and the characteristics of the leader (see figure 9.6). Effective leadership results when these three components fit together well. Effective exercise leadership requires a behavioral style that fits the goals and needs of the participants. Likewise, it is important for coaches to assess the age and

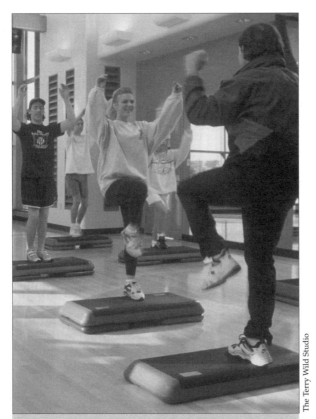

Individual adherence to exercise programs is improved through group involvement and social support.

The Terry Wild Studio

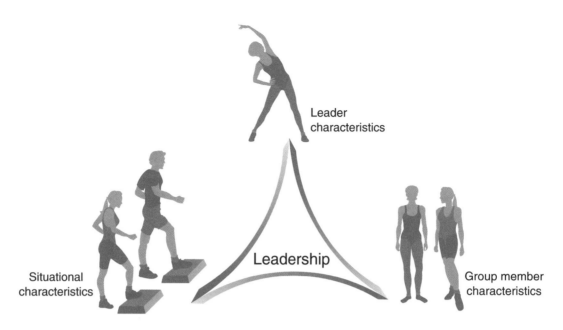

Figure 9.6 Interactional leadership: Effective leaders understand the need to adapt their leadership style based on the needs of the group members and the situation or environment.

abilities of their athletes in relation to situational demands and then modify their behavior to be appropriate in this situation.

Keys to gaining influence and earning respect as an effective leader include exuding self-confidence and competence; demonstrating interpersonal skill in communicating effectively; engaging in appropriate goal planning and commitment; and being a positive role model in terms of professionalism, emotional control, and lifestyle management. Because the public looks to health professionals as role models for healthy lifestyles, it is important that leaders in the health professions (including physicians) engage in positive health habits including regular exercise. Programs that prepare health providers for physical activity counseling are likely to be more effective if they initially focus on the exercise habits of health-care providers and various strategies for modeling healthy lifestyles to clients.

Effective leaders influence the behavior of other people. A key factor in this influence is the ways that leaders communicate and provide feedback. Feedback and reinforcement, although seen as extrinsic motivators, can be used in a positive way to enhance people's feelings of competence, which then serve to increase their intrinsic motivation. This area, called **behavior modification**, has been developed from animal research in psy-

chology and deals with how the use of reinforcers influences human behavior.

The fundamental assumption of behavior modification is that behaviors are strengthened when they are rewarded and weakened when they are punished or unrewarded. Many potential reinforcers exist in the physical activity environment (e.g., trophies, money, status, weight loss, fitness, popularity). What is important is how individuals perceive reinforcers that they receive from leaders. If feedback and rewards are seen as controlling, then they only serve to enhance extrinsic motivation and will actually weaken intrinsic motivation. In sport, extrinsic rewards that are used to control athletes such as college scholarships, trophies, and all-star selections often decrease intrinsic motivation. Incentives such as weight loss and prizes for attendance may be motivating to exercisers, but could be problematic if used to coerce or manipulate individuals. Behavioral contracts and attendance lotteries are examples of incentives used for exercise adherence, but research indicates that these inducements alone do not have a lasting effect on exercise behavior. It is important that rewards and feedback are used not to control athletes or exercisers, but rather to make them feel that they've earned praise and reward through their effort and competence (Smith, 1998).

Reinforcement may be used by leaders to enhance the perceptions of competence and feelings of worthiness of physical activity participants.

Moreover, it is important to praise and reward the right behaviors. When young children first attempt physical skills, their coaches or teacher should reinforce these mastery attempts. Research supports the effectiveness of a mastery goal orientation as opposed to an ego or outcome goal orientation. Hopefully, children will learn to value individual improvement and mastery in physical activities, which serves to enhance their perceptions of competence, control, and self-worth. Exercise motivation is enhanced by this personal mastery approach and feedback that is tailored to help the individual gauge his or her competence and improvement based on personal performance and fitness standards.

> Think about individuals who have significantly influenced your life with their leadership skills. Why were they effective? What were their leadership styles, and what type of reinforcers did they use to guide your behavior?

Aggression

The social processes of competition in Western society are often seen as a precursor to aggression in sport. Why do fights break out in hockey matches? Why does crowd violence often erupt at soccer matches? Aggression is behavior directed toward inflicting harm or injury on another person. A main source of aggression in competitive situations is the inevitable presence of frustration.

Frustration often results when a person's goals are blocked, and in competitive sport, the main objective is to block the goal achievement of the opponent. Social learning theory views aggression as a learned behavior that develops as a result of modeling and reinforcement. Ice hockey players are glorified for fighting with opponents, and baseball players are encouraged and even expected to charge the mound and aggress against the pitcher as a result of being hit by a

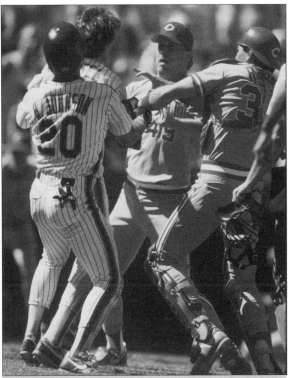

Violence and aggression occur in sport due to frustration and social learning, such as watching sport role models engage in aggressive acts.

© Ron Vesely

pitched ball. Children learn aggressive behaviors at an early age. Research also links aggression to cognitive levels of moral reasoning. Athletes have been shown to have lower moral reasoning skills when compared to nonathletes, and athletes have been shown to view aggression as more legitimate when compared to nonathletes (Bredemeier, Weiss, Shields, & Cooper, 1986).

It is popularly believed that competition and/or exercise reduces aggressive impulses in humans by providing a release or purging of aggression (called catharsis). However, research does not support this claim, but rather shows that aggressive tendencies *increase* after competing, engaging in vigorous physical activity, or watching a competitive event. Thus, competitive and physical activity participation and spectatorship do not serve as a catharsis for aggressive responses.

Aggression, or behavior intended to harm another person, has been shown to be socially learned behavior and is related to lower levels of moral reasoning.

Physical activity participation does not "blow off steam" or purge individuals of aggressive tendencies.

Gender Socialization

The social processes of **gender** formation and maintenance have been studied extensively with important implications for physical activity behavior (Gill, 1992). Gender is defined as social and psychological characteristics and behaviors associated with being male or female. A popular myth is that differences in the thoughts, feelings, behaviors, and physical performance capacities between males and females are based on the biological sex differences of being born female or male.

This biological explanation for differences between males and females ignores the social complexity and variations in gender-related behavior and performance. For example, it is popularly assumed that males can naturally throw a baseball harder and farther than females because males are stronger. It is also assumed that males are better long distance runners than females because of greater muscular and cardiovascular endurance. However, there is substantial overlap between male and female performance on all motor skills. This means that although the most highly trained male is stronger than the most highly trained female, some females are stronger than many males. Thus, although our society loves to assume that all females and males are stereotypically grouped according to popular beliefs about limits of physical activity performance, males and females actually are more similar than they are different. And most of the gender differences that are apparent in physical activity behavior are based not on biology, but rather on the differential socialization patterns of girls and boys, which typically advantage boys in terms of opportunity, support, and expectations for physical activity proficiency.

Besides perceived strength and motor proficiency differences, gender differences are also assumed and have been found in various psychological characteristics such as self-confidence, aggression, and competitiveness. The gender differences that are documented develop over time and are influenced by rigid gender socialization and stereotypical expectations of conformity to sociocultural norms for distinct female and male

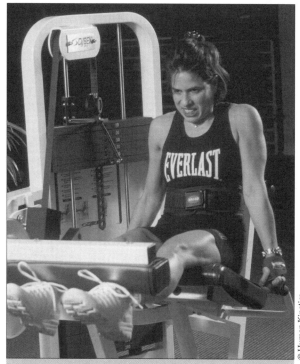

Strict socially defined gender expectations have limited females' participation in certain physical activities.

© Human Kinetics

behaviors. Much of the gender research has neglected to consider socialization and thus has reinforced existing and limiting gender stereotypes.

Consider how this occurs. If coaches believe that female athletes are less skilled and competitive, their behavior toward these athletes will reflect this belief. This "self-fulfilling prophecy" can be a vicious cycle that allows stereotypical ideas about females and males to limit their achievement in various areas. If you had a daughter and a son and had to predict which ice sports they would become involved in, you would probably say figure skating for the daughter and ice hockey for the son. And you would probably be right!

Boys, more than girls, value sport and perceive the need to be competent at sport and physical activity. Sport is a very sex-typed area; popular culture views it as more appropriate for males than females. This view exerts powerful socialization influences on young girls when they are deciding whether to participate in sports. It is no coincidence that girls become less active in sports and physical activity at puberty when society gives them the message that they now should focus on more "appropriate" activities in preparation for womanhood. This disadvantages many women who in later years wish to engage in physical activity yet lack the requisite motor skills, knowledge, and confidence. Physical activity leaders must understand this aspect of socialization and provide classes and individual counseling to allow women to develop knowledge and confidence in their physical capacities. Child-care responsibilities represent a major barrier to women's participation in exercise, and unmarried women report participation in significantly more vigorous activity than married women (Marcus, 1995). Overall, gender expectations and prescribed societal roles influence the physical activity participation of females and males quite differently.

Most gender differences develop through socialization based on stereotyped expectations for gender conformity and sociocultural norms that specify distinct female and male behaviors.

Developmental Concerns in Psychology of Sport and Exercise

Because human beings undergo constant physical and psychosocial development, it is important to examine the psychological implications of physical activity participation from a developmental perspective. Ideally, a life-span approach to the study of physical activity behavior allows us to understand how participation in physical activity relates to the psychological characteristics and responses of individuals at different stages in their lives.

Considerable research has examined the psychosocial aspects of children's participation in physical activity. In the United States, an estimated 25 million children under the age of 18 years are involved in physical activity programs. These early sport experiences can have important lifelong effects on the psychological development of children. Parents' activity levels, beliefs about exercise, education, and encouragement are all strong determinants of exercise behavior in children. Most children cite multiple reasons for wanting to participate in physical activity, but most are intrinsic such as having fun and learning skills (Gould & Petlichkoff, 1988). Most children withdraw from physical activity

because of interest in other activities, yet often cite some negative factors such as lack of fun and too much pressure. As we saw in chapter 2, the sharpest age-related decreases in exercise participation is late adolescence when young adults begin to make the transition to independent living. Physical fitness and aerobic activities have been linked to improving self-concept in children far more than participation in competitive sport (Gruber, 1986). This may be due to the immediate feedback derived from fitness training and a feeling of physical mastery that is often a more long-term occurrence in sport participation. Physical activity programs that are beneficial for children emphasize fun, challenge, skill and fitness improvement, and social affiliation to match their participation motives (Weiss, 1991).

Successful physical activity programs for children emphasize fun, challenge, skill and fitness improvement, and social affiliation to match their participation motives.

Although most children who participate in physical activity do not experience excessive anxiety, stress can be a problem for certain children in specific situations (Scanlan, 1986). Children with low self-esteem; high trait-anxiety; and frequent worries about failure, social evaluation, and adult expectancies are at risk for stress in their physical activity participation. Also, situations that maximize pressure and importance such as championship events may cause increased stress in children.

An important consideration for adult physical activity leaders is the modification of physical activity to make it more developmentally appropriate. Modified competitive games have been shown to increase enjoyment and skill development of children. An example of this would be the "coach-pitch" modification in youth baseball. Children at a young age lack the skills to pitch a ball effectively, so a modified game in which the coach pitches to batters increases the number of hits, defensive activity, learning, and enjoyment. Modifying activities so they are developmentally appropriate is an excellent way to ensure success. Positive experiences in physical activity as a child are crucial in developing the skills, knowledge, and habits for a healthy lifestyle in adulthood.

Think about a physical activity that you enjoy. How could this activity be modified to optimally appeal to and benefit children? How about teenagers? Senior citizens? Explain your reasoning for each answer.

Sport and exercise psychology specialists have spent very little time studying the psychological aspects of physical activity participation for older adults. Diseases of the cardiovascular system cause over half of the deaths of individuals over the age of 65. By 2020, one of every six Americans will be over 65 years old. Because cardiovascular disease risk factors are present in almost epidemic proportions in older individuals, physical activity and other health-promotion intervention strategies aimed at older adults represent a critical social need for the new millennium. Such strategies also reduce disability in the elderly, thus providing them a greater quality of living in their later years. Major causes of disability in this age group are strokes and falls that result in fractures. Losses in strength, flexibility, and balance increase the risk of falling in elderly people, which again directly supports the need for systematic physical activity to enhance neuromuscular control in this age group (Hagberg, 1994). Decreasing cardiovascular disease risk factors through exercise also reduces the chance of strokes in the elderly.

Many misconceptions exist about older adults' capabilities to remain physically active. Research has documented both physiological and psychological benefits of physical activity for older adults. Physical activity has been shown to increase the maximal oxygen consumption (a measure of cardiovascular function), reduce blood pressure, and increase muscular strength and lean body mass in older adults. As with younger persons, physical activity also has been shown to increase feelings of well-being and self-confidence and reduce anxiety and depression in the elderly (Willis & Campbell, 1992). Specific exercise prescriptions for older adults should emphasize cardiovascular and strength activities, while also including flexibility and balance components to offset common risk factors for falls (Hagberg, 1994). Physical activity programs should be specially adapted to meet the needs of older adults

who often seek social affiliation and who need to retain a basic level of physical competence and a positive psychological outlook during this stage of their lives.

Physical activity can slow the physiological aging process by increasing muscular strength and cardiovascular fitness and reducing blood pressure in older adults.

Intervention Techniques for Physical Activity

Often called mental training or psychological skills training, intervention techniques are used to learn cognitive skills (e.g., self-talk) and behavioral strategies (e.g., goal setting) that can enhance physical activity behavior. Intervention techniques may be used to increase exercise adherence, improve sport performance, develop important life skills for young people participating in physical activity, aid in rehabilitation from injury and disease, and enhance career transition and retirement from sport. Exercise interventions are most effectively administered by health promotion specialists, in both community-based and individualized interventions. Worksite-based exercise interventions are a promising approach to increasing levels of physical activity and have developed as a result of the rising cost of providing health insurance for employees (Marcus, 1995). Sport psychology interventions are typically conducted by professionals with graduate degrees in sport psychology, yet a growing trend is the education of coaches in the use of intervention techniques who then can implement mental training with athletes as part of their overall physical training program.

Intervention techniques in sport and exercise psychology are used to increase exercise adherence, enhance sport performance, develop life skills, aid in injury rehabilitation, and ease career transitions and retirement from sport.

An important goal of intervention strategies is to maximize the chances of achieving an inner state of well-being and enjoyment termed "flow" (Csikszentmihalyi, 1990b). Exercisers speak of "runner's high" or that elusive state in which physical activity is effortless and immensely enjoyable. Athletes train to achieve the ultimate high of "being in the zone" and enjoying the ultimate thrill of sport characterized by peak performance. Actual flow experiences and peak performances are rare, and we typically stumble onto them without any planned mental training. However, psychological skills training in physical activity can be used to help athletes and exercise participants learn ways to maximize their chances of achieving flow or peak performance.

Think back to a time you experienced flow. Describe the activity that you were doing and what the experience felt like. What made it different from other experiences? How long did it last, and why do you think it went away when it did?

Goal setting is a basic technique used to focus on specific attainable behaviors presented as reachable yet difficult. Research indicates that goals are most effective if they are difficult and systematically monitored and evaluated. Simply setting goals at the beginning of a season or exercise program will not facilitate development unless these goals become the constant focus of attention. Other effective goal setting practices include the use of short-term goals as progressive steps toward reaching a long-term goal, and an emphasis on performance or controllable goals as opposed to outcome goals such as winning a race. Flow occurs when our abilities match the challenge of the situation; effective goal setting can help individuals achieve flow by allowing them to plan and focus on specific challenges that push them to achieve based on personal ability levels (see figure 9.7). Specific performance goals allow competence and success to be personally defined and achievable for everyone.

Another popular intervention technique is self-talk, or personal statements that we all make to ourselves. Many variations of this technique

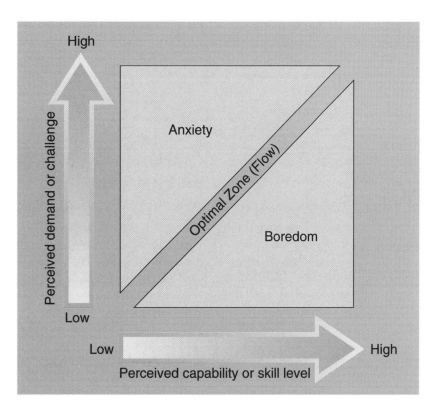

Figure 9.7   Flow or peak experiences occur when our ability meets the challenges of the situation. Personal goal setting is helpful in creating personal challenges to enhance flow.

exist (e.g., cognitive restructuring, systematic desensitization, thought-stopping, stress inoculation), but the basic premise is that the things we say to ourselves drive our behaviors. The goal of effective self-talk is to engage in planned, intentional productive thinking that convinces our bodies that we are confident, motivated, and ready to perform. Athletes are taught to identify key situations or environmental stressors that cause them to "choke" and then plan and mentally practice a refocusing plan that can be used to focus attention appropriately in that situation (Orlick, 1986). Exercisers can use self-talk to strengthen their commitment to completing workouts by telling themselves that they feel strong, by telling themselves that they are gaining health benefits, or by seeing their bodies as finely tuned machines. Productive self-talk is critical in maintaining self-confidence, which has been shown to be a major predictor of exercise adherence and sport performance.

Attentional control and focusing is perhaps the most important cognitive skill for any type of physical activity. In sport, performance is dependent on the cues that athletes process from themselves and the social and physical environment. In exercise, learning how and when to focus on one's body (called "association") as well as distract oneself (called "dissociation") such as with music or visual imagery can enhance the exercise experience and help performance. Attentional control strategies such as "centering" (Nideffer & Sagal, 1998) allow individuals to select relevant cues and design physiological (e.g., deep breathing) and psychological (e.g., feeling strong, quick, and confident) triggers to focus attention optimally.

Imagery, a mental technique that "programs" the mind to respond as programmed, uses all the senses to create or recreate an experience in the mind (Vealey & Greenleaf, 1998). Jack Nicklaus, perhaps the greatest golfer of all time, says that hitting a golf shot is 50% mental picture. Research has demonstrated that imagery enhances motor performance, and although it cannot take the place of physical practice, it is better than no practice at all. The use of imagery by elite athletes is widespread and is often cited as an important mental factor in their success. Novice athletes can use imagery to create positive mental blueprints of successful performance, while exercisers can use imagery to visualize their muscles firing and

getting stronger when training for fitness. Exercisers can also use imagery to "dissociate," or to direct attention away from the repetitive exercise activity to visualize motivational or pleasant things. Many runners like to use personal audiotape or compact disc players when they run to help them create pleasant mental images.

Individuals use physical relaxation techniques to teach them to control their autonomic functions including muscular and hormonal changes that occur during physical activity. These techniques allow them to engage in physical activity with much greater mastery and control over the responses of their bodies to environmental stimuli. Such physical relaxation techniques include breathing exercises, muscular tension–relaxation techniques, and various types of meditation. Momentary relaxation prior to exercising is effective to facilitate smooth, coordinated muscular effort. Individuals can learn how to regulate physiological arousal by reducing their heart and breathing rates to induce a more relaxed state. Obviously, physical relaxation techniques can be used in conjunction with goal setting, imagery, and self-talk to optimize both physical and cognitive readiness to engage in physical activity.

The goal of physical relaxation training is to teach individuals how to control the responses of their autonomic functions when faced with stressors in physical activity environments.

Conclusions From Overview of Knowledge

You've now been exposed to a variety of areas studied in sport and exercise psychology. And your "tour" of knowledge was not exhaustive, meaning that it didn't cover all the topics in this area of study, the purpose was to provide you with a glimpse of the knowledge that researchers and practitioners have developed over the years in this subdiscipline of physical activity. You should now have a better idea about such things as how exercise influences our mental health, why intrinsic motivation is critical in fueling exercise and sport behavior, and how professionals in the subdiscipline can use intervention techniques to enhance sport performance and exercise adherence.

To cap off the chapter, the next section presents a "focus topic," or an area that is typically of popular interest in sport and exercise psychology. Due to the public fascination with athletes' abilities to perform under pressure, the topic of "choking" is presented to help you gain a basic understanding of this common, and dreaded, phenomenon in sport.

Focus Topic: "Choking" in Sport

Remember the scenario presented at the beginning of the chapter in which you are crouched in the starting blocks of an Olympic race? Let's now examine a typical performance issue—"choking"—that occurs in sport so that you'll know how to avoid choking if you ever find yourself in that situation. We'll pool our knowledge from the chapter to develop the right "mental skills recipe" to help you perform your best.

Why Do People "Choke?"

Choking is a popular term for performing poorly in stressful situations due to a lack of mental skill. Basically, choking occurs when you focus your attention on the wrong things. Athletes choke because they lose control of their thought processes, and their minds do not allow their bodies the freedom to perform effectively. Our minds and bodies are connected so intimately that even with years of physical training and the development of outstanding physical skill, a lack of mental skill at a pressurized moment in competition can interfere with our bodies' abilities to perform what is usually a simple task (e.g., kicking a short field goal, shooting a free throw, executing a gymnastics vault). Thus, choking begins with our thoughts, but also affects our physical responses by creating tension in our muscles, or, excessive physiological arousal.

Choking is the opposite of peak performance or flow. Peak performance and flow are characterized by a lack of self-consciousness or ego-involvement. When we are in flow, we're not thinking about what other people think of us. Research on achievement goals indicates that athletes are more confident, less anxious, and perform better when they are focused on the specific task as opposed to being ego-focused on demonstrating ability or achieving a favorable outcome such as winning. Peak performance and flow involve intrinsic motivation and total immersion in the activity itself—as opposed to focusing on the pressure of achieving the outcome. Thus, people that rely on extrinsic motivation are prime candidates to choke because they tend to focus all attention on extrinsic rewards such as winning or gaining approval from others.

Choking occurs at both the cognitive and physiological levels. Previously in the chapter you learned that every athlete has a unique individual optimal arousal zone. Arousal and anxiety include both cognitive and physical components; thus, athletes need to understand their optimal arousal zone with regard to both mental and physical activation (Martens, Vealey, & Burton, 1990). Choking, or catastrophic performance declines, occurs when the cognitive and physical components of arousal interact in a certain way (Hardy, 1990). Think of it as a bad chemical reaction. Many times athletes will be able to perform effectively at high levels of physical arousal, but choking occurs when the cognitive arousal is increased to a point at which it interacts with physical arousal to hurt performance.

→

Arousal theory also demonstrates that high levels of arousal may be good or bad depending on whether they are perceived as stressful. Many athletes perform better at extremely high levels of arousal; they perceive this as exciting and optimally challenging (Kerr, 1985). This is because they perceive low stress in that particular situation. Athletes choke when they experience high levels of arousal coupled with high levels of stress, or perceived threat, which creates overstimulation and anxiety.

All of these aspects of choking provide clues as to how to prepare mentally to avoid it. So let's go to work and plan the strategies you would follow to win your first Olympic gold medal and reign as "world's fastest human"!

Overcoming the "Choke"

Mental preparation begins with thorough physical preparation. To perform successfully in pressure situations, athletes must be able to relax and trust that their training and physical preparation achieved through numerous repetitions will provide them with a sound automatic performance base. Self-confidence to perform well in sport doesn't come from hope; rather, it is earned by preparation and knowing that no shortcuts in training have been taken. Thus, returning to the scenario at the start of this chapter—when you are waiting in the blocks for the race of your life—your mind must be clear of any doubts about your physical preparation and physical ability to perform at an optimal level.

Coupled with this thorough physical preparation, you must have set appropriate and effective goals with respect to performance expectations. One of the biggest contributors to choking is thinking about the outcome or importance of competition while performing. Setting specific performance goals that allow you to focus on the process of performing provides the attentional focus needed to perform optimally. The goals you have set for yourself as a sprinter for this race might be to keep your body low and drive your arms hard for an effective start from the blocks and then to keep a disciplined form or technique, which will allow you to achieve your maximum acceleration quickly.

Prior to this race and over your years as a competitor, you have engaged in self-reflection to better understand your optimal arousal zone with respect to both physical and cognitive activation. You know what your optimal zone is, and you have a competition focus plan that allows you to get centered into it. This plan includes a detailed race plan for the thoughts and feelings that you will program into your mind and body in the hours and minutes leading up to the race, including the use of imagery to see and feel yourself running strongly and efficiently. It also involves trigger words that you use to keep your thoughts positive about the race. You have also mentally rehearsed a refocusing technique that you can use at any time prior to the race to rid yourself of distracting thoughts and feelings. You are now ready for the performance of your life!

Mental training to optimize physical activity experiences is not infallible. It is unrealistic to think that athletes can avoid choking totally. John McEnroe, the great tennis champion, has said that choking is inevitable—that at some time every athlete falls victim to the mental pressure of the situation. Athletes should acknowledge that choking can occur and should then be prepared in case it happens. Optimizing mental skills does not mean that athletes can control everything that happens to them, but it does means is that they can learn to respond in productive ways when bad things do happen.

Helping People Get Started with Exercise

- Introduce them to light and enjoyable exercise (minimal risk of discomfort or injury).
- Help them establish personalized and realistic goals (avoid comparison to others).
- Use the "shaping" technique by rewarding small achievements along the way to reaching a goal (progressive, graduated exercise goals).
- Avoid situations in which the individual may feel vulnerable or have lapses in confidence (such as when activity is viewed as "inappropriate" or sex-typed).
- Use immediate, informational feedback, provide encouragement, and help them to regulate their own confidence by practicing productive self-talk.
- Physically guide them through movements in which they initially lack confidence.
- Gradually encourage them to take control of their exercise behavior through self-monitoring and self-regulation once they have gained skill and become knowledgeable.

Modified from Smith & Biddle 1995.

Choose a physical activity that you like to do. Plan a "centering" technique that you can use easily to help yourself gain the focus you want to have during this activity. To do this, jot down two or three physical behaviors that are personally effective in helping your body feel ready for the activity. Then, jot down two or three key focus thoughts that you will use to prepare yourself to think productively while doing this activity.

Physical Behaviors

_____

_____

_____

Focus Thoughts

_____

_____

_____

Wrap-Up

Sport and exercise psychology, as a young science, has only begun to scratch the surface of understanding the thoughts, feelings, and behaviors related to participation in physical activity. But the knowledge base that has developed over the last three decades is impressive as research continues to study personality, motivation, group processes, developmental concerns, and intervention techniques related to physical activity. Researchers and practitioners in the subdiscipline are committed to extend and apply this knowledge to enhance participation in physical activity for all individuals.

If you are especially interested in what you've learned so far about sport and exercise psychology, you might want to take an introductory sport or exercise psychology course and browse through some of the leading journals in the subdiscipline, such as the _Journal of Sport and Exercise Psychology_, the _Journal of Applied Sport Psychology_, and _The Sport Psychologist_. You might also want to talk to a professor about career opportunities in the subdiscipline of sport and exercise psychology. We all cannot be Olympic athletes, but we all can engage in meaningful physical activity to derive personal fulfillment and optimal health and well-being.

Study Questions

1. What is the focus of study in sport and exercise psychology? How is this subdiscipline similar to and different from motor behavior and the sociocultural study of physical activity?

2. Identify several questions that would be studied by sport and exercise psychologists based on the three main goals of the subdiscipline.

3. What was significant about Coleman Griffith's early work in sport psychology? Why did the subdiscipline not emerge again until the 1960s?

4. Identify the six research methods used in sport and exercise psychology and provide one example for how each method is used in the subdiscipline.

5. Does sport "build character"? Why or why not? Does exercise participation improve mental health? If so, how?

6. Explain why intrinsic motivation is a better source of motivation than extrinsic motivation. How can leaders in both exercise and sport contexts enhance intrinsic motivation in participants?

7. Explain the concept of optimal arousal zone and discuss how this differs across individuals and types of activities. How does arousal differ from stress?

8. Explain cohesion in groups and discuss how cohesion can facilitate sport performance as well as exercise adherence. What are some ways that cohesion can be developed and nurtured in groups?

9. Discuss several popular myths about the relationship between aggression and exercise/sport participation.

10. Identify some special concerns regarding physical activity participation for children. Similarly, describe some issues regarding physical activity for older adults.

11. Why is flow the goal of intervention strategies in physical activity? Describe how various intervention techniques may be used to enhance flow and peak experiences in physical activity.

10

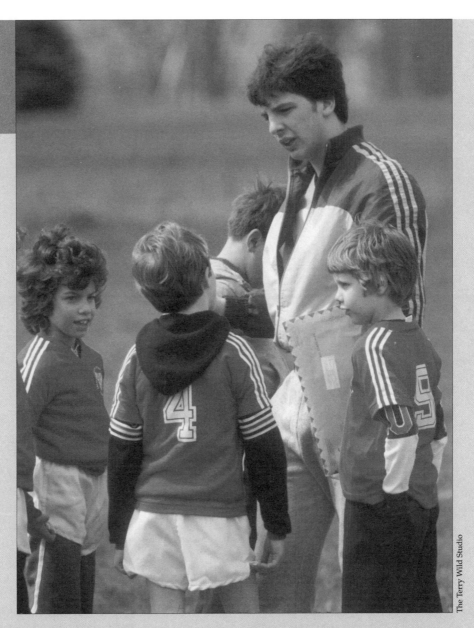

The Terry Wild Studio

Pedagogy of Physical Activity

Kim C. Graber and Thomas J. Templin

In this chapter . . .

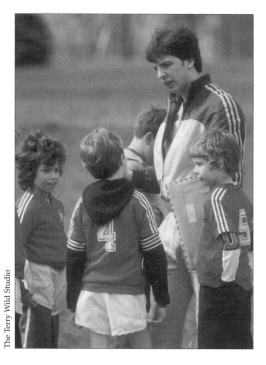

The Terry Wild Studio

Standing before the 24 young strangers assigned to your community soccer team, your heart begins to beat faster and you have a hard time catching your breath. While you have been looking forward to volunteering as a coach, you are now wondering if you have gotten in over your head. Your anxiety increases as you discover that the children you are talking to are less interested in your directions than they are in giggling and chatting with one another. You also realize that the practice facility is less than adequate, and the two soccer balls that have been provided will not be enough to keep all these youngsters occupied. As you strive to look calm and controlled, you wonder how much time you should spend talking and how much time the children should spend practicing. How can you gain the attention and respect of the players to make them want to listen and learn? Will your methods work?

Why Pedagogy of Physical Activity?

As a participant of physical activity, you probably were concerned primarily with improving your performance, playing well during competition, and enjoying the experience. You may have felt proud of your ability, hard work, and dedication in the case of an especially successful season or event. The truth of the matter is, if your performance improved, if you played well during competitive events, and if you enjoyed the experience, your instructor or coach probably was largely responsible. That is, he or she likely planned effective practice sessions, executed appropriate instruction, kept participants actively engaged in appropriate tasks, maintained a positive learning environment, and provided useful feedback.

Effective instructors understand their subject and know how to convey it appropriately. Expert instructors in river rafting, for example, know which techniques should be used to propel a raft when the river is smooth as opposed to when it is at its most dangerous. They understand when to expect a change in conditions of the river and how to maneuver from one type of water to another safely and effectively. They also know which techniques are most appropriate for novices and which are best for experts. They convey instructions in a manner that is understandable and provides the best practice opportunities for learners to accomplish new skills.

Pedagogy cuts across the entire physical activity field.

The subdiscipline of pedagogy of physical activity involves the scholarly study of teachers, coaches, and instructors of physical activity; the study of how learners acquire knowledge; and the study of curriculum. In the past two decades, pedagogical scholarship has become increasingly rigorous and progressively more lively. Pedagogy is now viewed as a viable and important topic of scholarly inquiry.

The pedagogy of physical activity also has the potential to inform the work of individuals who pursue careers in other subdisciplines described in this text. For example, if you are studying exercise physiology to become a fitness trainer or physical therapist, you will better understand how to provide appropriate instruction and feedback to your clients if you understand effective pedagogy. If you are interested in sport and exercise psychology and you understand the significance of how the learning environment is structured—and the role of the teacher or coach in establishing that environment—you will be better able to motivate your students (sometimes referred to as achievement goal theory).

As the scenario at the beginning of the chapter suggests, to teach others successfully in the development of physical activity requires a back-

ground in and knowledge about pedagogy of physical activity. Without a background in pedagogy, teachers and coaches tend to try to "wing it," which can sometimes work out fine in the short run, but which often leads to wasted time and effort—and stress for the coach or teacher. In the opening scenario, you, the volunteer coach, feel anxious and stressed because of unanswered questions. How will you get and keep the children's attention? How much time should you spend talking and how much time should players spend practicing? Will your methods work? A person with a background in pedagogy knows the answers to these questions. The knowledgeable coach knows that the best way to get and keep players' attention is to establish rules and procedures for good behavior, including teaching the players start and stop signals that will be noticed easily on the soccer field. The coach with a background in pedagogy knows that practicing a skill correctly and in gamelike situations is more important than listening to a 20-minute lecture on soccer techniques.

Pedagogy is often defined as "the art or science of teaching." For our purposes, we'll modify that definition a little and say that pedagogy focuses on *teaching behaviors* and *producing learning in students.* While the distinction between teaching and producing learning might not be immediately clear, what it comes down to is focusing on the student rather than the teacher. Instead of approaching each class with the question, What am I going to teach today? effective teachers instead ask themselves, What are my students going to learn today? This latter approach can lead to improved interaction between student and instructor and thus to a better education for students.

So, ideally, those who pursue pedagogy as a career choice are concerned with producing some type of learning in students (or clients). Whether you want to become a public school teacher, coach, aerobics instructor, golf teaching professional, fitness director, or rafting guide, you need to know the pedagogy of the pursuit. Sometimes this pedagogical knowledge is gained through an accredited agency or program, such as an education department at a university; other times the required knowledge might be acquired through working with a mentor, such as a personal fitness trainer or a specialist in river rafting or horseback riding. Ideally, though, all would-be coaches or physical activity instructors should supplement what they have learned about teaching their specific pursuit with further information from the knowledge base that concerns itself with the study of the theories and methods of teaching physical activity.

 CHAPTER OBJECTIVES

In this chapter we will focus on these key topics:

▌ What background knowledge you already have about pedagogy of physical activity

▌ What a physical activity pedagogue does

▌ The goals of pedagogy and two models for the study of teaching

▌ Historical breakthroughs in the acquisition of new knowledge and how the subdiscipline evolved

▌ Insights into how research on teaching is conducted

▌ What past and current research is telling us about the pedagogy of physical activity

Reflect on your own experience by answering the following questions:

1. Who stands out in your memory as the best teacher or coach you've ever had?

2. What qualities did this teacher or coach have that made him or her effective?

3. Who stands out in your memory as the worst teacher or coach you've ever had?

4. What weaknesses did this teacher or coach possess, or what qualities did he or she lack, that made him or her ineffective?

5. What do you think are the most important traits that a teacher or coach should possess?

What Background Knowledge Do I Already Have?

Research has demonstrated that undergraduate students who are interested in pedagogy often believe that they already know all there is to know about teaching and have little more to learn (Lanier & Little, 1986). This belief can be attributed to the many pedagogical *experiences* and observations of *professional practice* that you have already encountered while participating in physical activity or working as a coach, camp counselor, or supervisor in a recreation center. Consider that you have spent approximately 13,000 hours as a student. Add to these the hours passed in other learning environments, such as summer camps, recreational sport programs through school or the park district, or private instruction, and you'll find that you've accumulated many strong beliefs about teaching methods (Lortie, 1975; Schempp, 1989).

Experience accumulated before the start of formal instruction within a discipline is often referred to as **pretraining** and can significantly influence a student's orientation. For example, if you had excellent rapport with a coach who was particularly insightful and generous with his or her time, you may aspire to emulate those characteristics. On the other hand, you will probably try to avoid acquiring traits or behavior that you found unhelpful in your own experience.

Most students spend about 13,000 hours of their young lives in schools, where they are exposed to many types of teachers, coaches, and instructional methods. A student's accumulated experiences and impressions will influence his or her values and beliefs about teaching.

Despite the logic of emulating someone whose qualities you admire, there are drawbacks to relying *only* on past experience. Since teachers influence different students in different ways, you can't assume that your own positive experience with a particular instructor was shared by everyone. For instance, say you were a starter on your high school's basketball team. Because of your status, your physical education teacher allowed you to skip class on game days, singled you out to demonstrate new basketball skills to classmates, and gave you more opportunities than others to play basketball during class. Such positive personal experiences might lead you to believe that the pedagogy was sound. You may believe that athletes *should* be released from class prior to a game, that better players *should* demonstrate their skills for the benefit of their classmates, and that higher-skilled students *should* receive more opportunities for activity than lesser-skilled students. However, despite your personal experience, in reality all of these beliefs may be mistaken, as they are based on unsound, unfair, or unsupported teaching principles.

Although it is probably human nature to accept and imitate the behavior of people you respect and reject that of those you do not respect when forming your own pedagogy, it is best to analyze the available research about teaching and learning and base your behavior and values on this analysis. To some degree you will always refer to personal experience when making decisions about instruction and designing curriculum, but this experience should never be your only criterion. We will discuss this later in the chapter, in the section "Overview of Knowledge in Pedagogy of Physical Activity."

You may even have some background knowledge of pedagogy of physical activity from your own previous *scholarly study*. Perhaps you have already taken an introduction to education course in which you learned about classroom teaching methods. Many of these same methods are applied to physical activity settings. Or perhaps you have learned some drills and practice techniques from Web sites or "how-to" books to help you perform better in the physical activities you most enjoy. These practice techniques were likely developed by expert teachers and coaches, so you may have gained a sense of sound pedagogical principles.

All instructors will be influenced by past experiences and beliefs they acquired during pretraining, but the best instructors base their programs and teaching methods on sound pedagogical precepts.

This chapter will introduce you to the study of pedagogy of physical activity, often referred to as sport pedagogy. Because most of the research on pedagogy of physical activity has focused on teaching in public schools, much of this chapter will focus on that research. However, it is important to realize that many of the findings can be transferred to other instructional arenas such as coaching, working as a wilderness guide, teaching aerobics, or giving golf lessons. Thus, when we refer to teachers in this chapter, we usually mean the individuals responsible for client or student learning in any of the many instructional settings.

Figure 10.1 shows how pedagogy of physical activity fits into the scholarly study of physical activity. Similar to the subdiscipline of psychology of sport and exercise (chapter 9), the subdiscipline of pedagogy influences the three dimensions of the field introduced early in the text. First, as a result of our past experiences in physical activity, we in the subdiscipline have come to enjoy movement and wish to help duplicate those desirable experiences for others. Second, the scholarly study of pedagogy allows the generation of new knowledge (such as when particular instruction is most effective for producing learning in students). And third, through practicing the profession, instructors are able to impart research-based knowledge to students to help them learn and to create enjoyable experiences in physical activity.

As you read this chapter, think of your own educational experiences thus far, asking yourself whether you received effective instruction and why or why not. Consider how you might incorporate some of the findings from research into your own pedagogy, particularly when these findings contradict your own experiences as a student.

What Does a Physical Activity Pedagogue Do?

Similar to the other subdisciplines described in this book, experts in pedagogy have many career options. Generally, most elect to obtain certification and become teachers and coaches in public schools. Based on state certification requirements, individuals elect a grade level in which

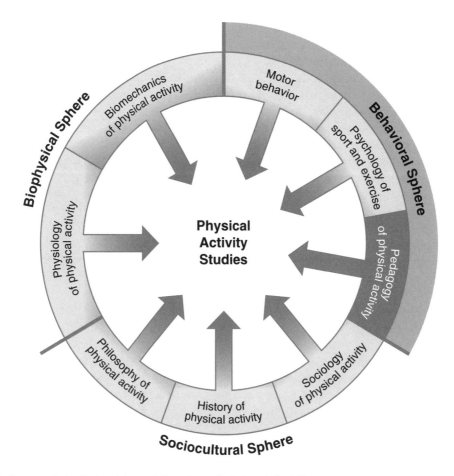

Figure 10.1   Pedagogy of physical activity and the other scholarly subdisciplines.

they intend to teach and enroll for courses that specifically address how to instruct children of that particular age. While many individuals choose to work at the elementary level because they enjoy interacting with young children and appreciate the enjoyment that youngsters experience while engaged in physical activity, others decide to work in middle or high schools because they also wish to coach. As a means of supplementing their salary in the summer months, many teachers also work as camp counselors, swim instructors, and recreation leaders.

Some individuals who obtain certification decide that they are better suited to teach in corporate fitness centers or community recreation centers than in the public schools. Others may elect to become specialists, such as wilderness experts or golf professionals. Regardless of the area that they select, most individuals with a background in teaching acknowledge the importance of the pedagogical knowledge they acquired during

teacher education, and sometimes maintain roots in the profession by attending professional conferences for teachers or maintaining membership in educational organizations.

Most professors of pedagogy have been employed at one point or another as teachers in public schools. Many elect to work at the university or college level because they want to improve teacher education and enjoy preparing teachers. An increasing number of professors also have a desire to engage in research. These individuals design studies intended to help us better understand the work of teaching and how to promote effective instruction that leads to student learning. In addition to preparing future teachers and conducting research, professors also are responsible for presenting papers at professional conferences; collaborating with teachers in the public schools; remaining informed about state certification requirements; and serving on departmental, college, and university committees.

Goals of Pedagogy of Physical Activity

The subdiscipline of pedagogy derives knowledge and principles from many other disciplines. For example, when conducting studies and writing research reports, educational researchers might refer to sociology, psychology, motor learning, exercise physiology, anthropology, or history. The specific study of teaching physical activity, however, draws primarily from knowledge derived from research on classroom teaching and teachers. Although this research has several goals, a primary aim is to discover or create effective teaching practices and uncover knowledge related to student learning.

Researchers in pedagogy of physical activity usually focus on one of two areas: teaching or teacher education. Research on teaching pertains to the teaching and learning process that occurs in educational settings, such as public and private schools, aerobics classes, sport clinics, and so on. A typical study might try to determine if students learn better through one method of instruction than another. Another study might look at how many times an instructor provides feedback to individual students during class and whether that feedback is specific or general.

Research on teacher education encompasses such things as the study of teacher educators (professors) and teacher certification programs. For instance, a researcher might look at which elements of an undergraduate teacher education program most influence the teaching beliefs and behaviors of the program's graduates. Although knowledge about how teachers learn to teach can be of great value in education, here our focus will be on teaching itself rather than teacher education. Accordingly, throughout this chapter we'll explore the body of knowledge derived from the research on teaching literature.

Research on teaching is concerned with the scientific study of the processes of teaching and learning, and is deeply rooted in what happens in general education. Current methods of research on teaching are based on one of two conceptual frameworks: the *Four Principal Variables* framework and the *Four Types of Knowledge* framework.

Four Principal Variables

The Four Principal Variables conceptual framework uses a model developed by Dunkin and Biddle in 1974. This model suggests that the teaching/learning process is a complex interaction between four principal variables (see figure 10.2).

The first variable, presage, consists of instructor characteristics that may have an effect on the pedagogical process. The study of presage variables focuses on examining *teacher formative experiences*, which are those experiences a future instructor has prior to entering a formal certification program such as teacher education. Such studies may examine ethnicity, gender, and social class to try to determine what types of individuals elect teaching or coaching as a career. Presage variable studies may also include examining *teacher training experiences*, for example, by comparing the effects of fifth-year teacher certification programs to those of traditional four-year programs. Finally, presage variable studies also involve the study of *teacher properties*. Here, researchers attempt to assess the personality characteristics of a teacher, such as enthusiasm, to learn the effect of such characteristics on the teaching process.

The second principal variable, context, concerns the conditions of the instructional environment, some of which the instructor can control, but much of which cannot be altered. Because the conditions in which individuals teach and learn certainly affect achievement, these variables are important to consider. Context variables may profile *student formative experiences*, such as student background characteristics. For instance, students coming from single-parent or impoverished families may be studied to try to determine the influence of these backgrounds on the classroom environment. Some researchers focus on *student properties* by examining standardized achievement test results. Others study *school and community factors,* comparing, for instance, rural schools with urban schools or focusing on such issues as busing. Finally, *classroom contexts* may be investigated for many different variables, such as class size, available equipment, or access to computer technology or instructional films.

The third principal variable, process, involves the events and activities in the instructional environment and all that is done by instructors and

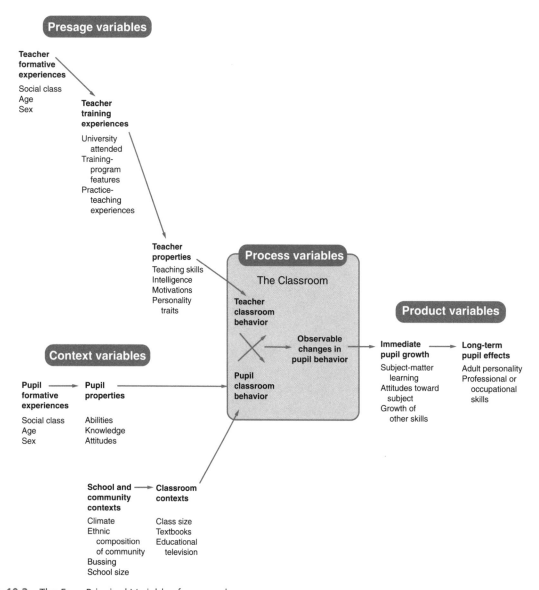

Figure 10.2 The Four Principal Variables framework.

Reprinted, by permission, from M.J. Dunkin and B.J. Biddle, 1974, *The study of teaching* (New York: Holt, Rinehart and Winston), 38.

students. One dimension, *teacher classroom behavior*, focuses on behaviors such as how instructors discipline students, how equipment is organized, when class instruction commences, and how students are organized. In another dimension, *student classroom behavior*, researchers examine students to study such variables as whether students are responding to instructions as intended by the instructor, if students appear to be listening, or how students interact with their peers.

The fourth category in the model, **product variables**, concerns instructional outcome—that is, student achievement or performance as it relates to either learning the subject matter or the stu-

dents' attitudes toward the subject. *Immediate student growth* can be measured through sport skills tests, paper and pencil exams, standardized achievement tests, or interviews with students. Such instruments allow investigators to determine whether students have acquired knowledge or what their feelings are toward the subject. *Long-term student effects* refers to whether adults retain what they learned as students and how that learning has influenced their adult lives and professional careers.

The Dunkin and Biddle model illustrates that pedagogy is a complex process influenced by many variables interacting simultaneously. The model also shows that individual variables cannot be interpreted and understood in isolation, with no regard to other variables. A new method of coaching that appears successful in a rural community with 20 homogeneous students, for example, may not be successful in a multicultural urban setting.

Four Types of Knowledge

Twelve years after the Dunkin and Biddle model was introduced, another framework for understanding and delineating pedagogical research was developed, in part, by Shulman (1986) (see figure 10.3). He believed that instructors bring different types of knowledge to the learning environment, which significantly influences the teaching and learning process. It appears that for the foreseeable future, researchers will continue to contemplate and investigate the different types of knowledge that instructors possess. Researchers interested in studying knowledge might look, for example, at how coaches modify a volleyball drill based on the age group being coached. Or they might be interested in comparing the instructional behaviors of an experienced, knowledgeable golf professional to those of a novice teacher.

Categories of the four basic types of knowledge are as follows:

1. *Curriculum knowledge* concerns what instructors know about the development and design of educational programs. For instance, a public school teacher with curriculum knowledge might advocate one curriculum for younger elementary school students and a different curriculum for older elementary school students.

2. *Content knowledge* refers to what an instructor knows and understands about the subject matter he or she is teaching. Instructors may acquire content knowledge about an activity such as aerobics through participation in a fitness clinic, during professional activities courses at a university, or as a result of reading a recent textbook.

3. *General pedagogical knowledge* refers to knowledge about the pedagogical process. For example, a fitness clinic instructor with general pedagogical knowledge understands that feedback should be specific rather than general and that clients can't learn without adequate opportunity to engage in appropriate practice.

4. *Pedagogical content knowledge* is a combination of general pedagogical knowledge and content knowledge. Possessing this form of knowledge allows instructors to make their subject matter more comprehensible for students. It includes "overarching conceptions of what it means to teach a particular subject, knowledge of curricular materials and curriculum in a particular field, knowledge of students' understanding and potential misunderstanding of a subject area,

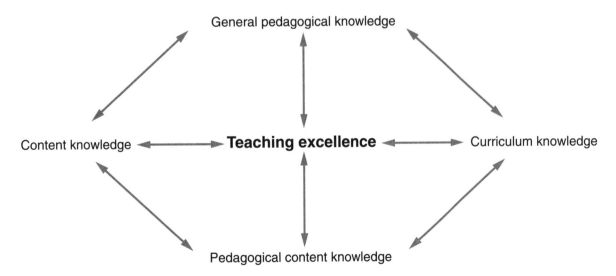

Figure 10.3   The Four Types of Knowledge framework.

and knowledge of instructional strategies and representations for teaching particular topics" (Grossman, 1989, p. 25).

What the Two Models Have In Common

A common thread that runs through both models is the search for attributes leading to effective instruction. This search is guided by a variety of questions, has been refined over time, and is constantly expanding in ways that lead researchers and instructors to reexamine their previous understandings of what constitutes effective ways to teach. Although not all of the research that you will be introduced to in this chapter can be grouped into these two frameworks, they do provide a good starting point for understanding the goals of most pedagogical investigations, as outlined in the following list.

Goals of Pedagogy

1. To understand how the four principal variables (presage, context, process, and product) interact with and influence the teaching and learning processes

2. To understand how instructional knowledge is developed, conveyed, and understood by learners

3. To discover how students learn best

4. To uncover those teaching behaviors that foster and encourage student learning

5. To understand how the workplace affects what teachers and students are able to accomplish

History of Pedagogy of Physical Activity

Until the 1960s most research in teaching physical activity was rudimentary and did not take advantage of the powerful ideas about teaching already discovered in classrooms (as opposed to gymnasiums). By the 1970s physical education programs in universities began to "splinter" into many subdisciplines, and those professors who sought to study teaching in physical education began to ask much more sophisticated research questions and use modern techniques to analyze their data. Instructors and researchers in physical education began to illuminate the teaching and learning process in ways that enabled the development of valuable new approaches to the study of teaching.

As the body of research has expanded and become more refined, the study of pedagogy has earned and been given greater respect. Up until this point in history, research on the pedagogy of physical activity has concentrated primarily on the school physical education setting, although much of the research impacts the work of any teacher of physical activity—from aerobics instructors to tennis professionals to outdoor adventure guides. Initially spurred by such work as Dunkin and Biddle's classic text, *The Study of Teaching* (1974) and Lawrence Locke's classic review of sport pedagogy, "New Hope For a Dismal Science" (1977), a cadre of researchers who study physical activity has engaged in the enthusiastic pursuit of new knowledge (Mitchell, 1992). In addition, these investigators have begun to make better use of ideas and methods from classroom research, thus allowing researchers to make valuable connections between what happens in the classroom and what transpires in physical activity settings.

Since the early 1970s the body of knowledge in pedagogy has progressed through a series of developmental stages, resulting in increasingly sophisticated research that is more applicable to physical activity.

While the most influential research on teaching effectiveness has emerged since the late 1970s and has focused primarily on physical education teachers in the public schools, it is worthwhile to understand the earlier stages that brought us to where we are today. Basically, pedagogical research has gone through four significant developmental stages: (1) the Search for Teacher Characteristics, (2) the Search for the Perfect Method, (3) Descriptive Analytic and Process–Product

In Profile

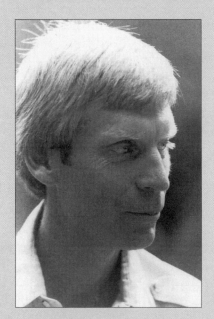

Daryl Siedentop

As a professor at The Ohio State University, Daryl Siedentop has significantly influenced the development of sport pedagogy and school physical education from the early 1970s to the present. Siedentop's contributions display a cycle of scholarship over nearly three decades from the development of a play education curriculum model, to experimental supervision research aimed at changing teaching behavior in physical education, to descriptive-analytic research on teaching through the development of the Academic Learning Time-Physical Education (ALT-PE) concept and research instrument, to application of Doyle's ecological model to physical education, to the evolution of the play education theory into a sport education curriculum model that is used worldwide.

Siedentop is the author *Physical Education: Introductory Analysis*, an early book in which he set forth and developed the "play education" curriculum theory from which his sport education model, and his book *Sport Education: Quality PE through Positive Sport Experiences* eventually emerged. He received the International Samaranch Award for excellence in sport pedagogy for his text, *Developing Teaching Skills in Physical Education*. Through all his contributions, Siedentop has not only influenced generations of university physical education teacher educators through doctoral education, but importantly, generations of preservice and inservice teachers. With the direct purpose of improving teaching and curricula in school physical education, Siedentop has been an exemplary teacher of teachers. Along with a mere handful of other scholars, Siedentop is recognized as one of the leading sport pedagogues in the world.

Research, and (4) Specialized and Diversified Research.

Stage I—Search for Teacher Characteristics

This first stage includes the majority of scholarship that occurred prior to the 1960s (Graham & Heimerer, 1981), when investigators were primarily concerned with understanding the personal characteristics of teachers, students, and administrators, all who appeared to influence learning. Studies focused on presage variables, as described earlier in the Dunkin and Biddle (1974) model. Teacher variables such as gender, age, years of experience, appearance, and interpersonal skills were surveyed. In this early stage, the emphasis was on gathering, rather than implementing, information.

Stage II—Search for the Perfect Method

Research did little to inform the work of practitioners until the early 1980s. At this time a second stage emerged as research interest shifted and investigators became interested in comparing different methods of instruction to determine which methods were more effective (Graham & Heimerer, 1981). For example, Templin and Kollen (1981) compared two methods of teaching swimming to students at two high schools. Such studies were commonly referred to as "method A versus method B" and were often criticized for not controlling important variables. Results from this research were suspect due to incomplete descriptions of the methods employed and the design of the instructional setting.

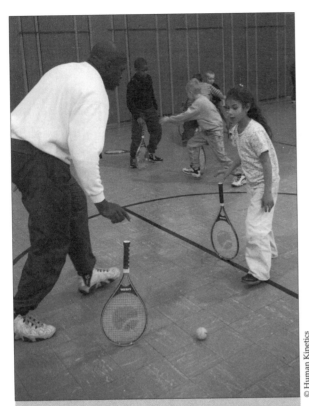

© Human Kinetics

While it may be true that the most effective teachers are well liked by their students, student achievement, not popularity, is the main goal of such instructors.

Stage III—Descriptive Analytic and Process–Product Research

Based on studies conducted in the classroom (Brophy & Good, 1986; Rosenshine & Furst, 1973) and critical assessment of research conducted in physical education (Nixon & Locke, 1973), research was rapidly advancing toward a third stage, *descriptive analytic research*. Bill Anderson's work in the late 1970s provided the initial thrust in pedagogical research when he described the behaviors of teachers and students in the classic monograph *What's Going on in Gym* (Anderson & Barrette, 1978). Studies that followed were often called *process–product research* or "teacher effectiveness research," in which researchers tried to relate teacher behaviors (process) to student achievement (product).

Although the results from early research were inconsistent (Lee, 1996), several interesting insights did emerge from these studies. For example, researchers called attention to such factors as minimal instruction time and levels of teacher competence (Lee, 1996). As an outgrowth of this research, investigators began to focus on areas such as **academic learning time**, "a unit of time in which a student is engaged in relevant physical education content in such a way that he or she has an appropriate chance to be successful" (Siedentop, 1991, p. 25).

Stage IV—Specialized and Diversified Research

Process–product research continues today, but investigators have progressed into a fourth stage, in which research interests are highly specialized and diverse. Some researchers use a modified process–product format as they design research on such topics as the study of academic learning time. Other investigators focus on instructor knowledge, student thought processes, or curriculum development. These researchers might study how knowledge is constructed and implemented or focus on what a student thinks while learning a motor skill. Still other researchers do sociological analyses of teachers and schools to learn, for example, the life history of teachers; or they study such issues as why individuals elect to become teachers, how students influence an instructor's behavior, and why the influence of pretraining may have greater impact on teacher behavior than an entire program of teacher education course work. Finally, some investigators are interested in studying social issues such as teaching responsibility to students, teacher sexual orientation, or teaching inner-city students.

Current methods of investigation allow researchers to study the learning environment in ways that were not possible several years ago.

As pedagogical researchers continue to address new questions, the body of knowledge expands, demanding the development of new methods of investigation and new theoretical frameworks for interpreting the results. If you'd like a more detailed account of the history of pedagogy of physical activity or research on teaching, refer to the work of Bain (1997), Graber (in press), and Lee (1996).

Historical Time Line

1885	The Association for the Advancement of Physical Education (AAPE) is founded.
1887	The *American Physical Education Review* becomes the first periodical of the AAPE.
1899	The first national convention of the AAPE in Boston results in recommendations for the conduct of physical training in schools.
1901	The Committee on Teacher Training offers guidelines for admission to and requirements within physical education training in colleges and universities.
1910	Debates rage at the national convention of the AAPE about the role of teaching hygiene at the expense of physical education.
1916	The Committee of Promoting Physical Education in the Public Schools is established by the AAPE.
1916	The Women's Athletics Committee is founded.
1927	A curriculum research section is initiated in the AAPE.
1930	The AAPE ceases publication of the *Review* and starts two new journals: the *Journal of Health and Physical Education* and *Research Quarterly*.
1930	Ruth Savage writes on the characteristics of "good" teaching in the first issue of *Research Quarterly*.
1937	The AAPE becomes the American Association of Health and Physical Education and affiliates with the National Education Association. One year later, the organization is renamed the American Association for Health, Physical Education, and Recreation.
1940–1945	Preparedness for war becomes a central thrust of physical education.
1956	Youth fitness becomes a national concern; the President's Council on Youth Fitness is created; national fitness testing is initiated.
1960–1985	Descriptive analytic research on teaching emerges, and observational systems for studying teaching are developed. Flanders Interaction Analysis System paves the way for descriptive analytic research, which is first published by Anderson and Barrette in 1978.
1970	Research on teaching and teacher education in sports emerges as a scholarly subdiscipline known as sport pedagogy.
1972	Title IX of the Educational Amendments Act becomes law.
1974	Dunkin and Biddle develop their model for the study of teaching.
1974	*Research Quarterly* establishes Curriculum and Instruction as a subsection.
1976–1985	The study of academic learning time becomes a major focus of research.
1981	The first issue of the *Journal of Teaching in Physical Education* is published.
1983	The first sport pedagogy meeting is held at Purdue University, sponsored by the Big Ten Committee on Institutional Cooperation.
1986	The first meeting of the International Association for Physical Education convenes in Heidelberg, Germany.
1986	A special interest group on research on learning and instruction in physical education is established within the American Educational Research Association.

| 1987 | *Strategies* is published by the American Alliance of Health, Physical Education, Recreation and Dance |
| 1999 | A special conference focusing on exemplary teacher education is sponsored by the National Association for Sport and Physical Education |

Other Significant Events

Since the late 1970s several significant events have influenced the pedagogy of physical activity. First, doctoral programs have produced graduates who, while contributing to the growing body of literature, have become teacher educators who have influenced the next generation of teachers (Mitchell, 1992). Second, major professional associations have formed special interest groups for those interested in studying the pedagogy of physical activity. For example, the American Alliance of Health, Physical Education, Recreation and Dance (AAHPERD) formed the Curriculum and Instruction Academy. Third, since its first publication in 1981, the *Journal of Teaching in Physical Education* has provided scholars with a forum to share their work with others. Published stud-

Sport Pedagogy Journals

- International Journal of Physical Education
- Journal of Physical Education, Recreation, and Dance
- Journal of Teaching in Physical Education
- Physical Educator
- Quest
- Sport Education and Society
- Strategies

Selected Education Journals That Publish Sport Pedagogy Research

- Action in Teacher Education
- American Educational Research Journal
- College Student Journal
- Educational Technology
- Elementary School Journal
- High School Journal
- Journal of Educational Research
- Journal of Research and Development in Education
- Teaching and Teacher Education
- Journal of Teacher Education

National and International Associations for Sport Pedagogy

- American Alliance for Health, Physical Education, Recreation and Dance (AAHPERD)
  - National Association for Sport and Physical Education (NASPE)
    - Curriculum and Instruction Academy (C & I is a division of NASPE)
- American Educational Reseach Association (AERA)
  - Special Interest Group: Research on Learning and Instruction in Physical Education (SIG is a division of AERA)
- National Association for Physical Education in Higher Education (NAPEHE)
- Association Internationale des Ecoles Superieures d'Education Physique (AIESEP)
- United States Physical Education Association (USPE)

ies in that journal have significantly influenced how teacher educators instruct future teachers and how teachers view their work.

Where Are We Now?

At the time of this writing, we are at a difficult point in the history of our public schools. School funding is rapidly diminishing, physical education programs are being eliminated, and curricular areas such as science and math are emphasized at the expense of other subjects. The elimination of physical education from schools where teachers who roll out the ball and provide no instruction is justified. Dismantling such programs might help increase the recognition and credibility of the many strong teachers and exemplary programs existing today. Such high-quality programs will be valued as an integral part of the school and will not be in the same jeopardy as the weaker programs. These exemplary teachers and programs will lead us well into the new century.

In the same light, fitness clubs and community recreational programs with strong reputations are filled with children and adults who are concerned about physical fitness and pursuing sport. A 1990 federal report entitled "Healthy People 2000" emphasized the need for lifetime physical activity; such a goal depends partially on physical activity instructors to help redefine the manner in which physical activity is conducted and sport is perceived. The pedagogy subdiscipline should continue to grow and prosper, particularly as instructors who have "retired on the job" (Siedentop, 1991) leave the ranks and are replaced by energetic newcomers who have better access to the current body of knowledge.

Quality physical activity programs in schools, recreation centers, parks, country clubs, and athletic settings have the potential to set the pace for the next century.

Research Methods in Pedagogy of Physical Activity

While researchers in pedagogy of physical activity use many techniques for collecting data, most of them use one of two general types, representing different **paradigms** (or research models). One of these is the **quantitative paradigm** (also called the positivistic paradigm) in which researchers use surveys, questionnaires, or direct observation instruments (Schempp & Choi, 1994) to come up with numbers or statistics to support their findings (although they sometimes supplement their data with interviews and observations). An example would be a study in which investigators attempt to determine how much time a week students spend being physically active during physical education class.

The second kind of research falls under an interpretive or **qualitative paradigm**. Researchers who employ this paradigm are generally less interested in the statistical analysis of data than they are with understanding events from participants' points of view. These researchers often observe the research setting, conduct interviews with research participants, and analyze documents associated with the study. An example of this type of research would be investigators asking students questions to try to determine their motivations for participating in mountain biking, football, or taekwondo.

One of the most significant differences between the two methodological frameworks resides within the process of "seeking truth." The quantitative (or positivistic) paradigm involves defining research questions in advance, forming hypotheses about anticipated results, developing a precise research design, and designing time lines and data collection techniques to which the researcher must closely adhere. It is assumed that such controlled designs will answer research questions as precisely as possible. Further, this paradigm requires the investigator to be objective and remain neutral.

In contrast, the qualitative (or interpretive) paradigm allows for the development of initial research questions that are open to change or modification as the study progresses and the researcher becomes more familiar with his or her central topic. Although data collection techniques are frequently developed in advance, they may remain open to development as the study unfolds and the investigator becomes increasingly sensitive to what phenomena are most relevant to the research questions. This framework acknowledges that there is no absolute truth but subscribes to an orientation that truth is perceived differently by different individuals and that what transpires in one environment is not necessarily indicative of what might occur in another environment.

If you were to design a research study, what research question would you most like to answer? How might you go about answering the question?

Pedagogical researchers have engaged in considerable debate about which paradigm for data collection is the best or the most appropriate. Some positivistic researchers believe that quantitative methods provide the most reliable data because results can often be generalized to other research settings. For example, if a research study indicates that students learn best if they are provided with clear and explicit teacher feedback, after employing the appropriate statistical analyses, analysts could determine with a fair degree of certainty that the same results would occur in other instructional settings. In contrast, many interpretive researchers believe that quantitative methods are inappropriate for studying human beings because statistics don't allow for individual viewpoints, beliefs, and voices to be heard. These investigators are less concerned with whether the results of their studies are generalizable and more concerned that the results reflect the many facets of the research setting and the many different voices of the participants. Interpretive investigators care as much about discovering which method of instruction appears to hold the most promise as they do about the feelings of participants toward that method of instruction. Discovering why individuals are more receptive to a particular method might help explain why one method is more effective than others.

Both paradigms have provided researchers with many techniques for collecting data in physical activity settings. Positivistic (quantitative) researchers have observed and coded student behaviors to determine how long students are actively engaged in appropriate learning tasks versus how much time they spend listening to instructions, being placed on teams, and being organized into drills. Such researchers have also observed and coded instructor behaviors to ascertain how their time is spent, which clients receive most of their attention, how much feedback they provide, and whether or not they exhibit equitable behaviors. They have also sought to determine if one instructional method may produce greater student learning than another.

To examine student thought processes, interpretive (qualitative) researchers ask learners to recall what they were thinking about while performing a motor skill. Some interpretive investigators have instructors recall significant pedagogical events by asking them to write statements that address a specific question, or they may show these instructors a photograph and ask them to describe what the picture brings to mind. Others talk to learners informally, either one on one, in group interviews, or both, to discover their feelings about their teachers, coaches, or the activities they are being asked to perform. Occasionally, interpretive researchers might even participate in the research setting themselves.

Even while leaning toward one paradigm, many researchers employ a combination of the quantitative and qualitative methods during the course of their data collection.

Regardless of which research method they prefer, more and more investigators agree on at least one thing: that "a body of knowledge is only as good as the methods used to build it" (Schempp & Choi, 1994, p. 41). Thus, researchers realize the importance of determining the exact question they are trying to answer *before* deciding on the most appropriate means of collecting data. In some cases the positivistic paradigm will be appropriate, and other times the interpretive paradigm will hold the most promise of yielding the most useful data.

If you are interested in learning more about the different research techniques that fall under the two paradigms, read the work of Schempp and Choi (1994) and Silverman (1996).

Overview of Knowledge in Pedagogy of Physical Activity

In this section you will get a glimpse of the broad wealth of knowledge thus far acquired about teaching in physical activity settings. You will become acquainted with the types of research questions being addressed and learn new ways to view teaching effectiveness. Our primary goal here is twofold: to offer insight on (1) what instructors need to know about effective pedagogy and (2) what instructors need to know about the workplace environment. As we discuss these issues, we will ask you to stop reading now and then to consider your own educational experiences and compare them to what has been learned through evolving research. Further, your general understanding of pedagogy will be improved through a broad discussion of the research done in physical activity settings and a presentation of noteworthy studies done so far. Whether you aspire to teach physical education in a school, be a personal trainer at a fitness club, coach youth sports, teach swimming, or do any number of possible careers in teaching and coaching, you can learn much from pedagogical research—it applies to you.

What Instructors Need to Know About Effective Pedagogy

Although research has the potential to inform teachers how to teach most effectively, the majority of teachers do not subscribe to research journals—nor do they attend the same professional conferences as researchers. Instead, in the majority of cases, the knowledge informing teaching practice is derived primarily through a teacher's past experiences as a student in the public schools and other physical activity settings, through certification programs, informal discussions with other instructors, and in-service workshops and conferences focusing on the practitioner rather than the researcher.

In addition to what they learn from experiences outside actual instructing time, teachers also acquire much of their pedagogical expertise in the form of **professional practice knowledge** (sometimes referred to as craft knowledge by researchers), which is simply the knowledge accumulated through formal study and on the job. Over hours, weeks, and years of instructional experience, teachers learn (often the hard way!) which techniques work well with students and which do not. Instructors and coaches often refer to their professional practice knowledge when explaining their instructional decisions to others.

From the outset, beginning instructors will be influenced by their own instructional experiences and acquire new techniques grounded in professional practice knowledge. But, as we warned early in the chapter, as valuable as personal experience can be, it is a serious mistake for teachers or coaches to look to personal experience as their only guideline to how to teach or coach. Enough scholarly research has now been done

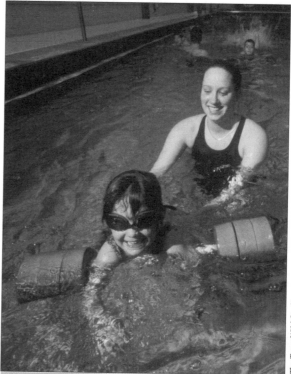

Among many other avenues of gaining knowledge about teaching, instructors learn by comparing their own techniques to those of their colleagues.

The Terry Wild Studio

that *any* teacher, no matter how experienced, can learn from research.

Although the available research sometimes seems inaccessible to instructors—because it can be difficult to understand or does not apply directly to their situations—there's no question that scholarly study has significantly influenced the way physical activity is instructed. More teachers than ever are concerned with such issues as managing time, reducing off-task student behaviors, and promoting quick lesson transitions. Instructors now have a vocabulary for talking about pedagogy that was not present until late in the 20th century. This all indicates that teachers are gradually becoming aware of the research on effective teaching and making attempts to incorporate the results into their own practice.

Although professional practice knowledge is a powerful source of information, such knowledge is not a substitute for thoughtful consideration of the available research literature on effective teaching.

Does More Experience Mean More Effectiveness?

Thinking back on your educational experiences thus far, make a list of your past teachers and coaches and assign each of them a corresponding letter (A, B, C, etc.) as an identifier, not as a grade. Then place the teacher's or coach's letter in the appropriate place on each of the two continuums below. (If you don't know how experienced an instructor was, take your best guess.)

Teacher/coach experience

| No experience | 1 year of experience | 4–10 years of experience | 10+ years of experience |

Teacher/coach effectiveness

| Very ineffective | Average effectiveness | Very effective |

After you've plotted each teacher and coach on the continuums, observe how, in your experience, teacher/coach effectiveness does or does not seem to have been influenced by experience.

Ten Important Factors to Consider in Effective Pedagogy

- Appropriate Practice, p. 336
- Active Learning Time, p. 337
- Class Management and Discipline, p. 338
- Accountability, p. 339
- Specific Feedback, p. 340
- Knowledge of Curriculum, p. 340
- Hidden Curriculum, p. 342
- Equity, p. 342
- Addressing Individual Student Needs, p. 343
- Instructor Expectations, p. 344

The next section of this chapter will describe ten important factors of which instructors should be aware when teaching physical activity. Whether you are teaching baseball skills in physical education class, coaching soccer in a youth sport league, teaching the V step in dance aerobics, or correcting someone's golf swing, each of these factors is important to determining the success that your students may achieve.

Appropriate Practice

Your experiences in physical activity settings were probably very similar to those that we all experienced as children. If such is the case, your teachers probably had you play dodgeball, kickball, "steal the bacon," and other such games. Upon entering secondary school, you may have received a few days of instruction before spending most physical education class periods playing softball, basketball, football, volleyball, soccer, and the like. If you are a person now interested in pursuing a career in the physical activity field, you probably had above average skills in these games and sports—you might have enjoyed eliminating other students in dodgeball or scoring the winning goal in soccer. Such memories probably remain satisfying for you and likely influenced your interest in a career in physical activity.

Unfortunately, your positive experience in physical education class was not shared by all of your classmates. For those students who were less skilled—the ones you were quickly eliminating from games such as dodgeball—physical education class was, at best, supervised recess and, at worst, an opportunity for embarrassment. For the majority of these students, there was no instruction available and thus small chance of improving their skills. Think about it: Did you acquire your athletic expertise by participating in physical education class? Or did you acquire skill through extracurricular activities organized by coaches (or parents) who were determined to help you improve your level of playing ability?

Despite the best intentions of instructors (some of whom cite time and space constraints as primary restrictions to aiding student learning), it is sometimes difficult for any of us to defend physical education class as an opportunity to improve skill level. For example, if a student spends one or two days practicing a volleyball bump pass before being expected to perform the pass correctly during a game, how much chance

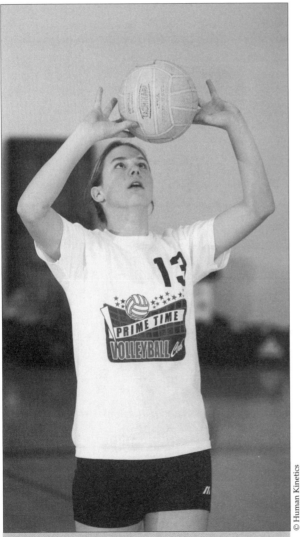

What would be the most appropriate way to practice setting a volleyball?

is there for the student to succeed? Consider that serious volleyball players spend hundreds of hours developing their skills. As another example, think back to when you played volleyball in physical education class. When practicing the volleyball set, were you ever asked to set the ball against a wall? If so, you were practicing a skill with minimal value, as the trajectory of the ball as it rebounds from a wall is quite different from that experienced during game play. Despite the good intentions of your teacher, you were not performing a well-designed drill.

As was pointed out in chapter 3, for students to succeed at any skill, they must be exposed to *appropriate practice*. When designing activities, instructors need to consider whether drills simulate actual game situations. For example, the most appropriate method of practicing a volleyball set is to practice setting the ball to a target area from a position in which the volleyball is bump-passed to the setter, not tossed. This drill closely resembles a gamelike situation.

For practice to be appropriate, students must practice the skill correctly. In one study (Silverman, 1990), middle school students were instructed over a seven-day time span on both the volleyball serve and the forearm bump pass. The results indicated that for both skills, "appropriate practice trials were positively related to achievement and inappropriate trials negatively related to achievement" (p. 305). In other words, students only learned during appropriate practice.

Active Learning Time

Do you recall the many times as a student you were asked to wait in line for a turn? If you're like many students, you sometimes may have had to wait over half the class for an opportunity, say, to bounce once or twice on a trampoline. Or maybe you played volleyball with 11 others on your side of the net, waiting minutes at a time for a chance to touch the ball. If this sounds familiar, you're not alone in your experience. For various reasons, thousands of students each year receive inadequate opportunities to practice and learn new skills.

Based on research conducted in the classroom (Brophy & Good, 1986), time on task has been clearly linked to student achievement. "Time on task," also called **engaged time**, is defined as the time students spend actually doing physical activity or sport. Engaged time in physical activity settings is traditionally very low, the research indicating that students in physical education classes only spend approximately 30% of class time engaged in physical activity (Anderson & Barrette, 1978; Metzler, 1979, 1989). The rest of the time they spend waiting (33%), in management and transition activities (22%), and receiving information (25% or less). Compounding the problem of low engaged time is the limited actual time in which students are *appropriately* engaged (performing correctly with frequent success). Such time is often called academic learning time or **functional learning time**. Unfortunately, academic learning time typically consumes only 10 to 20% of an entire class period (Siedentop, 1991).

Often, the problem of inadequate learning time is caused by limited resources or facilities. For instance, if a tennis professional at a park district or country club has twelve clients in class and has access to only six rackets and one court, obviously, all of the clients will not receive adequate

learning time. As instructors gain experience, they learn how to make the best of what they have to work with—for example, our tennis professional might have four of his twelve clients play doubles, two serve as referees, two act as line judges, and the remaining four perform drills in the space bordering the court. Of course, many activities require no specific court or equipment and relatively little space; these activities optimize academic learning time. For example, clients in aerobics classes can be engaged for up to nearly 87% of instruction time (Claxton & Lacy, 1991).

Class Management and Discipline

Probably the most common concern among new instructors is class management and discipline. *Class management* involves organizing students in such a way that learning is most likely to occur, whereas *discipline* involves teaching rules, enforcing them when they are broken, and rewarding exceptional behavior. Regardless of their experience level, instructors can never prepare for all the situations they might encounter in their edu-

Think back to your days in physical education class and recall a class in which only a small percentage of your time was spent engaging in physical activity. What might have accounted for your low percentage of active learning time? Lack of equipment? Poor class management? Listening to the instructor talk? Waiting in line?

Do you recall any classes in which you were engaged in active learning for a high percentage of class time? What did this instructor do differently in order to increase your active learning time?

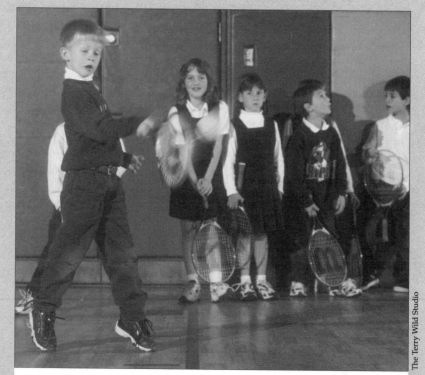

Students do not learn while waiting in line.

The Terry Wild Studio

cational setting. How do you handle a student who refuses to take a time-out? How do you deal with an aggressive parent who insists that his son pitch for his Little League team?

The best that instructors can do is to learn to take proactive measures that tend to decrease potential difficulties. Among others, George Graham (1992) has excellent ideas for ways to create a positive learning environment. In general, he suggests using the first few classes or practices of the new instructional period to establish and implement rules and procedures for good behavior. For example, in a physical education class students need to learn the new teacher's signals, such as start and stop signals, and other signs to look or listen for during class that tell them to behave in a certain way or that a particular behavior choice is good or poor. If such lessons are learned early, the entire school year will run more smoothly for the class. As another example, before the season begins Little League coaches should educate all who are involved—players, parents, spectators—about both the league rules governing play and their own private rules governing the team. They need to not only describe the rules but also explain the reasons behind them.

🔑 As a rule, instructors can best assist students as they learn rules and routines by (1) having high expectations, (2) being firm but warm, (3) developing clear rules, and (4) describing how rules will be enforced.

In a study of seven effective elementary specialists, instructors were observed teaching students the stopping and starting signals for class by using the signals a total of 346 different times during the first few days of instruction (Fink & Siedentop, 1989). After the first few classes, most students were behaving appropriately; those who did not follow the signals were promptly reprimanded. By implementing this routine during the first few days of every unit, these teachers quickly constructed an environment in which learning could take place.

Unfortunately, many instructors still do not understand that good management and discipline lead to a better learning environment. Because they believe they will have better control and be able to watch more closely if only one student performs at a time, they make students wait idly for their turns. These instructors don't understand that when young students are bored, with nothing to focus on but standing in line, they will fall easily into off-task behavior, often creating discipline problems. Effective instructors know that when students are appropriately engaged, and when the lesson moves along briskly, discipline problems are reduced and students have greater opportunity to learn.

Accountability

Recalling your own experiences as a student on an athletic team, do you remember being asked to perform a dozen push-ups, only to stop as soon as the coach turned away? Some students try to manipulate their teacher's or coach's expectations to suit their own purposes. In an eye-opening study of public school physical education, students were observed hiding from the teacher and acting as though they were actively engaged (Tousignant, 1981). The investigator referred to these students as competent bystanders—well-behaved students who consistently avoided participation without being noticed.

Unfortunately, instructors often allow learners to manipulate their expectations. In fact, some teachers even negotiate expectations with learners (Siedentop, 1991). For example, a camp counselor may ask a student to practice catching pop flies with another student. Within a few minutes, the counselor may notice that the students are also catching and throwing grounders. Instead of insisting that the students stick to the drill, the counselor is satisfied that they are participating and not causing trouble. The counselor's choice to say nothing, however, reinforces the students' choice to create lessons of their own.

🔑 Students manipulate the learning environment when they engage in off-task behaviors or become competent bystanders. By ignoring off-task behavior, instructors encourage further manipulation.

Students learn accountability through clearly stated and consistently enforced expectations. One instructor behavior for promoting student accountability is called "with-it-ness." Instructors demonstrate their with-it-ness by knowing what's happening in the learning environment and by demonstrating this awareness by communicating, verbally or otherwise, with the students. They hold students accountable for their actions, which makes the students less likely to try to manipulate the learning environment.

Specific Feedback

In addition to providing clear instructions, teachers and coaches must also provide clear, specific feedback. Unfortunately, instructors often provide too many instructions, and students either become bored and stop listening or cannot remember all that was said. In contrast, during practice, instructors seldom provide students an adequate amount of feedback that is correct, prompt, and specific.

The research and our own experiences indicate that instructors make several mistakes when providing feedback. First, feedback is often incorrect. For example, instead of correctly diag-

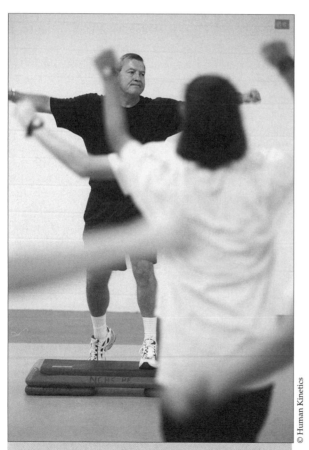

Even in exercise settings it is important for instructors to demonstrate "with-it-ness."

© Human Kinetics

nosing a problem as lack of trunk rotation during an overhead throw, a coach may tell an athlete to face the target. Second, some instructors do not time their feedback so that the learner receives prompt help when practice trials are defective in form or produce unsuccessful results. Practicing incorrect performance for an extended period has predictably negative results! Furthermore, teachers provide less feedback during game play (Rink, 1983). Feedback provided during game play, however, can be valuable; it gives all students information about ways to improve. If this form of feedback were not important, coaches would not videotape games for later analysis with athletes. Third, feedback is seldom specific. Although encouraging students with, "Good job," may be motivating, it does not convey what specifically was "good" about their performance.

🔑 Instructors can increase the probability that instruction will be effective by providing appropriate learning activities; maximal active learning time; and feedback that is correct, prompt, and specific.

Many researchers have dedicated their careers to studying feedback. Although researchers in motor learning have studied feedback for years, their research occurs in a laboratory. Fortunately, an increasing number of pedagogical researchers have become committed to collecting data in gymnasiums and playing fields. There are, however, inherent difficulties with collecting data in an "uncontrolled" environment (as opposed to a laboratory where conditions are carefully controlled). This has resulted in mixed findings (Lee, Keh, & Magill, 1993), some of which indicate that in real class settings a significant relationship does not always exist between feedback and learning (Silverman, 1994). As more studies are conducted and research design increases in sophistication, however, it may be possible to inform instructors about how to provide feedback in ways that more reliably support learning.

Knowledge of Curriculum

It is becoming increasingly important that instructors are knowledgeable about alternative forms of curriculum. In fact, many of these alternatives

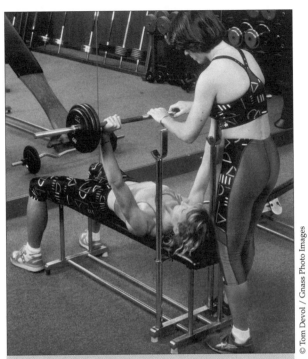

Feedback should be correct, prompt, and specific.

© Tom Devol / Gnass Photo Images

are currently being touted as the wave of the future (Locke, 1992). You and the majority of your classmates were likely exposed to a traditional curriculum in which instructors designed activities with little student input and employed a teacher-dominated approach. Although a traditional approach can be effective if taught by a creative teacher, the alternatives that follow offer strong promise and can be implemented in many different environments. The first six alternatives are discussed in greater depth in an excellent text by Siedentop, Mand, and Taggart (1986).

Effective teachers are concerned about implementing curricular models that are interesting to students and produce the greatest opportunity for student learning.

The first, the *multiactivity* or *elective* curriculum, allows learners to choose one activity from a wide selection of activities. They are encouraged to develop skills that will transfer into a lifetime interest in that activity. Although this form of curriculum requires an adequate number of instructors and ample facilities, it is currently

emphasized in many park districts, YMCAs, schools, and colleges.

The second alternative, the *fitness curriculum*, emphasizes developing cardiorespiratory fitness, muscular endurance, muscular strength, flexibility, and knowledge about the body and how it responds to exercise. Students participate in strength training and engage in cardiorespiratory activities such as running, swimming, circuit training, and aerobics.

Sports education, the third curriculum model, appears to hold much promise, particularly as a means of improving secondary physical education (Siedentop, 1994). In this model, teachers treat students as athletes. Students are formed into teams and not only learn how to play, but also assume some responsibility for roles as managers, coaches, trainers, officials, statisticians, and tournament administrators. Learners appear to enjoy this form of curriculum (Hastie, 1996; Taggart & Alexander, 1993) and probably receive higher amounts of functional learning time because of their eagerness to improve.

A fourth type of curriculum, *wilderness and adventure education*, introduces learners to such activities as canoeing, backpacking, camping, white-water rafting, climbing, first aid, skiing, and new and cooperative games.

The fifth, the *social development model*, is concerned with teaching students self-control and responsibility and draws heavily on the pioneering efforts of Hellison (1995). Learners are provided with a ladderlike model that employs six different levels ranging from "irresponsibility" (Level 0) to "going beyond" (Level 6). As discussed in chapter 2, this model holds particular promise in environments in which students have not had opportunities to develop personal responsibility and positive social skills.

Finally, the *conceptually based program*, the sixth curriculum alternative, is designed to emphasize learners' cognitive development through the teaching of sports and activities. This model stresses problem solving, critical thinking, and knowledge acquisition at a higher level. For example, students may be asked to analyze the biomechanics of a volleyball serve or design an individual fitness program that emphasizes principles of exercise physiology.

In addition to the models described, experts have created a variety of other curricular models, such as movement education for children, that have proven successful in many activity programs. Regardless of the model you select, it should maximize the opportunity for students to engage in relevant, meaningful, and appropriate activity. Developing knowledge about the different approaches will enable you to make the most informed decisions.

Hidden Curriculum

One aspect of curriculum that you probably have not considered is the powerfully influential **hidden curriculum**. This form of curriculum represents the learning that instructors and students are unaware of (Dodds, 1983). Once instructors or students become aware of what is being learned, the curriculum is no longer hidden. For example, if physical education teachers favor athletes by allowing them to participate without the proper uniform, other students learn that athletes have superordinate status. If teachers allow students to participate in dodgeball without any consideration of students who are less skilled and afraid of balls, some students may learn that physical education is painful, risky, and unpleasant. If teachers insist that all students receive equal amounts of practice and playing time, students may come to believe that everyone should have a fair opportunity to learn. If teachers encourage students to discover answers to their own questions, students may discover that learning is a shared enterprise.

🗝️ The hidden curriculum, in which instructors and learners are unaware of what is being learned, is often more powerful than the explicit curriculum.

While the hidden curriculum sends strong messages to learners—both negative and positive—instructors often find it difficult to detect (Sarason, 1971). For this reason, instructors are responsible for continually questioning all elements of their instructional behaviors and searching out those that, silently and without notice, work against the goals of effective instruction.

Equity

The learning environment in which physical activity occurs is often an inequitable environment in which some students are provided with less (or more) attention from instructors and coaches due to race, gender, physical ability, physical appearance, and socioeconomic status. Despite measures such as Title IX and Public Law 94-142, students continue to be disadvantaged for reasons beyond their control.

In physical activity settings, one of the most common forms of discrimination is against students with less ability. Elimination games, for example, are commonly employed in a host of different physical activity environments. Students with the lowest levels of skill are usually the first eliminated, even though they are the ones most in need of practice. Further, these students are often ridiculed by classmates. If you were low skilled, how would you feel when it was your turn to roll on a scooter during a relay race, particularly if your team was in the lead?

🗝️ Teachers must ensure that low-skilled students will not be ridiculed or embarrassed.

You may have unknowingly formed beliefs due to the hidden curriculum in your physical activity experiences. Take a moment to think about what you learned in physical activity classes—whether it was in school physical education, dance or martial arts classes, or after-school sports—that has little to do with the techniques you were being taught.

Do you believe that varsity athletes should receive special treatment? That only boys or girls can excel at certain sports? That if students don't like physical activity it is okay for them not to participate in physical education classes?

How did you learn these things? What hidden curriculum was present in your experiences?

In 1984 Patricia Griffin published the results of a fascinating study in which she described six patterns of female involvement during coeducational physical education classes. The six patterns—what Griffin called athletes, JV players, cheerleaders, lost souls, femme fatales, and system beaters—break down this way:

- Athletes—those few who are highly skilled
- JV players—those whose ability level ranges between average to low skilled and who are often ignored by teammates
- Cheerleaders—those who are low skilled but enjoy the excitement of the game
- Lost souls—those who are low skilled and usually fail during their attempts to participate
- Femme fatales—those who vary in skill level but create discipline problems, describe the game as "stupid," and choose not to participate
- System beaters—those who are typically absent

If you are female, do you see yourself in this list? Although Griffin's study was conducted over 15 years ago, her descriptions of female behaviors during physical activity are far from obsolete. It remains true that far too few instructors make efforts to ensure that girls encounter an equitable, enjoyable, and successful experience in physical activity.

Regardless of teachers' intentions, if they favor some students over others, they are discriminating. Such results are destructive and professionally unacceptable. If teachers or coaches have any personal biases against particular races, genders, sexual orientations, or religions, they must check those opinions at the door before entering the learning environment. All students deserve an equal opportunity to learn.

Addressing Individual Student Needs

Consider the many instances in which you may have had difficulty paying attention during a high school or university lecture because you were concerned with a test in another class, upset over the break-up of a personal relationship, or feeling ill after a late night of partying. Students enter the learning environment with a host of problems that are bound to interfere with their ability to learn. Studies have shown, for example, that students' grades typically decline when their parents undergo conflict or divorce. In some areas such as inner cities, learners are faced with a myriad of serious problems (gang involvement, poverty, lack of adequate nutrition) that get in the way of or even prevent learning. As a result, instructors are often confronted with a need to address the emotional and material needs of students, with far less time for concern about physical activity (Ennis, 1994).

As described in the section on curriculum, Hellison (1995) has developed a model for practitioners who work with "at-risk" youth. The results have been encouraging. Students who have encountered the model have become progressively more responsible for their own behaviors, and their instructors feel that these students have developed greater empathy toward their classmates (Hellison & Templin, 1991).

It is important to recognize that each learning environment and group of learners is different. For example, instructors employed in high socioeconomic status areas may encounter fewer immediately obvious emotional problems in students, yet students from wealthy families still undergo tremendous struggles. Regardless of the environment, instructors must address the individual needs of students by employing techniques to meet the needs of all learners, such as

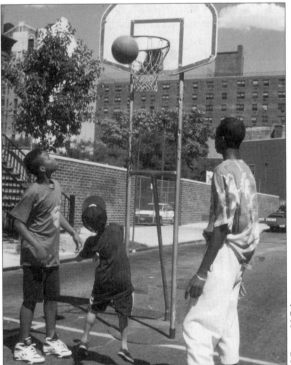

What would you need to know about this environment to design a learning environment that meets the needs of these students?

© Frances M. Roberts

Expectations significantly influence the learning process. They may concern a group of students or an individual, and they typically center on student performance or behavior. When expectations influence instructor behavior, and subsequently student behavior, the term **self-fulfilling prophecy**, also known as the **Pygmalion effect**, becomes relevant. For example, if a swim instructor believes that a particular child cannot achieve and subsequently ignores her, the lack of interaction with the instructor causes a void in the child's opportunity to learn. As a result, she may begin to believe that she is incapable, even though this may be far from the truth. If the child performs poorly, the instructor believes that his initial impressions were correct. Even if the child performs well, the instructor may believe that luck was responsible. In contrast, if the instructor expects the child to be a high achiever, he may provide additional support to enhance her achievement. The child may begin to believe that she is skilled and act accordingly. In essence, the Pygmalion effect can cut in either direction, with negative or positive results.

When first meeting someone, we commonly form an initial impression of the person. Similarly, instructors probably cannot help quickly developing impressions of students. These impressions are based on physical appearance, past observations, a student's or player's reputation as an athlete, or information derived informally from others. It's important, of course, to remember that forming impressions is a subjective process and leads to many false conclusions. We all can think of times when our first impressions proved to be very wrong. More important, if the impressions *are* negative and are communicated to students, the impressions will not be helpful in encouraging learning—even if they prove to be accurate!

Teacher characteristics can affect the ways in which impressions/cues about students are interpreted. For example, a teacher may be attracted to a student because he or she reminds the teacher of a difficult period earlier in life. As a result, the teacher may provide that student with extra support. The teacher chooses to do so because he or she needs to perceive the student as capable; failure by the student would only remind the teacher of his or her own vulnerability.

Second, learner attributes are also likely to influence a teacher's behavior. In one study of mainstreamed classes, Martinek and Karper (1981) discovered that elementary school teachers had low expectations for the social relations that developed between mainstreamed students and their classmates. In another study, teachers expected highly attractive students to perform better in physical activities and to be more socially adept with their peers than less attractive students (Martinek, 1981).

Third, social context is equally likely to create impressions about performance. Martinek and Karper (1986) discovered that physical education teachers held higher expectations for highly skilled students when those students were engaged in individual or competitive activities. They expected lower-skilled students to perform better in cooperative activities (and less well in individual activities). Further, teachers provided more technical feedback to high-ability students during individual activities, and more empathy (and lower expectations) to less-skilled students during competition. By trying to hold what they regard as "reasonable" expectations, teachers risk communicating the message to some students that, "You probably will not do very well," and the corollary, "So I don't expect you to try very hard." Good intentions aside, those subtle messages are devastating to learning.

The effects of expectations can have particularly unhappy results for students who are perceived as low achievers (Martinek & Johnson, 1979; Martinek & Karper, 1984). Feelings of helplessness often become a part of these students' personalities (Martinek,

→

1991). When this occurs, students are referred to as having acquired **learned helplessness** and may be observed to exert little effort, become abusive, blame others, or quickly concede to failure (Martinek & Griffith, 1993, 1994; Walling & Martinek, 1995). Fortunately, researchers are now better able to diagnose students who have acquired learned helplessness and are able to provide instructors with suggestions for improving the self-concepts of these learners.

As you stand before children who eagerly wait to learn soccer under your direction, how do you anticipate that your expectations will mold their performance? If you hold reasonably high (and appropriate) expectations, particularly for the quality and extent of their effort, and especially for those whom you may be most inclined to ignore, you may witness surprising results.

The authors gratefully acknowledge Tom Martinek for his assistance and contributions to this focus topic.

Key Pedagogical Principles

Provide appropriate practice.

Provide a high amount of academic learning time.

Always be concerned about class management and discipline.

Hold learners accountable.

Provide clear, specific feedback.

Develop a knowledge of different curricular models.

Keep an eye out for the hidden curriculum.

Ensure an equitable learning environment.

Address the individual needs of learners.

Consider how your expectations influence students.

Be prepared to encounter workplace conditions that may range from superb to less than ideal.

varying their instructional styles. Some students, for instance, learn better with less direct instruction, while others need greater direction. Whether an instructor is employed in a school or in another physical activity environment, he or she must recognize that students bring the baggage of their personal lives to class.

All learners carry personal problems into the learning environment at one time or another. Instructors need to be aware of this and be ready to adjust their teaching approach as necessary.

What Instructors Need to Know About the Workplace Environment

We all have been exposed to physical activity settings that are excellent. Typically, these settings have good facilities and outstanding instructors. They are a joy to attend and significantly contribute to our quality of life. Learning is fun and we come away with an expanded set of skills. Teachers in this type of setting are highly motivated and thrive in a workplace that promotes their effectiveness. In essence, factors promoting a high quality of work life are present: respect from clientele, worker participation in decision making, collegial support and stimulation, a high sense of efficacy among teachers, resources to perform effectively, and a common sense of vision within the organization (Stroot, 1996). Regrettably, the quality of life for teachers in other settings may be just the opposite. Settings that are underfunded, poorly maintained, underequipped, and that have no vision often produce unmotivated teachers.

The quality of the workplace often can determine the success and satisfaction of both employees and clientele. Understanding the influence of the workplace or the context in which one is employed is very important to the instructor of physical activity. Like other workplace settings, physical activity settings such as schools, fitness centers, YMCAs, or private golf clubs contain a host of contextual factors that one must understand and cope with in order to be successful. Social, psychological, political, economic, and other organizational factors may emerge on a microscopic level (within the work setting or individual class). For example, having access to a power base along with having the moral and financial support of colleagues and administrators within an activity setting is critical for an instructor. Also, having support and adequate resources certainly helps define a positive workplace.

Larger influences outside of the workplace may affect what transpires within the workplace as well. Issues related to family, population demographics, civil rights, health care, drugs and violence, educational reform and policy, or advances in information technology may influence what occurs in the workplace (Tyson, 1996). How instructors cope with contextual factors influences their success as instructors and, ultimately, the success of learners.

Although researchers have yet to examine the influence of the workplace in nonschool physical activity settings (e.g., fitness clubs, community recreation centers), researchers have shown considerable interest in examining the environment in which physical education teachers are employed. Many of the findings will be interesting to all instructors of physical activity, regardless of the setting in which they work. Some findings are positive, while others offer unflattering portraits of the workplace.

Life and Work in the Physical Education Setting

Teacher effectiveness and satisfaction are often linked to the characteristics of the work setting. Understanding the specific nature of any workplace is important as one contemplates working within a given activity arena. In 1975 Lawrence Locke's study of the ecology of the gym gave us our first understanding of the complexity of the physical education setting. This research showed that (1) teacher behavior is characterized by diverse activity and isolation from other adults; (2) differences among students influence teacher effectiveness; and (3) the curriculum of physical activity is distinctly different from that of other subjects relative to space, activities, and relationships.

This study was followed by many investigations that examined the culture of the physical education setting. These studies illustrated the positive and negative aspects of school physical education—what life in the gym is like for teachers and students. They have suggested that while elementary physical education (where it exists)

is in a relatively healthy state, secondary physical education suffers from a variety of difficult social and political problems—some of which appear now to be reaching a point of crisis.

In contrast to the exciting and profitable learning settings observed in most elementary schools, secondary physical education settings have been described as supervised recess, in which embarrassment, humiliation, discomfort, and student inactivity appear to be the norm.

In reporting the results of an extensive study of high schools, O'Sullivan and her colleagues (1994) characterized the state of secondary physical education as follows:

1. Teachers and students share similar views of the purpose of physical education—to expose students to lifetime activities. However, differences emerge when defining how fitness connects to physical education.

2. Fitness activities have little relationship to the development of health- or skill-related fitness.

3. Teachers spend too much time on class management activities suggesting the absence of well-planned, meaningful, and engaging activities for students.

4. Teacher autonomy is born out of benign neglect—physical education teachers are viewed as marginal figures in the overall school hierarchy.

5. Teachers have limited goals for students.

6. Teachers' sense of self-worth is validated through activities outside of physical education, such as coaching and officiating.

7. Gymnasiums are well-managed and happy places even in the absence of great levels of student achievement.

8. The curriculum of physical education is consistent among teachers—traditional sports and activities are most valued.

9. Instruction is described as casual, the premium on learning is mostly absent, and students with lower skill levels enjoy class less.

10. Student evaluation is not based on the measurement of performance but on compliance with behavioral standards (e.g., following the rules and rituals established in the class).

11. More than half of the students like physical education less and perceived it as less important than other subjects. Parents are in agreement with this assessment.

Overall, these findings reflect the dysfunction of many secondary physical education sites and represent a strong call for the restructuring of physical education at this level and the provision of alternative systems of physical education.

This research supports previous findings (Locke & Griffin, 1986) and vividly depicts the malaise that exists within American society relative to the role of secondary physical education. Cases of struggle appear to be more commonplace than profiles of excellence. Griffin (1986) summarized the various obstacles to excellence as (1) a lack of teacher or program evaluation; (2) a lack of formal incentive or reward for good teaching; (3) a lack of professional support for teacher and program development activities; (4) inadequate facilities, equipment, and scheduling; (5) failure to include teachers in decision making; (6) compliance and smooth operations being valued over teaching competence; (7) acceptance of mediocrity; and (8) isolation. In discussing these obstacles, Griffin stated, "in most cases, the schools did not intentionally limit what could be accomplished. . . . Instead, they practiced benign neglect. The tendency of everyone to ignore physical education presented what seems to have been the most formidable obstacle to excellence" (p. 58). In essence, physical education as a subject area at the secondary level seems to be perceived as superfluous to student learning, and the physical education teacher holds an occupational status that has been described as marginal.

In contrast to some of these negative characterizations of school physical education, we know that there also are positive examples of excellence in the schools. For example, the American Alliance of Health, Physical Education, Recreation and Dance annually recognizes elementary, middle, and secondary school teachers of the year for excellence in teaching. These teachers and

---

Contrasting Dimensions of Physical Education

Obstacles to Excellence

- Lack of program evaluation
- Lack of rewards
- Lack of professional development for teachers
- Inadequate equipment, facilities, and scheduling
- Failure of including teachers in decision making
- Compliance valued over teaching competence
- Acceptance of mediocrity
- Isolation

Models of Excellence

- Innovative instructional strategies
- Novel curriculums
- Integration with other subject areas
- Unique strategies to promote learning progressions
- High profile public relations programs
- Supportive colleagues and administrators
- Adequate funding
- Exemplary class-management strategies
- Involvement in professional development activities
- After-school programs for students and adults
- Modeling of athletic skill and fitness
- Promotion of equitable learning

---

others described in the literature (Anderson, 1994; Graham, 1982; Templin, 1983) provide exemplary physical education. Excellence is documented through (1) innovative instructional strategies, (2) novel curriculums, (3) the integration of physical education with other subject matters, (4) unique ways to promote learning progressions, (5) high-profile public relations programs, (6) supportive colleagues and administrators, (7) adequate funding, (8) exemplary classroom management strategies, (9) involvement in professional development activities, (9) after-school programs for students and adults, (10) the modeling of athletic skill and fitness, and (11) the promotion of equitable learning settings. These teachers demonstrate a sincere interest and enthusiasm for teaching, a genuine concern for students, and a continued desire to grow and develop as teachers. The settings in which they are employed are not unlike other physical activity settings (e.g., fitness clubs, private golf and tennis clubs, recreation centers) in which the welfare of participants or customer service is a high priority.

(key icon) Research on school physical education has revealed both positive and negative dimensions of the school environment.

Workplace Conditions

Although research on the influence of workplace conditions in nonschool physical education settings is limited, a number of studies of school physical education reflect the power of various factors to influence the teaching and learning process. Typically, these are represented as political, organizational, and personal/social factors. For example, the economic conditions of a school often influence what facilities and equip-

ment are at the disposal of teachers and students. As a result, some schools are able to offer a wide variety of curricular opportunities for students, whereas other schools are more limited. Figure 10.4 illustrates the factors most likely to influence workplace conditions.

(key icon) Workplace conditions have the potential to facilitate or constrain the instructor of physical activity.

Within the school context, teachers' success and satisfaction, or lack thereof, is linked to many variables. Class size, for example, has the potential to influence what material a teacher is able to cover, the amount of feedback he or she can provide to individual students, and the degree to which students receive ample opportunities to practice. School policy may dictate how often students receive instruction or how they will be

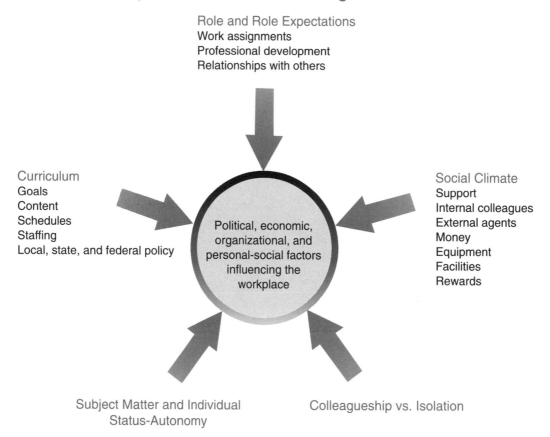

Workplace Conditions Influencing the Teacher

Role and Role Expectations
Work assignments
Professional development
Relationships with others

Curriculum
Goals
Content
Schedules
Staffing
Local, state, and federal policy

Political, economic, organizational, and personal-social factors influencing the workplace

Social Climate
Support
Internal colleagues
External agents
Money
Equipment
Facilities
Rewards

Subject Matter and Individual Status-Autonomy

Colleagueship vs. Isolation

Figure 10.4 Workplace conditions influencing the teacher.

Conditions That Have a Negative Impact on Physical Education Teachers

Conditions	Impact on instructors
Curriculum content	Teachers at both the elementary and secondary level often teach too many physical activities and too many classes in a day to be effective. Teachers often feel disempowered to determine the curriculum in terms of time allocation and number of activities.
Class size	Class size is generally quite large in physical education—well beyond the size of other classes.
Staffing	Physical education teachers are often isolated and left alone to fulfill instructional demands.
Policy	Local and state policies often require the minimum in physically educating students at the elementary and secondary levels. Grading policies dictate a teacher's instructional approach.
Students	Physical education teachers who are preoccupied with the control of disruptive students feel less effective. Student gender, ability, and other characteristics greatly influence a teacher's effectiveness.
Status/rewards	Physical education teachers are often perceived as marginal faculty relative to the overall goals of a school. Administrators, parents, and students perceive physical education as less important than other school subjects. Physical education teachers who receive strong support from administrators, colleagues, students, and parents feel more successful in their work. They often believe they are more appreciated for their work in coaching than in teaching. Teachers do feel a sense of accomplishment from student progress.
Facilities	Teachers often express the need for better facilities and equipment to enhance their instruction.

graded. The box above is a list of the conditions that Tyson (1996) suggests a physical education teacher encounters, along with a description of how they negatively influence the work of the instructor.

Working Toward Positive Work Settings

These examples from physical education research suggest the important role that context has on pedagogy regardless of the physical activity setting. Whether one is an aerobics instructor in a fitness club or a golf professional on the golf range, positive conditions influence the success of the teacher and learner. The degree to which you are able to thrive in an environment that is less than ideal often depends on your ability to employ various coping strategies. Compliance, compromise, and attempts to redefine the context in which you work often call for skilled decision making—sometimes at the risk of alienation

from others. You may challenge the norms of the setting in trying to overcome problems related to a particular situation. Challenging the status quo is always risky, but persistence and a commitment to improve your teaching or the instructional setting may reap positive results. At the other extreme, you can give up, ignore the problem, or even relocate to another setting. Regardless, you must learn to adapt to the conditions of the physical activity settings in which you work.

The complexity and shifting interaction of various conditions are what shape a stimulating, frustrating, challenging, and rewarding career. The bottom line is to be prepared to work and to understand the challenges and rewards that are inherent in any workplace. The ideal setting is one in which teachers are rewarded for excellence. Such settings exhibit a social order that is caring, supportive, and politically positive—in which politics and economics do not hinder your ability to perform good work. The social order is healthy if individuals work collaboratively toward the achievement of goals. Such a setting values and rewards teaching. Finally, a good work environment will facilitate both progress and the continuing struggle to improve. Positive work settings and good teachers usually go hand in hand for the benefit of students. This is true whether you teach in a school, YMCA, recreation center, or other activity setting.

Wrap-Up

The objective of this chapter was to introduce the knowledge base in pedagogy of physical activity. Exciting developments have occurred over the past two decades, and new knowledge will continue to emerge as researchers ask more sophisticated questions and develop new methods for collecting data. The information in this chapter is but a small sample of the types of knowledge currently available to those in pedagogy.

If you are considering embarking on a teaching or coaching career, you will need to know much more about pedagogy than we are able to discuss here. You will have greater success if you consistently and objectively reevaluate your current beliefs in light of new research-based knowledge about effective teaching. As a member of the next generation of instructors, you can make a difference.

Study Questions

1. How do the experiences you acquired as a student of physical activity connect to the examples of effective and ineffective teaching discussed in the chapter?

2. What methods of researching the pedagogy of physical activity seem best to you? Why? What are other methods and their advantages and disadvantages?

3. Describe which historical events you believe had the greatest impact on the evolution of research on teaching. What research questions require further investigation?

4. In order to reduce management time, what routines are most important for students to learn? Which routines would you emphasize? Describe how you would implement those routines.

5. Explain the implications of competent bystanders in the physical activity setting. Describe one personal incident in which you either acted as a competent bystander or observed another student doing so.

6. Why is most teacher feedback ineffective? Provide one example of feedback that is too general or inappropriate and one that is most likely to be effective.

7. Which curricular framework would you choose to implement as an instructor? Why?

8. Describe the implications of the hidden curriculum. What did you learn from the hidden curriculum as a student in physical activity settings?

9. Define the Pygmalion effect and describe the implications of teacher expectations on student learning. How would you interact with a student who is experiencing learned helplessness?

10. Describe conditions that enhance and constrain teacher effectiveness and satisfaction in the physical activity setting.

11. Describe the pros and cons of working in the following settings: (a) secondary school physical education, (b) elementary school physical education, (c) health and fitness club, (d) children's recreation center baseball program, and (e) two other physical activity settings of your choice.

PART III

BIOPHYSICAL SPHERE

In this part . . .

11

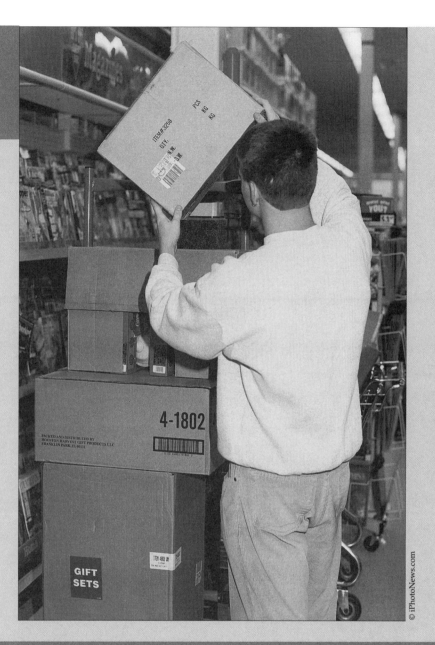

© iPhotoNews.com

Biomechanics of Physical Activity

Kathy Simpson

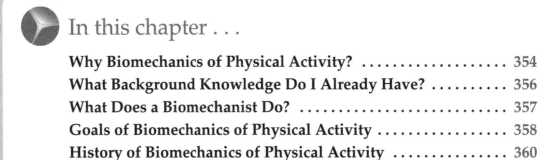

In this chapter . . .

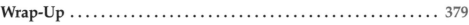

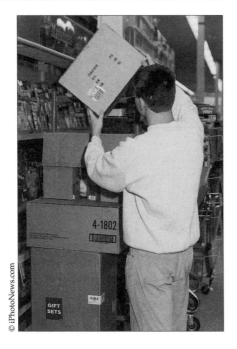

While at work in the storeroom of a discount store, your supervisor tells you to place boxes of clothes onto shelves that are above your head. Lifting a box, you realize that the boxes must weigh 60 pounds! How are you going to lift all those boxes without hurting yourself? Should you: (1) keep your back straight when you lift the boxes, (2) keep the boxes close to your body when lifting, (3) use portable steps to reach the shelves, and/or (4) wear a back/abdominal support?

Why Biomechanics of Physical Activity?

If you have ever been involved in organized sports or physical activity classes, such as dance or swimming, you probably were taught that your degree of success was related to your technique. Employers who are concerned about worker productivity and costs due to worker injuries also teach their workers how to perform tasks. In both cases, the principles of biomechanics—that is, how basic mechanical laws affect human movement—are at work.

To answer the questions in our opening scenario of how to lift the boxes effectively and safely, we need to consider the forces acting on you and particularly on your back. From biomechanics research we know that to prevent muscle injury, you should use your lower back muscles as little as possible. You also want the least amount of force applied to the other tissues in your back and spinal column. So, should you keep your back straight while you lift? Research tells us that you do want to keep your back in natural alignment, but not as straight as a board, in order to avoid putting excessive pressure on the lower-back vertebrae and vertebral disks. Keeping small boxes (those small enough to put between your legs) close to your body when lifting allows you to use the strong muscles of your legs, which will require less effort and also take the stress off your lower-back muscles. Since lifting a box above chest height forces you to arch your back, which puts a lot of pressure on the vertebrae and the vertebral disks, yes, you should use portable steps designed for this purpose.

Whether or not you should wear an abdominal support is much more controversial. The results from studies are inconclusive or contradictory to one another (McGill & Norman, 1993). At the very least, industrial workers who wear abdominal supports should be given training on their use, so that the supports are worn correctly and not used to replace good lifting techniques.

This example illustrates one application of biomechanics of physical activity. **Biomechanics** of physical activity is defined as the study of the movements and the structure and function of human beings using the principles and methods of mechanics of physics and engineering (Atwater, 1980; Hatze, 1974; Winter, 1985). These principles are concerned with forces and motion. According to the laws of physics, our ability to move, speed up, or slow down our bodies depends on how forces act on us. We can't move our body or body parts without some **force** being exerted, either internally as a result of muscle contraction or externally by other people, objects, or the environment (e.g., gravity, wind, water). For example, in our opening scenario, you couldn't lift the box unless you applied a force to the box. Furthermore, forces can act directly on our bodies not only to move us, but also to injure us if the amount of force is too high, if the force is applied too quickly, or if the force is applied for too many repetitions. In the opening scenario, lifting improperly could generate excessive forces on the vertebrae of your lower back. When you get an injury, such as a broken bone or an ankle sprain, forces are most likely to have caused this injury.

We have defined physical activity in this text as intentional, voluntary movement directed toward achieving an identifiable goal. In this chapter, we explore how biomechanists apply physical laws and principles, especially those involving forces and mechanical energy, to the production of physical activity. Furthermore, we will investigate the effects on our bodies of the forces that are generated during physical activity, as these forces influence the structure and function of tissues for better (e.g., stronger bones) or for worse (e.g., injuries).

Biomechanics is the science that applies the mechanical principles of physics and engineering to the motion, structure, and functioning of all living systems, including plants and animals. Biomechanists in the field of physical activity, however, are principally concerned with the biomechanics of physical activity, which uses the basic mechanical principles that govern the motion of all living beings to investigate human movement and the structure and function of the human body.

You may encounter other situations in your life that involve biomechanics. Consider how you would go about determining solutions to the following situations if you were a layperson versus a biomechanist or other type of kinesiologist with biomechanics training: You are working with a soccer team of six-year-olds and teaching the children how to kick a field goal. As a former soccer player, you rely on your knowledge of what your volunteer coaches taught you about kicking a soccer ball. However, the kids seem to be struggling with getting the ball to go very far, and you aren't sure what to tell them to improve their kicking ability. Now, assume that you are a coach with good biomechanical training. Knowing biomechanical principles related to generating force will enable you to teach them how best to move their bodies to generate the necessary force to kick the ball. When observing each child's technique, you can concentrate on the movements that can be improved to generate more force and increase accuracy, and ignore other parts of the technique.

As another example, you decide to help your friend who is recovering from a muscle injury buy a home weight machine to perform strength exercises. As a friend, you might suggest a machine that was featured in a sports magazine or the equipment that looks the most impressive. As a biomechanist, fitness specialist, or physical therapist trained in biomechanics, however, understanding how different machines provide resistance (e.g., hydraulics, rubber bands, or weight stacks attached via pulleys) will help you decide what equipment will work your friend's muscles optimally. Furthermore, by knowing that the leverage and the force of muscles change throughout a movement, you'll seek the machine that can best work the muscles throughout an entire exercise.

You can see from these examples that people with a background in biomechanics can use their knowledge of how the human body moves in regard to how forces act on the body or within the body to enhance performance, improve fitness, and reduce injury potential.

 ## CHAPTER OBJECTIVES

In this chapter you will learn about these key topics:

- What background knowledge you already have about biomechanics of physical activity
- What a biomechanist of physical activity does
- The goals of biomechanics of physical activity
- How biomechanics of physical activity emerged within the field of physical activity
- How biomechanists engage in research and analyze movement
- What is known from biomechanics research about how forces and physical laws of nature affect performance and movement

What Background Knowledge Do I Already Have?

Through your physical activity experiences, scholarly study, and observations of professionals in the field of physical activity, you have already gained some knowledge of biomechanics. Let's look first at some examples from your past *experiences* in physical activity. If you have ever wondered if certain shoes work well for running because they absorb impact forces, while others give you more stability for tennis, you have considered the very issues that biomechanists have investigated for the footwear industry. All of your life you have been learning how forces act on you and how the laws of physics affect your every movement. Think of how difficult it is for a young child to learn to stand, walk, throw a ball, or jump as high as possible. These tasks are easy for you—you've learned how gravity, friction, air resistance, and other forces shape your movements. Although you may or may not be able to consciously articulate the principles that govern forces and motions, every time you move or maintain balance, you are making use of these principles to accomplish your movement or to remain stationary.

Some of your *scholarly studies* also have provided you with background information in biomechanics. Biomechanics of physical activity applies the principles of physics and engineering to physical activity. Thus, if you have taken courses in biology, anatomy, physics, and math (algebra, trigonometry, and geometry), you already have much of the background knowledge needed to begin the scholarly study of biomechanics.

Finally, you have probably learned biomechanical principles from physical activity *professionals* without even knowing it. Perhaps your track coach taught you how to push hard to get out of the blocks fast during a sprint start. Your coach may have told you, You have to push back with your foot to move your body forward, to teach you how to make good use of Newton's Law of Action–Reaction. Or, when visiting a retirement facility and seeing adults who appear unstable while walking or standing, you may have observed that a clinician applies stability principles derived from physics; for example, the client may be taught how to use an assistive device such as a cane. Or, perhaps, as a student assistant, working with an athletic trainer, you have watched the athletic trainer observe the mechanics of a pitcher to assess if abnormal force loading to elbow tendons may be the cause of a developing injury.

As you can tell from the examples we have given, biomechanics is relevant to the biophysical sphere of scholarly study (see figure 11.1). The scholarly study of biomechanics provides the opportunity to learn how to apply physics and engineering to many physical activity or other biologically based situations, from clinical rehabilitation of physically compromised patients to elite athletic performance enhancement.

Physical activity and the structure and functioning of the human body are influenced by the laws of physics that govern forces and their effects on motion. The application of physics and engineering principles to physical activity and the structure and functioning of the human body is the realm of the human movement biomechanist.

What Does a Biomechanist Do?

Career opportunities in biomechanics include such positions as researcher, clinical biomechanist, performance enhancement specialist, ergonomist (industrial task analysis specialist), and university professor. A researcher working in an industrial biomechanics laboratory performs experiments to solve problems of interest to employers. For example, a biomechanist employed by a footwear corporation might work with

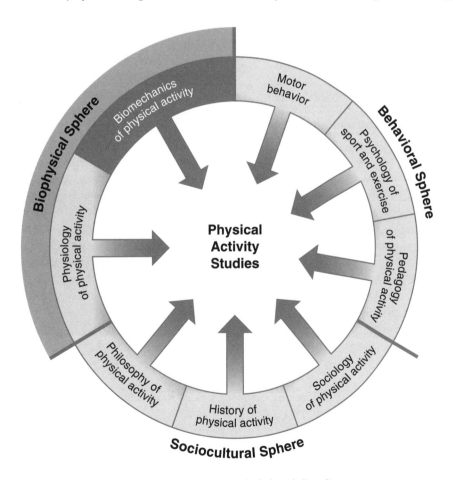

Figure 11.1 Biomechanics of physical activity and the other scholarly subdisciplines.

engineers to understand the interaction among the structure of people's anatomy, how people move, and the forces that act on people in order to design better footwear. A researcher working in a veteran's hospital laboratory may help physicians and therapists understand how to best help diabetic patients who have undergone foot amputation to regain normal walking patterns after having been fitted with artificial limbs.

A performance enhancement specialist might work with coaches of elite athletes or professional teams to improve performance. One biomechanics company works with golfers and tennis players who come to the company's facilities to have their techniques analyzed.

Ergonomists work in research and development departments as part of a team of individuals designing equipment such as gardening tools, airplane controls, factory machines, sports equipment, and so on. As we saw in chapter 2, ergonomists may also work for ergonomics-focused corporations, conducting job site analyses to determine, for example, if the tasks or equipment can be modified so that the workers will suffer from fewer injuries and fatigue less easily.

Clinical biomechanists may work in medical settings, such as research hospitals that have biomechanics laboratories, as an integral part of a patient's functional assessment and evaluation of treatment. The Shriner's Hospital in Greenville, South Carolina, is one such hospital. Teams consisting of a surgeon, physical therapist, and biomechanist often work together to determine whether a child with cerebral palsy requires surgery. The biomechanist's responsibility is to perform the gait (walking) analysis and to interpret the findings for the surgeon and physical therapist.

The university professor not only teaches biomechanics to a variety of physical activity and/or health-allied professionals, but also performs research to help us better understand the basics of how the structure and function of our bodies helps us move (muscle mechanics) or how forces produce injury (e.g., investigating causes of ligament tears). Other research may be more directly applied to determine, for example, what ankle brace, if any, a volleyball player should wear to prevent an ankle sprain.

Biomechanics of physical activity is a growing subdiscipline. In addition, many people who benefit from biomechanics are other physical activity and health-allied professionals. Some of the most common applications of biomechanics include

- improving performance in sport, dance, activities of daily living, and other physical activities;
- reducing or preventing injury during work, at home, while exercising, or in sport;
- improving movements of individuals with pathologies in clinical situations;
- increasing a performer's health via an exercise or training regimen; and
- assisting with the design of sport and exercise equipment, artificial limbs, occupational equipment, and training and rehabilitation devices so that performers can move not only more effectively but also more safely.

Does a career in biomechanics interest you? If so, ask yourself the following: Do you like analyzing people's movement techniques? Do you find yourself trying to figure out a better way to perform a task? Do you like the idea of applying the physics and math you've learned to a movement situation? Or does investigating the internal structures of the body, for example, tendons, to determine how they function to produce force or to absorb force safely, appeal to you? If you answered yes to these, look up the American Society of Biomechanics Web site (**http://asb-biomech.org/**) for information about biomechanics, jobs, graduate programs, and biomechanists to contact.

Goals of Biomechanics of Physical Activity

The goals of the subdiscipline of biomechanics of physical activity can be broken down into two major areas, general and applied (Contini & Drillis, 1954). The goal of the general area is *to understand how the basic laws and principles that govern the motion of human beings affect human motion and the structure of the human body.*

The applied area refers to making use of the theories underlying biomechanics and applying them to specific situations such as activities of daily living, art, dance, exercise, sport, and medicine. Therefore, the second goal is *to understand the relationships between mechanical laws and principles and techniques of specific movements, for example, a golf swing, running, or lifting hospital patients, in order to improve the outcome of a performance.* Questions biomechanists might ask include: Is it true that someone who has excellent technique is a great performer? How can people move their bodies to generate more force to jump higher, run faster, leap higher? How can an occupational task, such as harvesting grapes, be changed to reduce fatigue and improve worker output?

The third goal of biomechanics is to *understand the interactions between the human user and the mechanics of equipment or assistive devices in order to improve performance effectiveness and safety.* Questions biomechanists in this area might ask include: What type of dance floor will enhance performance? How can garden equipment be modified to improve the effectiveness and safety of completing a gardening task such as pruning?

These are the types of questions asked by biomechanists working in the field of **ergonomics**, or **occupational biomechanics**. As pointed out in chapter 2, ergonomics is a branch of biomechanics that has evolved from industrial engineering problems and not from physical education/activity institutions. Ergonomics is the use of a biomechanical approach to design the workplace by fitting the workplace to the worker (Chaffin & Andersson, 1991) and not the other way around. Configuring factory equipment so that industrial tasks, such as lifting boxes, can be performed with the least amount of fatigue and potential for injury is one application. Ergonomists also concentrate on determining the best designs for office furniture to reduce fatigue, overuse, and other medical problems, such as carpal tunnel syndrome. Companies specializing in ergonomic analyses of industrial tasks may include ergonomic engineers, biomechanists, and physical and occupational therapists specially trained in ergonomics.

The fourth goal of the subdiscipline is *to understand how injuries due to forces can be prevented.* Many assistive devices, such as shoe inserts, foot-ball pads, and walking canes, are designed to prevent injury. Biomechanists working in this area ask such questions as: Will placing a vibration device on a tennis racket reduce tennis elbow injury? Does stretching before exercising prevent injury? Do particular knee replacement designs improve the stability of the lower extremity during activities such as walking or lowering oneself into a chair? Is movement technique related to injury causation?

Based on the relationships observed between golf movement technique and injuries, sports medicine physicians (Rizzo & Trigg, 1994) realize that poor technique can create chronic wrist and shoulder problems for golfers, due to excessive forces being applied to the tissues of the these body regions. If you were an injured golfer, you might not understand why you were performing the motions that caused the injury. Maybe you didn't know how to rotate your trunk effectively, thereby limiting your ability to produce clubhead force. As a result, you compensated by trying to develop more force using your arms, thus straining the shoulder region.

Goals of Biomechanics of Physical Activity

To understand

1. How the basic laws and principles that govern the motion of human beings affect human motion and the structure and function of the human body

2. The relationships between mechanical laws and principles and techniques of specific movements in order to improve the outcome or effectiveness of a performance

3. The interactions between the human user and the mechanics of equipment or assistive devices in order to improve performance effectiveness and safety

4. How to prevent injuries caused by forces

As you can see, the goals of biomechanics are applicable to many areas of physical activity and allied health areas. Although biomechanics of physical activity is a subdiscipline of kinesiology, it is also very closely related to the subdisciplines within physics called mechanical physics and engineering. Biomechanics of physical activity applies the laws and principles of physics, engineering, and biology to investigating phenomena of human beings.

🔑 Although biomechanics of physical activity is a subdiscipline of kinesiology, the guiding principles and concepts of biomechanics come from mechanical physics, mechanical and biological engineering, and biology.

To better understand biomechanics and its relationship with these other areas, it is helpful to look at a brief history of biomechanics of physical activity.

History of Biomechanics of Physical Activity

Many Americans were first introduced to the term *biomechanics* in the 1980s during the 1984 and 1988 Olympics. The first national effort to improve the performances of elite athletes and potential future Olympians by using an interdisciplinary scientific approach at a central location occurred at the newly built United States Olympic Commission Training Center in Colorado Springs. Short television features demonstrated how biomechanical and physiological analyses were used to improve the techniques and training programs of athletes who came to the center. In addition, biomechanists at this time were involved in the development of high-technology footwear and other sport equipment. Biomechanics research gained recognition as magazines featured articles about training and equipment during the fitness explosion taking place in the United States during this time.

Although *biomechanics* is an unfamiliar term to many people, biomechanics has been around for a very long time—some say since humans first made tools (Contini & Drillis, 1954). We will see that biomechanics of physical activity, however, is relatively young. Several historical events and individual scholarly activities led to its development and still influence the philosophies and methods biomechanists use today to investigate human movement problems.

Early Beginnings

Greek philosophers were among the first in the European world to practice so-called scientific thinking using observable data as opposed to basing conclusions on emotions. Aristotle (384–322 B.C.E.) is considered to be one of the first biomechanists as a result of his observations of animal motion and the walking patterns of humans (Fung, 1968).

The contributions of Leonardo da Vinci (1452–1519) show the influence of the scientific awakening that occurred during the European Renaissance. Da Vinci is credited with developing the modern science of anatomy and with the first systematic examination of mechanical principles of human and animal movement (Hart, 1963).

It was not until the last quarter of the 19th century and the first quarter of the 20th century, however, when the industrial revolution brought many new inventions, that objective instruments such as cameras were developed for measuring movements. The development of biomechanics (then called "kinesiology") in physical education, sport, and dance began in the very late 1800s and early 1900s. Two Swedish men (Posse, 1890; Skarstrom, 1909) interested in gymnastics were among the first in the United States to formally apply the term *"kinesiology"* to the analysis of muscles and movements in a physical education setting (Atwater, 1980). Some departments continue to apply this term to biomechanics courses, which can cause confusion since *kinesiology* is also used as the name for the larger discipline. In this chapter, whenever "kinesiology" is used to refer to the subdiscipline of biomechanics it will be placed in quotation marks.

Researchers in the 1920s, including some from areas outside of physical education, had the tools and interest to investigate the mechanics of locomotion (e.g., Fenn, 1929), the efficiency of human movement in sport and industrial settings (Amar, 1920), and the energetics of running (Furusawa, Hill, & Parkinson, 1927; Hill, 1926). Mechanical analyses of basic movements were not emphasized as part of the formal training of dance and physical educators, however, until the 1920s when Ruth Glassow and her students at the University of Illinois and later at the University of Wisconsin (1930) began classifying activities into categories such as locomotion, throwing, strik-

In Profile

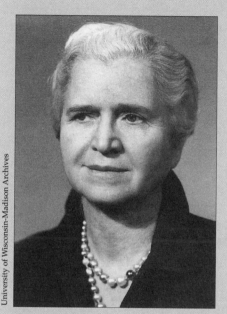

University of Wisconsin-Madison Archives

Ruth Glassow

In 1924 when Ruth Glassow began as an assistant professor of physical education at the University of Illinois at Urbana-Champaign, she was assigned to teach a "kinesiology" class (Atwater, 1980). She discovered that most textbooks at the time were focused on the simple analysis of muscle actions, mostly for gymnastics movements. She began investigating the basic principles of movement and how those principles could be applied to a variety of movements (Atwater, 1980; Cooper, 1977).

For 32 years at the University of Wisconsin-Madison, Glassow and a group of associates classified movement skills into various categories and determined the mechanical principles thought to underlie the effective performance and teaching of these skills. During her research, Glassow was a pioneer in using motion pictures for analyzing skills. Glassow, similar to other professionals during this time, also was a leader in generating knowledge in other areas— physical education measurement and evaluation, child growth, motor development, and motor learning. Glassow's work led to the publication of *Fundamentals of Physical Education* (1932) and *Measuring Achievement in Physical Education* (Glassow & Broer, 1938), and *Kinesiology* (Cooper & Glassow, 1963), a text for physical educators. Glassow was honored in 1964 with the Luther Halsey Gulick Medal, the highest honor awarded by members of AAHPERD.

ing, balance, and so on, and applied fundamental principles of mechanics and physics to the skills in each category (Atwater, 1980; Cooper, 1977; Widule, 1980).

Several leaders in the 1930s supported the use of "kinesiology" to understand human movement in physical education and orthopedics. The work of Glassow continued to expand at the University of Wisconsin (Widule, 1980; Glassow, 1932). Thomas Cureton, a professor of applied physics and mechanics at the YMCA College in Springfield, Massachusetts, taught the mechanics of sports and physical activities at Springfield College, wrote articles that supported the need for more applied "kinesiological" research (Cureton, 1932), and performed research primarily in swimming (e.g., Cureton, 1930). Charles McCloy, a leading researcher in many areas of physical activity, identified specific mechanical principles that influenced movement (see McCloy, 1960 for a review of his work). As a professor of orthopedic surgery, Arthur Steindler also profoundly influenced the study of "kinesiol-

ogy". According to Atwater (1980), one of his legacies was to coin the word *biomechanics* and give it a definition (Steindler, 1942), although Nelson (1970) believes Europeans may have started using this word first.

These early investigators had a profound effect on physical education through their articles, books, and research because they were among the first to encourage physical education/activity professionals to identify and use biomechanical principles. Their influence was exponential because many of their students became the core of college professors who were trained to teach future physical activity specialists and college professors (Atwater, 1980). As a single example, Katherine Wells studied under Steindler and McCloy (Chaffin & Andersson, 1991) and went on to write a basic textbook (Wells, 1950) that not only presented mechanical principles underlying basic movements, but also discussed applications of biomechanics to physical and occupational therapy, corrective exercises, and the performance of daily living skills.

Several societal events prompted the development of other forms of biomechanics. Following World War I, for instance, researchers in France and Germany applied biomechanics to improve prosthetic devices for war veterans who had lost limbs. This stimulated the beginning of the physical medicine areas, including physical therapy. Interestingly, the rebuilding of industry in Europe after World War II also involved biomechanical analyses of work movements, particularly in Russia and Germany (Contini & Drillis, 1966). Thus, ergonomics was born. In addition to helping war victims of World War II, physical medicine research regarding pathological gait (walking) was also used to help victims of the polio epidemics (Atwater, 1980).

An increase in biomechanics research related to human factors design occurred in the 1950s. Human factors engineers design equipment based on how people process information and how they respond to the information when performing a task. For example, an automotive human factors engineer would incorporate knowledge of how drivers react when an unexpected object appears in the road in order to design the brakes and steering wheel correctly. During this time, the new automotive, space, and aviation transport industries (Contini & Drillis, 1966) and the armed services (Thomas, 1969) needed to know the sizes, shapes, weights, and so forth, of people, particularly men, in order to design seats, cockpits, and instrument panels to fit these users.

The Era of Contemporary Biomechanics

The study of biomechanics of sport and other physical activities continued to grow mainly out of college physical education programs. In the 1960s biomechanical conferences were organized, professional organizations were created, and graduate-level university programs were established in the United States (Atwater, 1980). Biomechanists (then still termed "kinesiologists") promoted the scientific study of physical activity within the primary professional and scholarly organization, the American Association for Health, Physical Education and Recreation (AAHPER). The Kinesiology Section (renamed the Kinesiology Council and now known as the

Biomechanics Academy) was finally recognized officially in 1965. The first international professional association (the International Society of Electromyographical Kinesiology) was also formed during this period.

The 1970s saw a rapid expansion in number and scope of national (e.g., the American Society of Biomechanics) and international professional organizations (e.g., the International Society of Biomechanics) and university programs in biomechanics. Interest in this area was also demonstrated by people in areas outside of biomechanics. A symposium on sport mechanics, for example, was sponsored by the Applied Mechanics Division of the American Society of Mechanical Engineers, while biomechanics research related to sports medicine was welcomed at the American College of Sports Medicine meetings. Dance "kinesiology" also evolved during this time.

Since then, the university programs and professional organizations related to biomechanics have continued to expand. More colleges and universities offer not only courses in biomechanics but also undergraduate- and graduate-level specializations in this area as well. Many other biomechanics organizations exist around the world. Technical journals, to mention only a few, include the *Journal of Biomechanics*, the *Journal of Applied Biomechanics*, and *Clinical Biomechanics*.

Contemporary research themes that have been emerging and are projected to continue to flourish include the following:

- Understanding movement challenges encountered by people at all phases of life and those with particular physical activity impairments
- Refining current mathematical models as well as generating new mathematical models in order to predict and prescribe physical activities (e.g., simulating gait to test the effect of different knee ligament surgeries)
- Understanding the biomechanics of injury—its treatment and prevention

Other biomechanical areas of research believed by Charles (1994) to be emerging include the following:

- Control biomechanics: an approach that combines neuromuscular physiology and

Historical Time Line

1890 Baron Nils Posse is possibly the first to use the term *"kinesiology"* (Posse 1890).

1909 With Posse, Skarstrom was among the first to formally apply the term *"kinesiology"* to the analysis of muscles and movements in a physical education setting (Atwater, 1980).

1912 Wilbur Bowen publishes *The Action of Muscles in Bodily Movement and Posture*. This book, with its various names, authors, and editors, has had the longest history of any kinesiology textbook. Currently it is called *Kinesiology and Applied Anatomy* by P.J. Rasch et al.

1924 Ruth Glassow at the University of Illinois begins classifying activities into categories (such as striking, locomotion, and balance) and applying mechanical analyses to these categories. She continued her work for several decades at the University of Wisconsin.

1935 Arthur Steindler's book, *The Mechanics of Normal and Pathological Motion in Man* is published. He also taught classes in "kinesiology" to physical education and orthopedic medical students (Atwater, 1980).

1950s Continued expansion of the number of textbooks, types of research methods, number of research publications, and topics researched.

1963 First on a trial basis (1963–1964), the Kinesiology Section was formed and officially recognized in 1965 (and renamed the Kinesiology Council) within AAHPER. Initially its philosophy was to encompass all scientific areas of human movement. Currently it is known as the Biomechanics Academy within AAHPHERD.

1965 The International Society of Electromyographic Kinesiology is one of the first organizations to bring together "kinesiological" scientists (biomechanists) from all over the world.

1967 The First International Seminar on Biomechanics is held in Zurich, Switzerland.

1968 The first issue of the *Journal of Biomechanics*, the first international journal to focus on mechanical principles in biological systems, is published.

1970 Indiana University hosts the first meeting in North America on biomechanics for physical educators and biomechanists.

1973 The International Society of Biomechanics is formed.

1976 The American Society of Biomechanics is formed.

Some data from Atwater 1980.

motor control to understand the mechanisms that generate and control movement

- Ecological biomechanics: synthesizing biomechanics and psychology to investigate how human movement is organized based on laws related to energy considerations and the tendency for systems to seek equilibrium and stability

- Synergistic biomechanics: synthesizing biomechanics and art, based on the concept that human movement involves more than mechanics

Research Methods in Biomechanics of Physical Activity

Biomechanics research has greatly benefited from technological advances. Even in the early 1990s many biomechanists spent hours manually tracking thousands of frames of film in order to analyze the motion of a performer. Now it is possible to use special cameras that can track the motion of the performer in just minutes! What other tools do biomechanists use to accomplish the goals of biomechanics? How do biomechanists perform gait analyses for patients, research the cushioning properties of newly designed shoes, analyze the performance of Olympic athletes to help them improve, and perform research to answer fundamental questions about how and why we move? Any time a biomechanical question is approached, whether by an allied health professional, a coach, or a biomechanist, a somewhat common analysis process is used to answer the question of interest.

In chapter 2 we saw how a clinician might conduct a general analysis of a patient. To give you a sense of how a practitioner such as a teacher or physical therapist might conduct a more thorough analysis using biomechanics, first we will go through the simplified steps of an analysis (figure 11.2). Then, we will use some of these steps in the section, "Overview of Biomechanics of Physical Activity."

Step 1: State Performance Goals

Let us assume that you want to determine whether a new prosthetic design will improve the running speed of a man who has lost part of a lower limb. As shown in the model, it is first necessary to identify the overall goal(s) of the movement in conjunction with the participant's goal(s) for performing the movement. Your performer may want to be able to jog 20 minutes for exercise, with the amputated limb performing as naturally and effortlessly as the intact limb. Or the runner may want to be able to run a 10K race as fast as possible.

Step 2: Consider Influencing Factors

Next, you must understand the characteristics of the performer and understand the uniqueness of the individual in terms of physical and other characteristics. Thus, your performer may be motivated to function as well as possible using a new prosthesis or may be hesitant to try a design that potentially could produce tissue damage to the residual limb. The strength and length of the amputated limb are very important physical characteristics of the performer. The environment would also influence performance (e.g., the prosthesis and running surface).

Step 3: Understand Motions and Mechanics

In this step you must understand the motions and mechanics involved in your performer's movement. Running requires that the performer collide with the ground, then propel the body upward and forward through the air. When the leg is not on the ground, it must be pulled through in preparation to place it back on the ground again. Thus, the prosthetic design should allow the performer to produce the necessary propulsive force, to impact safely with the ground without producing excessive pressure on the stump, and to swing the prosthetic leg forward in a natural manner.

Step 4: Determine Relevant Biomechanical Principles and Movement Techniques

The fourth step is to determine what mechanical principles are most relevant to the performer's movement goals. In addition, you need to determine what movement techniques and prosthetic equipment designs would help you capitalize on using these mechanical principles to the best benefit. Newton's laws, principles related to energy, and fluid mechanics are examples of principles you could choose from.

Because you realize that the amputated limb is lacking muscles of the lower leg and foot, the prosthetic limb will have to provide some of the propulsive force needed. Thus, you might be interested in the principles related to storing and releasing energy, similar to what happens when a spring is compressed and then is allowed to regain its shape. A prosthesis does exist that uses a spring in the foot. Another lower leg prosthesis containing carbon fibers uses a shaft that can be bent to store and release energy. A principle related to Newton's Law of Acceleration is helpful to apply to the performer—when forces are applied to the performer over a period of time, then the performer will gain momentum. Thus, when the ground applies propulsive forces to the performer he increases his momentum.

Movement analysis model for practitioners

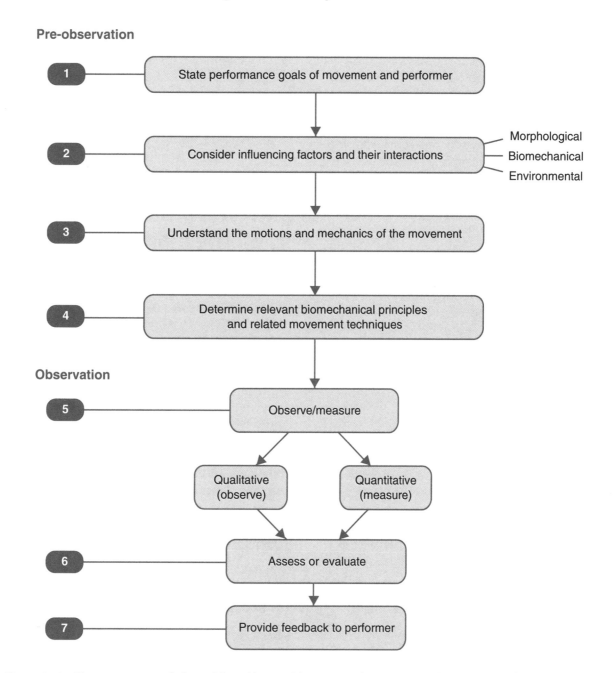

Figure 11.2 The movement analysis model used by practitioners to evaluate or assess the movement of a client. Each step of the analysis is labeled by number.

Step 5: Observe/Measure

For the step of observing and measuring (step 5), the analysis process diverges, depending on what you (the kinesiologist, biomechanist, or allied health specialist) are trying to accomplish with the performer. Oftentimes, you will observe the qualities of the performer's movements. In doing so, you are performing a **qualitative analysis**. Thus, if you were a prosthetist, physical therapist, or a coach working with the individual with a prosthesis, you would watch to see if the prosthetic limb swings excessively outward, or listen to hear if the prosthetic limb side is hitting the ground too hard.

However, if you are a biomechanist who is performing research to determine what prosthetic design works best you will need to obtain numerical data using biomechanical instrumentation. If you are a clinician, such as a physical or occupational therapist or an athletic trainer, you may also wish to obtain numerical data using biomechanical instrumentation to provide evidence that the prosthesis selected is the most appropriate prosthesis for the client. As a fitness instructor, you may wish to measure the improvement in running speed of the performer over several months. If a tool is used to measure and evaluate quantities related to space, time, motion, force, or energy during a performance to answer other questions such as, Does this new shoe model control pronation? or Is the performer effectively creating enough force to jump far enough? this is termed a **quantitative analysis**. Later in this chapter, we explore the instrumentation used for quantitative applications.

Step 6: Assess or Evaluate

After obtaining the qualitative and/or quantitative data for your performer, you must interpret the meaning of the findings in relation to the performance goals and the biomechanical principles and related movement techniques. If you were determining the optimal prosthetic design for your performer that will enhance running velocity, for example, you may have measured the amount of knee flexion that occurred when the prosthetic side limb was in contact with the ground. When comparing one prosthetic design (A) to another design (B), you observed that the knee angle values of design A were much closer than B's values to the angles generated by the nonprosthetic limb. Your assessment: Design A allowed more knee flexion than B during the landing phase, allowing for a more effective reduction of impact forces. Therefore, you recommend that design A rather than B be used for this participant.

Step 7: Provide Feedback

The last step in this process involves providing the performer qualitative and/or quantitative

feedback. As a physical educator, fitness instructor, coach, or other professional working to enhance the performance of your client, you may provide feedback about the performer's technique while the performer is learning or refining skills. If you were a clinician, you might choose to provide feedback to clients regarding technique or improvement in accomplishing tasks as they heal during a rehabilitation process or adapt to new equipment (e.g., orthotics or artificial limbs).

Overview of Knowledge in Biomechanics of Physical Activity

Knowledge in the subdiscipline of biomechanics of physical activity is largely generated from conducting biomechanical analyses. In order to give you an idea of what biomechanists have learned through research, we will investigate some fundamental concepts, research findings, and research methods via a more in-depth look at three of the steps of the analysis model (figure 11.2) that are so integral to the subdiscipline: step 4, determining the relevant biomechanical principles and movement techniques; step 5, measurement methods; and step 6, assessment and evaluation of the performer.

Applying Biomechanical Principles

Biomechanical researchers attempt to answer research questions using biomechanical principles. For example, they might ask, What causes stress fractures to the lower leg of military recruits? Is it excessive impact forces? However, before you can apply various principles to a movement situation or a research question, you must first identify the forces that are acting externally and internally on your performer. Let's start by looking at external forces.

How Do External Forces Act on Performers?

Figure 11.3a depicts the forces acting on a road racer who uses a specially designed wheelchair. See if you can identify all of the forces that act on the performer before proceeding. Figure 11.3b shows the answers.

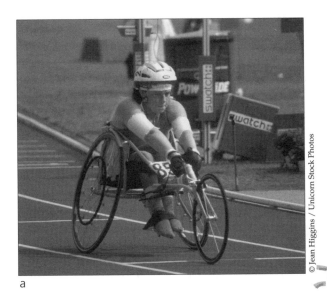

a

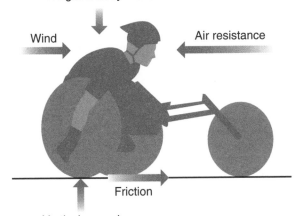

b

Figure 11.3. (a) See if you can identify the forces that are acting on a racer who uses a racing wheelchair. (b) These forces are identified here.

We all know that gravity pulls us toward the earth. The force of gravity—known as weight—is pulling the performer and the wheelchair downward. This means that the ground must be holding up the wheelchair and performer, suggesting that the ground can create force. While the wheelchair/performer causes a downward action, the ground reacts by pushing upward; hence, the ground is producing a **ground reaction force**. Also, notice that when the performer pushes on the wheel, the wheel pushes against the ground in a backward direction. The ground reacts by pushing forward, thus allowing the wheelchair and the performer to be propelled forward. This is another example of a ground reaction force.

A ground reaction force is generated any time you push against the ground (action) because the ground pushes back (reaction). Ground reaction forces (GRFs) can be created in any direction—sideways, vertically, forward, and backward. Whenever you're touching only the ground, without GRFs you couldn't go anywhere! You must push against the ground so it can move you in the opposite direction. Later in this chapter, we will explore how findings of GRF research have been used to evaluate footwear designs and to investigate causes of overuse injuries suggested to be due to vertical impact forces.

Think about a physical activity you often do—walking, cycling, basketball, volleyball. What are the effects of ground reaction forces on your movements? In what directions are these GRFs created?

Friction creates ground reaction forces in all directions but the vertical direction. Are friction forces involved in the wheelchair racing example? Most definitely! When you push against the ground in a direction parallel to the ground—left, right, backward, or forward—the ground can create ground reaction forces in the opposite directions because friction forces are created.

Air resistance also is acting on this racer, but this is often a negligible force. However, the faster a performer is moving in the air or the water, the greater the fluid forces are that act against him or her. This explains why a sprint racer who moves extremely fast might wear special clothing to reduce air resistance, whereas a slower, long-distance recreational racer would not.

The most common forces acting on a human performer include gravity, ground reaction forces, friction, and fluid resistance (air/water). A biomechanical researcher or practitioner must know what forces are relevant to the movement or research question.

How Do Internal Forces Act on Performers?

Forces also can act inside our bodies (internal forces) and affect the tissues that these forces act on. When a limb rotates, ligaments can be stretched by the inertia of the moving limb. When a person lands on the ground after jumping upward, the bones of the leg are compressed due to the vertical-impact GRFs pushing upward on the body and the inertia of the body's momentum pushing the body downward. Excessive internal forces can cause injury when they act on tissues such as ligaments, tendons, and bones. Therefore, tissue biomechanists are interested in the internal force loading on body tissues in order to understand the etiology of injury, how to design appropriate prostheses and body replacement parts, and how to increase force production by tissues such as muscles.

Figure 11.4 shows examples of some of the kinds of mechanical loading that forces produce and corresponding examples. Injuries can occur

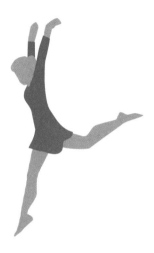

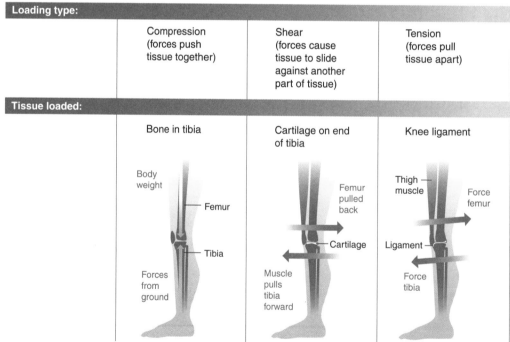

Loading type:		
Compression (forces push tissue together)	Shear (forces cause tissue to slide against another part of tissue)	Tension (forces pull tissue apart)
Tissue loaded:		
Bone in tibia	Cartilage on end of tibia	Knee ligament

Figure 11.4 Some of the types of force loading applied to human tissue (compression, shear, tension) during landing from a dance leap. Compressive loading: The shin bone (tibia) near the knee joint undergoes compression due to various forces that compress this portion of the bone. Shear loading: If the femur is pulled back and the tibia is pulled forward, the two bones are sliding past one another, causing shearing on the cartilage protecting the end of the tibia. Tensile loading: Concurrently, when the two bones are sliding in opposite directions, a knee ligament that is attached to the femur and the tibia is being stretched/pulled, thereby undergoing tension. This ligament prevents the bones from sliding too far apart.

when the magnitude and rate of loading of the forces involved or the number of repetitions involved in various movements are too great. Tissue biomechanists often measure internal forces to answer their research questions; for example, how much force can be applied to ankle ligaments before an ankle sprain will occur?

Compressive loading, which occurs when forces act to push together or compress an object, is one example of an internal force that tissue biomechanists may study. Let's explore the findings of a research study investigating internal forces that occur when a dancer lands after a leap (Simpson et al., 1997a; 1997b). During the landing, the femur (upper leg bone) pushes against the tibia (shin bone), thereby producing compressive forces of up to 16.8 times the dancer's body weight! To generate these high compressive forces, not only do the vertical GRFs contribute to the tibia being pushed upward with the inertia and weight of the body pushing the femur downward, but the strong thigh muscles also pull the two bones together.

A second finding of these studies demonstrate shear loading, another type of internal force loading. The ends of the dancer's tibia and femur slide (shear) in a forward/backward direction against each other. For the dance landing, shearing is due largely to thigh muscles attached to the front of the tibia, which slide the tibia forward. The maximum magnitude of this shear force is 5.1 times the dancer's body weight.

To prevent the tibia from shearing too far forward, one of the knee ligaments that is attached to both the femur and the tibia inside of the knee resists this action. This knee ligament becomes stretched, demonstrating a third kind of internal force—tensile loading.

As another example of research related to compressive force loading, runners and physical activity specialists have been concerned that, over a long period of time, high impact forces and/or a high rate of loading of these forces can contribute to the development of osteoarthritis (degeneration of the cartilage covering the ends of bones at a joint). This is believed to be due to the high-impact forces that act to produce high compressive loading in the lower extremity. In a review of the research about the effect of exercise and joint structure on the risk of developing osteoarthritis, Lane (1995) observed that with low-impact activities, the risk of developing osteoarthri-

tis in joints that were aligned correctly was not increased. However, athletes that had some type of joint abnormality or injury and highly competitive athletes appeared to be at risk for developing osteoarthritis. Even obese individuals who are not athletic may be predisposed to osteoarthritis due to excessive compressive loading on their weight-bearing joints. For every kilogram of extra body mass (2.2 lb of weight), investigators found a 9–13% increased risk of developing osteoarthritis (Cicuttini, Baker, & Spector, 1996).

It should be noted that although laboratory (e.g., Radin et al., 1985) and clinical evidence (e.g., Chadbourne, 1990) links excessive compressive and shear forces to various force loading (e.g., joint degeneration or stress fractures), it is not clear how injury occurs. Is it excessive force that causes injury? Certainly if the magnitude of force exceeds the maximum strength of the tissue, for instance, maximum ligament strength, the tissue will be damaged. However, researchers have shown that the number of times a tissue is loaded repetitively (e.g., the number of miles a bone in the foot is compressively loaded during running) reduces the amount of force it takes to produce an overuse injury. It is not known how many repetitions can occur before an overuse injury occurs. This would be very helpful to know; athletes could train more safely if they knew how many miles/week they could run without risking a stress fracture in their feet or legs.

Injuries can occur during impact situations when the magnitude of force applied to tissue exceeds the maximum strength of the tissue or the forces are applied to the tissue too quickly. Also, overuse injuries can occur to tissues when submaximal forces are applied to the tissue if the number of repetitions is excessive. However, it is not known how many repetitions are required during actual physical activity to produce such an injury.

To further explore tensile loading (remember the dancer's stretched knee ligament), consider pitching. Much work has been done by a team of biomechanists and orthopedic surgeons at the American Sports Medicine Institute to determine why pitchers get injured. From motion measurement data, it has been observed that elite pitchers reach peak angular velocities about the shoulder joint of 7,000 degrees/second (Dillman, Fleisig, & Andrews, 1993)! Imagine the stress that is placed on the shoulder and elbow joints when trying to decelerate the arm during the follow-through phase. In addition, the arm's inertia wants to pull the arm out of the shoulder joint. The amount of tensile force that acts on ligaments, tendons, and other connective tissue that resists the arm being pulled out of the shoulder joint (Fleisig, Barrentine, Escamilla, & Andrews, 1996) is equivalent to hanging from a bar with one arm while holding up one of your massive friends.

In conclusion, we must have an external force acting on us to make us move. In the previous description of external forces, such as ground reaction forces and friction forces, we used another physical law of nature called the Law of Action–Reaction. Internally, physical laws of nature also apply. Muscles pull on bones in order to make our limbs move. Ligaments, bones, and other structures also can determine how our limbs can move based on the laws of physics. Let's now take a more in-depth look at step 4 of the analysis process to explore how a few of these physical principles—whether related to external or internal forces—can be applied to human movement situations and biomechanical research.

How Do Physical Laws of Nature Shape Our Movement?

Whenever a physical activity practitioner or biomechanist is faced with improving performance, testing a theory about how we move, or evaluating a patient's movement, one of the most important questions to answer during the movement analysis process is, What biomechanical principles are most relevant to the performance of this movement? Remember, in step 4 of the analysis process described earlier, biomechanical principles refer to the mechanical principles and laws of nature that affect any living being. Having identified the most relevant principles for a given movement, a physical activity specialist, clinician, or biomechanist can determine how best to apply the principles to the individual performer in terms of movement techniques and/or equipment. These laws also apply to internal biomechanics, that is, what occurs inside the body.

An important skill for a physical activity specialist, biomechanist, or health-allied rehabilitative specialist is to be able to identify the relevant mechanical principles that apply to the movement of interest or to a phenomenon occurring inside the body.

To demonstrate how the mechanical laws of nature are used by biomechanists, we will examine some of the applications of Newton's laws to movement. The physical laws first described by Sir Isaac Newton affect the movement of any living being on earth. The Law of Inertia states that a body that is at rest or in motion will stay at rest or in constant motion until an external force acts on the body. This applies to many movements in which the performer is traveling through the air, for example, the long jump, dance leaps, basketball layups, and so forth. (In many of these movements, air resistance is so minimal that it can be considered negligible.)

Once the performers leave the ground, the Law of Inertia explains why they will continue to move forward with constant velocity until they hit an external object, such as the ground. These performers can do nothing to change how fast they move horizontally in the air. Performers who are trying to achieve maximal horizontal distance (e.g., the long jumper or a dancer leaping) must concentrate on generating as much velocity as they can while they are still on the ground. Indeed, the velocity at takeoff has been found to be one of the most important factors to the success of movements whereby the goal is to achieve maximal horizontal distance (Hay, 1993a).

Any performer who leaps into the air must have motion in the vertical direction. How does the Law of Inertia apply to motion in this direction? Because gravity is an external force acting on the performer, the vertical motion will not remain constant. Indeed, performers who leap into the air upward and forward will continue to move forward at a constant velocity until they land, but they will be slowing down vertically until the peak of the jump, at which point they fall back to earth.

The Law of Action–Reaction is another biomechanical principle that is very important to any performer who wants to move. It is humanly impossible to move forward without some force acting on you in the horizontal direction; unless you have something pushing you, you won't move an inch. This law states that for every action, there is an equal and opposite reaction. As shown in figure 11.5, if you push back against the ground (action), the ground will push back (reaction). Therefore, performers who want to move forward, backward, sideways, or upward as quickly as possible must learn how to push against the ground effectively so that the ground can push on them and make them move.

🔑 Examples of mechanical principles that apply to any movement include Newton's first and third laws of motion: the Law of Inertia and the Law of Action–Reaction.

💡 How does the Law of Inertia and the Law of Action–Reaction apply when you (a) run to the net while playing tennis, (b) make a jump shot in basketball, and (c) lift another person (helping them to stand)?

Several other principles help explain how best to apply force to create motion or slow down motion. Some mechanical principles can explain how rotation of a person or an object is created. Whenever a force is applied to cause an object to rotate, it is called a torque or a moment. When muscles contract (see figure 11.6), they almost always cause a limb or other body part to rotate at a joint; hence, muscles can create moments when they contract. Other principles help explain the behavior of objects as they travel through a fluid substance such as air and water. These principles help explain why a pitched baseball or softball can drop, rise, or curve, and how swimmers or bicyclists can best create propulsive forces and reduce fluid forces that slow them down.

🔑 When a force causes a limb or the entire body to rotate, it is called a torque or a moment.

Biomechanical Instrumentation and Other Tools

In step 5 of the analysis process we mentioned that biomechanical instrumentation and other tools could be used during a quantitative analysis. We will now explore the various types of tools used to measure biomechanical quantities.

What simple tools besides a tape measure can you think of that can be used to measure or observe time, movements in space, or force

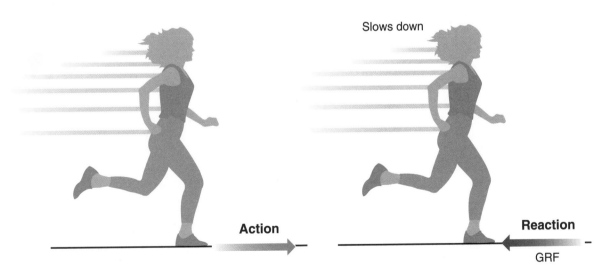

Figure 11.5 When a runner wants to move forward and upward into the air, the runner pushes down and backward (action). The ground creates a reaction by producing forces of equal magnitude that act in the opposite direction to the action. These forces produced by the ground are called ground reaction forces (GRFs).

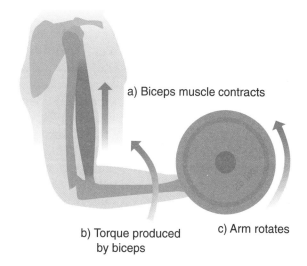

a) Biceps muscle contracts

b) Torque produced by biceps

c) Arm rotates

Figure 11.6 When muscles contract, they can make a limb rotate. Thus, they produce a torque on the limb.

quantitatively? The following are some of the instruments that may have come to mind: stopwatches or metronomes to measure time, barbells and free weights to measure how much force a person can exert, a bathroom scale to measure how much force is being pushed against it, or a video camera to capture the motion of a per-

former. From the video images, a movement specialist can measure height, lengths, and distances that a limb traveled or the length of a step taken during a dance step. A protractor can be used to measure how many degrees a limb rotated. For example, from a videotape of a fitness walker, we could evaluate with a protractor whether the walker was landing with the foot at a 40-degree angle as suggested (Yanker, 1983, p. 44).

Motion Measurement Devices

Motion measurement technology is used to track the motions of any body segment (the jaw, for example) or the entire body. Body positions, velocities, and accelerations can then be determined. One method is to use digital, video, or other camera-based technology to trace the motion of reflective markers placed on points on the human body in order to track the motion of the various body segments (figure 11.7).

Another kind of motion measurement technique uses markers placed on the body that emit signals, such as light-emitting diodes (LEDs). The signals from the markers are captured by some type of sensor to track movement. The U.S. military uses sensors to establish the position of pi-

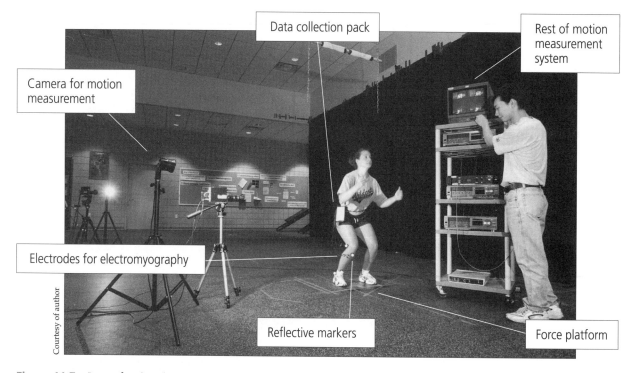

Data collection pack

Rest of motion measurement system

Camera for motion measurement

Electrodes for electromyography

Courtesy of author

Reflective markers

Force platform

Figure 11.7 Parts of various instrumentation systems. Motion measurement components include the video camera, reflective markers, other hardware, force platform, and electrodes for electromyography (EMG), and data collection pack.

lots' heads when flying. Magnetic fields are emitted by special markers on pilot helmets.

Feedback about performance techniques from motion analyses has been helpful to many elite and professional athletes in areas such as pole vaulting, gymnastics, golf, and professional baseball. This technology is used in the private sector by companies that offer services such as golf stroke analyses (Mann, Griffin, & Yocom, 1998). Motion measurement equipment is also used to analyze movements observed in occupational and clinical settings.

Instrumentation Used to Measure Forces

Measuring quantities related to force can tell us what is causing motion or injury. To measure how much force is being placed on a joint, a ligament, or an object requires attaching tiny force-measuring devices (force transducers) to tissues or artificial transplants inside the body. Because of the practical limitations of implanting devices inside the body, most knowledge about the strength of biological tissues, such as ligaments or bones, has, until recently, come from studies with cadavers.

Clinical strength-measuring devices also use transducers to measure how much force a patient can exert. Transducers are devices that convert one form of energy (e.g., mechanical) into a measurable signal. Force platforms have been used to measure how much force the ground exerts on a performer (ground reaction forces) who pushes or lands against it. Force platforms are metal plates that contain transducers that transmit electrical signals that correspond to the magnitude of force exerted on it by a performer (see figure 11.7). Usually the force platform is embedded flush to the surface. Knowledge about ground reaction forces are helpful to biomechanists for many purposes, such as the evaluation of new models of footwear or the evaluation of a patient's gait.

Pressure is the amount of force applied to a given amount of surface area. High pressure against human tissue can cause injury. If too much pressure is placed on an area of the foot of a diabetic person who cannot sense discomfort, for example, the skin in that area can deteriorate and become infected. By placing a pressure-sensitive insert inside the shoe, biomechanists or clinicians can measure the pressure exerted on the bottom of the foot. A diabetic patient who is at risk for foot infections, for example, can have an indi-

vidually tailored shoe evaluated to be sure that there are no zones of high pressure (Cavanagh, Simoneau, & Ulbrecht, 1993).

As another example, the pressure distribution of the foot can be evaluated when a person is wearing a special shoe insert (orthotic) to correct the functional problems resulting from an anatomical deformity. Pressure devices are often used inside the body to measure forces applied on joint replacements to determine the pressure distribution on the intact bone or to determine the loading on the replacement.

No matter how sophisticated it might be, instrumentation often does not permit biomechanists to measure muscle forces directly. Often motion and force platform data are used to calculate estimates of muscle forces using physics and engineering methods.

Another method of estimating muscle forces involves measuring the electrical activity of the membranes of the muscle cells (fibers) when they are stimulated by nerve cells to contract. This

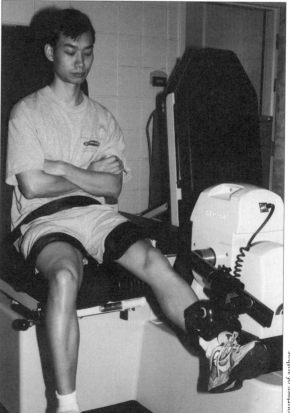

The strength-measuring device contains a force transducer to measure the amount of force the thigh muscles can generate.

Courtesy of author

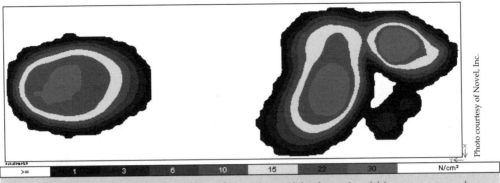

| | | 1 | 3 | 6 | 10 | 15 | 22 | 30 | N/cm² |

Photo courtesy of Novel, Inc.

Pressure distribution of bottom of foot for patient with ulceration (skin worn away down to flesh) under the big toe. The different shades represent different amounts of pressure. The middle of the heel, ball of foot, and big toe exhibit the greatest pressure zones.

method, called electromyography (EMG), requires placing electrodes on the surface or inside of muscles (see figure 11.7) where the muscle fiber membranes are most likely to be stimulated by nerve cells. When the participant performs the movement of interest, such as walking, the electrical activity in the muscles is picked up and amplified. The measured amount of electrical activity can then be converted into an estimated amount of force that the muscle produced during the movement. Although it is difficult to obtain accurate muscle force estimates using this method, EMG is being used for this purpose in complex mathematical models and for simulating movements.

EMG also has been helpful in identifying the muscles that are active during a particular movement. This also helps identify what muscles should be targeted for strength, power, or endurance training. Conversely, EMG studies of exercises can be performed to determine what muscles are being trained during an exercise. Clinicians can also use EMG to determine whether a muscle is functioning correctly. Individuals with movement disorders can also learn how to substitute the use of other muscles for a nonfunctioning muscle. Knowledge about muscle activity has led to the development of 'stimulated' walking, in which spinal-cord-injured patients can wear a device that stimulates various muscles with electricity at the right time to produce the necessary muscle forces to allow the person to walk (Kobetic, Marsolais, Samame, & Borges, 1994).

Think up a question that is of interest to you that could be answered using biomechanical analysis; for example, can people jump higher when wearing basketball shoes than when wearing cross-training shoes? How could you answer this question if you could design an experiment that uses biomechanical instrumentation?

Assessment and Evaluation of a Performer: Biomechanical Profiles

Notice that step 6 of the analysis process is to assess and evaluate the performer. In this section we will focus on the use of biomechanical profiling as an example of how this can be accomplished by practitioners who work with clients, such as athletes or patients undergoing rehabilitation. Two applications of profiling in biomechanics are discussed: performance enhancement including the issue of the existence of a "correct" technique for performing a movement, and the clinical application of comparing a patient's performance to normative performance values.

What Is a Biomechanical Profile?

An issue that has always been important since the first human began analyzing movement is determining the "best" way to perform a movement. Do elite athletes have better movement technique than novices? Do elite athletes generate more force or power than novices? The biomechanical and other characteristics representative of a group of performers—for example, elite athletes, athletes with disabilities, or novices—are called **profiles**. Profiles are used to compare one group of performers with another for a variety of purposes. One application of profiles would be to devise methods to help novice athletes improve performance by examining how elite athletes move, produce force, and otherwise exploit the laws of physics to produce an optimal performance.

Generating profiles of average individuals is useful to clinicians for comparative purposes, too. How do individuals with a particular dysfunction or disease move differently from average people? What does the torque pattern of a group of leg muscles look like if there is a suspected knee problem compared to the muscle torque pattern of a normal knee?

Profiles, or a set of biomechanical and other performer-related characteristics of a given group of individuals, provide information for comparisons with other groups of individuals, for example, individuals with dysfunctional movements versus those with average functional movements, skilled versus novice performers, injured versus noninjured clients, and so on.

Profiling is used in two primary areas: for performance enhancement in sports and for rehabilitative and other purposes.

Profiling and Performance Enhancement in Sports

If you have ever participated in an athletic activity, have you ever asked yourself, How can I improve my movement technique to perform better? Determining the "correct" technique for a sport or other movement has always been an important topic for biomechanists, coaches, and athletes.

Typically if you're like many people trying to find the best technique, you might observe how the very best athletes perform and attempt to copy their movements. Similarly, a biomechanist might determine the biomechanics of elite athletes to determine the optimal technique. This profile strategy is called the "elite athlete model" because it is assumed that elite athletes are successful as a result of using ideal technique.

Hay (1993b) investigated the techniques of elite long jumpers and found that they reach their maximal speed when running toward the takeoff board at the second-to-last step prior to takeoff. Elite jumpers slow down a little to be able to get the body in the correct position for takeoff. However, jumpers don't want to slow down too much because the faster the jumper can take off, the greater the distance jumped. In fact, for many competitive events that involve projecting the body (e.g., the long jump) or an object (e.g., a javelin), elite performers often generate more velocity to project the body/object than less skilled performers (Berg & Greer, 1995; Hay, 1993b).

Although profile databases can be very helpful in determining the biomechanics that underlie differences between elite and novice athletes, movements are shaped by factors related to the performer (see step 2, movement analysis model). For this reason it would be unreasonable to expect that the technique used for a given movement should be identical for people of different sizes, strengths, and anatomical variations.

You might assume that a very good long-distance runner would not perform wasted motions that would require energy but not help him or her move forward quickly. Cavanagh and Williams (1987) filmed runners using high-speed cameras and measured oxygen consumption (estimate of energy used) while the runners ran on a treadmill at a set speed. They were surprised to find that the best runners were not necessarily those who used the least amount of oxygen. Nevertheless, some evidence did show that the runners' technique affected their oxygen consumption. Runners who used less oxygen displayed less vertical oscillation, kept their arms from swinging in a large arc, and demonstrated other motion differences that may have represented subtle differences in muscle activity. Cavanagh and Williams concluded that each individual was naturally adopting a movement pattern based on that individual's anatomical and physiological characteristics. Therefore, while some movement techniques should enable performers to accomplish their movement goals, the techniques must be selected with the individual in mind.

Biomechanical profiles have helped researchers and coaches determine what movement techniques are related to performance effectiveness. Researchers also have found that the characteristics of each individual must also be considered when attempting to enhance performance.

Profiling as Used for Rehabilitative and Other Purposes

Clinicians supervising the rehabilitation of clients' injured tissues or helping patients perform everyday activities at a functional level are interested in the movement patterns of people who do not have injuries or dysfunctions. The movements of "average" people rather than elite athletes are assumed to be the norm in this profiling model. When we use biomechanical values of the general population rather than values of elite athletes, we are using a "normative" model.

Because walking is one of the most important and common movements that a client needs to be able to perform on a daily basis, we will use it as an example. For a movement such as walking, clinicians obtain normative values for movement characteristics such as speed, step length, cadence, and amount of knee and hip flexion, by measuring the values of many people and then averaging their scores. These normative values are considered to represent the profile for this population. These values then can be used when evaluating the movements of people with some type of movement impairment. A medical rehabilitation team may want to know if a patient's hip replacement surgery was effective by comparing the patient's step length and cadence to the normative values. If the patient is found to walk with shorter steps and at a slower cadence than other people who are similar to the patient in age, then the rehabilitation specialists and the surgeon can determine reasons and solutions to improve the patient's walking ability.

You can see that normative values would be helpful for clinicians faced with helping a client with a medical problem, for example, a stroke. By comparing the post-stroke patient's gait with the step cadence value for people of his or her age group, the clinician can determine whether the patient is functioning adequately.

Normative values, however, must be based on a population that is very similar to the client. As Craik and Dutterer (1995) noted, a variety of factors influence walking performance beyond the physical makeup of the individual's body—the age, ethnicity, experience, and physical activity level of the individual, as well as the environment in which the person walks and the person's purpose for walking. Older people may walk more slowly than younger adults, but this can be due more to factors other than age (Craik & Dutterer, 1995), such as general health, medications, strength, and so on. Finally, as we mentioned earlier, people can show many subtle differences in their movement patterns yet be able to walk at the same speed, cadence, and step length (Winter, 1991). Thus, the biomechanically smart clinician looks for a pattern of unusual values (e.g., lack of hip flexion, short time on ground when supporting the affected leg, or shifting the weight toward the nonaffected side while walking) and for reasons for these unusual values before deciding that a problem exists.

Athletic trainers who evaluate and rehabilitate injured athletes find that the normative values for athletes are different from the values for the general population. A dancer needs more flexibility than the general population, for example. Instead of using population norms, the trainer may be able to obtain preseason measures for strength and flexibility. Then, if an athlete becomes injured—for example, a football player hurts his knee—the team doctor may allow the athlete to return to competition if the player's leg strength is within 90% of the preseason value.

Generating more accurate and useful normative biomechanical values in clinical applications will remain a very important biomechanical issue in the future. The same is true for improving the profiles for occupational tasks in order to reduce the risk of job-related injuries. Ergonomists will continue to refine the profiles for tasks such as lifting, typing, and assembly-line tasks.

Biomechanists are very interested in the development of profiles containing normative biomechanical values so that clinicians can better evaluate injuries, movement disorders, and improvements in functioning. Ergonomists will continue to refine profiles of various populations for evaluating the performance of occupational tasks.

Anyone who participates in a physical activity that involves striking the ground with the foot, such as walking, running, tennis, or aerobics, has been faced with the issue of what type of footwear to wear.

The maximum amount of GRF that hits the foot during the peak of the collision phase of various activities (derived from biomechanical studies using force platforms to measure ground reaction forces, or GRFs) are shown here:

- Walking—1 to 1.3 times body weight (BW) (Winter, 1991)
- Running—2.0 BW for jogging barefoot to 7.9 BW for sprinting with spikes (see review by Nigg, 1983, p. 21)
- Low-impact aerobics and bench-step aerobics—1 and 1.6 BW, respectively (Khalil, Abdel-Moty, Rosomoff, & Rosomoff, 1993; Ricard & Veatch, 1990)
- Gymnastics—9 to 14 BW (e.g., Panzer, 1987)

A 240-pound fitness walker would therefore strike the ground with 240 to 312 pounds of force. A 100-pound gymnast could impact the ground with a peak force of 1,400 pounds during a back somersault. Placing this much stress on the body is very strenuous on the tissues of the performer over time. As mentioned earlier, researchers have observed signs of joint degeneration and other problems due to excessive impact-force magnitudes and the rapid rate of impact loading that create high compressive forces and loading rates (Noyes, DeLucas, & Torvik, 1974; Radin, Yang, Riegger, Kish, & O'Connor, 1991), although the relationship between impact force and injury hasn't been demonstrated clearly.

Many motions of the foot and leg occur during the landing phase of these activities. The foot, thigh, and lower leg flex to absorb these enormous amounts of force and to gain balance. In addition, these body segments are designed to rotate in many directions, and when the foot is on the ground, the foot has to be able to handle the rotations of the body while at the same time remaining fixed to the ground. Therefore, footwear must not only protect the body from impact forces, but also provide stability so that the foot doesn't roll excessively inward or outward or the leg doesn't twist too much at the knee joint.

Therefore, choosing the right shoe for physical activity is very difficult for most people. Footwear is not only divided by activity (e.g., running versus aerobic shoes), but also can be further specialized by other factors. For example, tennis shoes vary in their ability to provide stability. One model of tennis footwear may be great for baseline players, and another model might be better for players who like to run up to the net. To add to the confusion, extra features may be built into the shoe only to make the shoe look more appealing. Also, within the same line of footwear several models may vary in cost. Does a higher cost mean extra protection against injury? If you become a physical activity specialist, you will be asked constantly by your clients, "What shoe should I buy?" This section will help you understand some of the basic biomechanical concepts related to footwear.

Let's look at the issue of reducing vertical impact forces, which may reduce the chance of an overuse injury such as a stress fracture to a bone of the foot or lower leg. Figure 11.8 shows two typical vertical GRF-time curves exhibited by runners who land differently. The left curve demonstrates an impact peak that occurs soon after the runner touches the ground (F1). Runners who land with this style, mostly heel strikers, will want to reduce this peak. For runners who exhibit the curve shown on the right, mostly runners who land more flatfooted, the peak value (F2) may represent the maximum force to be reduced by footwear. The slope of either curve represents the rate at which

→

impact forces are being applied to the runner. For any style of runner, reducing the rate at which the vertical GRF-time curve rises is desirable, as the rate at which forces are applied to bone also is related to bone failure (e.g., Radin et al., 1985; Radin, Yang, Riegger, Kish, & O'Connor, 1991).

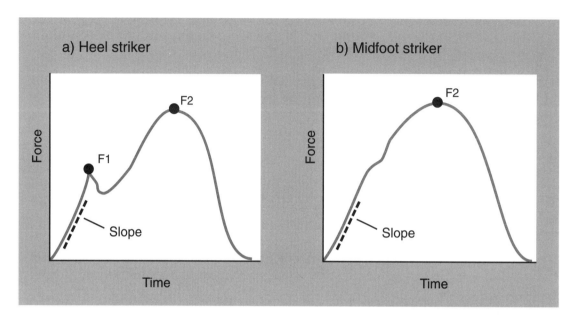

Figure 11.8 Vertical GRF-time curves of runners: (a) the pattern typically produced by runners who strike the ground heel first; (b) the pattern typical of runners who initially land more flat-footed with more of the force concentrated at the middle of the foot toward the outside edge. Biomechanists are interested in maximum impact force (F1) for a rearfoot striker, peak force (F2) for a midfoot striker, and the maximum slope of either curve that occurs between the beginning of the curve and F1 or F2. The steepness of the slope indicates how rapidly impact forces are being applied to the body. Forces that are applied at a rapid rate to bones and joints have been associated with bone injuries and cartilage degeneration.

Biomechanists have proposed that softer midsoles would absorb more of the impact forces than harder midsoles (the midsole is the middle layer of the sole that can contain several different materials for different purposes, such as cushioning and foot support). However, it is not clear if using a softer midsole material reduces impact forces or the rate of force application. Several studies (e.g., Nigg & Bahlsen, 1988; Snel, Delleman, Heerkens, & van Ingen Schenau, 1985) have shown that the impact peaks actually decreased when individuals wore harder compared to softer shoes. One explanation is that runners naturally tend to land softly when they perceive that the shoe and/or surface is hard (Robbins & Waked, 1997). Some argue that softer midsoles may not allow participants to perceive the actual magnitudes of impact forces.

This issue continues to puzzle footwear designers who want to protect their running customers from excessive loading yet "create favorable consumer impressions about the cushioning properties of their shoes" (Valiant, 1995). Think about this issue the next time you put on a new pair of shoes and start noticing how nice and cushy they feel.

Another area that concerns footwear biomechanists is stability. Clinically, considerable evidence suggests that excessive rearfoot pronation (heel rotation such that the inside of your ankle rolls toward the ground) is related to injury. For example, runners who came to clinics complaining of shin splints and inflammation of the Achilles tendon and other lower leg tendons and ligaments demonstrated excessive pronation

(Gehlsen & Seger, 1980; Nigg, Stacoff, & Segesser, 1984; Viitasalo & Kvist, 1983). Conversely, many runners who show excessive rearfoot motion do not suffer from injury (Williams, 1993). Williams notes that shoe companies claim that substantial control is needed, but no one knows how much pronation is natural or excessive.

For lateral cutting movements found in court sports, ankle sprains are a problem (Fiore & Leard, 1980), as the foot tends to roll excessively inward. By manipulating the sole design and the height of the upper, the lateral stability provided by footwear may be improved (Stacoff, Steger, Stussi, & Reinschmidt, 1996). Motion measurement analysis has shown that higher-cut shoes are better at reducing the amount of ankle rolling.

Because many factors influence a person's predisposition to injury, decisions about footwear can be frustrating. Experts have attributed the majority of running injuries to training errors such as too much distance, anatomical factors, muscle imbalances, shoes, and surfaces (see the review in Williams, 1993). Indeed, the training regimen and surfaces that a performer runs on are apt to be much more important factors in the prevention of injury than the shoes the performer wears. If a person runs on a very hard surface many hours each week, it wouldn't matter what shoes he or she wore; the shoes won't prevent injury if the runner is predisposed to impact-related injuries. In addition, little difference in energy absorption exists among shoe models (Shorten, 1993). In summary, to avoid injury, people should buy a good pair of shoes designed for a particular activity, replace them frequently, and train smart.

Footwear may help prevent certain types of injuries for those individuals predisposed to injury. However, for running, many other factors, such as the hardness of the surface, amount of training, and anatomical factors, heavily influence a person's predisposition to injury.

Wrap-Up

Whether or not you realize it consciously, the physical laws of nature act on you at all times. Biomechanists as well as other physical activity specialists can apply the principles of these mechanical laws to enhance performance; reduce injury; evaluate the effectiveness of a movement technique for athletic performance or for daily functioning; or select the proper sport equipment, tool, or occupational equipment. The theoretical knowledge regarding how mechanical principles influence our movements and the structure and function of the human body can be applied to occupational, sport, exercise, daily task, and clinical rehabilitation situations. Furthermore, an understanding of the theoretical knowledge of biomechanics as well as the use of biomechanical research methods are helpful to professionals in other subdisciplines of kinesiology, such as motor behavior, exercise physiology, and pedagogy of physical activity.

For more detailed information about biomechanics, you might browse the books and journals listed in the reference section for this chapter or search the web for biomechanics titles. To join in discussions about biomechanical issues with biomechanists, consider subscribing to one of the biomechanics listserve groups (to subscribe to Biomch-L, type **listserv@nic.surfnet.nl**). Each time you learn more about a particular physical activity, be aware of the evidence or rationale presented to convince you to try a particular movement technique or piece of equipment. Is it based on knowledge of mechanical principles and biomechanics research? Be an informed performer and smart consumer.

Study Questions

1. What is the definition of biomechanics of physical activity?

2. How has biomechanics been studied throughout various periods of time? When did biomechanics emerge as an independent subdiscipline?

3. Prior to the use of the term *biomechanics* what was this subdiscipline called?

4. Who is thought to have coined the term *biomechanics*?

5. In what types of settings do biomechanists typically work?

6. What are the most common forces acting on a human performer?

7. For each applied goal of biomechanics, provide an example of how this goal is relevant to a possible occupation of interest to you, for example, working as a physical therapist in a hospital setting. First provide a specific description of the profession and career setting. Then for each applied goal of biomechanics, list the goal and describe an example of how you, if in this career setting, would help various clients achieve the biomechanical goal.

8. Pick a movement. Determine the performance goals and influencing factors for that movement as if you were doing a movement analysis.

9. Pick a simple movement. For each of the types of loading discussed in the text (compressive, tensile, and shear), identify one or more tissues undergoing that type of loading.

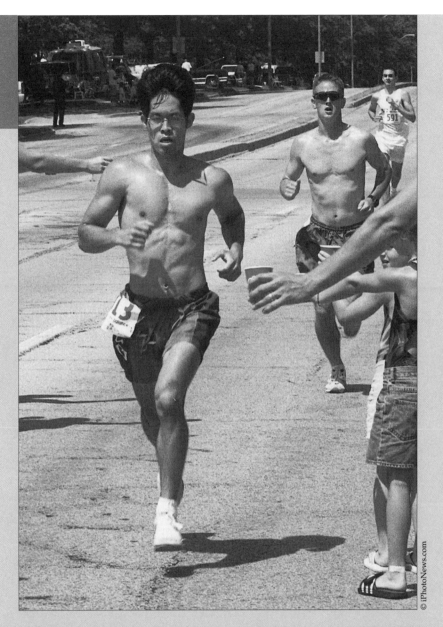

© iPhotoNews.com

Physiology of Physical Activity

Emily M. Haymes

In this chapter . . .

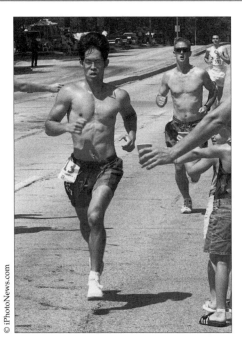

You are a recreational runner who regularly trains mainly by running on the local high school track. At the encouragement of a friend, you run in your first 10K road race. The race course finishes with a long downhill run which you run at a pace faster than your normal training pace. The next day you notice that your leg muscles are very sore, especially when walking down stairs. Why? Is the soreness due to some sort of physiological change? Did you damage the muscle while running?

Why Physiology of Physical Activity?

Our opening scenario is a good example of why people study physiology of physical activity. Running downhill for the first time is usually followed by muscle soreness 24 hours later. Students of physiology of physical activity know that this type of muscle soreness, known as **delayed onset muscle soreness**, is due to muscle damage that will repair itself over the next week. We often experience such soreness after unaccustomed physical activity that requires muscles to contract while they are lengthening. Running and walking downhill or down stairs are two examples of this type of activity. Another example is lowering a weight. The first time we do this type of strenuous activity, some of the muscle fibers are likely to tear and will have to be repaired. This is a normal physiological process that will result in a muscle fiber that is more resistant to tearing.

When students who have never studied physiology of physical activity are asked why their muscles are sore several days after exercise, they usually have no idea. Some may have heard that it is due to lactic acid accumulation inside the muscle. But they are wrong! In exercise physiology courses, students learn what happens inside muscle fibers during contractions and the role played by the cardiovascular system in removing lactic acid from the muscle during and immediately after exercise. Students also learn how techniques developed in histology (the study of tissues) and biochemistry (the chemistry of living organisms) can be used to examine muscle damage.

Although many of us may never participate in competitive running events, we all participate in various types of physical activities. Did you ever wonder why your heart is beating faster when you finish swimming several laps or after running to class, or why your muscles begin to fatigue after several repetitions of lifting a weight? These are just a few of the questions that have intrigued students of physiology of physical activity. Often called exercise physiology, the physiology of physical activity is the study of the acute physiological responses to a bout of exercise and the changes in physiological responses that occur as a result of repeated exercise bouts. It evolved as a specialization from physiology, which is the study of the body's functions. Students of exercise physiology examine not only what happens to the body during exercise but also how the responses occur. For example, the students discover that the heart beats faster as running speed increases and also learn about the mechanisms that control heart rate during exercise.

 Physiology of physical activity, often called exercise physiology, is the study of acute physiological responses to physical activity and the changes in physiological responses

to chronic physical activity. At your institution, either term may be used to designate what is essentially the same subdiscipline of kinesiology.

Knowledge of the principles of physiology of physical activity serves as the foundation for the development of conditioning programs for various sports, fitness programs for people of all ages, and rehabilitation programs for those with injuries or chronic diseases. Exercise physiology also serves as a foundation for understanding why physical activity is beneficial in reducing the risk of chronic diseases as well as the amount of energy used in different work-related physical activities required in the military and industry.

CHAPTER OBJECTIVES

In this chapter you will learn about these key topics:

- What background knowledge you already have about physiology of physical activity
- What a physiologist of physical activity does
- The goals of physiology of physical activity
- How physiology of physical activity evolved as a subdiscipline of both physiology and physical activity
- What types of research methods are used by exercise physiologists in studying physical activity
- What research has shown us about physiology of physical activity
- How physical activity can influence both fitness and health status

What Background Knowledge Do I Already Have?

Your previous physical activity experiences, your academic studies, and your observations of physical activity professionals in action have already given you some foundation for the study of physiology of physical activity.

From participating in physical activity—that is, *experiencing* physical activity—you have discovered physiological principles for yourself. You might not know the underlying physiological mechanisms, but if you have ever wondered why your body responds the way it does to physical activity, you have begun to explore the physiology of physical activity!

Perhaps you have noticed that the more intense your exercise, the faster your heart beats and the deeper and faster you breathe. Maybe you have recognized that lifting weights builds muscle strength and bulk. If you have participated in a physical activity over the long term—playing a full season of soccer or basketball, bicycling or running several days a week for six months, or taking aerobics classes for several months—you have probably realized that your body adapted to an initial level of physical activity and that to continue improving you had to run more laps and bike more miles at a faster pace, do more sit-ups, or add more intense cardiovascular and muscular work to your routine. All of these experiences have given you some knowledge of physiology of physical activity, even if you don't know the underlying physiological reasons for these responses.

Think about how your body feels after a bout of exercise. What physiological changes can you pinpoint? Consider your breathing pattern, heart rate, skin temperature, or muscle fatigue. Which change intrigues you the most? What do you suppose causes this change in your physiology?

More than likely, you have gained some background knowledge of physiology of physical activity through *scholarly study*. You probably have already taken a basic biology course in high school or college in which you learned about cell structures and functions. You also may have taken a general chemistry course in which you learned about atoms, molecules, and chemical reactions. An understanding of how cells function and the roles certain chemicals play in the body will as-

sist you in learning about the physiology of the human body and how the body responds to physical activity.

And finally, by observing physical activity *professionals* in action, you may have picked up on some physiological principles. Perhaps you have an older friend or relative who attended cardiac rehabilitation sessions after having had a heart attack. In all likelihood, an exercise physiologist oversaw the program and made recommendations regarding your friend's or family member's exercise levels. Your family doctor may have suggested that you or a member of your family exercise more regularly to improve health and fitness. This doctor's recommendations were based not only on what the medical profession has learned about exercise, but also on what physiologists of physical activity have discovered in their research about how the body responds to physical activity. Perhaps you had a coach who encouraged you to eat certain foods prior to competition—to carbo load before endurance events or to drink a lot of liquid on a hot, humid day. Your coach was applying research done by physiologists of physical activity.

You can see from figure 12.1 that physiology of physical activity is considered a subdiscipline of the biophysical sphere, along with biomechanics of physical activity. While biomechanists apply principles of physics and engineering to many physical activity situations, exercise physiologists apply principles of biology and chemistry to understand how the body responds to physical activity.

What Does a Physiologist of Physical Activity Do?

The term *exercise physiologist* is usually reserved for those who have completed a master's or doctoral degree in exercise physiology. Many exercise physiologists with doctorates are employed by colleges and universities where they teach courses in exercise physiology, anatomy and physiology, exercise testing and prescription, and nutrition and sport; conduct laboratory research on various problems such as the effects of conditioning programs on sport performance or reducing the risk of chronic diseases; and write research grant proposals that are submitted to federal

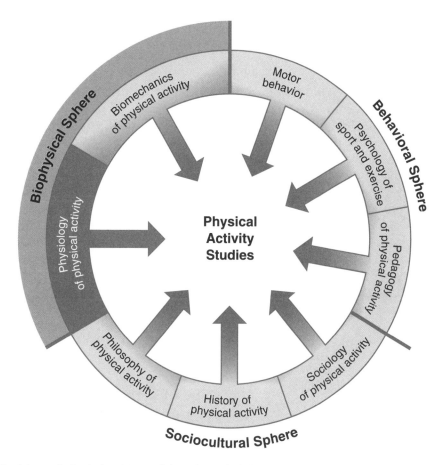

Figure 12.1   Physiology of physical activity and the other scholarly subdisciplines.

agencies (e.g., the National Institutes of Health) or foundations (e.g., the National Science Foundation) that support research on physical activity. Some exercise physiologists are employed by the military and NASA to conduct research on specific problems (e.g., preventing heat illnesses during basic training or using physical conditioning in the space shuttle to prevent bone loss).

Are you interested in a career in exercise physiology? If so, what interests you the most about the subdiscipline? Would you like to work with general recreational exercisers, athletes, cardiac rehabilitation patients, or in a laboratory doing research? You may want to visit these online sources: **www.acsm.org** and **www.acefitness.org.**

Exercise physiologists with master's degrees are frequently employed in corporate fitness or hospital-based wellness programs where they conduct exercise testing and design and conduct physical activity programs for employees or clients. Others choose to specialize in *clinical exercise physiology* and are employed by hospitals in cardiac rehabilitation programs to conduct exercise testing and supervise patient exercise programs.

Goals of Physiology of Physical Activity

In a 40th anniversary lecture at the American College of Sports Medicine's annual meeting, Brooks (1994) described the two primary goals of exercise physiology as "either the use of exercise to understand human physiology, or the use of physiology to understand human exercise." Scientists who use physical activity to understand human physiology are usually classified as basic scientists. These scientists conduct research to find out as much as possible about physiological mechanisms. They may use exercise, for example, to study blood pressure regulation. Their findings are then put to use by applied scientists to solve specific problems. Applied scientists looking to understand certain physiological phenomena or to solve certain problems in exercise physiology will use physiology to understand physical activity. They may, for example, use what basic scientists have discovered about muscle glycogen changes to understand maximal exercise performance. The goals of applied scientists may be further subdivided into the use of physiology to understand sports, fitness, and the health benefits of physical activity.

Basic scientists use physical activity to understand human physiology; applied scientists use physiology to understand physical activity.

Use of Exercise to Understand Physiology

Basic scientists' use of exercise as a tool to understand the functioning of different body systems originated in the larger and older discipline of physiology. Most of the early research was focused on the effects of exercise on the functions of organs and systems. Exercise physiologists have examined the functional responses and structural adaptations of the cardiovascular, respiratory, muscular, and endocrinological systems to different types of physical activities. Recently, research interest has focused on the responses of the reproductive, skeletal, and immune systems to acute and chronic exercise. Physical activity has proven to be a very useful tool in understanding physiological control mechanisms. For example, researchers have learned much about the role of the nervous system in the control of the respiratory system from experiments using both active and passive movements of the limbs.

The discipline of biochemistry (i.e., the chemistry of living organisms) is closely related to exercise physiology. Investigators looking to examine the fuel sources used by muscles during exercise, for example, used research techniques developed in biochemistry and physical chemistry. The use of the muscle biopsy needle by Bergstrom and Hultman (Hultman, 1967) to examine muscle glycogen concentration during exercise resulted in one of the most important advances in exercise physiology. Biochemical techniques also have been used to develop our understanding of lactate production and use of energy stores during physical activity.

Our understanding of how cells function has been greatly enhanced by research in molecular biology, one of the newest subdisciplines of biology. Molecular biological techniques are used by scientists in determining how genes regulate protein synthesis. Exercise physiologists use molecular biological techniques to help them understand how muscle protein synthesis is turned on and off by increased and decreased muscular activity (Booth, 1989).

Use of Physiology to Understand Exercise

The application of physiological techniques to understand and improve human exercise performance has been a major goal of exercise physiology since its inception. Some of the earliest studies conducted by applied scientists in the Harvard Fatigue Laboratory examined the physiological responses to strenuous exercise and training (Dill, Talbott, & Edwards, 1930; Margaria, Edwards, & Dill, 1933). The basic concepts of maximal oxygen intake, oxygen debt, and lactate production were first described early in the 20th century (Hill & Lupton, 1923). During the last 50 years applied exercise physiologists have used physiological techniques to understand and improve sport performance and physical fitness, and to understand and document the health benefits of physical activity. These three areas are discussed in the following sections.

Goals of Physiology of Physical Activity

1. To use exercise to understand human physiology
2. To use physiology to understand human exercise

3. To use physiology to improve sport performance

4. To use physiology to improve physical fitness

5. To use physiology to understand the health benefits of physical activity

Use of Physiology to Improve Sport Performance

Sport physiology has been defined as the application of "the concepts of exercise physiology to training the athlete and enhancing the athlete's sport performance" (Wilmore & Costill, 1994). Examples of the types of research conducted by sport physiologists include studies of distance running performance, overtraining in swimmers, and the effects of dehydration on wrestlers. Sport physiologists also make use of information and techniques from other disciplines and subdisciplines to enhance performance. One example is the relationship between carbohydrate intake and performance in endurance events. Sport physiologists may use information gleaned from nutrition research on the carbohydrate content of different foods to manipulate the diets of athletes to enhance glycogen storage and improve performance.

Sport physiology is the application of physiological concepts to the training of athletes.

Sport physiologists are especially concerned with the effects of the environment on sport performance. Data from sport physiology studies has been used to develop guidelines for the prevention of heat illness in sports. Prior to the 1968 Summer Olympics in Mexico City (2,200 meters [7,218 ft] above sea level), leading exercise physiologists conducted numerous studies on the acute effects of and acclimatization to altitude. Sport governing bodies used the knowledge gained from these studies to prepare their athletes for Olympic competition.

Use of Physiology to Improve Physical Fitness

Understanding the physiological determinants of physical fitness and how training programs im-

prove fitness is another important goal of exercise physiology. Interest in improving physical fitness in the United States was stimulated in the 1950s by two events—a study reporting that American children were less fit than European children and President Dwight D. Eisenhower's heart attack (Berryman, 1995). These two events led to the development of numerous training programs for improving physical fitness. Research conducted by many investigators over the past four decades has resulted in recommendations on the optimal intensity, frequency, and duration of training programs for improving physical fitness.

Exercise physiologists' interest in understanding fitness spans the entire life span. Although studies of fitness in youth and young adults have dominated, recent interest concerning the effects of physical activity and training in the elderly has increased. Such studies provide linkages between exercise physiology and the disciplines of human growth and development and gerontology (the study of aging). The influence of heredity on physical fitness components and trainability has recently attracted considerable research interest among exercise physiologists. Much of this interest has been stimulated by the work of Claude Bouchard and his colleagues with identical twins.

The physiology of fitness is also closely linked with psychology and the subdiscipline of exercise and sport psychology. Understanding why some people adhere to training programs and others drop out has led to various strategies for motivating people to become physically active. The perceived exertion scales developed by Borg (1973) are another example of the linkage between exercise physiology and psychology. As we saw in chapter 4, Borg developed numerical scales that allow people to report how easy or hard they perceive they are working. These scales have proven to be very useful in monitoring exercise intensity without additional equipment because an individual's perception of exercise intensity is directly related to heart rate.

Use of Physiology to Understand the Health Benefits of Physical Activity

Another major goal of exercise physiology is to understand the relationship between physical activity and disease prevention. Although exercise has been thought to have health benefits for over a century, the first scientific evidence to support this belief was not reported until the 1950s (Paffenbarger, 1994). Many studies have examined the relationship of physical activity and physical fitness to coronary heart disease, and much is known today about the role of exercise in reducing the risk factors for coronary heart disease in men. Less is known about the relationship of physical activity to heart disease in women. Understanding the role of physical activity in preventing other diseases such as non-insulin-dependent diabetes, osteoporosis, and cancer is attracting much research attention at the present time.

Sometimes exercise physiologists are interested in the big picture—how physical fitness can prevent disease in large populations. In such cases, exercise physiologists might collaborate with specialists in epidemiology, using two different types of studies—longitudinal (comparing the same group of people over several time periods) and cross-sectional (comparing different groups of people).

Physiologists who study the role physical activity plays in disease management and rehabilitation are known as clinical exercise physiologists. Students training in this area must also become familiar with basic concepts in several medical specialties such as cardiology and pulmonary medicine and work under the direction of a clinician.

History of Physiology of Physical Activity

Physiology of physical activity evolved from physiology in the 18th century after Antoine Lavoisier discovered that animals use oxygen and produce carbon dioxide (U.S. Department of Health and Human Services, 1996). As a result, scientists began exploring how humans respond to physical activities and daily work tasks (e.g., lifting loads).

Early History

One of the first studies to report the physiological responses to physical activity appeared in the late 18th century. Investigators discovered that the oxygen consumption of a person lifting a 16-pound (7.3 kg) weight was 2.5 times greater than that of the same person at rest (Dill, 1974). In 1871 investigators at Columbia University conducted another early physiological study of physical activity. They studied a single subject before, during, and after walking more than 300 miles (482 km) in five days and found that he lost body protein (muscle mass) during the prolonged walk (Dill, 1974).

Technological developments in the late 19th and early 20th centuries stimulated research in exercise physiology. The Haldane gas analyzer allowed physiologists to measure the amount of oxygen, nitrogen, and carbon dioxide in expired air, and the Tissot spirometer allowed them to measure accurately the volume of air expired.

The first exercise physiology laboratory in the United States was established in the Department of Anatomy, Physiology, and Physical Training at Harvard in 1891 (Berryman, 1995). Development of the motor-driven treadmill and the cycle ergometer in 1913 allowed researchers to control more precisely the amount of work done during an exercise test. Research conducted at the Carnegie Nutrition Laboratory by Francis G. Benedict and colleagues in the early part of the 20th century was the first to use the cycle ergometer and motor-driven treadmill to determine how much energy was expended during walking, running, and cycling (Dill, 1974).

One of the early contributors to our understanding of the physiology of physical activity was August Krogh of the University of Copenhagen. Krogh developed one of the first cycle ergometers, which he used to study the physiological responses to exercise. He received the Nobel Prize for physiology in 1920 for his research on the regulation of microcirculation (Åstrand, 1991). His research with Johannes Lindhard on the relative contribution of fat and carbohydrate to energy expenditure is a classic that exercise physiology students still read today; it established that carbohydrate diets improve the efficiency of exercise (Krogh & Lindhard, 1920). During the 1920s and 1930s Krogh's laboratory attracted three young physiologists, Erling Asmussen, Erik Hohwü-Christensen, and Marius Nielsen, who were to make major contributions to our understanding of the physiology of physical activity.

The work of A.V. Hill, Joddrell Professor of Physiology at University College, London, in the 1920s was a major stimulus of much of the early research in exercise physiology. He received the Nobel Prize for his work on energy metabolism in 1921. Many of the basic concepts of exercise physiology concerning oxygen consumption, lactate production, and oxygen debt were presented in a classic paper by Hill and Lupton in 1923. In 1926 Hill visited the United States where he presented a series of lectures at Cornell University, Ithaca, New York, and the Lowell Institute in Boston. During his trip to Boston he visited Arlie Bock's research laboratory at Massachusetts General Hospital. Bock had become well known for his work on blood gases during exercise and had pioneered the arterial puncture technique (Dill, 1985). Working with Bock were L.J. Henderson and a postdoctoral fellow named David Bruce Dill, who were instrumental in founding the Harvard Fatigue Laboratory.

The Harvard Fatigue Laboratory (1927–1946) had a profound influence on exercise physiology research in the United States and Europe.

Two laboratories that developed in physical education departments also had a major impact on research in exercise physiology. Peter V. Karpovich established an exercise physiology laboratory at Springfield College in 1927 (Kroll, 1982). Karpovich became particularly well known for his research on the effects of ergogenic aids on physical performance and as one of the founders of the American College of Sports Medicine. Thomas K. Cureton, Jr., established an exercise physiology laboratory at the University of Illinois in 1944. This laboratory became well

In Profile

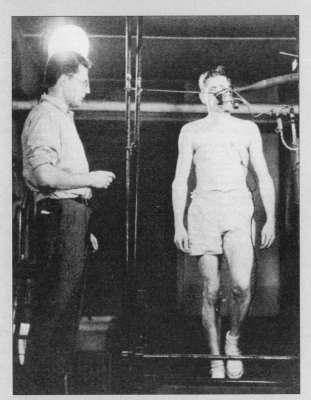

Harvard Fatigue Laboratory

The Harvard Fatigue Laboratory, founded in 1927, was the brainchild of L.J. Henderson, a physical chemist. David Bruce Dill was the director of the lab. The lab included a room containing a treadmill borrowed from the Carnegie Nutrition Lab (see photo), a large gasometer, a room for basal metabolism studies, an animal room, and a climatic room (Dill, 1967). Among the areas of research undertaken by this lab were environmental studies conducted at high altitude, in the desert, and in steel mills.

Although the Harvard Fatigue Laboratory was in existence only until 1946, it had a profound effect on exercise physiology research in the United States and Europe during the second half of the 20th century. Many young investigators received their formative training in the laboratory as postdoctoral or doctoral students, including Ancel Keys, R.E. Johnson, Sid Robinson (on treadmill in photo), and Steve Horvath. Among the many international scientists who spent time in the lab were Lucien Brouha, Belgium; Rodolfo Margaria, Italy; and E.H. Christensen, Erling Asmussen, and Marius Nielsen, Denmark (Dill, 1967). All of these investigators went on to establish their own laboratories and were responsible for training many of the leading investigators in physiology of physical activity over the past 50 years.

known for its studies on physical fitness. Many of the leading investigators of the physiology of fitness received their training in Cureton's laboratory.

Significant Events Since 1950

Two of the most important events that have stimulated research on the physiology of physical activity since 1950 occurred in England and Sweden. In 1953 Jeremy Morris and colleagues published their study on coronary heart disease and physical activity in which they found that London bus drivers had a significantly higher risk than conductors on double-decked buses (Morris, Heady, Raffle, Roberts, & Parks, 1953). Although the original study was widely criticized for failure to control for other variables (e.g., obesity, hypertension), it was responsible for stimulating interest in epidemiological research on physical activity, physical fitness, and chronic disease (Paffenbarger, 1994). Morris's research also stimulated studies of the effects of fitness and endurance training on risk factors for coronary heart disease (e.g., serum cholesterol, blood pressure).

The introduction of the biopsy needle for sampling muscle glycogen during exercise by Jonas Bergstrom and colleagues in Sweden in 1966 led to research on human muscle energy sources (e.g., ATP, creatine phosphate), muscle mitochondria, and muscle fiber types by other investigators who were interested in the biochemistry of exercise. Prior to that time, researchers had conducted studies on muscle metabolism during exercise on animal models. Two of the early scientists to use the biopsy technique to study muscle metabolism during exercise were Bengt Saltin and Phil Gollnick. Their studies have made major contributions to our understanding of the acute and chronic effects of exercise on human muscle fiber composition and metabolism. These studies also were responsible for stimulating much of the present-day interest in the cellular responses to exercise.

In 1954 a group of physiologists, physical educators, and physicians who were interested in promoting scientific research on sport, health, and human fitness founded the American College of Sports Medicine (ACSM). Joseph B. Wolffe, a cardiologist, was elected the first president of ACSM. In 1969 ACSM began publishing *Medicine and*

Science in Sports, which was the first scientific journal in the United States dedicated to sport science. The name of the journal was subsequently changed to *Medicine and Science in Sports and Exercise* in 1980. ACSM has had a significant impact on the direction of exercise physiology in the United States. In the early 1970s ACSM established a certification program in clinical exercise physiology, and the first edition of its *Guidelines for Graded Exercise Testing and Exercise Prescription* was published in 1975. The first ACSM Position Stand on the prevention of heat injuries during distance running was also released in 1975.

Interest in the anthropometric (body measurements) and physiological characteristics of Olympic athletes began with studies conducted at the 1928 Summer Olympics in Amsterdam by members of the newly formed Fédération Internationale de Médecine du Sport (FIMS) (Park, 1995). The selection of Mexico City as the site of the 1968 Summer Olympic Games stimulated not only scientific studies on the effects of altitude on sport performance but also a more general interest in the use of exercise physiology to improve sport performance. The U.S. Olympic Committee established its Sports Physiology Laboratory at the Olympic Training Center in Colorado Springs in 1978.

Although the first reports of amenorrhea (i.e., fewer than three menses per year) among women athletes appeared in the 1970s, the first study reporting low bone densities in amenorrheic athletes was not published until 1984 (Drinkwater, Nilson, Chesnut, Bremner, Shainholtz, & Southworth, 1984). This study by Barbara Drinkwater and her colleagues stimulated much interest in the role of exercise and sport in the development of amenorrhea, bone loss, and osteoporosis. It also marked a more general shift in interest toward the role of physical activity in women's health issues.

Two of the most important events in the 1990s involved the release of official statements by U.S. government agencies on the role of physical activity in the prevention of chronic diseases. The first followed an NIH Consensus Development Conference on Physical Activity and Cardiovascular Health held in December 1995. Among the consensus development panel's conclusions were that "physical inactivity is a major risk factor for cardiovascular disease" and "moderate levels of physical activity confer significant health benefits" (NIH Consensus Development Panel on Physical Activity and Cardiovascular Health, 1996). The second statement was the first Surgeon General's Report on Physical Activity and Health by the U.S. Department of Health and Human Services in 1996 (see chapter 2). The report concluded that regular physical activity, in addition to reducing the risk of heart disease, also reduces the risk of diabetes, hypertension (high blood pressure), and colon cancer, and helps control body weight (U.S. Department of Health and Human Services, 1996).

Both the National Institutes of Health (NIH) and the surgeon general concluded that moderate physical activity is beneficial in reducing the risk of chronic diseases (i.e., heart disease, diabetes, hypertension, and colon cancer).

Research Methods in Physiology of Physical Activity

In order to understand the physiological responses and adaptations to physical activity, researchers developed and standardized specific research techniques and methodologies. Research in exercise physiology primarily involves using quantitative techniques to measure changes in physiological responses. However, researchers realized early on that studies conducted in different laboratories could only be compared if the techniques were standardized. For example, investigators wanting to compare oxygen uptake (e.g., volume of oxygen used) of cyclists tested at the U.S. Olympic Training Center in Colorado Springs and at the Florida State University in Tallahassee must first reduce gas volumes (e.g., volume of gas inhaled and exhaled) to a standard

Historical Time Line

1777	Antoine Lavoisier discovers that animals use oxygen and produce carbon dioxide.
1891	The first exercise physiology laboratory in the U.S. is established at Harvard University.
1910s	F.G. Benedict conducts research on energy expenditure during exercise at the Carnegie Nutrition Laboratory.
1920	August Krogh wins the Nobel Prize for research on microcirculation.
1921	A.V. Hill wins the Nobel Prize for research on energy metabolism.
1927–1946	The Harvard Fatigue Laboratory conducts research on exercise and environmental physiology.
1953	Jeremy Morris publishes research on coronary heart disease and physical activity.
1954	The American College of Sports Medicine is founded.
1966	The first research using muscle biopsy technique to measure muscle glycogen is published.
1969	*Medicine and Science in Sports* begins publication.
1975	*Guidelines for Graded Exercise Testing and Exercise Prescription* is published.
1980	*Medicine and Science in Sports* becomes *Medicine and Science in Sports and Exercise*.
1984	The first studies reporting amenorrhea related to low bone density in women athletes are published.
1995	The NIH Consensus Development Conference on Physical Activity and Cardiovascular Health is held in Bethesda, Maryland.
1996	The first Surgeon General's Report on Physical Activity and Health is released.

temperature and pressure (STPD) at both sites because gas volumes are affected by both temperature and pressure. At higher altitudes such as Colorado Springs, the gas volume will be larger due to the lower barometric pressure (Boyle's Law—the volume of a gas is inversely proportional to its pressure when the temperature of the gas is constant). For this reason, researchers always correct gas volumes to sea level barometric pressure (760 torr) when calculating oxygen uptake.

Ergometers

In order to standardize the measurements of exercise intensity, researchers developed specific types of exercise equipment called ergometers. Cycle ergometers and motorized treadmills are the two most commonly used ergometers in exercise physiology. Both have their advantages and disadvantages.

Cycle ergometers are useful for comparing subjects at the same absolute exercise intensity regardless of body weight. This is especially helpful when conducting research at submaximal (low to moderate) exercise intensities. Physical work can also be calculated easily with a cycle ergometer. Blood pressure measurements and blood sampling during exercise are easier to ob-

tain while cycling because the arm is stationary. The major disadvantages of the cycle ergometer are that peak oxygen uptake is generally lower and fatigue occurs earlier because only the legs are used.

🔑 Cycle ergometers and motorized treadmills are used to standardize the intensity of exercise.

Motorized treadmills allow subjects to be tested during walking and running at different speeds. Exercise intensity at a constant speed can be increased by increasing the slope (grade) of the treadmill. For studies of moderate to heavy exercise, treadmills are preferable to cycle ergometers because running is more strenuous than cycling for most people. Researchers have to account for subjects' body weight when using the treadmill, however. Obviously, a heavier person walking or running at the same speed and grade as a lighter person will work harder since body weight is lifted with every step. Measuring blood pressure and sampling blood are more difficult on the treadmill, especially during running, because the arm is moving.

Other types of ergometers are used in some settings. Arm ergometers are used to study up-

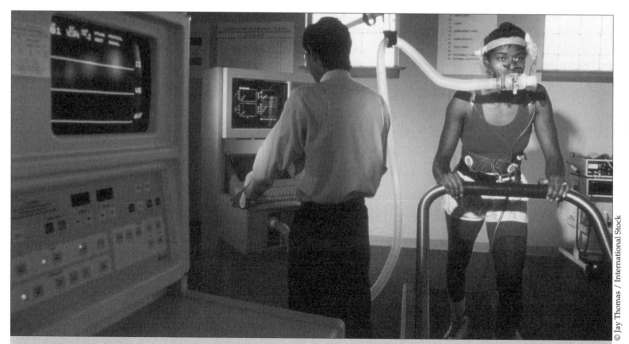

Using the treadmill to control the exercise intensity while testing a subject.

© Jay Thomas / International Stock

per body exercise. The swimming flume, developed in Sweden, has been used to study the physiological responses to swimming. Rowing ergometers are particularly useful in studying oarsmen.

Some research studies must be conducted "in the field"—that is, outside of a laboratory, in subjects' natural exercise environments. Such studies can prove useful, but they present some difficulties for researchers. Controlling physical activity intensity and environmental conditions is much more difficult in field studies. Fortunately, such studies have become more feasible in recent years as a result of the development of low-cost battery-powered monitors that store heart rates.

Oxygen Uptake

The most commonly used research method in exercise physiology is the measurement of oxygen uptake. This requires measuring the volume of oxygen and carbon dioxide in expired (exhaled) air. Early investigators collected the expired air in Douglas bags and analyzed the gas concentrations using chemical (Haldane or Scholander) analyzers. The volume of gas in the bag was then measured in a Tissot spirometer. Such analysis was tedious and time consuming. Investigators in modern laboratories measure gas concentrations with electronic analyzers, and gas volumes with flow meters or pneumotachometers. When these devices are interfaced with computers, they provide nearly instantaneous and continuous information on oxygen uptake.

By measuring oxygen uptake, researchers can obtain valuable information on how the muscles use oxygen and how much energy is expended during physical activity. The most widely accepted method for determining the cardiorespiratory (aerobic) fitness state of an individual is to increase the intensity of exercise progressively until a plateau in oxygen uptake is observed. This plateau represents **maximal oxygen uptake**. Physiologists also use submaximal exercise tests to estimate cardiorespiratory fitness. These tests don't require individuals to work to achieve maximal oxygen uptake (an arduous task for some people), but rather use the relationship between heart rate and oxygen uptake to estimate oxygen uptake at the age-predicted maximal heart rate (this is determined by subtracting the person's age from 220).

Maximal oxygen uptake is the most commonly used indicator of cardiorespiratory fitness.

Body Composition

Body composition is measured in most exercise physiology laboratories in order to determine the percentage of body fat in individuals. The gold standard for determining body composition in humans is the hydrostatic weighing technique, also known as **underwater weighing**, in which the individual is weighed while completely submemged underwater. This technique makes use of the Archimedes Principle that the weight of the water displaced by an object is equal to the volume of the submerged object (density = mass/volume). Once body density has been determined, equations derived from chemical analyses of human cadavers are used to estimate the amount of body fat.

The hydrostatic weighing technique is the most widely accepted technique for determining body density and body composition.

Physiologists have developed numerous other techniques for estimating body density including measuring total body water using isotopes (e.g., deuterium), subcutaneous fat thickness with skin-fold calipers, tissue impedance with bioelectric impedance analyzers (BIA), and bone mineral density with dual energy X-ray analyzers (DXA). Skin-fold thickness measurements are the most commonly used technique because the calipers are relatively inexpensive, portable, and can be used to screen large numbers of subjects in a short period of time. Skin-fold measurements are made at several sites, usually three or more, and either the thickness of individual sites or the sum of all sites is used in an equation to estimate body density.

Biochemical Methods

Exercise physiologists also use biochemical methods to examine changes at the tissue and cellular levels during and following physical activity. These invasive techniques include taking blood samples and muscle biopsies. Blood samples are obtained from either venipuncture of superficial

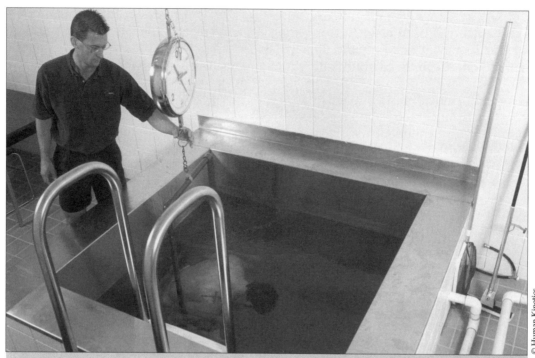

Person having his body density measured using the hydrostatic weighing technique.

arm veins or finger pricks, depending on the size of the sample needed. Monitoring changes in the concentration of various blood constituents is useful in determining energy substrate utilization, acid–base balance, dehydration, immune function, and endocrine responses to acute and chronic physical activity.

One of the most commonly used biochemical techniques in exercise physiology is the measurement of blood lactate from fingertip samples taken during exercise as an indicator of anaerobic metabolism. Once blood samples are obtained, exercise physiologists use appropriate chemical equipment such as centrifuges, spectrophotometers, pH electrodes, high-pressure liquid chromatography (HPLC), and radioimmunoassays (RIA) to analyze the samples.

Physiologists use muscle biopsies obtained before and after exercise to examine changes in energy substrates (e.g., glycogen, triglycerides), lactate production, and enzyme activity. Chemical methods used to analyze tissues help them determine muscle fiber types in the biopsy samples. Examination of muscle tissue samples under an electron microscope is useful in determining structural changes following different types of training as well as structural damage after exercise.

Magnetic resonance spectroscopy (MRS) is one of the newest techniques used in studying skeletal muscle metabolism during exercise. In this technique, a person contracts the muscles of a limb (i.e., one leg) inside a large doughnut-shaped magnet. This noninvasive technique is used to measure continuously two high-energy phosphate compounds, **adenosine triphosphate** (ATP) and phosphocreatine (PC), during physical activity. MRS has proven to be a useful technique for studying the relationship of energy supply and muscular work as well as the potential causes of muscle fatigue (Kent-Brown, Miller, & Weiner, 1995).

What one aspect of your sport performance or physical fitness would you like to improve? If you were to enter a training program to improve this aspect, which research method would you use to measure the physiological changes related to your performance or fitness level before the training and after the training?

Animal Models

The effects of physical activity on some organs cannot be studied easily in human subjects. Examples include the brain, heart, liver, and diaphragm. Researchers use animals (e.g., rats) to examine both the functional and structural changes that occur in response to single and repeated bouts of exercise. Animal treadmills and running wheels monitor the quantity of exercise.

One of the major advantages in using animals in physiological research is that both the subjects and the environment can be more carefully controlled than is possible with human subjects. Another advantage is that some experimental techniques not approved for human use can be used to study physiological responses. An example would be the injection of radioactive isotopes of iron to study changes in tissue iron stores with training. Use of animals with genetic abnormalities has also proven useful in examining the effects of exercise on certain clinical disorders such as obesity and hypertension. Most of the studies that have applied the techniques of molecular biology to examine exercise have used animal models.

One major criticism of animal research is that not all physiological and chemical mechanisms observed in animal species are identical to those observed in humans. There is some truth to this assertion. For example, growth hormone produced in humans is not identical to that of any other species. Changes in tissues due to training also may differ among species. Investigators must be careful to select the animal, usually a mammal, that most closely reflects human responses to physical activity.

Regardless of whether researchers have used humans or animals to study the physiological responses to exercise, our knowledge of the physiology of physical activity is based on the results of thousands of research studies that have been conducted over the past century.

Overview of Knowledge in Physiology of Physical Activity

Physiologists have studied responses to single and repeated bouts of physical activity exten-

sively over the past century. Much of this research has centered on three body systems: the muscular, cardiovascular, and respiratory systems. The influence of environmental factors such as temperature, diet, and altitude on physiological responses and performance has also been examined carefully. This overview will first examine how physiological systems respond to physical activity and then discuss other factors that influence physiological responses.

Skeletal Muscles

The only way your body can move is by contracting muscles. The muscles you use to perform any form of physical activity, from lifting a stack of books to running a road race, are skeletal muscles, which are under the control of the nervous system. Each muscle is composed of many muscle cells, which are called muscle fibers. Inside the muscle fiber many myofibrils run the length of the fiber. The myofibrils contain the contractile elements that shorten to move your bones during physical activity. Three main types of muscle fibers have been identified in human skeletal muscles.

Physical activity (movement) can occur only when skeletal muscles contract.

Muscle Fiber Types

Did you ever wonder why some people can run extremely fast for short distances (e.g., the length of a football field) while other people are much better at running long distances (e.g., a marathon)? It is very likely that muscle fiber types in the leg muscles of these individuals are different. Muscle fiber types are classified according to the speed at which they contract as fast twitch (FT) and slow twitch (ST). Fast-twitch fibers are further subdivided according to the energy system they use (these are explained in greater detail in the next section). Fast-twitch fibers that use anaerobic (without benefit of oxygen) energy systems almost exclusively are named fast glycolytic (FG) fibers, while fast-twitch fibers that use both aerobic (also called oxidative) and anaerobic (also called glycolytic) energy systems are called fast oxidative glycolytic (FOG) fibers. Slow-twitch fibers primarily use aerobic energy systems. Characteristics of the three fiber types are presented in table 12.1.

During light- to moderate-intensity exercise such as walking to class or jogging, slow-twitch fibers are recruited first. Because these fibers fatigue very slowly, light to moderate physical activity can be sustained for prolonged periods of time. As the intensity of activity increases, FOG fibers are recruited next with the FG fibers recruited at the highest intensities (e.g., an all-out sprint). Although the FG fibers produce much greater force and power, they fatigue rapidly. Thus, the highest intensities of physical activity can be sustained for only short periods of time (less than one minute).

Energy Sources

In order for a muscle to contract, it must have an adequate energy supply. Three different energy systems are used to supply the energy we need during physical activity: the ATP-phosphocreatine system, the glycolytic system, and the aerobic system. The ATP-phosphocreatine system is used during the first 10 to 15 seconds of activity, the glycolytic system is used for maximal exercise lasting 1 to 2 minutes, and the aerobic system is the primary source of energy in activities lasting more than 2 minutes.

ATP-Phosphocreatine System. No work can be completed without a source of energy to drive it. This principle applies to machines as well as human muscles. The primary source of energy for muscle contraction is a high-energy phosphate compound called adenosine triphosphate (ATP). When a muscle fiber contracts, ATP is split into adenosine diphosphate (ADP) and an inorganic phosphate (P). During rapid muscle contractions, ADP can combine with phosphocreatine (PC), another high-energy phosphate compound stored inside the muscle fiber, to resynthesize a single molecule of ATP. The newly synthesized molecule of ATP can then be split to release the energy needed for another muscle contraction.

$$ATP \longrightarrow ADP + P + energy$$
$$ADP + PC \longrightarrow ATP + Cr$$

Because the quantities of ATP and PC stored in muscle fibers are relatively small, high-intensity exercise cannot be supported by the ATP-PC system for more than 10 to 15 seconds (figure 12.2). We use this energy system when we sprint down a basketball court.

Glycolytic System. But suppose you want to run a longer distance (e.g., around a 400-meter track)

TABLE 12.1
Muscle Fiber Type Characteristics

Characteristics	Fiber type		
	Slow twitch	Fast oxidative glycolytic	Fast glycolytic
Contraction speed	Slow	Fast	Fast
Force	Low	High	High
Mitochondria	Many	Many	Few
Capillaries	Many	Many	Few
Myoglobin	High	High	Low
Anaerobic capacity	Low	High	High
Aerobic capacity	High	Moderate	Low
Fatigue	Slowly	Intermediate	Rapidly

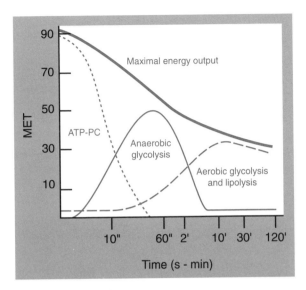

Figure 12.2 Relative contribution of the ATP-PC, anaerobic glycolysis, and aerobic glycolysis and lipolysis energy systems over time during physical activity.
Reprinted, by permission, from J.S. Skinner and D.W. Morgan, 1985, Aspects of anaerobic performance. In *Limits of Human Performance. The Academy Papers No. 18*, edited by D.H. Clarke and H.M. Eckert (Champaign, IL: Human Kinetics), p. 32.

as fast as you can. Because you deplete the phosphocreatine during the first 15 seconds, another source of energy must also be used. Muscle fibers also store glycogen, a complex carbohydrate composed of long strands of glucose molecules. During activity, glucose is released from glycogen and is broken down by enzymes (e.g., biological catalysts) to form pyruvic acid in a pathway known as glycolysis. The glycolytic pathway does not require oxygen and is therefore anaerobic. If inadequate oxygen is present inside the muscle fiber, some pyruvic acid will be converted to lactic acid. The breakdown of a single glucose molecule to lactic acid results in a net increase of 3 ATP molecules, which, as you know, are the energy units for muscular work. However, because muscles cannot tolerate excessive buildups of lactic acid, activities requiring anaerobic glycolysis can continue for only 1 to 2 minutes (see figure 12.2). If you have ever experienced a burning sensation in your muscles while exercising strenuously, it was because you were producing lactic acid. Examples of activities that are likely to produce lactic acid are riding a bicycle uphill and swimming 100 meters as fast as possible.

🔑 The anaerobic breakdown of glycogen produces lactic acid.

Aerobic System. If, on the other hand, you were engaging in prolonged physical activity, such as running a 10K race or hiking up a mountain, you would need energy from yet another system at your disposal. Energy for these kinds of activities is produced by aerobic glycolysis and lipolysis (see figure 12.2). In the presence of oxygen, pyruvic acid enters the muscle **mitochondria** and is broken down completely in a process called the Krebs cycle. Hydrogen ions are removed during this process and enter the electron transport system where they are used to resynthesize ATP. The aerobic breakdown of a single glucose molecule in this system will produce carbon dioxide (CO_2) and water (H_2O) and results in a net increase of 38 ATP molecules—quite an increase from the 3 molecules created in the glycolytic system.

$$C_6H_{12}O_6 + 6\ O_2 \longrightarrow 6\ CO_2 + 6\ H_2O + 38\ ATP$$
(Glucose)

The length of time muscle glycogen can continue to supply energy is determined by the amount of glycogen stored in the active muscles and the intensity of the activity. High-intensity activities (e.g., 80–90% of the maximal heart rate) deplete muscle glycogen stores more rapidly than moderate-intensity activities (e.g., 60–79% of the maximal heart rate). Muscle glycogen stores are depleted in approximately 90 minutes during high-intensity exercise. Soccer is an example of a high-intensity sport in which muscle glycogen stores are very low at the end of a match. If the muscle glycogen in fast-twitch muscles is depleted, the athlete will not be able to sprint in the latter part of the match.

Blood glucose can also be used by skeletal muscles for energy production. Glycogen stored in the liver is broken down to glucose, which enters the blood and is used by most cells of the body as a source of energy.

During light and moderate activity (e.g., walking), fat is a major contributor of energy for muscle contraction. The greatest amount of energy stored in the body is stored as fat. Fats (triglycerides) are stored in adipose tissue located throughout the body, and small quantities of fat are located in the muscles. Triglycerides are broken down (lipolysis) to free fatty acids and glycerol that enter the blood. Fatty acids can enter the muscle fiber where, in the presence of oxygen, they are broken down to carbon dioxide and water in the mitochondria. The amount of energy released in this process that can be used to resynthesize ATP depends on the length of the fatty acid. A single molecule of palmitic acid, which is an example of a 16-carbon fatty acid typically found in adipose tissue, will yield approximately 129 ATP molecules. This is more than three times the amount of energy released from a single glucose molecule.

$$C_{16}H_{32}O_2 + 23\ O_2 \longrightarrow 16\ CO_2 + 16\ H_2O + 129\ ATP$$

As you can see, lipolysis, or the breakdown of fats, offers by far the most energy of the three systems to allow you to undertake prolonged bouts of light to moderate exercise. Because you have large amounts of stored body fat that can be mobilized and used for energy during light to moderate physical activity, you can walk or hike for many hours without becoming fatigued. Table 12.2 summarizes the use of the different energy systems during sports and physical activities.

 In the presence of adequate oxygen, fatty acids are a major contributor of energy for muscle contraction.

Think of the sport, exercise, or leisure activity you participate in most frequently. Which energy systems do you use primarily during this physical activity, and at what point in your activity is each system used?

Adaptations to Anaerobic and Aerobic Training

Repeated exercise bouts that are anaerobic in nature (i.e., high-intensity, short-duration activi-

TABLE 12.2
The Different Energy Systems Used During Sports and Physical Activity

ATP-PC system

- Initial, high-intensity physical activity
- Used during the first 10–15 seconds
- Used in any sprint up to 100 meters (e.g., basketball, soccer, football, field hockey, softball)

$$ATP \longrightarrow ADP + P + energy$$
$$ADP + PC \longrightarrow ATP + Cr$$

Glycolytic sytem

- Kicks in after ATP-PC system cannot support the activity
- Primary source of energy during first 1–2 minutes of high-intensity exercise
- Used in the following sports events: 400- and 800-meter run, 100- and 200-meter swimming events, 500- and 1000-meter speed skating events, Alpine skiing events

Aerobic system

- Primary energy system used during prolonged continuous light and moderate intensity activities
- Uses both carbohydrates and fats as energy sources
- Used in walking, jogging, distance running (e.g., 5000 meters and longer), cycling, swimming laps, triathlons, cross-country skiing

$$Glucose \longrightarrow CO_2 + H_2O + ATP$$
$$Fatty\ acids \longrightarrow CO_2 + H_2O + ATP$$

ties such as sprinting) increase the activities of enzymes (proteins that act as biological catalysts) involved in the ATP-PC and glycolytic systems. Increased activity in key muscle enzymes such as creatine phosphokinase (CPK), phosphofructokinase (PFK), and lactate dehydrogenase (LDH) suggests an increased capacity to resynthesize ATP during high-intensity exercise of short duration. CPK is the enzyme that catalyzes the resynthesis of ATP from PC, while PFK and LDH are the key enzymes in the glycolytic pathway. This is why coaches include activities such as wind sprints to increase anaerobic capacity during the training season for many sports (e.g., field hockey, soccer, basketball).

Repeated bouts of aerobic activities (endurance training) result in several structural changes within the muscle. Both the size and number of mitochondria in the muscle fibers increase with endurance training. In addition, the activities of key oxidative enzymes in the Krebs cycle, electron transport system, and fatty acid oxidation increase. This means that the muscle has a greater capacity to use the aerobic energy system and fatty acids as a source of energy following endurance training. Another important adaptation is an increased blood supply to the muscle fibers as the number of capillaries increases. This adaptation increases both the oxygen and nutrient supply to the muscle fibers. The end result is that aerobically trained muscles are better able to sustain physical activity for prolonged periods of time. This is why swimmers and distance runners train over long distances in the early part of the training season.

Adaptations to Resistance Training

Muscular strength is defined as the maximal amount of force exerted by a muscle group. The maximal amount of force developed is affected by the speed of the muscle contraction. Less force can be developed during high-velocity movements than during slow contractions. In some physical activities, the ability to develop force rapidly is critical to performance. For example, a volleyball player must rapidly extend the legs in jumping to block a spike at the net. Muscular power is the product of the force times the speed of movement. The ability of a muscle to repeatedly exert force over a period of time is known as muscular endurance.

Resistance training programs to improve muscular strength may use isometric (tension is produced without the muscle changing length), isotonic (muscle changes length without changing tension), or isokinetic (muscle changes length at a constant rate of velocity) exercises. An example of an isometric contraction is when you put the palms of your hands against a wall and push as hard as you can. Lifting a free weight (e.g., barbell) is an example of an isotonic contraction. Resistance training equipment that allows you to set the speed of movement is isokinetic. Regardless of the type of exercise used, the muscle group must be overloaded progressively for strength to increase. Progressive overload requires that the muscles exert near maximal force with each contraction. This is known as the overload principle.

🔑 Muscles increase in strength as a result of progressive overload.

If you were interested in using resistance training to improve your performance in a given sport, obviously the type of training you use should match the sport techniques as closely as possible. The exercises you choose will determine how well, or whether, you improve in your techniques. Strength gains will be greatest over the range of movement and velocity of the resistance exercises used (Morrissey, Harman, & Johnson, 1995). If your sport requires you to move at high speed, higher-velocity isokinetic or isotonic training would be more beneficial than low velocities or isometric training.

Think about the physical activities you participate in on a regular basis. How many of these activities require physical strength? Which type(s) of resistance training would be most beneficial in improving strength for these activities? Why?

Muscular strength increase is believed to be due to two factors: an increase in muscle size and neural adaptations. An increase in muscle size as a result of resistance training is due to the increase in size of individual muscle fibers (hypertrophy).

Although evidence from studies of resistance training in cats suggests that muscle fibers split and increase (**hyperplasia**) (Gonyea, 1980), researchers have not observed increased numbers of fibers in other animal species (Gollnick, Timson, Moore, & Riedy, 1981; Timson, Bowlin, Dudenhoeffer, & George, 1985). Neural adaptations that may occur include recruitment of additional muscle fibers (motor units), better synchronization of muscle fiber contraction, and reduction in neural inhibition.

Cardiovascular System

As you recall, skeletal muscles draw from various energy systems in order to perform the work we require from them. The aerobic system, which is used for sustained physical activities, is limited primarily by the availability of oxygen. The transport of oxygen to all tissues is a primary function of the cardiovascular system, which is composed of the heart, blood vessels, and the blood. It responds immediately to physical activity in several ways in order to increase the supply of oxygen to skeletal muscles. Both the volume and distribution of blood flow change during physical activity. In addition, chronic physical activity results in several important physiological adaptations in cardiac function that improve endurance.

Cardiac Output

Cardiac output is defined as the amount of blood pumped out of the heart per minute. It is a function of both the heart rate (number of heart beats per minute) and **stroke volume** (amount of blood pumped per beat). Resting cardiac output is remarkably constant in adult humans at approximately five liters per minute.

cardiac output = heart rate × stroke volume

5,040 ml/min = 72 beats/min × 70 ml/beat is an example of the cardiac output in a healthy young adult.

During physical activity cardiac output increases as the use of oxygen by the muscles increases. Oxygen uptake (written as $\dot{V}O_2$), or the amount of oxygen used by muscle tissues, increases in direct proportion to the intensity of exercise until maximal oxygen uptake ($\dot{V}O_2$max) is reached. The amount of oxygen delivered to

the tissues depends on how much oxygen is in the blood and how much blood the heart is pumping (cardiac output).

$$\dot{V}O_2 = \text{cardiac output} \times (\text{arterial} - \text{venous}) \text{ oxygen content}$$

As your muscles take up more oxygen, your cardiac output increases. At lower exercise intensities, this increase is due to increases in the amount of blood pumped per beat (stroke volume) and the number of beats per minute (heart rate). As your exercise intensity increases above 40% of $\dot{V}O_2$max, however, your stroke volume plateaus—that is, you have reached the limit of how much blood your heart can pump per beat. Your heart rate continues to increase along with oxygen uptake, however, until you achieve your maximal heart rate (see figure 12.3). At this point, you have also reached your limit for oxygen uptake. So, as you can see, maximal oxygen uptake appears to be limited primarily by the heart's capacity to pump blood, the maximal cardiac output.

Cardiac output and $\dot{V}O_2$ increase during physical activity in direct proportion to the intensity of the activity until maximal cardiac output is reached.

Because $\dot{V}O_2$max and maximal heart rate are reached simultaneously, the fitness instructor can

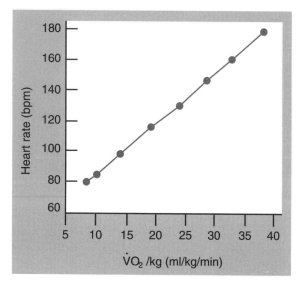

Figure 12.3   Relationship between heart rate and $\dot{V}O_2$ during a graded exercise test.

use submaximal exercise tests to estimate $\dot{V}O_2$max. This is very useful in exercise testing and prescription as it does not require the client to exercise to fatigue.

Blood Flow Distribution

When you are at rest, most of your blood flow (cardiac output) is distributed to your brain and internal organs (e.g., liver, kidneys) with only 15% going to your skeletal muscles. When you become physically active, more blood is needed in your muscles in order to supply oxygen and nutrients and to remove waste products. The onset of activity stimulates your sympathetic nerves to constrict (vasoconstrict) blood vessels in regions of your body where less blood flow is needed and dilate (vasodilate) blood vessels in your skeletal muscles and heart. During heavy exercise, two-thirds of your blood flow is distributed to your skeletal muscles by shifting blood flow away from your kidneys and digestive organs. Because blood flow to the kidneys is reduced, formation of urine decreases. This is the reason why it is difficult to obtain urine samples immediately following exercise.

Cardiovascular Adaptations to Training

When you consider a training program, you are usually looking to improve your strength and/ or endurance in a particular sport or physical activity, a simple goal. Exercise physiologists, however, consider what this means to the various body systems. As you learned earlier, it involves training your muscles and using the various energy systems that fuel the work of those muscles to best effect. Training also involves working with your cardiovascular system.

Your ability to exercise at moderate to heavy intensities for prolonged periods of time is referred to as your aerobic or cardiorespiratory endurance. One of the best indicators of aerobic endurance is your $\dot{V}O_2$max, which is also known as maximal aerobic power. You can increase your maximal aerobic power with endurance training. Much of the improvement in your $\dot{V}O_2$max is due to an increase in stroke volume—the amount of blood pumped per beat. The cardiac muscle of your heart actually increases in size and contracts more forcefully in response to endurance training. As a result of training, you will have an increased stroke volume both at rest and during exercise, and your heart rate will be reduced. In other words, you will be able to pump more blood with less work!

Of course, you will want to know if your training regime was successful. Exercise testing before and after an endurance training program is important for two reasons: (1) it establishes your baseline fitness level, and (2) it allows you to determine the effectiveness of the training program. A graded exercise test, in which intensity is increased progressively, is one way to test the efficacy of your training program. At each stage of the test you should notice that your heart rate is lower than it was before you started training (see figure 12.4). This is because with training, your heart rate has become more efficient. Your stroke volume has increased and your heart rate has decreased in order to provide the most appropriate cardiac output for a given exercise intensity. However, your *maximal* cardiac output increases primarily due to the increase in maximal stroke volume—you can pump more blood at the maximal heart rate. Most studies indicate there is little change in maximal heart rate after training.

Following endurance training, stroke volume increases and heart rate decreases at a given exercise intensity.

Your endurance training regime will also result in an increase in the number of capillaries in

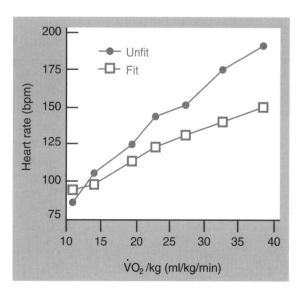

Figure 12.4 Comparison of the heart rate responses of fit and unfit subjects during a graded exercise test.

your skeletal muscles. This means that you can receive more blood and therefore more oxygen in your working muscle fibers during activity. Researchers have discovered that, following training, the difference in the amount of oxygen in the arteries (which move blood from the heart) and veins (which move blood back to the heart) is greater, suggesting that the muscles are extracting more oxygen from the blood. The increase in muscle capillaries may be responsible for the increase in oxygen extraction.

Determine your resting heart rate by counting your pulse for 15 seconds and multiplying by 4. The average heart rate is 70 beats per minute. Is your resting heart rate less than 70 beats per minute? Based on the amount and types of physical activities you participate in daily, can you explain why your resting heart rate is above or below 70 beats per minute?

Despite your best efforts at fitness training, you may find that others remain far ahead of you in gains, some seemingly without even trying. This brings us to a discussion of the other factors that affect maximal aerobic power. One is your genetic makeup. Studies of the $\dot{V}O_2$max of identical and fraternal twins have shown variation between identical twins pairs but much greater variation between fraternal twin pairs (Bouchard et al., 1986). In other words, individuals with identical genes (e.g., identical twins) are more alike in maximal aerobic power than fraternal twins who do not have identical genes. Another factor that influences maximal aerobic power is age. $\dot{V}O_2$max begins to decrease after the age of 30 due to a decrease in maximal heart rate and therefore maximal cardiac output. The decline in $\dot{V}O_2$max with aging may also be due in part to a decrease in physical activity, as researchers have observed that athletes who maintain their training levels experience a slower decline in $\dot{V}O_2$max (Hagberg, 1987).

Respiratory System

As you now know, the cardiovascular system is the transport system carrying oxygen to skeletal muscles to do the work of physical activity. But where does that oxygen come from? The respiratory system has the job of regulating the exchange of gases (including oxygen) between the external environment (air) and the internal environment (inside the body). In order for this exchange to occur, air must be moved from the nasal cavity or mouth through the respiratory passageways to the alveoli within the lungs. Once the fresh air enters the alveoli, oxygen can diffuse into the blood in the pulmonary capillaries, and carbon dioxide can leave the blood and enter the lungs to be exhaled into the environment. The process of moving air in and out of the lungs is known as **ventilation**. Gases follow pressure gradients in moving into and out of the lungs and blood, always moving from a region of higher pressure to one of lower pressure.

Ventilation During Physical Activity

The amount of air exhaled per minute is known as the minute volume (V_e). It is the product of the amount of air exhaled per breath (**tidal volume**) and the number of breaths per minute (respiratory frequency). The minute volume of a person at rest is approximately 6 liters per minute.

$$V_e = \text{tidal volume} \times \text{frequency}$$
$$6000 \text{ ml/min} = 500 \text{ ml/breath} \times 12 \text{ breaths/min}$$

Not all of the air you inhale with each breath actually reaches your lungs; some remains in the respiratory passageways. When you take a deep breath (increase your tidal volume), more air will reach the **alveoli** of your lungs where gases are exchanged with the blood than if you take several shorter breaths. While both breathing patterns may result in the same minute volume—that is, the same amount of air will exit your lungs—the deep-breathing pattern will allow more air to reach the alveoli for gas exchange before being exhaled.

At the beginning of physical activity, you may notice that your breathing increases rapidly during the first minute until it reaches a plateau. Researchers believe the stimulus comes from sensory **receptors** in the moving limbs (e.g., muscle spindles, joint receptors) as well as the motor cortex (i.e., the part of the brain that stimulates muscles to contract). At low exercise intensities, the increase in minute volume (air exhaled) is due primarily to an increase in the amount of air exhaled with each breath; the number of breaths remains constant. At higher exercise intensities, however, both respiratory frequency and tidal volume increase—you take more frequent and bigger breaths.

🔑 Ventilation increases rapidly at the onset of physical activity and also increases as a function of the exercise intensity.

As your level of exercise intensity increases, your breathing also increases, steadily at first, and then much more rapidly at higher intensities (see figure 12.5). The point at which your breathing begins to increase rapidly is known as the **ventilatory threshold**. Ventilatory threshold occurs at exercise intensities between 50 and 75% $\dot{V}O_2$max. Because this point corresponds with a decrease in blood pH and an increase in the amount of carbon dioxide exhaled, researchers believe that the ventilatory threshold reflects the point at which the blood can no longer meet the oxygen needs of the tissues. As a result, the respiratory system speeds up to remove more carbon dioxide from the cardiovascular system. Does this surprise you? The respiratory system is relatively insensitive to the blood oxygen content. It is the carbon dioxide content of the blood that is driving the system.

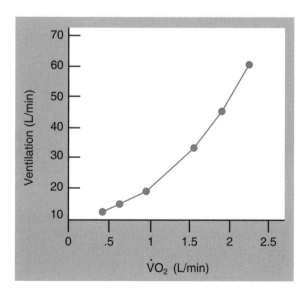

Figure 12.5 Relationship of ventilation to $\dot{V}O_2$ as the exercise intensity is progressively increased during a graded exercise test.

After you have been training for a while, your maximal ventilation—the amount of air entering and leaving your lungs—increases when you exercise. This increase appears to be due to increases in both tidal volume and respiratory frequency—you're taking deeper and more frequent breaths. Moreover, your ventilatory threshold, or the point at which your breathing really increases, occurs at a higher exercise intensity after training.

Temperature Effects

In addition to studying the three primary body systems that affect physical activity, exercise physiologists have also studied the influence of environmental factors on our experience of sport and exercise. One such factor is temperature variation. Our bodies have complex and effective ways of dealing with temperature changes in the outside environment.

During muscle contractions much of the energy released by the splitting of ATP is converted to thermal energy (heat). This heat-generating process is known as **thermogenesis** and is used to help maintain the body's internal temperature at approximately 37 °C (98.6 °F). Humans are able to regulate their internal (core) temperature so that it remains relatively constant over a wide range of environmental temperatures (Haymes & Wells, 1986).

Thermoreceptors located in the brain and the skin respond to changes in temperature by sending nerve impulses to the hypothalamus in the brain, which in turn stimulates the appropriate heat loss or heat conservation mechanisms. If the body temperature is increasing, heat loss is increased by stimulating the sweat glands to produce sweat and the superficial blood vessels in the skin to vasodilate. Vasodilation of skin blood vessels brings warm blood to the surface where some of the heat can be dissipated directly to the environment via **convection**, but only if the temperature of the air is below that of the skin. Body heat is also lost through the evaporation of sweat. In order for sweat to evaporate, heat must be supplied to change it from a liquid to a gas.

🔑 Muscle contractions produce heat, which helps maintain the body's internal temperature.

In cold environments, heat conservation mechanisms are stimulated by a decrease in body temperature. Vasoconstriction of superficial blood vessels shifts blood flow away from the skin into deeper blood vessels. Such a shift in blood flow increases the distance between the warm blood and the skin surface, and the thickness of the tissue insulation. The subcutaneous fat layer underneath the skin is a very effective insulator in the cold. Shivering is also stimulated by a drop in body temperature. During shivering, superficial muscle fiber contractions produce heat, which increases body temperature.

Effects of Exercise

When you begin to exercise, the heat produced by splitting ATP increases the temperature of your active muscles. Blood flowing through these regions of the body is warmed and distributes the heat to other regions of your body. As your core temperature rises, thermoreceptors sense the change in temperature and relay this information to the thermoregulatory center in the hypothalamus. Once your body reaches a threshold temperature, your skin blood vessels begin to vasodilate and you begin to sweat. In thermoneutral environments (i.e., comfortable ambient temperatures), your core temperature reaches a plateau in 20 to 30 minutes (see figure 12.6). The higher the intensity of your physical activity, the higher your core temperature will be when it reaches a plateau.

> During physical activity increased heat production by skeletal muscles stimulates vasodilation of skin blood vessels and sweating.

Have you ever wondered why you sweat more profusely during physical activity in warm environments? When air temperatures approach or exceed skin temperatures, the body's mechanism of bringing warm blood to the surface to cool doesn't work; the air isn't cool enough to be of any help. In this case, the evaporation of sweat becomes the major avenue of heat loss. In hot, humid environments, heat loss through evaporation is also limited. This results in a higher body temperature (see figure 12.6). The risk of heat illness (e.g., heat exhaustion, heat stroke) during physical activity rises as air temperature and humidity increase.

We tolerate physical activity in cool environments better because our bodies can lose heat from blood close to the skin as well as from the evaporation of sweat. In cold water, however, heat loss from the skin increases dramatically because water is an excellent conductor of heat. Submersion in cold water stimulates shivering and an increase in metabolic rate. Swimming in cold water also elevates the metabolic rate, which may lead to an earlier onset of exhaustion. Similarly, individuals whose clothing becomes wet during physical activity in cold environments lose heat more rapidly and will begin to shiver also. Such individuals will fatigue sooner and are at risk of hypothermia (below normal body temperatures).

Effects of Acclimatization

While athletes are at greater risk of heat illness in warm environments, they can accustom their bodies to exercising in such environments. This process is called acclimatization. Repeated exercise bouts in warm environments result in several physiological changes. One such change is that the onset of sweating occurs at a lower core temperature. This means that an athlete will begin to sweat earlier during physical activity. As a result, core and skin temperatures will be lower. Heart rate also decreases due in part to an expansion of blood fluid volume that occurs with

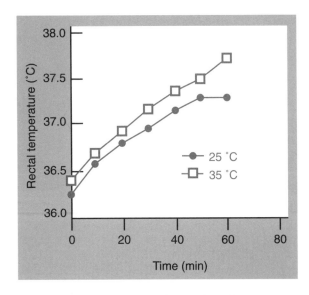

Figure 12.6 Increases in body core (rectal) temperature during exercise in thermoneutral (25 °C; 77 °F) and warm (35 °C; 95 °F) ambient temperatures.

acclimatization. Athletes expecting to compete or simply exercise in warm environments will find that they will be better able to tolerate physical activity for prolonged periods after acclimatization. Moreover, their risks of heat illness will be reduced.

Less is known about acclimatization to cold environments because there have been few studies of cold-acclimatized individuals. The best evidence of cold acclimatization in an active population comes from research conducted on Korean women divers who dive in cold water throughout the winter. Prior to 1977 the women divers wore cotton bathing suits while diving in 10 °C (50 °F) water. These women divers did not shiver until their body temperatures were much lower than those of women who were nondivers. During the winter months, the women divers also had significantly elevated resting metabolic rates compared to their rates during the rest of the year (Hong, 1973). These physiological adaptations allowed the women to continue diving during the winter months.

Nutritional Effects

Nutritional intake is another environmental factor studied by physiologists of physical activity. The energy sources our muscles use, such as glycogen and fatty acids, are derived from our intake of important nutrients from our diet. While most of us have enough stored fat to sustain low-intensity activities for many days, we need shorter-term energy sources, such as carbohydrates, for moderately heavy endurance activities. Because the amount of carbohydrate stored in the body is less than one pound, daily carbohydrate intake is crucial to athletic performance. We will explore the role of carbohydrates as well as that of two other nutrients, water and iron.

Carbohydrates

Carbohydrate is stored as glycogen primarily in skeletal muscles and the liver. During high-intensity physical activities, muscle glycogen stores are the primary source of energy. Normal muscle glycogen stores will be depleted in approximately 90 minutes of continuous exercise at 75% $\dot{V}O_2$max. The amount of glycogen stored is directly related to the carbohydrate content of the diet.

Coaches and athletes know that diets that are very high in carbohydrate (70% or more of the calories) and that are consumed for two or three days will increase muscle glycogen storage. This technique is known as carbohydrate loading and is used by some endurance athletes prior to competition. Carbohydrate loading is most effective in activities lasting more than two hours (e.g., marathons). Research has shown no apparent advantage to carbohydrate loading for activities lasting less than one hour.

> The amount of glycogen stored is directly related to the carbohydrate content of the diet.

Liver glycogen is the primary source of blood glucose, which many cells use for energy, particularly the cells of the nervous system. When the liver glycogen stores are depleted, blood glucose levels fall. Low blood glucose levels are often associated with fatigue in prolonged exercise. Consumption of carbohydrate drinks containing 6–8% carbohydrate by weight during prolonged exercise has been shown to improve performance and delay the onset of fatigue (Coggan & Coyle, 1991). Drinks containing a higher concentration of carbohydrate (greater than 10% by weight), however, will delay gastric emptying, which may lead to gastric distension and distress (Davis, Burgess, Sientz, Bartoli, & Pate, 1988).

Muscle glycogen stores may be depleted during intermittent physical activity characteristic of many sports. Depletion of the glycogen stores could have a negative impact on performance. For example, soccer players were found to deplete their muscle glycogen stores during the second half of a match. Those players with depleted glycogen stores covered less distance and spent more time walking and less time running during the second half (Saltin, 1973). Some athletes with low carbohydrate intakes (i.e., less than 50% of the total calories) may progressively deplete their glycogen stores through daily training. In order to maintain adequate glycogen stores, physically active individuals should consume a diet containing 55–60% of the total calories as carbohydrate. Consumption of foods high in carbohydrate immediately following exercise is also beneficial because it has been found to increase the rate of muscle glycogen synthesis (Ivy, Katz, & Cutler, 1989).

Fluid Intake

Water makes up 55–60% of the human body. During physical activity some of this water is lost through sweating. When you exercise on a warm day, even just walking to class, you will notice that sweating increases. Especially in warm environments, fluid replacement is extremely important because the volume of sweat lost can be substantial.

Sweat loss decreases body fluids both within and between cells, as well as decreasing **plasma volume** (the fluid portion of blood). When the fluid volume of blood is decreased, less blood is returned to the heart, which reduces the amount of blood in each heartbeat (stroke volume). In order to compensate for the reduced stroke volume, the heart rate increases. If fluid losses are not replaced, the sweat rate will fall, causing an increase in body temperature. Such a situation puts individuals at greater risk of developing heat illnesses, especially heat exhaustion.

Inadequate fluid intake during physical activity will result in an elevated body temperature and a greater risk of developing a heat illness, and possible decrements in performance.

Failure to adequately replace fluids can also lead to decrements in performance in some physical activities. For example, Armstrong, Costill, and Fink (1985) found that running velocities at distances ranging from 1,500 to 10,000 meters (approximately 1 to 6 miles) were reduced 3–7% following a 2% decrease in body weight. Short, high-intensity activities such as sprinting are less likely to be affected by **hypohydration** (decreased hydration) than more prolonged events.

To ensure adequate fluid replacement during physical activity, you should drink fluids (e.g., water, carbohydrate-electrolyte drinks) at regular intervals (every 15–20 minutes). This is important during many types of physical activity including hiking, bicycling, aerobics classes, and working outdoors.

If you play a sport such as soccer or field hockey, fluid replacement during play is difficult because the rules do not allow time-outs except for injury during competition. Drink additional fluid prior to a match and during half-time in these sports to reduce the fluid deficit. Following activity you should continue to drink fluids even though you may not feel thirsty. Unfortunately, thirst is not an accurate indicator of hypohydration. During activities lasting less than one hour there is no advantage to consuming carbohydrate-electrolyte drinks. In more prolonged activities, fluids containing a small amount of carbohydrate are more likely to be beneficial in enhancing fluid absorption and maintaining blood glucose.

Write down all of the food and drink you consumed during the previous day. How many servings of foods high in carbohydrate (e.g., grains, pasta, fruits, vegetables) did you consume? How many servings of foods that are good sources of iron (e.g., meats, cereals enriched with iron) did you consume? How many cups of fluid did you drink?

Iron Intake

As you know, physical activity cannot take place without the transport of oxygen-carrying blood to the muscles. The blood is able to transport oxygen with the help of iron. Oxygen essentially "rides" on the iron atoms in the **hemoglobin** found in red blood cells. Each hemoglobin contains four iron atoms that bond with four oxygen molecules. A person with no iron stored in the body cannot synthesize hemoglobin, which results in lower levels of hemoglobin in the blood. As hemoglobin concentrations fall, the amount of oxygen transported to the tissues decreases. Eventually, the person becomes anemic. Anemia is defined as a hemoglobin concentration below 12 grams per deciliter of blood in women and 14 grams per deciliter in men. Both maximal oxygen uptake and endurance are reduced in anemic individuals (Celsing, Blomstrand, Werner, Pihlstedt, & Ekblom, 1986).

Depletion of iron stores can lead to anemia, which reduces maximal oxygen uptake and endurance.

Iron deficiency is one of the most common nutritional deficiencies in the United States, especially among adolescent girls and women. The average woman consumes only two-thirds of the recommended dietary allowance of 15 milligrams of iron per day. Iron depletion is fairly common among adolescent and adult female athletes (Clarkson & Haymes, 1995). However, the incidence of iron deficiency anemia among female athletes is no greater than among women in the U.S. population. The most likely causes of iron depletion in physically active women are inadequate iron intake and excessive blood loss through the menses. Low iron intake in female athletes is most commonly observed in those who restrict their caloric intake (e.g., gymnasts) and those who consume diets that are low in meat (e.g., runners) (Clarkson & Haymes, 1995). Heme iron found in meat, fish, and poultry is more highly absorbed from the gastrointestinal tract than the nonheme iron found in other food sources. Most women can prevent iron deficiency by consuming iron-rich foods in their daily diet.

Physical Activity, Fitness, and Health

One of the most important benefits gained from a lifetime of physical activity is the improvement in physical fitness. Although there are many characteristics of physical fitness, it is usually limited to cardiorespiratory endurance, muscular strength, and muscular endurance. Fitness has been defined "as the ability to perform moderate to vigorous levels of physical activity without undue fatigue and the capability of maintaining such ability throughout life" (American College of Sports Medicine, 1990).

The American College of Sports Medicine (1990) recommends that adults take part in physical activity 20–60 minutes per day and 3–5 days per week at 60–90% of maximal heart rate to improve cardiorespiratory endurance. Exercise intensities that are 60–80% of maximal heart rate (50–74% $\dot{V}O_2$max) are usually perceived as being moderate exercise, while exercise intensities of 80–90% of maximal heart rate (75–84% $\dot{V}O_2$max) are considered heavy exercise. Activities that are aerobic and can be maintained for prolonged periods are best for improving cardiorespiratory endurance. These activities include running, hiking, walking, swimming, cross-country skiing,

Think of a physical activity that you participate in on a regular basis. How many minutes per day do you participate in this activity? How many days per week do you participate in this activity? Have you ever counted your heart rate immediately after this activity? If so, how high was it? If you haven't done this before, the next time you participate in this physical activity, measure your heart rate immediately after exercising. Calculate what percentage this exercise heart rate is of your maximal heart rate (220 – your age).

bicycling, aerobic dancing, stair climbing, and rowing. Sports such as soccer, field hockey, and tennis also help develop cardiorespiratory fitness because they are high-intensity, intermittent activities carried out over prolonged periods of time.

The recommended amount of physical activity for improvement in cardiorespiratory endurance is 20–60 minutes of activity at 60–90% of maximal heart rate, 3–5 days per week.

Effects of Age on Fitness

While research has shown that maximal oxygen uptake ($\dot{V}O_2$max) does decline with age at the rate of approximately 10% per decade, the decrease is smaller (5% per decade) in individuals who remain physically active (Hagberg, 1987). The decline in cardiorespiratory endurance in older individuals may be due in part to a reduction in the intensity and duration of physical activity. Master athletes who maintain their training intensity experience little change in maximal oxygen uptake as they age.

$\dot{V}O_2$max, which is used as the primary indicator of cardiovascular endurance in adults, increases in absolute terms (liters per minute) with growth in children. Since body mass is increasing with growth, more oxygen is required to supply the active tissue. When $\dot{V}O_2$max is expressed per kilogram of body weight, however, it remains relatively constant or decreases during growth

(Bar-Or, 1983). Results of several studies of children suggest that $\dot{V}O_2$max per kilogram does not increase with training in prepubescent children until the peak of the growth spurt is achieved (Zwiren, 1989). This does not mean, however, that children's endurance does not improve prior to puberty. Improvements in children's endurance with training may be related to improvements in other factors such as running economy and anaerobic capacity (Rowland, 1989).

Physical Activity, Fitness, and Coronary Heart Disease

Many of us participate in physical activities under the assumption that higher levels of fitness are associated with improved health status. This generally held assumption is based on research conducted by exercise physiologists. Blair, Kohl, Paffenbarger, Clark, Cooper, and Gibbons (1989) found that individuals who are the most fit have a lower relative risk of developing or dying from cardiovascular disease or cancer than those who are less fit. They based their determination of physical fitness on a cardiovascular endurance test.

Participation in physical activities, as opposed to levels of fitness, also reduces the risk of cardiovascular disease and colon cancer. Paffenbarger (1994) estimated that engaging in moderate-intensity physical activities added approximately 1.5 years to life. Using the number of calories expended walking, stair climbing, and in leisure-time sports weekly as an index of physical activity, Harvard alumni had a 46% lower risk of dying from cardiovascular disease if they used 2,500 calories or more per week in physical activities (Paffenbarger, 1994). Participants in moderate-intensity activities (e.g., brisk walking, swimming, cycling) had a 37% lower risk compared to those who did not participate in leisure-time sports.

High levels of physical fitness lower the risk of developing and dying from cardiovascular disease. Regular participation in moderate-intensity physical activity also reduces the risk of cardiovascular disease and colon cancer.

Increased cardiovascular endurance is associated with a reduction in several coronary heart disease (CHD) risk factors, including elevated blood lipid levels (cholesterol and triglycerides),

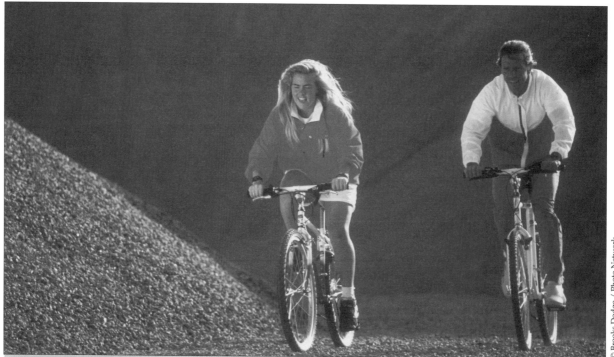

Participation in physical activity can reduce the risk of cardiovascular disease and colon cancer.

© Brooks Dodge / Photo Network

hypertension (high blood pressure), smoking, physical inactivity, and obesity. Elevated total serum cholesterol and low-density lipoprotein (LDL) cholesterol levels increase the risk of CHD, while elevated high-density lipoprotein (HDL) cholesterol is associated with a lower risk of CHD. Physical activity programs that increase cardiovascular endurance usually result in an increase in HDL cholesterol (Durstine & Haskell, 1994). Increases in fitness are accompanied by decreases in blood triglyceride levels as well. Total serum cholesterol is less affected by moderate and heavy exercise programs, but some studies report LDL cholesterol is reduced following endurance training.

> Increases in cardiovascular endurance are associated with an increase in HDL cholesterol and a reduction in blood triglyceride levels.

Physical activity and fitness also play a role in reducing the risk of hypertension, or high blood pressure. High blood pressure (systolic blood pressure greater than 160 mmHg) increases the risk of CHD approximately threefold. In hypertensive individuals, an acute bout of moderate physical activity that lasts more than 30 minutes will reduce blood pressure for several hours (Hagberg, 1989). Endurance training lowers blood pressure in hypertensive individuals by approximately 10 mmHg. Lower-intensity exercise programs (50–60% of maximal heart rate) are as effective in reducing blood pressure as those of higher intensity (American College of Sports Medicine, 1993). Among individuals with normal blood pressure, those who are more physically active have lower blood pressures than those who are less active. Fit individuals are also less likely to develop hypertension.

Physical Activity, Weight Control, and Obesity

Researchers in physiology of physical activity have added to our understanding of the process by which the body burns calories and uses energy. They have learned that the metabolic rate—the rate at which the body uses energy—increases in direct proportion to the intensity of activity. From their research we know that daily physical activity helps us control body weight. We also know from their research how many calories we burn when we participate in various intensities of activity.

Lower-intensity activities such as walking at 3 mph will increase the resting metabolic rate (1 calorie per kilogram per hour) threefold. For a 70-kilogram (154-lb) person, this would be the equivalent of four calories per minute. A person who walked two miles per day would expend an additional 160 calories each day or 1,120 calories per week. Higher-intensity activities such running at seven miles per hour increase the resting metabolic rate tenfold, which is the equivalent of 12.5 calories per minute. Running two miles per day would expend an additional 214 calories each day or 1,500 calories per week. Total energy expenditure is also dependent on the duration of physical activity. Running four miles per day would increase energy expenditure to 428 calories.

Moreover, energy expenditure doesn't come to a screeching halt at the end of an exercise bout. Tests have shown that the metabolic rate remains elevated during recovery from physical activity. Thus the total energy expended due to a single bout of exercise will be somewhat greater than the energy cost of the activity.

> Energy expenditure during physical activity is directly proportional to the intensity and duration of the activity.

While some of us are looking to maintain our body weight with exercise, others are looking to lose body weight and body fat. Regular participation in endurance activities leads to reductions in body weight and body fat. The recommended exercise dose for weight loss is a minimum of 20 minutes of activity that expends 300 calories per session at least three days per week (American College of Sports Medicine, 1990). Lower-intensity exercise (200 calories per session) is also beneficial in reducing body weight if the person exercises more frequently.

When caloric intake exceeds caloric expenditure, the excess calories are converted to fat and stored in the adipose tissue. Sedentary individuals are more likely to be overweight or obese, a condition that puts them at increased risk of developing CHD (Willett et al., 1995). Reducing body weight has been found effective in lowering serum triglycerides and reducing blood pressure in hypertensive individuals.

Low levels of physical activity are also associated with a higher risk of non-insulin-dependent diabetes (NIDDM) (Paffenbarger, 1994). Individuals with NIDDM are less sensitive to blood insulin levels (insulin resistance). Because insulin is necessary for cellular uptake of glucose, blood glucose levels are elevated in NIDDM. Physical activity increases the cells' sensitivity to insulin and cellular uptake of blood glucose. Participation in daily physical activities is beneficial not only in reducing the risk of NIDDM but also in helping individuals with NIDDM regulate their blood glucose levels.

Now that you have some basic knowledge about the physiological systems and some of their responses during physical activity, we will examine how exercise physiologists can put this knowledge to use in designing training programs for several different purposes.

Focus Topic: Training

Training is defined as repetition of an activity that produces adaptations in one or more physiological systems (physical performance capacity). Three principles determine the training responses: overload, specificity, and reversibility. The principle of overload means that for training to occur, the intensity of the activity must be greater than what is normally experienced by the physiological systems. For example, for an older sedentary individual, beginning an exercise program with brisk walking may be sufficient to overload both the cardiovascular and muscular systems.

The principle of training specificity means that adaptations occur only in the muscles used and are specific to the activity used. In the opening scenario you had trained by running on a level track. Following a long downhill run, you experienced delayed onset muscle soreness because the leg muscles were not trained to contract eccentrically (i.e., while lengthening). Another example of this same specificity principle is the weightlifter who trains by lifting the heaviest weight three to five times; this person is increasing the strength of the muscles but not their endurance. The principle of reversibility means that when you stop overloading the systems, the training adaptations are lost.

People train for two main reasons—to improve performance in a sport or to improve their fitness and health. The training specificity principle is extremely important when training to improve performance in a specific sport because the athlete must engage the energy systems predominantly used in the sport. Recall the three energy systems (the ATP-PC system, the glycolytic system, and the aerobic system) that were discussed earlier. Most distance events (e.g., 10K races, marathons, and triathlons) primarily use the aerobic energy system. Therefore, runners, swimmers, cyclists, and triathletes training for these events should emphasize endurance training that involves the aerobic energy systems. Three types of training are used to improve endurance: long, slow distance; interval training; and high-intensity, continuous exercise.

Long, slow distance training is performed at a moderate exercise intensity (70% of the athlete's maximum heart rate) over a distance that is longer than the competitive event (Powers & Howley, 1990). The purpose of interval training is to stress the aerobic system; intervals must last at least one minute with rest intervals between them at a ratio of 1:1. The intensity of exercise is higher in interval work bouts (85% of the maximum heart rate). In high-intensity, continuous training, the athlete trains at an inten-

→

sity that approximates the lactate threshold (i.e., intensity where blood lactate concentration increases rapidly) for 25 to 50 minutes (Powers & Howley, 1990).

Many sports (e.g., basketball, football, soccer, tennis) are intermittent in nature and rely primarily on the ATP-PC energy system to supply energy. Training to improve performance in these activities requires not only training to improve neuromuscular skills but also training to improve ATP production using the ATP-PC system. This requires high-intensity interval training with short work bouts (e.g., 10 seconds) interspersed with recovery intervals at a ratio of 1:3 (e.g., a 15-second sprint followed by a 45-second recovery). Recovery may be either complete rest or slow walking between work bouts.

Sports that require 30 seconds to 2 minutes of sustained high-intensity effort rely primarily on the anaerobic glycolysis energy system. These sports include 400- and 800-meter running events and 100- and 200-meter swimming events. High-intensity interval training with work intervals lasting 30–90 seconds should be used to stress the anaerobic glycolysis energy system. Usually the work-to-recovery ratio for intervals is 1:2 with the recovery interval being rest, walking, or slow jogging.

While training to improve performance is used by athletes of all ages, training to improve fitness and health is the goal of many physically active individuals. In order to improve cardiorespiratory fitness, the recommended training intensity is at 60–80% of maximum heart rate for 20–60 minutes per day. The recommended training frequency is 3–5 days per week; higher frequencies of training (greater than 4 days per week) are accompanied by a higher incidence of musculoskeletal injuries.

One of the most common reasons for stopping an exercise training program is being injured (Pate et al., 1995). For this reason, exercise programs designed to improve fitness and health should begin with moderate-intensity activities and gradually increase the intensity and duration of the activities as fitness improves. For example, an exercise program for sedentary adults may begin with walking at a speed of 3–4 miles per hour and gradually increase the duration from 20 to 60 minutes. The intensity would then be increased first to alternating walking and jogging and finally to jogging.

When you undertake a training program, you expect to improve either in a sport or in general fitness. Improvement depends on the intensity, duration, and frequency of training, the total length of the training program, and your initial fitness level. Greater intensities, duration (minutes per day), frequency (days per week), and total length of the training program will lead to larger increases in your cardiorespiratory fitness. However, you may observe a plateau in your rate of fitness improvement after several months of training. Increases in fitness are greatest for those with the lowest initial fitness levels and least for those with the highest initial fitness levels.

Many people have the mistaken impression that strenuous exercise (no pain, no gain) programs are required in order to gain the health benefits of physical activity. To the contrary, scientific evidence suggests that engaging in moderate physical activities on a regular basis also confers health benefits (Pate et al., 1995). Moderate-intensity physical activities include brisk walking (3–4 miles per hour), cycling less than 10 miles per hour, swimming at a moderate speed, badminton, table tennis, golf (pulling a cart), climbing stairs, and mowing the lawn with a power mower. The Centers for Disease Control and Prevention and the American College of Sports Medicine have recommended that "every U.S. adult should accumulate 30 minutes or more of moderate-intensity physical activity on most, preferably all, days of the week" (Pate et al., 1995). This does not have to be 30 minutes of continuous activity; it may include intermittent activities as well. The goal should be to accumulate activities that use approximately 200 calories over a 30-minute period. By emphasizing moderate instead of strenuous physical activities, experts hope that a higher percentage of the adult population, and women and older adults in particular, will engage in physical activity on a regular basis.

Wrap-Up

Physiology of physical activity is an exciting subdiscipline that seeks to study the body's acute responses to physical activity and the changes that occur with long-term physical activity. From changes in metabolism to cardiovascular responses to adaptations to heat and altitude, exercise physiologists have discovered the remarkable ways in which our body sytems work together when the body is physically active. In this chapter we examined the physiological responses to a single bout of physical activity and the changes that occur in physiological responses due to repeated bouts of activity. We also exam-ined the effects of environmental and nutritional factors on physiological responses and performance. Finally, we examined the relationship of physical activity to fitness and health.

If you are intrigued by what you learned in this chapter, you should consider taking courses in anatomy and physiology and exercise physiology. Many career opportunities exist in exercise physiology including health/fitness instruction in hospital-based, commercial, and corporate fitness programs; clinical exercise physiology specializations in cardiac rehabilitation programs; college or university teaching positions; and research positions in medicine, the military, and other government agencies.

Study Questions

1. Discuss the differences in goals of the basic scientist and the applied scientist in studying the physiology of physical activity.

2. Identify each of the following individuals and describe his contribution to the physiology of physical activity:

   a. August Krogh

   b. A.V. Hill

   c. David Bruce Dill

   d. Peter V. Karpovich

   e. Thomas K. Cureton

3. Why do exercise physiologists use cycle ergometers and treadmills in studying the physiology of physical activity?

4. What are the primary sources of energy used by skeletal muscles during physical activity? Describe each.

5. Describe the cardiovascular adaptations that occur as a result of endurance training.

6. Describe thermoregulation during physical activity in a warm environment.

7. What are the effects of a low-carbohydrate diet on performance in endurance activities?

8. Discuss the relationship of physical activity to coronary heart disease.

9. Explain why individuals who are physically active are better able to control body weight.

Practicing a Profession in Physical Activity

In this section . . .

Scholarly study

Experience

Professional practice

For some people, experiencing and studying about physical activity is an end in itself. Like psychology, English, or history majors, they may choose to major in kinesiology without any specific plans to carve out a career in the field. As the discipline of kinesiology becomes more organized, its popularity as a liberal arts subject grows. This is understandable given that the goal of a liberal education is to understand humanity in its totality, and that physical activity plays a profound role in helping us express our humanity.

But for most kinesiology majors, experiencing and studying physical activity is a means toward an end: a career in the physical activity professions. You probably have chosen your major with an eye toward working in a job centered around some aspect of physical activity. The array of careers open to kinesiology majors is vast: sport coaches; sport administrators; athletic trainers; physical education teachers; fitness trainers, consultants, and programmers; rehabilitation specialists in the fields of cardiology, physical therapy, occupational therapy; and many others. Each of these careers may require different areas of concentration in undergraduate course work, but all are anchored in an understanding of the spheres of physical activity experience and the spheres of scholarly study of physical activity.

Those working in the field of physical activity share something else in common: all are professionals and, as such, assume the same responsibilities and obligations of all professionals. Chapter 13 will stimulate your thinking about what it means to be a professional and suggest steps you can take now to guarantee your success as a professional.

While experts in the discipline of kinesiology generally recognize six spheres of professional practice, we will explore only four of them in this text: health and fitness, therapeutic exercise, instruction, and sport management. Chapters 14 through 17, authored by experts in each of these spheres, focus on specific careers in detail. These chapters may be your first exposure to the work world of physical activity, or they may serve to help you consolidate your thinking and affirm your commitment to a long-anticipated career. To help you organize your thoughts about the types of work and worksites available to kinesiology majors, we have grouped the many different types of work according to general objectives and goals, working environments, and qualifications for professionals.

Two of the six spheres of professional practice—scholarly study and artistic expression—are not covered in this section. It might surprise you that scholarly study can be an area of professional practice. Think back to the people who are responsible for compiling the spheres of scholarly study that were described in section 2. Who discovered all of this knowledge of physical activity? Most of them were professionals who devoted their careers to studying, researching, and teaching about physical activity at an advanced level, usually at a college or university (as a college professor), but possibly at a research or scientific lab (as a research scientist). These positions normally require a PhD in a specialized area in kinesiology. Since decisions about such careers are usually made much later in students' educational programs, we chose not to address them in this text. If, as you study about physical activity, you become interested in pursuing such work, don't hesitate to consult with your faculty advisor about steps you might take to prepare yourself for this career.

The other sphere not covered in this section includes physical activity careers in the area of artistic expression. Physical activity plays a vital role in dance, drama, music, painting, sculpting, and other artistic forms. However, training for careers in these areas normally is managed by art, music, dance, and drama departments rather than by kinesiology departments.

If you're like most of your peers, you may be uncertain as to which physical activity career you will pursue—if you plan to pursue one at all. This is normal and it shouldn't cause you any anxiety at this point. In fact, one of the objectives of this textbook and the course you are taking is to help you chart a course for your professional future. Reading and *studying* this section, however, should move you closer to selecting a career. As you do this, keep in mind that this will be only the first in a number of career choices you are likely to face over the course of your working years. Two, three, and even four changes in careers are likely for those entering the workforce at this time. Nevertheless, it's important that you make the most intelligent career choice possible, and this section will help you accomplish this important goal.

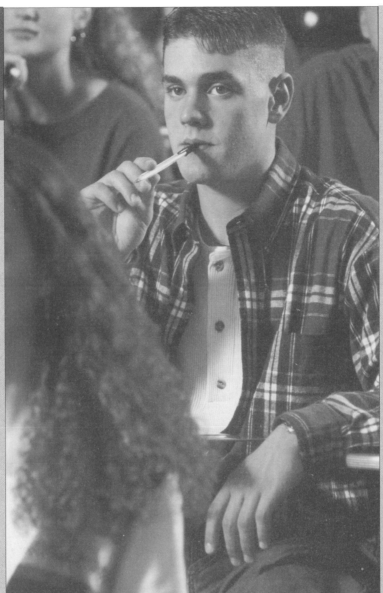

13

© Jay Thomas / International Stock

Becoming a Physical Activity Professional

Shirl J. Hoffman

In this chapter . . .

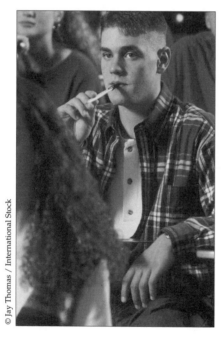

© Jay Thomas / International Stock

An award is bestowed on a physical education professor for "having provided 25 years of distinguished *professional* service to the university."

A director of a fitness center, aware that an employee is giving clients misinformation about nutrition and exercise, tells him that he is "not behaving in a *professional* manner."

A director of a community sport program tells her associate that he should join the North American Society for Sports Management "because it is the *professional* thing to do."

A physical therapist has a habit of coming to the clinic in dirty clothes and often fails to comb her hair or wear a clinical coat when treating patients. Her supervisor reprimands her for "not conducting herself like a *professional*."

An athletic trainer is praised by the athletic director for "possessing the highest *professional* standards."

A janitor at a local football stadium prides himself on the quality of his work, noting that he is regarded "as a valuable member of the janitorial *profession*."

A student, asked by a friend about his plans following graduation, said, "I don't know, right now life beyond graduation seems like the great black void." Unfortunately, he's not alone in feeling uneasy about graduating and starting a career. Many undergraduate students share the feeling. The world is filled with uncertainty, and nobody likes to leave his or her career to chance. If you have already committed to a specific career in the field of physical activity, you're likely to enjoy your study of kinesiology a bit more than students who have yet to make that commitment. But regardless of whether you have already made that commitment, it is a good idea to review all of the factors that bear on selecting a career, especially a career in the physical activity professions.

In most people's minds the purpose of a college or university education is to get a job, but what kind of job do you want? Will you be satisfied with just any type of work? Of course not. You came to college to earn a degree that will help you find a good-paying job that is respected by the community, a job that offers good working conditions and a reasonable amount of time off for leisure pursuits. You may want your job to count for something, to make a contribution to society. Your ideal job may be one in which other people benefit from your work, which is always a good feeling. You may want a job that is so enjoyable that you willingly put in extra hours in the evenings or on weekends. Ideally, it should be a job that not just anybody can do; it should require some thinking and skills that set you apart from the ordinary workforce. You may also want to be in a position to make most of the decisions concerning what you do and how you go about your work. (You surely remember previous jobs in which you didn't have much freedom to make decisions.) And last, but certainly not least, you want a job that involves physical activity.

If this describes the position you hope to secure following graduation, then the physical activity professions might appeal to you (see figure 13.1). This chapter is intended to help you decide whether a career in a physical activity profession is right for you.

 ## CHAPTER OBJECTIVES

In this chapter we will:

▌ Acquaint you with the characteristics of a profession

▌ Differentiate professional from nonprofessional work

▌ Explain the types of knowledge and skills essential for performing professional work

▌ Discuss what you need to do during your undergraduate years in order to gain entry into and succeed in your chosen professional field

▌ Help you know if you are suited for a career in a physical activity profession

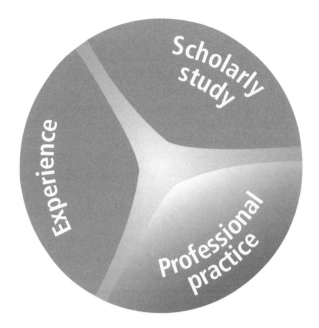

Figure 13.1 This chapter introduces the physical activity professions, one of three dimensions of kinesiology.

As you can see from the scenarios at the beginning of this chapter, the term *profession* is used in many different ways. But it actually has a very special meaning. A profession is a particular line of work or occupation, and a professional is a very particular type of worker. Teachers, doctors, lawyers, and physical therapists are professionals. Although they may describe themselves as professionals, janitors, housepainters, and craftspersons such as plumbers, electricians, and carpenters aren't. Knowing why this is the case will help you better understand the distinctive roles and responsibilities of the type of work to which you aspire.

A degree in kinesiology is the foundation for a career in the physical activity professions, a term designating all professions in which physical activity plays a central role, usually as a medium for therapy, education, health, recreation, or entertainment. Teaching physical education, coaching, being a fitness consultant or fitness director for a corporation, and serving as an athletic trainer or conditioning specialist for an athletic team are examples of positions in the physical activity professions. Some of these careers are similar with respect to general objectives, methods, educational requirements, working environments, and other factors. They can be grouped into relatively distinct spheres of professional practice in physical activity. Figure 13.2 depicts the major spheres of the physical activity professions. Keep in mind that these spheres represent very general categories; each is comprised of several different professional occupations.

Two things about the spheres bear mentioning. Although artistic expression forms a distinct sphere of professional practice, in most cases these careers are pursued through departments of dance, drama, and art rather than departments of kinesiology. For this reason, we do not deal with this sphere in any detail. Also, you will not find much in this section about careers in the scholarly study of physical activity. Careers in this sphere are mostly research or professorial positions in colleges or universities. Generally, they require a doctoral degree in one of the subdisciplines described in section 2. For most undergraduates, decisions about such careers are made late in the undergraduate program or during advanced study at the master's level.

The chapters that follow in this section describe some of the most popular physical activity professions that students graduating from kinesiology programs enter. The first step in deciding which of these exciting career paths you will follow is to familiarize yourself with what it means to be a professionals. By joining the ranks of professionals, you will share in some of the attributes, expectations, and obligations of those working in all professional fields, whether they be lawyers, counselors, clergy, physicians, or kinesiologists.

It is one thing to say you're a professional (like the janitor in the opening scenario), but it is quite another to actually become one. Do you know what sets professionals apart from nonprofessionals? Do you know the type of college preparation required of professionals? Do you know how one becomes a respected member of a profession, remains in good standing, or gets dismissed from a profession? Do you know the benefits and obli-

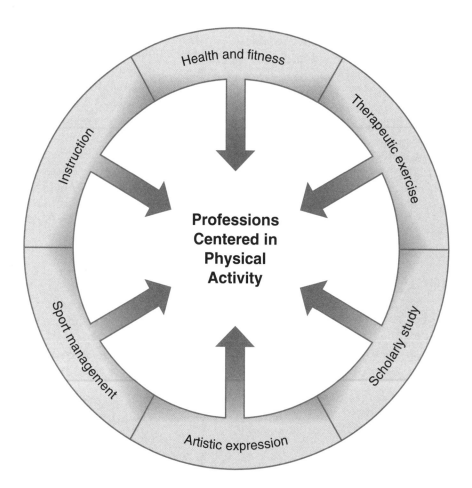

Figure 13.2 The spheres of professional practice centered in physical activity.

gations of being a professional? And are you able to recognize the traits future employers look for in students to determine who are most likely to become respected, qualified professionals? These are important questions for anyone seeking admission to the professions, and, if you're like most of your peers, you probably haven't given them a great deal of thought.

Learning about the skills and knowledge required for specific occupations such as teaching or coaching, health-fitness promotion or consulting, community sport leadership, athletic training, cardiac rehabilitation, and other careers will come later. Right now it is time to pause and take stock of your own interests, talents, and commitments, to find out if you really have what it takes to enter the workforce as a professional in the physical activity field.

What Is a Profession?

Often we use the term *professional* in an informal way to describe the quality of a person's performance. The work of a cabinetmaker may be described as "very professional," or a friend who is an excellent golfer may be described as "a real pro." Sometimes the term is used to describe those who play and/or teach a sport as a full-time source of income (e.g., *professional* baseball players, or tennis or golf *professionals* who teach at clubs) to distinguish them from those who play only part time and are not remunerated (amateurs). These hardly convey a complete picture of the formal definition of a professional. Normally, cabinetmakers or athletes are not thought of as members of a profession in the same way

we think of lawyers, physicians, teachers, counselors, physical therapists, rehabilitation specialists, or clergy as members of a profession. Surely, members of a profession are known for doing their work well, and for doing it full time and for pay, but this is hardly the whole story!

A cluster of attributes have been used to describe professional types of occupations (Greenwood, 1957; Jackson, 1970). Although some characterizations of a professional may seem a bit idealistic, they are still useful in helping us understand the distinctions of this type of work. You will discover that most types of work aren't easily classified as being completely professional or completely nonprofessional. Although some workers such as physicians may be located at the extreme "professional" pole, and common laborers may be located at the extreme "nonprofessional" pole, most types of work probably fall at some point on the continuum depicted in figure 13.3. In fact, some of the physical activity professions are termed *minor professions* or *semiprofessions* to underscore this point (Lawson, 1984).

Workers in the jobs positioned closest to the "professional" pole of the continuum

1. master complex skills that are grounded in and guided by systematic theory and research;

2. perform services for others known as clients or patients;

3. are granted a monopoly by the community to supply certain services to its members;

4. are guided by formal and informal ethical codes intended to preserve the health and well-being of their clients; and

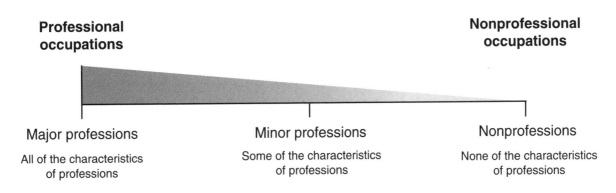

Figure 13.3   The professional continuum.

5. meet the expectations and standards prescribed by their professional subcultures.

Let's look more carefully at each of these characteristics.

🔑 Those who are preparing for a position in the physical activity professions should know what a profession is, the type of work professionals do, how one gains entry to and acceptance in a profession, the obligations of professionals, and the most important factors to be considered in preparing for a career in the physical activity professions.

Professionals Have Mastered Complex Skills Grounded in Theory and Research

Professionals are sometimes referred to as **practitioners**, a term signifying that they are "practicers" of a particular art or science. This underscores the fact that professionals are not merely gifted thinkers; they are also gifted doers. *Professionals establish their reputations by being able to bring about predetermined outcomes efficiently and effectively, usually on behalf of others.* Doing this requires skill; in fact, the expert skill of professionals is what sets them apart from other types of workers. We usually associate the concept of skill with expert motor performances—the speed of a world-class sprinter or the agility of a pro basketball player. Or we may consider professionals such as dentists or surgeons as being expert performers of **motor skills**. In most cases, however, the expertise of professionals is manifested in their cognitive, interpersonal, and perceptual skills. The **cognitive skills** of analysis, deduction, diagnosis, prescription, and high-level reasoning are particularly important. In fact, they are absolutely essential if professionals are to make expert decisions regarding their professional practices.

A workplace biomechanist must be able to analyze workers' movements in order to diagnose why a certain group of workers has a high injury rate, and then must be able to devise strategies for correcting the movements and reducing injury. An athletic trainer must be able to communicate well with athletes and motivate them to continue with their rehabilitation programs on days they do not feel like it. Each of these skills involves a systematic application of techniques, based in knowledge, in order to bring about certain carefully defined objectives. Becoming a professional, then, involves recognizing what steps need to be taken in any given situation, knowing the procedures for carrying out those steps, and having the skill required to do it.

How do physical activity professionals acquire these important skills? To a certain extent, these skills are based on knowledge acquired from having performed and watched others perform physical activity. Remember physical activity experience can be an important source of knowledge for kinesiology students. Most professionals have had a great deal of experience, either participating in or watching the physical activities that form the focus of their professional practice. For example, while not all elite soccer, basketball, or gymnastic coaches were elite performers of the sports they coach, most have spent time performing and watching the activity, and are familiar with and comfortable in the contexts in which the sports are played. (We talk more about the contribution of physical activity experience to your professional development later in this chapter.)

To a certain extent, the skills of the physical activity professional also derive from a knowledge of theory about physical activity. This **theoretical knowledge** is embedded in concepts and principles related to physical activity that come from the subdisciplines summarized in section 2. These concepts and principles comprise the body of **kinesiology theory**. But not all or even most of kinesiology theory may be directly applicable to the daily tasks performed by professionals. For example, learning how to calculate the optimal angle of the shot put's projection in biomechanics class may not be very useful information to a track coach, just as learning the details of pulmonary function in exercise physiology class may not be directly applicable to the athletic trainer's work.

This is not to suggest that kinesiology theory is unimportant. Because it focuses on broad principles about physical activity, it can have a potent, albeit indirect, impact on the way professionals think and on the skills they use to solve problems. This is particularly important because professionals are constantly required to adapt knowledge to new situations and to think in highly flexible ways. Bricklaying and carpentry— trades or crafts, not professions—also require the use of certain cognitive and perceptual skills, but they are almost always applied to a stable set of problems and contexts. Because one brick wall is pretty much like another, even laypersons can buy books on home repair and, simply by reading, serve as their own bricklayer. Professional work, on the other hand, involves solving a constantly changing set of problems that cannot be solved by reading simple manuals. Mastering theoretical knowledge of kinesiology helps professionals to ask intelligent questions about their work, and enables them to devise flexible strategies for solving problems, even those they may never before have experienced.

For example, a physical education teacher may observe an error in a student's motor performance that he has never seen before. By systematically applying his knowledge of movement mechanics, motor learning, and pedagogy, as well as by using a "diagnostic eye" developed through practice, he will be able to devise practice experiences to correct the error. Likewise, an athletic trainer confronted in an emergency with a rare injury may rely on her in-depth knowledge of biomechanics, exercise physiology, and other kinesiological concepts to determine the best course of emergency action.

But theoretical knowledge by itself may not be sufficient to guide the skillful behavior of professionals. Usually it must become part of **professional practice knowledge** before it is useful to the professional. You may think of professional practice knowledge as knowledge of how to perform some professional skill. Professional practice knowledge in medicine might be knowing how to diagnose various diseases, or in law, knowing how to conduct oneself effectively in court. Professional practice knowledge in kinesiology may be knowing how to help a class of 10-year-olds learn to perform a cartwheel, how to direct and project your voice in a crowded fitness facility, or how to tape an ankle if you are an athletic trainer. Many times, professional practice knowledge is merely knowing how to apply kinesiology theory, but it is more than this. Professional practice knowledge is an amalgam of theoretical knowledge and other information learned by professionals as they go about their day-to-day jobs. Most professionals, physical activity professionals included, learn much of what they know about "what works and what doesn't work" by systematically reflecting on their professional actions and the consequences of those actions. Obviously, this process is not performed in a vacuum; it always proceeds on the basis of a vast and complicated knowledge base about theory and the application of theory. Professional practice knowledge, often called "knowledge in action" (Schon, 1995), is demonstrated, not by answering questions on a true-false or multiple-choice test, but by showing how well you can perform a professional skill. In such cases the "know-how" is *in* the action itself.

For example, consider a high school American football coach whose team is five yards away from scoring the winning touchdown in the state finals. His inexperienced quarterback is nervous and anxious and sure that he will fail to make the play. There is no time to practice a play or implement some new coaching strategy. Instead, the coach finds just the right words to say, the right motivations to use, to get the quarterback focused and confident. Although it is fairly easy

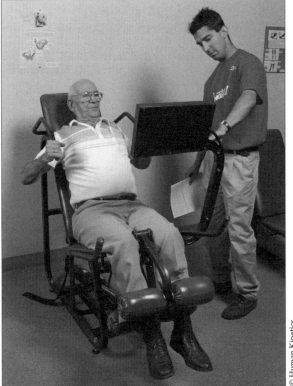

Professionals rely on a variety of different types of knowledge to carry out their daily tasks.

© Human Kinetics

to see that the coach is effective with his athletes and regularly produces winning teams, if asked how he motivates his players, he may find it very difficult to explain exactly what he does. Yet he clearly uses basic principles of sport psychology to accomplish his goals in combination with extensive knowledge acquired through trial and error in professional practice.

Finally, professionals also rely on **workplace knowledge** to perform relatively mundane tasks associated with their jobs. Usually this type of knowledge requires little formal education or training. For example, cardiac rehabilitation technologists must know how to monitor the cleanliness of the facility or how to schedule patients for examinations. They must know proper procedures for opening and closing the facility. Although such tasks are not professional in their scope and do not require highly sophisticated knowledge, they are important. A cardiac rehabilitation technician who does not maintain a clean testing facility, or ensure that the equipment is maintained in proper working condition, may soon find herself unemployed, regardless of the quality of her professional skills.

🔑 Professionals develop a range of cognitive, perceptual, and motor skills, anchored in theoretical, practice, and workplace knowledge, that enable them to achieve predetermined outcomes efficiently and effectively.

Professionals Perform Services for Clients or Patients

Most professional work takes the form of services that are performed for clients. **Service** connotes giving assistance or advantage to others, usually in a spirit of helpfulness and concern. Most professionals are conscious of their roles as service providers. In fact, those in nursing, criminal justice, family counseling, public health, recreation, and kinesiology increasingly refer to their professions as helping fields or **helping professions** (Lawson, 1998b). The beneficiaries of a professional's services are known as clients. (In the medical field, clients are patients; in teaching, they are students.) Professionals are in "the people business"; they like meeting and working with people, are comfortable in social settings, and are confident in their social skills. They derive great enjoyment from helping people meet their needs and accomplish important goals.

The notion of service comprises three important aspects. First, professionals are *committed* to providing service. It isn't uncommon to hear professionals describe their career as "a calling," suggesting that their primary motivation is to enhance the health, education, enjoyment, and general well-being of those they serve. In fact, concern for the well-being of clients often supersedes professionals' concern for their own comfort and satisfaction. You may have known physicians or lawyers who sacrificed lucrative practices in order to work in inner cities or Third World countries for poor and disadvantaged people. The same spirit is reflected in the teacher who volunteers her time to give remedial instruction to a student on the weekend, or the geriatric fitness leader who stays late following each session to give special attention to an elderly man too embarrassed to exercise with others present. Obviously, extreme financial sacrifices are not required of professionals, but harboring a spirit of wanting to help others is.

Reflect on the various jobs you have held and the different types of knowledge you have used in each. What workplace knowledge did you develop while on the job? For example, you might have learned how to use a time clock or a cash register, how to close a restaurant, certain abbreviations specific to your workplace, or which forms to fill out for certain requests.

Have you held any positions in which the knowledge you learned verged on professional practice knowledge? Maybe you taught swim lessons and got a feel for how to help young children brave the water. Or perhaps you volunteered at the local YMCA and observed how the program director chose and gave feedback to staff members. These types of knowledge will be essential as you develop in your profession.

Second, professionals render *expert* service. Being a professional means more than simply being willing to help. Professionals know how to determine a client's needs and how to initiate and evaluate an appropriate course of action to meet those needs. Because of this, professionals are granted a certain amount of autonomy to carry out their work. Their opinions are respected, and they have a great deal of freedom to make decisions about how they will help clients. Some professionals have more autonomy than others. Those in private practice tend to have more autonomy than those working in institutions such as hospitals, school systems, universities, the government, or the military where some degree of professional autonomy may be relinquished in order to satisfy the demands of the bureaucracy. The personal trainer in private practice may enjoy much more autonomy in decision making than the physical education teacher whose actions may be limited by school board policies, the dictates of a school principal, and the curriculum guide.

The third aspect of service is the fact that clients inevitably become dependent to varying degrees on the professional. This is not always desirable but it is inevitable, and the extent of such dependency varies widely. A dance student depends on his teacher to improve his technique just as a patient depends on her exercise therapist to design a program to help her recover from an injury. Unlike customers at a department store who usually have a clear idea of what they want and are able to evaluate the products they purchase, clients usually do not have the knowledge essential for judging the quality of the professional's conduct. Consequently, they can only have faith that the professional will keep their best interests a priority when making decisions. One of the most egregious violations of professional conduct is exploiting this vulnerability of clients. This is why the coach who orders an injured player back into the game, or a physical therapist who, not wanting to suffer financial loss, fails to refer a patient to a competitor even though the competitor may be better equipped to meet the patient's need, will quickly lose the respect of colleagues.

The touchstone of professional work is the delivery of expert services in order to improve the quality of life for others, always with priority given to the client's welfare.

Professionals Possess a Monopoly on the Delivery of Services

Professionals are valued by society because they provide a needed service unavailable through any other occupational group. If you need a cavity filled, you go to a dentist. If you need spiritual guidance, you may go to a member of the clergy. If you need to rehabilitate an injured knee in order to play basketball again, you may go to a sport physical therapist.

The physical activity professions came into existence and continue to flourish because they make a unique and valuable contribution to the health and well-being of society. People recognize the need for help in regaining or maintaining their health, becoming physically fit, increasing their proficiency in motor and sport skills, recovering from injuries, or organizing and coaching sport programs. No other discipline offers the knowledge and skills needed to prepare experts to help people meet this diverse range of needs as does kinesiology. In this sense, kinesiology and the physical activity professionals it prepares possess a monopoly on the delivery of physical activity services.

Professionals are valued because they alone have the knowledge and skills to meet a particular need or needs of the community.

Professionals Collaborate With Colleagues to Ensure High Standards and Ethical Practices

Professionals recognize that society has granted them authority to regulate their own conduct and expects them to do it. When standards of conduct by all members of a profession remain high, the needs of society are satisfied and the monopoly of the profession is protected. When the conduct of one professional violates accepted standards, it threatens all members of the profession by bringing into question the legitimacy of the monopoly. Thus, professionals have a vested interest in maintaining or improving not only the quality of their own practices but also the quality of service delivered by all members of their profession. In this sense, although professionals may work at clinics, schools, hospitals, or other agencies, they view themselves first and foremost as representatives of the profession as a whole.

Sometimes the quality of professionals' practices suffers because they fail to keep abreast of developments in their fields. Because the knowledge base for the physical activity professions is expanding continually, this can happen rather easily for exercise leaders, teachers, trainers, sport leaders, and other professionals. Professionals whose practices are not in accord with the latest information become a threat to all professionals in the field. A clinical exercise physiologist who fails to keep abreast of her field is in danger of recommending activities to clients that have been shown to be inferior or dangerous by recent research. Such a person may be accused of "acting unprofessionally."

As a way of ensuring that their knowledge and skills are not outdated, competent practitioners join professional organizations; regularly read professional books and articles; and attend conferences, workshops, and other meetings sponsored by professional societies. Unlike salespersons, business executives, or others in the commercial marketplace who tend to protect information from their competitors, members of a profession relate to each other as colleagues (literally "fellow workers") and willingly collaborate and share information in order to serve the best interests of their clients. If you want to be a top-notch professional, you must commit to educating yourself continually. Plan to join professional organizations and to read literature about your field regularly.

Operating on a less than adequate knowledge base is not the only way professionals breach standards of conduct. Professionals also can be sanctioned by their colleagues for unethical behavior in the workplace. Unethical conduct occurs when the behavior of a professional at the worksite comes into conflict with values held by his or her colleagues. In order to ensure that members clearly understand ethical expectations, professional organizations often publish a code of ethical principles and standards. The primary objective of such codes is to protect the

rights of clients. They may instruct professionals to describe and advertise their competencies accurately, describe the nature of the relationship that should exist between clients and professionals and between subordinates and professionals, and clarify matters involving financial transactions with clients. Figure 13.4 includes an abbreviated summary of ethical guidelines published by the Association for the Advancement of Applied Sport Psychology, which are intended to regulate the practice of sport psychologists who consult with athletes, as well as the actions of scientists who conduct research in sport psychology.

One way professions attempt to ensure that members understand the prevailing code of conduct and are competent to implement safe and effective practice is to license their members. A license is formal authority granted by law to practice a profession. Professions that require licenses can suspend a professional's license for any number of infractions, effectively terminating the professional's authority to practice.

Professionals have a vested interest in maintaining high standards of conduct for all practitioners in their profession. In order to accomplish this, professional organizations make available opportunities for continuing education by their members and publish guidelines specifying acceptable and unacceptable ethical conduct.

While the medical and legal professions have made effective use of licensing provisions to control the quality of professional services, relatively few physical activity professions are licensed. An exception is physical therapy. Athletic trainers are now being licensed in selective states, a trend that may soon move across the nation. Public school teachers are certified or licensed by state governing agencies. This doesn't mean that unethical or improper conduct by physical activity professionals goes unpunished. Usually, the appropriate sanction is administered at the local workplace, often in consultation with a professional organization. For example, a schoolteacher whose conduct violates ethical codes may be terminated by the local school board. A conditioning coach who administers illegal anabolic

The Ethics Code of the Association for the Advancement of Applied Sport Psychology (Abbreviated Summary)

Purpose: The Ethics Code provides a common set of values upon which members build their professional and scientific work. It has as its primary goal the welfare and protection of the individuals and groups with whom AAASP members work.

A. *Competence:* Members recognize the boundaries of their particular competencies and expertise. They maintain the knowledge required to perform the services they render. They provide only those services and use only those techniques for which they are qualified by education, training, or experience.

B. *Integrity:* Members are honest and fair. In describing or reporting their qualifications, services, products, fees, research or teaching, they do not make statements that are false, misleading, or deceptive. They avoid improper and potentially harmful dual relationships.

C. *Professional and Scientific Responsibility:* Members uphold professional standards of conduct and accept responsibility for their behavior. They are concerned about the ethical compliance of their colleagues' scientific and professional conduct. When appropriate, they consult with colleagues in order to prevent, avoid, or terminate unethical conduct.

D. *Respect for People's Rights and Dignity:* Members respect the rights of individuals to privacy, confidentiality, self-determination, and autonomy. They are aware of cultural, individual, and role differences, including those due to age, gender, race, ethnicity, national origin, sexual orientation, disability, language, and socioeconomic status.

E. *Concern for Others' Welfare:* Members seek to contribute to the welfare of those with whom they interact professionally. They are sensitive to real and ascribed differences in power between themselves and others, and they do not exploit or mislead other people during or after professional relationships.

F. *Social Responsibility:* Members are aware of their professional and scientific responsibilities to the community. They apply and make public their knowledge in order to contribute to human welfare. They strive to advance human welfare while protecting the rights of participants. They try to avoid misuse of their work, and they comply with the law.

Figure 13.4 Selected ethical principles and standards for members of the Association for the Advancement of Applied Sport Psychology.
Adapted, by permission, from M.L. Sachs, K.G. Burke, and S. Gomer, 1998, *Directory of graduate programs in applied sport psychology*, 5th ed. (Morgantown, WV: Fitness Information Technology, Inc.).

steroids to athletes may be fired by his university. Although the American College of Sports Medicine cannot suspend a cardiac rehabilitation therapist whose conduct puts a client at risk, the clinic director or other supervisor may decide to terminate the worker after consulting ACSM guidelines.

Professionals Adhere to Standards of Their Professional Subculture

Although professionals work in a variety of different locales and contexts, they tend to hold high expectations concerning the way members present themselves and relate to others. For example, professionals place a strong emphasis on politeness to colleagues as well as to those they serve. They tend to be well organized in their work, are not clock watchers, and don't hesitate to work extra hours when it is required. They dress according to accepted occupational standards and are attentive to matters of personal grooming and hygiene. A sport program director who comes to a board meeting in dirty and disheveled clothes, a cardiac rehabilitation technician who forgets to wear her lab coat, and a physical education instructor who teaches classes in street clothes are not dressed "professionally." The physical therapist who never combs or brushes his hair or the personal trainer who smells of body odor are all guilty of presenting themselves in an unprofessional manner. These are general expectations of professionals in any field.

In addition, physical activity professionals often are faced with a more specific set of expectations. For example, fitness leaders or physical education teachers may be expected to model the physically active life and to maintain a level of fitness appropriate for their age.

Different physical activity professions are likely to require unique types of knowledge, employ different types of skills, operate according to different standards and codes of conduct,

Is physical activity experience a daily part of your life? If not, you need to consider integrating it into your lifestyle. Do you smoke? Are you severely overweight? Although these are matters of personal choice, you should know that these and other unhealthy lifestyle habits could be impediments to your gaining employment or promotion in a physical activity profession.

require different languages and terminology, require different certification and continuing education procedures, and often involve different types of dress and on-the-job conduct. When an individual learns to accommodate to these pro-

Locating Occupations on the Professional Continuum

Now that we have studied the qualities and characteristics of a professional, where would you place the following occupations on the professional continuum? Locate each of the following occupations on the continuum by assigning each a numerical score. Assign occupations you believe should be located nearer the professional end of the continuum lower scores, and those nearer the nonprofessional end a higher score. (Scores for three occupations are provided in parentheses. These scores are for illustrative purposes only. Generally, physicians and lawyers are regarded as engaged in work that meets most, if not all, of the characteristics of a profession, while common laborers are regarded as engaged in work that lacks most, if not all, of these characteristics.) Be prepared to give reasons for the scores assigned to each occupation.

Professional				Nonprofessional
1	2	3	4	5

Physician (1)   *Laborer (5)*
Lawyer (1.3)

1. Physical education teacher in a public school
2. Exercise leader at a commercial fitness center
3. Cardiac rehabilitation specialist
4. Athletic trainer
5. Professional golf instructor
6. High school varsity football coach
7. Director of a corporate fitness program
8. University athletic director
9. Personal fitness trainer in private practice
10. Sport psychologist consultant to Olympic athletes

fession-specific expectations, he or she is said to have been "socialized" into the profession. Becoming socialized into a profession means learning how to conduct yourself according to the roles and responsibilities of the workplace. The ease, confidence, and efficiency with which professionals perform their daily activities and communicate with their clients and coworkers are good indications of how well they have been socialized into their professional roles.

Obviously, the sooner you become socialized into your profession, the more valuable you will be to an employer. This is one reason growing numbers of students in professional programs seek opportunities for volunteering in clinics, YMCAs, schools, and community agencies. Although usually not counted as course work, such extracurricular experiences can give you a head start in learning how to assume professional roles. Similar growth and leadership opportunities are available in student major clubs, athletics, student government organizations, and other on-campus activities.

🔑 Professionals should conform to the norms of the general subculture of their profession as well as to the norms and expectations of the specific subculture of their particular workplace.

How Do Our Values Shape Our Professional Conduct?

Personal values impact how we lead our lives, including how we approach our work. This might be a good place to stop and ask yourself about your values and how they might shape your professional philosophy and practices. Hal Lawson (1998a) has described two types of extreme value orientations that may characterize professionals in any field—mechanical, market-driven professionalism and social trustee, civic professionalism. Although these orientations are "ideal types," which is to say that most professionals don't fit completely into one category or the other, they can serve as reference points in helping you

determine how you want to operate as a professional

Mechanical, Market-Driven Professionalism

Mechanical, market-driven professionals tend to be fascinated with their professional methods and techniques, so much so that they sometimes lose sight of their clients' needs and desires. In many cases, their work becomes its own justification, valued by them and their colleagues regardless of whether it has any real benefits for society. The medical, nursing, and law professions sometimes are accused of this type of professionalism, but some of the physical activity professions can be guilty of this too.

Mechanical, market-driven professionals also are likely to serve their clients in a fragmented, compartmentalized fashion. That is, they view their professional contributions within the strict limits of their specialization and ignore the variety of relevant forces acting on the client, such as family disintegration, illness, or drug or alcohol dependency. These "other problems" tend to be dismissed as "somebody else's problem." Such professionals may treat clients humanely but with little feeling; they believe that an objective, "arms-distance" attitude is critical to professional success.

Because they are prestige conscious, mechanical, market-driven professionals devote much time to enhancing their status and competing with other professionals, even if it means sacrificing the quality of service given to their clients. They pride themselves on their expertise, viewing themselves as superior to those they serve and often encouraging clients to develop a dependency on them and their services.

Social Trustee, Civic Professionalism

Social trustee, civic professionals hold to a much different set of values. They believe that the worth of a profession is measured by its effectiveness in promoting the social welfare, enhancing social and economic development and democracy, and ensuring social responsibility and social justice. The actions of social trustee, civic professionals are guided not by a fascination with technology and technique or by a concern for status and prestige but by a vision of a good and just society. They operate according to this rule of thumb: "Healthy people and a good society first, me and my profession second in service of this greater good"(Lawson, 1998a, p. 7). They recognize that clients live in a multiplicity of worlds (e.g., work, school, family, church) and understand the ways in which worlds can interact to affect their clients' lives. Because of this they often work in teams with other specialists to achieve desirable goals. They make no pretense about being objective in their relationships with clients: their values are reflected in their professional practices. They don't view clients as being dependent on them, believing that the professional–client interaction can be a mutual growth experience in which each benefits from the other's knowledge and skill.

Consider the physical activity professionals you have come into contact with. Have you met mechanical, market-driven professionals? Social trustee, civic professionals? Which did you prefer? Which did you feel were more effective? Why?

Examples of Values Shaping Professional Conduct

Let's look at a couple of examples. A basketball coach of a large high school whose primary objective is to move on to the college ranks may operate as a mechanical, market-driven professional. His goal may be to produce a winning team, not for the satisfaction and educational rewards it can bring to his players, but because he considers establishing a creditable win-loss record as the best way to advance professionally. His career aspirations are the driving force in his life. He doesn't spend much time trying to develop the skills of those struggling to learn the game; in fact, as a physical education teacher he is known as a teacher who "throws out the ball" and retreats to his office to work on plans for the next game. Although some of his players have problems at home the coach doesn't have time to

listen to them; he tells them, What is important is how you perform on the basketball court, and it is my job to help you do this. If you're having problems in your personal life, go see the school counselor. He is well known for pushing his players to play when they are injured, for pressuring faculty into giving players passing grades, and for the caustic sarcasm he directs at players during practice and at officials during games. He justifies all of it because he has demonstrated that it produces winning teams.

A commercial fitness center director whose primary objective is to contribute to a good and just and physically active society—while still earning a livelihood—may operate as a social trustee, civic professional. Improving the health and well-being of the surrounding community through increased daily physical activity and lifestyle changes, while meeting reasonable financial goals, are this director's driving forces. She offers community-based programs at minimal cost to socially disadvantaged children or the elderly. She also encourages her fitness consultants not to induce dependency in clients but instead to teach them to become independent exercisers by taking advantage of seminars and opportunities to exercise at home or work. Fitness consultants treat clients as partners with shared responsibilities for improving their lifestyles. They relate to those they serve in a caring, sympathetic way and act as trained professionals who have earned the authority to make day-to-day decisions about how clients will be served. When the staff becomes aware of clients' personal problems such as spouse abuse, psychological disorders, obesity, or family neglect, they refer them to appropriate professionals. In addition, the director of this fitness center offers some free and discounted memberships to members of the community unable to pay full price.

Your personal values will influence how you act out your professional role. Mechanical, market-driven professionals value the profession, profit, personal prestige, and status over the rights and needs of clients. Social trustee, civic professionals value clients and the social good more than themselves or their profession.

How Are Physical Activity Professionals Educated for the Workforce?

Now that you've examined some of the general characteristics of the professions, it's time to consider what is required by way of formal education. By now you are aware that professional work requires advanced knowledge that can be obtained only through formal education at the undergraduate and graduate levels. Consequently, whether you will be qualified to enter the physical activity professions depends a great deal on the academic experiences you receive in college. If you're like most college students, you may not always understand why certain courses are required or understand what the purposes are of various phases of the curriculum. You might be interested to learn that kinesiologists themselves are engaged in a debate concerning the structure of the kinesiology curriculum. In fact, opinions among the faculty at your institution may vary widely. The curriculum model endorsed by the editors of this book incorporates the following five different, yet related, types of academic experiences essential for preparing kinesiologists for their professional roles:

- Liberal arts and sciences
- Course work in physical activity
- Course work in theoretical and applied theoretical knowledge in kinesiology
- Course work in professional practice knowledge and skills for particular professions
- Apprenticeship or internship experience at the worksite

The best professional preparation programs immerse students in all of these academic experiences.

Liberal Arts and Sciences

All college graduates, regardless of their career aspirations, are expected to be educated people. Used in this sense, *educated* means to have been exposed to great works of literature, to have learned about the historical development of human civilization, to have developed critical skills essential for analyzing arguments logically, to be able to determine the truthfulness of ideas and to identify the values embedded in them, to have developed sufficient knowledge about the arts to appreciate the richness they can add to one's life, and to have developed insights into the problems and prospects of their own culture and the culture of others. Accomplishing this goal requires courses in science, philosophy, history, literature, sociology, mathematics, art, music, and the dramatic arts, among others. This is why all colleges and universities require students to take courses in the liberal arts and sciences, sometimes also referred to as liberal studies.

It is called "liberal" education because only by immersing yourself in the arts and sciences can you "liberate" or free yourself from dependence on the thinking of others. Liberally educated people know how to educate themselves. They have developed a capacity for seeking the truth and for making intelligent choices when confronted by life's problems and opportunities. Admittedly, these are grand aims. In fact, you might wonder if producing an educated person in four years is possible. If you thought this, you're right on target. In fact, a liberal education is a lifelong process. Nobody is ever *completely* educated; everybody is always in the *process* of becoming educated. One of the hallmarks of educated persons is that they are aware of what they do not know and continually seek opportunities to expand their intellectual and cultural horizons by reading books and newspapers, attending concerts, patronizing the arts, and engaging in other lifelong educational activities.

Thus, the education you receive in college is just the beginning of your liberal education. Whether this initial immersion in the liberal arts and sciences has accomplished its purpose will be reflected in your level of interest in continuing to educate yourself after graduation. What types of books will you read? What kind of music will you listen to? How will you speak and write? Will your analysis of the claims of politicians and other public figures be logical and based in fact? Your approach to these and hundreds of other life experiences should bear witness to the fact that you are a liberally educated person. Of course, a liberal education is expected to have short-term effects too. The most important is to provide you with the broad-based knowledge and intellectual skills essential for undertaking more advanced study in your professional curriculum.

> A liberal education frees you from depending on others to do your thinking for you. It is the foundation on which all other educational experiences are constructed.

Course Work in Physical Activity

Kinesiology majors usually are required to enroll in physical activity courses, either as part of their liberal education requirements or in conjunction with their professional programs. As was noted in section 1, you entered college with a wealth of experiential knowledge about physical activity and no doubt found it to be a vehicle for learning much about yourself, others, and the world around you. But the physical activity experiences offered within the framework of a liberal and / or professional education should result in qualitatively richer experiences than the experiences you had before you came to college. Let's take a moment to consider how physical activity courses at the college level might affect you differently.

If you've already taken a physical activity course at your college, your first impression might have been that it wasn't all that different from physical education courses you took in high school. Both focused on sport, outdoor activities, or fitness. But even if the course of instruction seemed to be the same, what is different is *you*. As your liberal education continues to expand your horizons, your approach to physical activity should change as well. You should be a more intelligent analyst, a more persuasive critic, and a more astute observer of the world around you; this includes the world of physical activity as well as the world of ideas.

Will a liberal education make you a better performer of physical activity? Perhaps, but not necessarily. What it should do is cause you to approach the learning of a new skill or the task of improving your health and fitness in a more systematic and intelligent fashion, which may result in payoffs in terms of the outcomes produced. But the primary contribution of a liberal education should be to enrich your physical activity experiences, much the same way it should enrich your experiences of art, music, and litera-

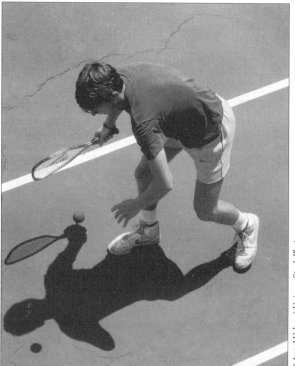

Your liberal education should enrich your physical activity experiences, making you a more intelligent analyst and astute observer of physical activity.

© Aneal Vohra / Unicorn Stock Photos

ture. A course in martial arts should attune you to the nuances of pace, tempo, and rhythm; a course in fencing should foster an appreciation of beauty, force, and form in movement. Your course work in physical activity may sensitize you to ethical and moral questions that might have gone unnoticed before you were exposed to a liberal education.

Physical activity courses may also be required as part of your kinesiology major. If you plan a career in teaching, coaching, or fitness leadership, the requirement may be quite understandable to you, but why require it for students in sport administration, physical therapy, or other professions in which physical activity performance is not part of the professional responsibilities? If you're struggling with this question, we suggest you think back on the general model of physical activity described in chapter 1, recognizing that knowledge gained through physical activity provides one of the three legs of the stool on which the discipline of kinesiology rests. Whatever profession you enter, performance of physical activity will be at center stage, and it is critical that you have acquired a wealth of firsthand physical activity experiences, not only to help you identify with physical activity problems confronted by your clients, but also to broaden and enrich your comprehensive understanding of the phenomenon of physical activity.

🔑══ College courses in physical activities are taken in conjunction with liberal studies and as an essential part of your professional preparation. As a result, you should develop the ability to examine your physical activity experiences from an informed, educated perspective and to integrate the knowledge learned from them into a coherent professional perspective.

Course Work in Theoretical Kinesiology

Section 2 gave you a general overview of the subdisciplines of kinesiology. These subdisciplines comprise what is often referred to as the theoretical knowledge of kinesiology. Theoretical knowledge is not only knowledge about sports and fitness, but also about physical activity in general. Obviously much of it is very applicable to professional practice. For example, theoretical knowledge about how the body responds to exercise (drawn from the subdiscipline of physiology of physical activity) is directly applicable to the work of a swimming coach or cardiac rehabilitation specialist. Other theoretical knowledge, in sport history, for example, or biomechanics, may not seem applicable immediately, but over time the knowledge may have a profound effect on how a professional thinks and, thus, operates.

Some professors would argue that students should not expect all of theoretical kinesiology to be immediately useful in their professional careers. This is not its primary purpose. From this perspective, courses in theoretical kinesiology (except the portions stemming from research about professional practice) should be viewed as similar to English, history, biology, literature, and other courses in liberal studies. Disciplines such as literature, philosophy, biology, and physics are not justified on the grounds that they prepare students for specific types of work, but because we believe they sharpen students' perspectives on

themselves and the world around them and help them develop new and creative ways of thinking. The argument can be made that physical activity is so critical to human life, that, like art, music, drama, and dance, it can teach us unique things about ourselves and our culture. Viewed in this light, theoretical kinesiology should not be expected to be any more immediately applicable to professional practice than should other liberal studies such as poetry or medieval history.

Figure 13.5 depicts the dominant view of theoretical kinesiology. The notion that theoretical kinesiology could stand alone as a separate discipline was originally conceived by Franklin Henry at the University of California at Berkeley (1964). Henry's view of the "academic discipline of physical education" was much narrower than the view presented in this text. For Henry, the discipline was limited to knowledge acquired through scholarly study of physical activity, what we refer to here as theoretical kinesiology. It did not include knowledge acquired through physical activity experience or through professional practice. Theoretical kinesiology consists of an assortment of knowledge about physical activity that has been gleaned from traditional disciplines in the humanities; biological, behavioral, and social sciences; and the arts. Whereas an introductory sociology course might offer scant coverage of the sociology of sport, and an introductory physics course might ignore the mechanics of motion, theoretical kinesiology focuses precisely on these topics. By extracting this neglected knowledge about physical activity from traditional disciplines, expanding it, and integrating it into a coherent course of study, kinesiologists have created a stimulating body of knowledge for students planning to enter the physical activity professions.

The evolution of theoretical knowledge of kinesiology has been an exciting development in the field of physical activity. But how much of this knowledge should be required of students embarking on careers in the physical activity professions? Should future athletic trainers, physical education teachers, or aquatic therapists be expected to master the entire theoretical body of knowledge of kinesiology? The sport management major may well ask why he must take courses in exercise physiology or biomechanics, and the student planning to be a conditioning coach may well ask why she should be expected

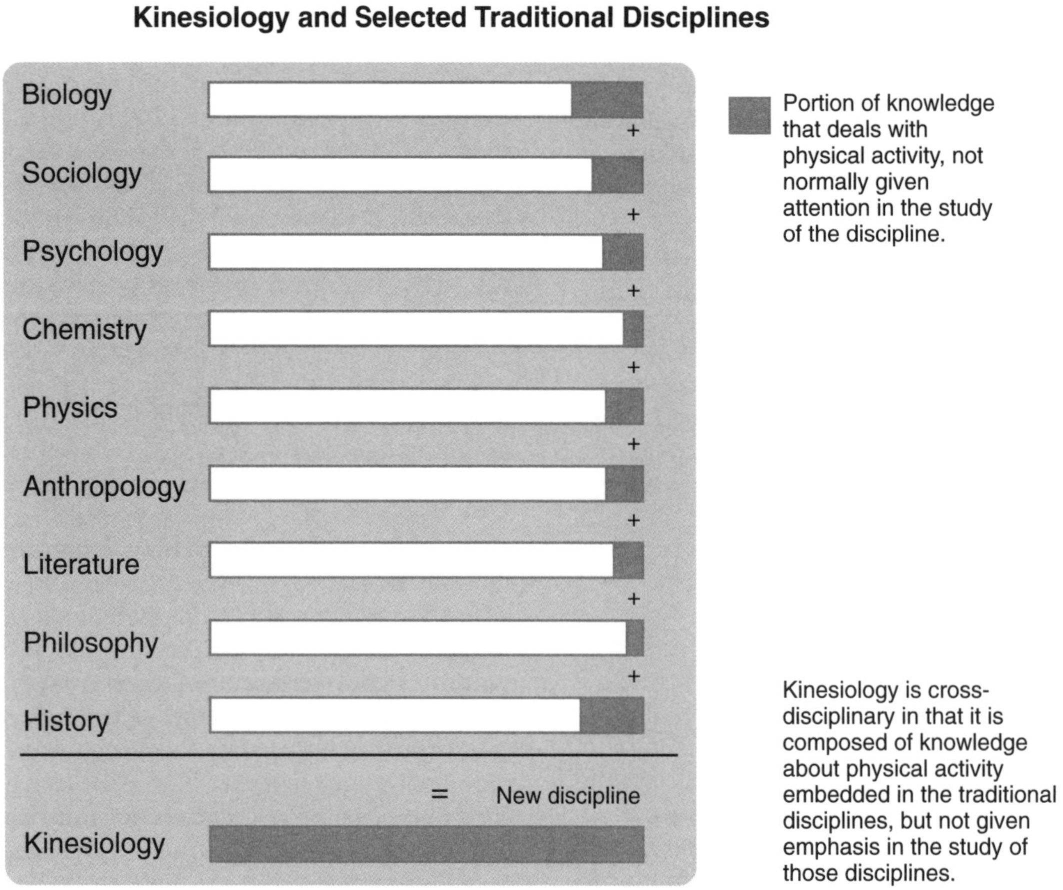

Kinesiology and Selected Traditional Disciplines

Figure 13.5   Theoretical knowledge in kinesiology.

to know about the history and philosophy of sport, especially when the concepts may not apply to the professional problems she will face in the workplace.

The answer to such questions has been a matter of vigorous debate among scholars for over 20 years. On one side are those who argue that kinesiology theory is not especially helpful to professionals, especially when no effort is made by professors to apply it to professional problems (Locke, 1990; Siedentop, 1990). On the other side are those who contend that all undergraduate kinesiology majors, regardless of their career aspirations, should be required to learn the body of theoretical knowledge of kinesiology (Newell, 1990a). They believe that by mastering such knowledge, physical activity professionals set themselves apart from nonprofessionals, thereby bolstering their monopoly on their profession and protecting physical activity professionals against threats of deprofessionalization. For example, the personal trainer who understands the mechanics

of energy systems or the physiology of muscle function will enjoy more professional respect than "fitness instructors" whose training consisted of a weekend workshop at the local gym.

Kinesiology theory is interesting in its own right; it may or may not be directly applicable to professional practice.

Another argument for requiring students to master theoretical kinesiology is that it ensures that all professionals in the field are united around a common core of physical activity theory, without which kinesiology might fragment into a number of completely different disciplines. Also, those who believe that all physical activity professionals should be required to study theoretical kinesiology argue that it actually might benefit future professionals in ways we do not fully understand. Just as a liberal education is believed to alter students' ways of approaching problems and opportunities in their lives, so an immersion in the theoretical knowledge of the discipline may equip physical activity professionals with general concepts and ways of thinking about physical activity that will assist them in solving the myriad problems they will face in professional practice.

What courses in kinesiology does your college or university require of all kinesiology or exercise science majors? What seems to be the rationale for the inclusion or exclusion of certain courses?

Because some disagreement still exists concerning the relationship of kinesiology theory to professional practice, course requirements in theoretical kinesiology tend to vary from institution to institution. Most undergraduate programs require students to take some courses in kinesiology theory regardless of their career aspirations. Table 13.1 lists courses required of all undergraduates at one university regardless of whether they plan to be physical education teachers, fitness consultants, athletic trainers, aquatic specialists, cardiac rehabilitation technicians, or community sport leaders.

Those entering the physical activity professions are expected to master kinesiology theory whether or not all of it is immediately applicable to their future occupations. As an extension of liberal studies with a narrowed focus on the phenomenon of physical activity, it represents a bridge between liberal studies and the physical activity professions.

Course Work in Professional Practice Knowledge

Your preparation as a professional wouldn't be complete if you didn't learn how to perform the essential skills of your profession. The point made earlier bears repeating: *Knowledge of kinesiology theory is not sufficient to prepare you for professional practice.* Physical education teachers need to master the difficult skills of planning and organizing lessons, communicating with and motivating students, and evaluating students' performances. They must be able to operate efficiently and effectively in the social context of the schools. These knowledge-based skills are learned by directly practicing how to be a professional by learning kinesiology theory developed through research about professional practice.

| TABLE 13.1 |||
| Required Courses in Kinesiology Theory* |||
Course	Credits	Year
Research and evaluation	3	2
History and philosophy of sport	3	2
Motor development	3	2
Motor learning and control	3	3
Psychology of sport	3	3
Sociocultural aspects of sport	3	3
Biomechanics of physical activity	3	3
Physiology of physical activity	3	3

*Courses required by all students in the Department of Exercise and Sport Science at the University of North Carolina, Greensboro, regardless of professional specialization.

Whereas most theories of kinesiology focus on the performance of physical activity and the sociocultural contexts within which physical activity is embedded, mastering professional practices centers on clarifying clients' needs and desires, analyzing impediments to the realization of these needs and desires, and implementing actions appropriate to the context and other relevant factors. Professional practice knowledge, an amalgamation of professional experience with research about professional practice, is systematically organized into practice theories. A practice theory may guide a professional in selecting the best way to perform cardiovascular tests on elderly persons at a nursing home with limited equipment, how to motivate a soccer player who is having academic difficulties and who misses off-season training sessions, or what type of balls and bats to use to speed the learning of children with autism.

Unlike kinesiological theory, practice theories and the skills of professional practice cannot be completely mastered simply by studying them; they are learned through action. They are acquired by "hands-on" practical experiences centered around solving real-life professional problems. You can learn *about* administering a stress test by reading a book, but you learn *how to* administer a stress test only by following up your reading with practical experience. By committing errors and receiving instructive feedback from your professors, you will gradually develop and sharpen your command of professional practice knowledge.

Knowledge of kinesiology theory alone will not equip you to perform the tasks required in your chosen profession. The competencies required in a profession are developed through course work that provides you with practice performing these skills.

These initial attempts at putting practice theories into action probably will be in relatively small classes on campus in which your performance will be evaluated more intensely than might have been the case in kinesiology theory courses. Your classmates may be used as simulated clients, and your initial attempts to perform professional tasks will be in the safe environment of the classroom where your mistakes will not lead to serious consequences. If you perform up to departmental standards in these courses, you will be certified to enter the final stage of your professional education: the apprenticeship or internship.

The Internship

An apprentice is a novice who learns how to perform a job by working closely with an experienced worker. Apprentices usually assist a veteran for little or no pay in return for the opportunity to learn the skills required to enter the full-time workforce. The term is used most commonly in connection with crafts or trades (plumbing, electrical contracting, carpentry) in which the apprenticeship is the only type of training offered for the job. In professional programs in colleges and universities, the apprenticeship phase is called an internship, and it is the culminating experience of four years of study. Unlike apprenticeships for the crafts or trades, internships for professional careers are preceded by a rigorous course of study.

In the physical activity professions the internship is known by a variety of names. It may be referred to as an internship in sport management and fitness instructor programs, as student teaching in physical education teacher education programs, and as clinical training in athletic training programs. Regardless of what it is called, the experience has the following two purposes:

- To teach you how to apply the knowledge and skills you have learned in your professional program to a real-life situation
- To test your level of preparedness to enter professional practice

For most students, this is the first opportunity to assume the role of a member of their chosen profession. It usually is the most challenging experience of the undergraduate years, and the most enjoyable. For these reasons, most students feel it is the most valuable experience of their undergraduate education.

The internship differs from traditional course work in three ways. First, it occurs at the worksite rather than at the college or university. This means that the subculture of the worksite rather than the subculture of your undergraduate department will dictate your conduct. You will be

The Challenge of the Internship

For most students, the internship is a challenging experience, the point in their college training in which they discover how much they've learned and how much they have yet to learn. The following accounts were offered by Clay and Sara, students studying to be physical education teachers, during their internships (student teaching).

Clay: "I really had no idea . . . the first couple of weeks was really hard for me to get adjusted to it. I feel more confident because I'm feeling a lot more respect from the kids. They're starting to treat me like a teacher. . . . I had just finished teaching a track unit and the last week we had a competition, and I didn't have to tell one person to dress out or show up to the class. Everybody did because they enjoyed having the competition and enjoyed doing the different events. A lot of them, whether or not they thought so, did improve. . . . I feel prepared to teach. Mainly, the students' response gives me the feeling like, Hey! I did come into the right profession."

Sara: "I finally started to be a little more relaxed and flexible. At the beginning, I was really regimented. We stuck to it [our plans] no matter what, whether it worked or not. That made me frustrated, it made the students frustrated, and I know that Ms. Green [the internship supervisor] was frustrated with me. But I finally kind of loosened up and at the end became a little more flexible. Ms. Green helped me develop my own style. It is not really set in concrete; I know it is going to change. I need to become more assertive and aggressive."

Students quotes reprinted from M.A. Solomon, T. Worthy, A. Lee, and J.A. Carter, 1991, "Teacher role identity of student teachers in physical education: An interactive analysis," *Journal of Teaching Physical Education* 10: 188–209.

evaluated not only on the knowledge you display but also on how well you conform to the rules of the workplace. If you were engaged in an internship at a conditioning program for a Division I athletic department, for example, you would need to pay attention to the local rules that govern the conduct of athletes and conditioning coaches in the training room. Is loud music acceptable? What are the dress expectations? Does the director of conditioning expect you to arrive 15 minutes before your scheduled starting time? What local terms are used to describe interventions, locations, or procedures? What safety measures are you expected to follow? What are the established emergency procedures? Does the supervisor like interns to show initiative, or does she prefer you to ask advice or permission before undertaking an action? These and other such considerations always must be taken into account in order to ensure success in the internship as well as later success in the profession.

A second way an internship differs from your regular course work is that your performance will be supervised on a day-to-day basis by an experienced professional who probably is not a member of the faculty in the department in which you are enrolled. A university supervisor may visit the intern site occasionally, but the primary overseer and evaluator of the quality of your work will be the professional to whom you are assigned. These on-site supervisors have been chosen because they are viewed by the faculty as good models for future professionals. At the same time you shouldn't be surprised if their opinions, philosophies, and methods of operation differ from those you learned in your professional course work. Being exposed to a variety of philosophies and methodologies will usually serve to expand your knowledge of the profession.

The third way the internship differs from typical course work is that you will be serving real, not simulated, clients. Your actions will have important consequences, and they can be serious. Serving real clients also means that you must learn the social graces expected of a professional. You will need to demonstrate poise, courtesy, alertness, and initiative. You will be expected to demonstrate a level of confidence that makes clients feel comfortable and encourages them to place their trust in you.

Tips for Future Interns

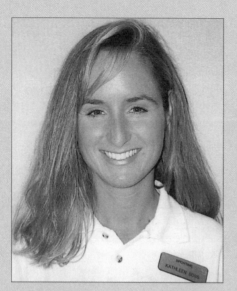

Kathleen Killion

Fitness Director of a Fitness Center

Kathleen Killion (who has a BS in exercise and sport science) is fitness director at Sportime, a large fitness center in Greensboro, North Carolina. In this 5,000-plus-member, 45,000-square-foot facility with 25 employees, Kathleen is in charge of fitness facilities and programming. Each year she oversees two to four interns in fitness and exercise leadership. She offers these tips to future interns:

My advice to every student is to make the most of your internship. If your department does not require an internship, ask for one. Changing your perspective from the outside looking in, to actually being in the role that you have studied to achieve, can have a significant impact on your future career. Use the internship as a bridge to your future. Students should remember that wherever an internship is offered, it is a place of business. Enter an internship in the same frame of mind that you might have beginning a new job. Share with your supervisor your long- and short-term goals, apply your knowledge of the field as a professional, take initiative, ask questions, be a team player, and always show your willingness to learn. Students should keep in mind that it is their responsibility to learn and be successful, not anyone else's. If you are not taught what you set out to learn, then teach yourself.

Internship requirements vary across institutions and professional specializations. If you are studying sport management, your internship may involve a semester of 20-hour weeks working in an athletic administration office where you might be required (like most professionals) to perform a range of duties, including mundane tasks such as handling mailings in the ticket office or answering the phone in the information office. You also might be given measured amounts of responsibility in performing the types of tasks that will be required of you as a sport management professional. If you are undertaking a student teaching experience in physical education, you may be required to spend an entire semester of full days in which you assume major responsibility for teaching classes. If you are an athletic training intern you will be responsible for logging an established number of clinical hours specified by the accrediting regulations of the National Athletic Trainers' Association (NATA), in a training room as well as traveling with an athletic team.

The internship is the culminating educational and evaluative experience for preprofessionals. As an educational experience it provides you with an opportunity to apply the knowledge and skills you learned in the undergraduate curriculum, while working under the supervision of a trained professional at an off-campus site. It is also an evaluative experience in that it tests your level of preparedness to enter your chosen profession.

Are You Suited for a Career in the Physical Activity Professions?

Now that you know something about the type of work professionals do and the educational experiences required to prepare you for such work, it's time to ask yourself how well suited you are for a career in the physical activity professions. The five-step approach depicted in figure 13.6 is intended to help you undertake this self-examination process.

Do My Attitudes, Values, and Goals Match Those of Professionals?

The first step is to consider how compatible you are with professional work generally, regardless of the particular field. Approach this task honestly and objectively. If you decide you're not well suited to a professional life, you should consider alternative careers.

Taking stock of your strengths, weaknesses, and potentials in relation to the personal attributes and preferences likely to be required in most types of professional work is an important first step. Nobody is in a better position to judge our attitudes, attributes, and preferences than we are, but sometimes our perceptions of ourselves can become a bit clouded. One way to bring our own attitudes into sharper focus is to compare them with those of our friends and peers. The results of a recent survey of over 275,000 freshmen entering 469 two- and four-year institutions in the United States (Reisberg, 1999) offer a convenient backdrop against which you can assess your own attributes and preferences.

If you are a typical undergraduate student, chances are that you believe helping others in difficulty is an important life objective (for 60% of freshmen it is), and you probably performed volunteer work during high school (74% of freshmen did) even though not required to do so. This suggests that you may be attuned to your civic responsibilities of helping others and improving society. This is a good start for a future professional! At the same time, a relatively small percentage (21%) of your peers indicate that they plan to continue to do volunteer work in college. This raises a yellow flag. If you don't plan to continue volunteer work in college, you need to remember that life's responsibilities and your personal commitments cannot be shelved during your college years. In addition, helping others is part and parcel of professional commitment. In fact, continuing to perform volunteer work throughout college, even if only for two or three hours per week, usually is interpreted by employ-

ers and graduate school admission officers as an indication that you understand the serious service responsibilities that come with planning a career in the helping professions.

Inevitably, this self-searching exercise will cause you to reflect on your major life goals. Based on the survey, chances are better than 50/50 that you decided to attend college in order to become an educated person (62% of freshmen), which is an admirable life goal for anybody seeking entrance into the professions. But, if you share the opinions of your peers, it is even more likely that you have your sights set on obtaining a high-paying job upon graduation (75%), being well off financially (74%), and becoming an authority in your field (60%). While there is certainly nothing wrong with setting your sights on financial success, being driven obsessively by the need for financial gain can create conflicts of interest in professional practice. Professionals, especially social trustee, civic professionals, are much more likely to identify service to humanity as their highest priority.

The fact that an overwhelming majority of your peers aspire to high-paying jobs but only some of them plan to prepare for graduate or professional school (49%) or would like to have administrative responsibility for the work of others (37%) indicates a serious misunderstanding about life in the professional workplace (Reisberg, 1999). High-paying jobs almost always come with some amount of administrative and supervisory responsibilities, and advancement in the professions is almost always linked closely to educational credentials. Generally, graduate degrees open up doors of opportunity routinely denied those who lack such credentials. Because educational standards for professional practice almost always rise over time, increasing numbers of undergraduate students will discover that a master's degree has become the minimal educational qualification for entering many of the physical activity professions.

Because professional work can have a vigorous, sometimes frenetic pace that may push you beyond the normal 40-hour week, stamina and robust health are especially important personal attributes for physical activity professionals. Moreover, most professional roles require effective oral communication, whether in speaking to small and large groups of people or in one-on-one interactions with clients. If you are among

Selecting a Career in the Physical Activity Professions

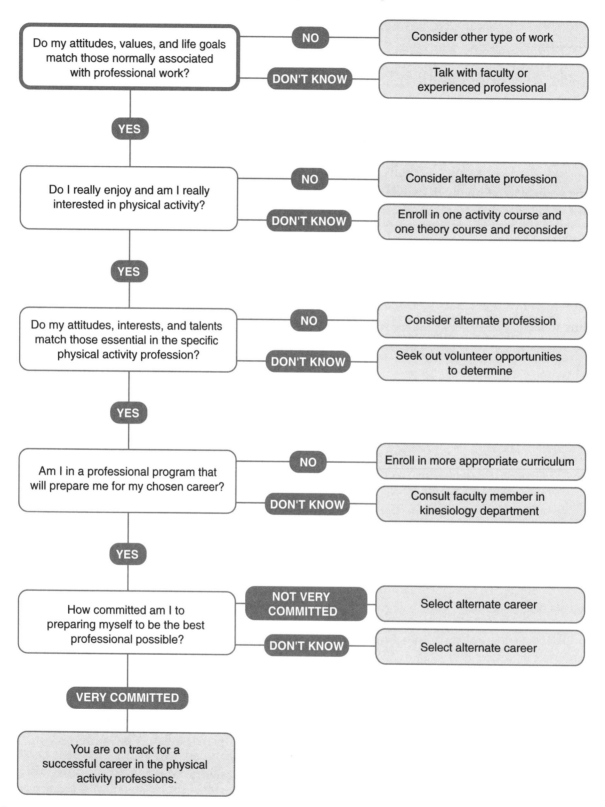

Figure 13.6 Careers in the physical activity professions are only for those committed to preparing themselves to be the best professionals possible.

the 69% of freshmen who rate themselves below average on public speaking ability, you should consider enrolling in a public speaking course at your college.

After giving the matter some thought, you may have concluded that you really aren't committed to a professional career. Perhaps you don't find working with people attractive, you don't particularly like helping to solve other people's problems, and you would rather work for a supervisor than take responsibility for acting on your own authority. Maybe the prospect of educating yourself continually to keep abreast of the professional literature, or constantly attending to the ethical ramifications of your work behavior, is not part of the vision you have for your own career. If so, it seems unlikely that you will be happy serving as a professional. We suggest that you continue to collect more information by reading the other chapters in this section of the book, talking to faculty members, and consulting with the career counseling center on your campus.

If, on the other hand, your self-analysis convinces you that you really would like a career in the physical activity professions, but also revealed some glaring deficiencies (fear of speaking before large groups, for example), consult with your faculty advisor about including academic experiences during your undergraduate years to bolster these weaknesses.

If you decide that your attitudes, values, and life goals match those normally associated with a professional career, you are ready to proceed to the next question in the decision model. If you conclude that you are not a good match for a professional career, seek advice from a faculty member or the career counseling center at your institution.

Am I Interested—Really Interested—in Physical Activity?

If what you have read about the professions excites you and matches your own interests and attitudes, the next step is to consider your degree of commitment to a career in the physical activity professions. It's natural to expect those who enter the physical activity professions to be more than merely interested in physical activity; they

should be *fascinated* by it. If you're not intrigued by performing, studying, and watching physical activity; if you aren't curious about the mysteries of body movement in all of its manifestations—biophysical, behavioral, and sociocultural—and if you're not prepared to apply your intellect and skills to exploring these mysteries, you probably are better off selecting an alternate profession.

The self-test in figure 13.7 is designed to help you gauge your own interest in physical activity. A total score of 22–30 suggests that your interest level is appropriate for a career in the physical activity professions. If you score from 16 to 21, you *may* be sufficiently interested, but it might be a good idea to give a bit more thought to your decision to enter the physical activity professions. You may want to enroll in one activity course and one theory course and then reconsider your career choice based on your enjoyment and achievement in those courses. If your total score falls below 16, it might be a good idea to talk with a career counselor about an alternative professional career.

Do My Attitudes, Interests, and Talents Lend Themselves to a Specific Physical Activity Profession?

The third step in this personal evaluation is to ask yourself if your attitudes, interests, and talents match the *specific* characteristics of the occupation you are considering. For example, if you envision a career in some aspect of therapeutic exercise or physical therapy, you should ask yourself if you enjoy interacting with sick and injured people. Obviously, most people—even medical students—require some time before they feel completely comfortable in medical environments, but you need to understand fairly early on your degree of comfort with the environments in which allied health professionals work.

If you like being around vigorous, healthy, active people, a career in physical fitness counseling, personal training, coaching, or athletic training would probably appeal to you. Do you have a special place in your heart for people with disabilities such as mental retardation, autism, blindness, cerebral palsy, deafness, or others? Would you find it challenging to help such people

Answer each of the questions by placing a check in one of the columns. Your total score for the ten questions is an index of your overall interest in physical activity. Score 3 for Yes; 1 for Somewhat/sometimes; and 0 for No.

	Yes	Somewhat/ sometimes	No
1. Do you regularly engage in a variety of different types of physical activity?			
2. Do you like to engage in *vigorous* physical activity?			
3. Are you a regular observer of sport, ice skating, or dance performances?			
4. When you watch dancing, ice skating, gymnastics, or diving, are you filled with a sense of wonder and appreciation?			
5. Do you feel comfortable in contexts in which people are engaged in physical activity (fitness centers, tennis courts, locker rooms, etc.)?			
6. When you watch athletic contests, do you find that you spend as much time appreciating the skill and grace of the athletes' movements as you do enjoying the drama generated by the game?			
7. Does the prospect of helping to improving another person's capacity to move efficiently and effectively excite you?			
8. Do you regularly read sport, fitness, or health magazines or newsletters?			
9. Would you say that physical activity experiences have played an important role in your life?			
10. Do most of your close friends lead physically active lives?			

A total score of 22–30 indicates a high interest in physical activity.
A total score of 16–21 indicates moderate interest.
A total score below 16 indicates insufficient interest for a career in the physical activity professions.

Figure 13.7   Assessing your interest in physical activity.

maximize their physical and mental potential? If so, a career in adapted physical education seems a reasonable goal. If you like being the center of attention, organizing and speaking to large groups of people, planning and monitoring and evaluating activities performed by others, and accepting responsibility for the actions of people younger than yourself, a career in teaching fitness, coaching, or physical education may be a good choice.

Does working at a desk dressed in business attire and adhering to a 9 to 5 workday appeal to you? If so, you might be well suited to a career in sport management. Are you more attracted to fluid and informal working environments in which you might have greater flexibility in your work schedule even though it may intrude on your weekends and evenings? If your answer is yes, then you might be better suited to more entrepreneurial types of professional positions such as that of personal trainer, professional sport instructor, or university professor. Chapters 14 to 17 will give you more complete descriptions of various physical activity professions to help you assess which careers may best suit you.

If you become convinced that your needs, interests, and attitudes do not match well with the specific professional occupation you had in mind, don't hesitate to explore other career possibilities within the physical activity professions. If, on the other hand, you're not sure, consider taking advantage of opportunities to volunteer at clinics, commercial or governmental agencies, schools, or at a variety of other physical activity settings. These will give you firsthand experiences in testing your compatibility with various working environments and will increase the probability that the career you choose will match your own interests, talents, and preferences. If possible, coordinate these volunteer experiences with your faculty advisor.

Is My College or University Program Well Matched to My Career Goals?

The fourth step is to determine whether the program in which you are presently enrolled will prepare you well for your chosen career. If, for example, you are most interested in a career in teaching and coaching, but your department offers only concentrations in exercise physiology, sport administration, and health promotion, the department's curriculum would seem a poor match for your career objectives. The same would be true if the program is slanted heavily toward the preparation of physical education teachers or professionals in the fitness industry and you are most interested in a career in sport management. If you have doubts about the fit between the course requirements of the program you are in and your career aspirations, don't hesitate to talk to a faculty member.

Perhaps your career goals have changed since you enrolled in your undergraduate program.

Although it would occur less often if students took the five-step approach being recommended here, changing career goals during the undergraduate years is fairly common. It is important to remember that switching majors or concentrations within the department (e.g., from physical education to exercise therapy) can delay your graduation for a year or more. It also can be inconvenient. If you decide to switch majors to an entirely new field, it may push your graduation even further into the future. Such a drastic change also will require you to become socialized into another department, get used to new professors, and form new alliances with classmates.

Though switching your major may be inconvenient, it is better to endure the delays and inconvenience than to continue training for a career in which you have little interest. If you are deep into your undergraduate program and find your career interests have changed to another physical activity profession, the best course of action might be to complete your present program and follow it up with a master's degree in your area of interest. Faculty members in your department will be ready and willing to advise you, even if it means referring you to other departments or even other institutions.

Asking questions about the pertinence of your program of study to your life goals is risky business. You may not like how you answer your own questions! But it is a vital exercise, one students too often ignore. Remember: those who reach career decisions early in their undergraduate years are more likely to enjoy their undergraduate studies and to appreciate their relevance, particularly in courses taken in their major.

How Committed Am I to Preparing to Be the Best Professional Possible?

At the first practice of the season, coaches often ask their teams the rhetorical question: How badly do you want it?, referring, of course, to the team's willingness to invest the time, energy, and hard work essential for winning the league championship. Now the question for you is, How badly do *you* want it? How much are you willing to invest to achieve success in your chosen profession? This last step in the process may be the most important because it supersedes all other questions in the process. You may have had little difficulty answering the questions up to this point, but if you aren't committed to success, there's really little point in continuing. Are you willing to commit to preparing yourself to be the best professional possible? Let's examine some of the ways in which such a commitment might be manifested.

Excellence in Academic Work

Graduating with a superb academic record is regarded by most employers as a baseline indicator of your level of commitment to becoming an outstanding professional. Obviously, some students are more academically gifted than others, but often, slight shortcomings in academic ability can be overcome by a special application of effort. In fact, few things make a more indelible impression on professors than a student's willingness to work hard to achieve academic success.

What types of behaviors suggest a willingness to work hard? Attending class regularly and on time, visiting the library regularly, and reading unassigned journal articles and books about the topics you are studying in class all are signs that you are taking your academic work seriously. And, believe it or not, most professors consider students who collar them after class with questions about the material in the day's lesson as being more committed than those who avoid them at all costs. Surprisingly, only 22% of freshmen students report seeking advice from their professors on a regular basis (Reisberg, 1999).

Perhaps the best predictor of your success in the physical activity professions is the level of commitment you make to preparing yourself to be the most knowledgeable and highly skilled practitioner possible.

Early Identification With the Professional Field

How early in the undergraduate program students identify with their chosen career is also a good indicator of commitment. In the chapters that follow, you will find many references to professional associations. Joining a professional association while still an undergraduate may be the most reliable indicator of commitment. Professional associations usually admit preprofessionals at reduced rates and offer reduced registration rates at conferences. Members receive the organization's publication and other information on a regular basis. Attending professional conferences is another indicator. Professional associations usually hold annual regional and national meetings that feature lectures, workshops, and exhibits of equipment used in professional practice. Attending these can be expensive, but then again, so can taking a spring break trip to the Florida beaches. Remember, when we make a commitment, we reveal our priorities.

Why is it important to identify with a profession while still an undergraduate? Because students who view themselves as members of the profession tend to approach their studies with a special excitement and vigor. Their orientation changes from that of a student who views courses as obstacles to obtaining a degree, to that of a professional who tries to extract from each course the knowledge and skills that will help him or her develop into the best qualified professional possible. When you identify with your chosen profession, you will seek out the advice of veteran professionals and observe them in practice. You will begin to establish a communications network with practicing professionals and will establish the habit of reading the journals in your field. You also will learn the language of the field and begin to feel comfortable around experienced professionals, even though you are still in the preparation phase of your career.

Another way to identify early with a physical activity profession is to obtain certification in an area in which you plan to work. Certifications are available from such groups as the American College of Sports Medicine, the National Strength and Conditioning Association, the American Council on Exercise, or the Aerobics Fitness Association of America.

Identifying early with the profession you plan to enter by joining appropriate professional organizations, attending conferences, establishing alliances with veteran professionals, and obtaining professional certifications will give you a head start on developing a successful career.

Becoming Engaged in College or University Life

Being engaged means being connected to what is happening around you. Next to academic performance, your level of engagement in your department, college or university, and community is regarded as one of the best indicators of your level of commitment to becoming a successful professional. Unfortunately, levels of student engagement on campuses appear to have declined in recent years, a trend that faculty and administrators find disturbing (Flacks & Thomas, 1998). Who are the engaged students? Engaged students are those who take responsibility for their academic experiences and for their professional futures. They are curious and are constantly testing their personal limits by seeking new ways to become involved in life experiences. They are active, energetic leaders who view the department as "their department" and seek out ways to participate in its operational life. They are likely to be leaders in their major clubs or student government on campus or coordinators of charity events or other community activities outside of the academic environment.

In addition to becoming engaged in extracurricular activities, it also is a good idea to become involved in academic-related activities. Does a professor need students to assist on a research project? Are volunteers needed as subjects in research studies? Does your institution sponsor undergraduate research assistantships? Will a professor sponsor you for work on an independent study of a topic of interest to you? Don't be afraid to register interest in such projects. Not only will it reflect a high level of commitment on your part, but also such projects offer excellent opportunities to develop the type of leadership skills and knowledge essential for success in the world beyond college.

Becoming involved in activities within and outside of your department is one indication of commitment to developing a successful career in the professions.

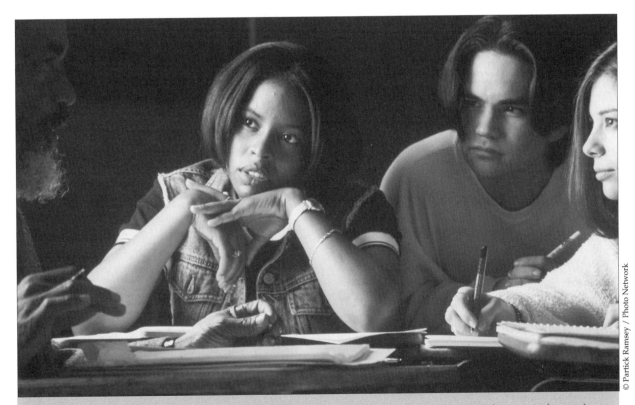

By becoming engaged in your department's activities, you will be showing your commitment to becoming a professional.

© Partick Ramsey / Photo Network

Participation in Volunteer Services

We have seen that the driving force of professionals, especially those in the helping professions, is a spirit of wanting to improve the quality of life for those in the community. Although it is easy for preprofessionals to say they want to serve others, nothing speaks more loudly than actions. If two students have approximately equal academic records, the advantage always will go to the student whose résumé displays clear evidence of volunteer service to community agencies. These might include such programs as Meals on Wheels, Boys and Girls Clubs, local food banks, Boy and Girl Scouts, shelters for the homeless, church-based programs, walk-a-thons for various charities, American Red Cross activities, and other community-based programs. When your volunteer experience is in an activity that bears some resemblance to the profession for which you are preparing, it has the added benefit of socializing you into your future profession. Volunteer work with physical therapy and sports medicine clinics, YMCAs and YWCAs, youth sport organizations, schools, Special Olympics, and other agencies associated with the physical activity professions are some potential volunteer opportunities that you might want to explore.

Attending Graduate School

Evidence of commitment to a profession may also be reflected in plans to pursue advanced graduate work. In professions such as physical therapy, a master's degree is a minimal entry degree, and the athletic training profession may require a graduate-level degree in the near future. Permanent certification for teaching physical education in many states requires a master's degree or its equivalence. You may not be prepared to think about graduate school at this early point in your undergraduate preparation, or you may have decided to delay that decision until a few years after you have graduated. For many, this may be

Whom Would You Hire?

You are the director of a large, comprehensive health-wellness rehabilitation center that operates under the auspices of a local community hospital. You are in the process of hiring an exercise specialist to oversee the exercise programs offered for health promotion. You have narrowed the choice down to two candidates. Of the following, whom would you hire?

Nick earned a 3.65 GPA in exercise science (or kinesiology) while working 25 hours a week as a waiter at a local restaurant. His work schedule prevented him from becoming involved in many on-campus activities outside of class except for the wrestling team where he was league championship three years in a row. He furnished excellent letters of reference from two coaches and his boss at the restaurant, all praising him as a bright, enthusiastic person with good "people skills." He is clearly well liked by the departmental faculty. One of Nick's professors noted that Nick received rave reviews by his internship supervisor and predicted that with experience he would develop into a first-rate professional.

Sam earned a 3.00 GPA in exercise science while working 10 hours each week in the campus recreation center where he served as a fitness consultant. He was secretary to the exercise science majors' club, organized a walk-a-thon to benefit homeless people, and spent two hours each week serving as a volunteer fitness leader for a program targeting disadvantaged children in an inner-city neighborhood. He has been a member of a professional organization for two years and took the initiative to become certified by the American College of Sports Medicine as an exercise test technologist. His letters of reference are from one professor, the director of the campus recreation center, and the director of the community-based program. All describe him as an "engaged" student with good people skills who has already begun to be socialized into the profession.

Whom would you hire and why?

a sensible plan. All things considered, however, making an early decision to continue with advanced graduate education in the physical activity professions is another indication of commitment.

Generally, master's programs in kinesiology offer advanced education in a number of specialized areas, although not all universities offer all specializations. A faculty member at your institution may be an excellent source concerning which institutions you might consider attending. Also, you may find posters or brochures advertising graduate study at various institutions posted in your departmental office. Normally, master's degrees require from 30 to 36 credit hours of work depending on the specialization. In most cases, full-time master's students are able to complete the requirements of the degree in one and a half to two and a half years. Master's programs that require a thesis have slightly fewer hours of course work, but require an in-depth research project that may take up to one year to complete. Some master's programs do not require a thesis but may require more course work than thesis programs. Sometimes nonthesis programs also require an internship. If you delay attending graduate school until after you have secured a position, and plan to do your graduate work by attending classes in the evenings, it may take you as much as four or five years to complete a master's degree.

> Volunteering regularly for service to a community agency is an indication that you share in your profession's commitment to service. Seeking in-depth, advanced education in graduate school may also be a sign that you are investing your interest and personal resources in a career in the physical activity professions.

The Decision-Making Process

By going through the decision-making steps in figure 13.6, you have embarked on an important process. If you responded affirmatively to all five questions, you are well on your way to a successful career in a physical activity profession. The next four chapters will give you an in-depth look at some of the professions you have to choose from.

If instead you hesitated at some questions or were not sure of your answers, the next four chapters may help you in your decision making. Use this as an opportunity to assess honestly and objectively whether you are suited to professional work, and especially to professional work in one of the physical activity professions.

Wrap-Up

Career decisions are among the most important decisions people make during their lifetime. Such decisions are not irrevocable; in fact, you likely will change your career several times over your working years. Nevertheless, nothing is to be gained by delaying your commitment to a career, and there may be much to lose. Students who make career commitments early are in a better position to benefit from their undergraduate education than students who have only tentative plans about the type of work they will do when they graduate. If you have decided to attain a degree in kinesiology by default (it didn't particularly excite you, but then, no other college major seemed any more appealing) and life beyond graduation looms like "the great black void," you should take steps to assess systematically your compatibility with a career in the physical activity professions.

Doing this necessarily involves learning what it means to be a professional and the types of work and work environments associated with each of the physical activity professions. It also involves making a realistic assessment of your level of excitement about and commitment to kinesiology and the physical activity professions. If this chapter achieved its goal, you will already have begun this self-examination process. Now it is time for you to learn more about the physical activity professions by studying the next four chapters. These chapters, written by experts in the professions being described, will provide specific information about what it is like to work in each of these areas. When you have finished, you should be in a good position to make this very important decision about your future career.

Study Questions

1. List three ways professional work differs from nonprofessional work.

2. What expectations might society have for professionals that it does not have for salespersons, garage mechanics, or carpenters?

3. Why is it important for professionals to attend professional conferences and read the professional literature?

4. List three differences that might be observed between a community sport program leader who adheres to mechanical, market-driven professionalism and one who adheres to social trustee, civic professionalism.

5. What is the value of the liberal arts and sciences to kinesiology majors?

6. What is the difference between theoretical kinesiology and professional practice knowledge?

7. Why is the internship an important experience in preparing kinesiology students for professional practice?

8. List five questions that all kinesiology students should ask themselves before deciding to major in kinesiology.

9. As an employer, aside from evaluating the college transcript, what other evidence might you take into consideration in determining how committed a candidate is to a career as a professional in athletic training?

10. If you decide to pursue a career as a physical education teacher during your second year of the kinesiology major after having entered as a sport management major, what is the best course of action to take?

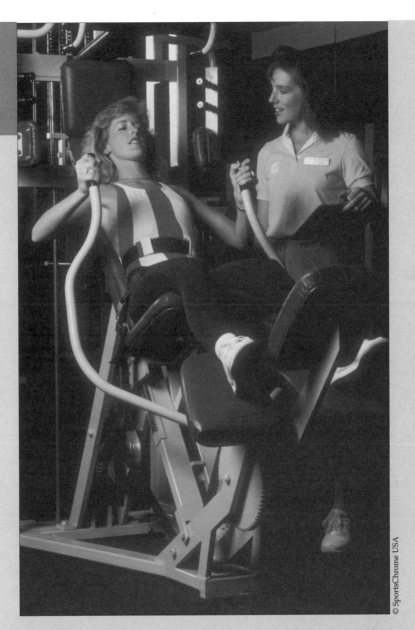

14

© SportsChrome USA

Health and Fitness Professions

Jeremy Howell and Sandra L. Minor

In this chapter . . .

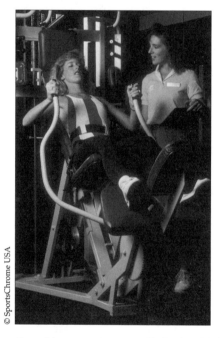

© SportsChrome USA

A personal trainer is hired by an executive who is overweight and out of shape. The executive wants to run a 5K in six months and is relying on the personal trainer to guide him in losing weight, gaining strength, and improving his cardiovascular endurance safely.

A group exercise instructor meets with the class members of a new session today and sees that two of the participants are over age 55. One of them tells him she has hypertension.

A health/fitness director realizes her facility should expand its programs next year in order to better reach less physically fit populations. What additional staff will she need to hire? What should their qualifications be? Will her budget allow this expansion?

In an interview with a health/fitness counselor, a client mentions that she is having trouble fitting her exercise program into her busy downtown executive lifestyle. She feels overwhelmed, irritable, and constantly exhausted. She also feels very guilty about not "working out." How will the health/fitness counselor begin to develop an exercise program that does not add to these health ailments of the client?

Health and fitness professionals face these types of situations every day in their careers. In each case, they must make decisions that will improve the health and fitness of participants and clients safely, while keeping within the goals and objectives of the facility or program they work for.

Health and fitness, one of the spheres of professional practice (see figure 14.1), is made up of many dynamic professions. The sphere of health and fitness professions includes such positions as group exercise instructor, fitness instructor, health/fitness counselor, personal trainer, health/fitness director, and an array of specialist positions, including health educator, clinical exercise specialist, and registered dietitian.

Although the scope of the professional work in this sphere is expanding to include a multifac-

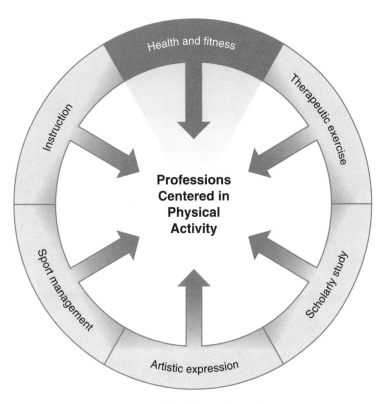

Figure 14.1   Health and fitness is one of the spheres of professional practice.

eted view of health and fitness, the core goal of these professions is to improve a person's physical functioning and physical health. Health and fitness professions have traditionally been conducted in worksite, clinical, commercial, and community settings, but in recent years the lines between these settings have become blurred as each type of program or facility has expanded its offerings to reach more people and impact their lives in more ways.

This expanding scope is opening up tremendous opportunities for kinesiology graduates and is making health and fitness positions some of the more exciting and dynamic careers people can enter. Our purpose in this chapter is threefold. First, we want to describe the new opportunities that exist for professionals in the health and fitness industry. Exactly what do health and fitness professionals do and where do they do it? Second, we want to analyze why these new opportunities are appearing at this time. What social forces are creating new possibilities for current kinesiology graduates? Third, we want to discuss how you can best take advantage of these new opportunities as you complete your education and move into your chosen career. What are the

educational requirements and experiences necessary to become an active, competent professional in this area?

 CHAPTER OBJECTIVES

In this chapter we will:

▋ Acquaint you with the wide range of professional opportunities in the sphere of health and fitness

▋ Familiarize you with the purpose and types of work done by health and fitness professionals

▋ Explain how the sphere of health and fitness is evolving and progressing, especially due to marketplace trends

▋ Inform you about the educational requirements and experiences necessary to become an active, competent health and fitness professional

▋ Help you identify whether one of these professions fits your skills, aptitudes, and professional desires

The World of Health and Fitness Professions

This is a very exciting time for those involved in the health and fitness professions. Despite the many studies demonstrating that the American public is not nearly as active as it should be (see chapter 2), the marketplace for physical activity professionals has never been better. This is because the health and fitness settings in which physical activities take place, and the jobs that physical activity professionals perform, are experiencing a remarkable expansion and transformation.

Take out a pencil and a blank sheet of paper and create three large vertical columns on your page. In the first column, write down a list of job titles that you associate with the term *health and fitness professions.* In the second column, next to each job title, list specific things that you think people in those jobs do. Now, in the third column, list the knowledge and skills that you think people in each job must have to perform their jobs competently. There are no right or wrong answers for this activity. We will ask you to refer to this list throughout the chapter and hope that you will find yourself adding to or deleting from your list as you read on.

Not since the jogging boom of the late 1970s have we witnessed the dramatic growth we are seeing today of a fitness and health industry that has embraced and promoted the relationship between exercise, personal responsibility, and prevention in quite specific ways (see Howell & Ingham, 2000). Today, scientific research and popular culture have popularized the notion that regular exercise can increase lean body mass, heart and lung function, immune function, blood vessels, blood flow, muscular strength, flexibility, bone density, balance, and self-esteem. Perhaps most important is the research that links physical activity to lowering the risk of death due to coronary heart disease, the leading cause of mortality in the United States. To emphasize this renewed national interest in health and fitness, the 1996 United States *Surgeon General's Report on Physical Activity and Health* (U.S. Department of Health and Human Services, 1996), developed in conjunction with the Centers for Disease Control (CDC) and the President's Council on Physical Fitness and Sports (PCPFS), details a decade of research studies on the health dangers of inactivity and an unhealthy lifestyle.

For those in the health and fitness professions, the surgeon general's report is an important document. No longer is physical activity just seen as a recreational activity. It is now firmly embedded in the national preventive health consciousness. Because of this, we are witnessing a new model of health in many fitness and health settings. Rather than fitness professionals just being asked to train, measure, and test people for improved athletic performance, they are increasingly having to develop individual exercise programs that are based on health and healthy lifestyle issues. This is the reason that we see increasing use of the term "wellness" and the creation of exercise programs that are connected to other physical, intellectual, emotional, social, and spiritual dimensions. This is a trend that will impact many of the jobs you might go into. And given the fact that we are living in a society that is experiencing a dramatic aging of the population, it is a trend that will be with us for quite a while.

In this chapter, we will first explain the traditional settings within which health and fitness professions occur as well as the most common professions. Then we will look closely at how the changing trends in society and culture are reshaping the health and fitness sphere of professional practice.

Health and Fitness Settings

The health and fitness industry is relatively young and is currently undergoing some very important changes. These changes have been experienced across all types of health and fitness settings and have resulted in expanded job descriptions and a greater number of positions for entry-level and experienced professionals. Traditionally, health and fitness professions take place in four primary settings, namely, worksite, commercial, clinical, and community. At one time, each of these settings had a distinct mission, set of objectives, type of programming, and target market. More recently, however, the various health and fitness settings have become more similar than dissimilar. Examples include commercial settings offering worksite health promotion programs, clinical settings operating for-profit fitness centers, and community settings providing medically based fitness programs in partnership with area hospitals. In summary, the lines between the various settings are no longer distinct.

🔑 Traditionally, health and fitness professions have taken place in four settings: worksite, commercial, clinical, and community. Recently, the lines between these settings have blurred, resulting in expanded job descriptions and a greater number of positions.

This section describes each type of health and fitness setting and provides an overview of the objectives, types of programs, and target markets for each setting. It also describes the changes that have occurred over time and the trends that we see emerging in the future.

Worksite Settings

Worksite health and fitness programs (often referred to as worksite health promotion programs) have experienced tremendous growth during the past decade. In the early 1980s worksite health and fitness programs were offered by less than 5% of employers. In the mid-1990s over 80% of all employers with more than 50 employees reported having some form of health and fitness program (O'Donnell & Harris, 1994).

Early worksite programs focused primarily on physical fitness, nutrition, weight control, stress management, and smoking cessation and were offered exclusively to employees of the sponsoring company. Pioneering corporations such as Johnson and Johnson, Coors Brewing Company, and Tenneco believed that health and fitness programs would help to reduce health-care costs, increase productivity and morale, decrease absenteeism, and improve their corporate image.

In 1992 the International Health, Racquet and Sportsclub Association (IHRSA) produced a booklet that described some of the significant data being reported in academic journals and trade

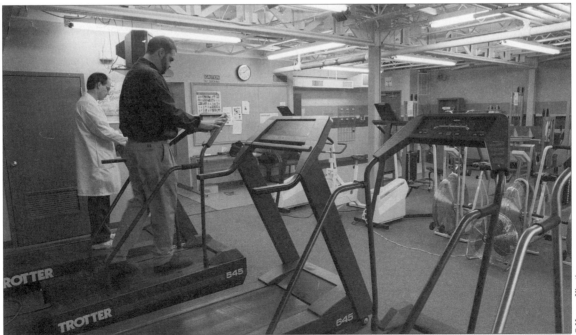

Like many companies, Supervalu in Champaign, Illinois provides their employees with a high-quality health and fitness facility.

© Human Kinetics

magazines supporting worksite programs. For instance, they reported that Tenneco found that the average annual medical claim was at least 50% lower for participants in its employee fitness program versus nonparticipants. Tenneco also found that employees who participated in their corporate fitness program were 13% less likely to leave than other employees. Similarly, Johnson and Johnson averaged a 30% return on investment from its Live for Life employee fitness program from 1978 to 1990. General Mills reported that in the first year of its TriHealtheon employee fitness program they received a payback of $3.10 per dollar invested. In the same vein, the Coors Brewing Company saved $1.4 million over six years due to reduced medical claims and absenteeism after beginning an employee fitness program. And in a study by Saatchi and Saatchi Advertising, 63% of employees enrolled in its fitness program said they believed that participating in the worksite fitness program improved productivity, and 75% thought it boosted morale and commitment (see International Health, Racquet and Sportsclub Association, 1992).

Employers have found that health and fitness programs can reduce health-care costs, increase productivity and morale, decrease absenteeism, and improve their corporate image.

As worksite programs continued to develop in the 1990s, additional services were added to increase employee awareness and help employees make healthy lifestyle changes. Examples of these services include health education classes, company health fairs, the distribution of educational materials, and the use of health risk appraisals to identify employee risk factors. More recently, worksite programs have expanded offerings even further to provide a work environment that *supports* healthy lifestyles in addition to helping employees *change* their lifestyles. In this expanded role, many worksite programs develop and implement on-site work policies regarding smoking behavior, the use of ergonomic work stations, and access to on-site child-care services. Other popular worksite programs include recreation activities, family and marital counseling, support groups, communication skills training, volunteer service opportunities,

meditation, travel and adventure activities, and Employee Assistance Programs (EAPs) (O'Donnell & Harris 1994). Also, in an effort to reduce the medical costs of all individuals covered by the company health plan, many worksite programs now promote health and fitness services to employee family members and retirees of the company.

Worksite programs have expanded program offerings to provide a work environment that *supports* healthy lifestyles in addition to helping employees *change* their lifestyles.

Another trend in worksite health and fitness programs is the building of increasingly elaborate health and fitness facilities as a way to recruit and retain new employees. Throughout the 1990s, as the job market in some industries became increasingly competitive for employers, the building of state-of-the-art, on-site health and fitness facilities became one way that employers competed for quality employees. Many examples of this exist in the computer software industry in the Silicon Valley area of San Francisco. Companies such as Oracle, EA Sports, Inc., and Applied Materials have incorporated extensive health and fitness facilities into their buildings. These days, when employees are job hunting, they are not only asking prospective employers about health insurance and retirement benefits but also wanting to know what types of health and fitness facilities and programs are provided by the company.

Another significant change that has occurred in worksite programs during the past decade is a shift from programs that are managed internally to programs that are managed by outside agencies. Many companies have established successful partnerships with outside commercial, community, and clinical facilities. The 1997 IHRSA annual "Profiles of Success" industry survey noted that the percentage of members of fitness and health clubs originating from corporate accounts had grown from 15.5% in 1995 to 23.4% (International Health, Racquet and Sportsclub Association, 1997). Many companies have found it more cost effective to "contract out" health and fitness programs to agencies with expertise in this area. As a result, corporate health and fitness programs are now often offered by outside agencies—even when the programs take place on site.

What are some of the objectives of worksite health and fitness programs? What is the target market for these programs (who are the participants)? What types of programs would you take part in if they were offered at your worksite? What skills do you think a health and fitness professional would need in order to create programs and activities in a worksite setting? Does this type of position interest you? If so, think about whether you have the skills and aptitudes needed for such a position, and make a plan to gain instruction in areas you need to improve.

Commercial Settings

Any description of the commercial setting must first begin with an acknowledgment that many different types of businesses fit into this category, and not all of them offer quality health and fitness activities delivered by qualified personnel. Fortunately, one of the most significant trends in the commercial setting is an increase in the number of high-quality health and fitness services being offered to members. Currently, more than 13,000 commercial health and fitness facilities and spas are in operation in the United States (International Health, Racquet and Sportsclub Association, 1997). Commercial health and fitness facilities typically operate with the objective of generating a profit. The manner in which this profit is generated places commercial health and fitness settings in two distinct categories: **sales-based facilities** and **retention-based facilities**. The following sections offer a comparison of these two business models.

Commercial facilities offer health and fitness programs similar to those offered in the workplace. Popular programs include fitness assessment and screening, nutritional counseling, personal fitness training, massage therapy, group exercise classes, spa services, wellness education classes, and corporate outreach programs. In ad-

dition, special population exercise programs for children, prenatal and postnatal women, older adults, and people needing physical therapy have increased in popularity.

The very nature of a for-profit business encourages innovation as a way to compete effectively for customers in the marketplace. As a result, the commercial health and fitness business is very dynamic and offers many opportunities for health and fitness professionals to get involved with a wide variety of programs.

Because commercial health and fitness facilities need to make a profit, they compete for customers, and this encourages innovative programming. Commercial health and fitness facilities are either sales based or retention based.

Sales-Based Facilities

Membership sales activities are the major focus in a sales-based health and fitness facility. These facilities rarely place limits on the number of memberships sold and offer highly discounted rates as a way of attracting a large number of new customers. Another common characteristic of a sales-based facility is the selling of long-term membership contracts. Within the industry, sales-based facilities are often referred to as operating under a "future service contract" philosophy. In order to receive the best possible rate, new members are often encouraged to make a long-term commitment in advance (usually up to three years) rather than paying for their membership monthly. As a result of this approach, sales-based businesses are not highly motivated to meet members' long-term needs or focus on retention activities such as offering high-quality programs run by qualified personnel. Instead, they often allocate extensive resources to advertising campaigns that offer very low joining rates.

Sales-based fitness facilities often use billboards and newspaper advertisements featuring slender, muscular young models, suggesting that exercise is only for individuals who are already fit and healthy. The result of such advertising is that individuals who would benefit *most* from health and fitness programs—those who are older, have special health concerns, or need to lose weight—are often discouraged from joining.

Moreover, people who are lured into sales-based facilities by what are frequently manipulative sales strategies often have a negative first experience of health and fitness facilities and are discouraged from getting involved with other programs in the future.

What do you think it would be like to be a professional physical activity specialist in a sales-based facility? Would you be likely to feel fulfilled and have a sense of helping people? Are professionals in a sales-based facility likely to adhere to a mechanical, market-driven professionalism or a social trustee, civic professionalism?

Retention-Based Facilities

Selling memberships is an important aspect of any commercial facility, but retention-based facilities make a sincere effort to meet the long-term needs of current members. These types of commercial facilities focus on delivering high-quality programs and services so that current members will continue their membership month in and month out, and will likely recommend the facility to others. Many in the industry refer to retention-based facilities as operating under a "voluntary dues" philosophy—that is, people pay dues voluntarily from month to month rather than paying one large membership fee up front.

Since retention-based facilities do not typically invest in extensive advertising, referrals from current members are essential to achieving the goal of profitability. Retention-based facilities place maximum limits on the number of memberships sold and only engage in sales activities to replace members who have left the club due to relocation or job changes. The greatest emphasis in a retention-based business is always on quality programming that meets members' needs. Because of the additional cost of offering quality programs and hiring qualified personnel, monthly dues in retention-based facilities tend to be higher than those in sales-based facilities.

What do you think it would be like to be a professional physical activity specialist in a

retention-based facility? Would you be likely to feel fulfilled and have a sense of functioning as a social trustee, civic professional (chapter 13)?

Unfortunately, retention-based facilities do not typically advertise the quality health and fitness programs they offer. Such facilities generally depend on word-of-mouth referrals to market their services, leaving the advertising market to the sales-based facilities. As a result, many people have a negative image of the commercial health and fitness industry. This point was well illustrated in a 1997 survey conducted by the International Health, Racquet and Sportsclub Association, in which members of the public indicated that they did not believe that a commercial health and fitness facility was capable of meeting their specific health needs.

Many of the most exciting and higher-paying job opportunities available in the health and fitness professions are in the commercial sector. Hopefully, in the future, retention-based facilities will spend more effort getting the word out to the public regarding the high-quality health and fitness programs they offer.

🔑 The credibility of the commercial fitness industry will improve when advertising begins to provide a more balanced image of health and fitness that is inclusive of all people regardless of age, race, ethnicity, body type, or current fitness level.

Think of some of the more popular commercial health and fitness clubs in your area. Are these facilities popular because of the advertising strategies they employ or because of the strong word of mouth that exists about the programs they offer? Do you think these facilities are sales based or retention based? What specific things are important to you in a health and fitness facility? What questions would you ask a sales representative if you wanted to join a commercial facility?

Clinical Setting

The clinical setting includes hospitals, outpatient medical facilities, and physical therapy clinics and represents one of the largest growth areas for health and fitness programs in the past decade. Currently, 25% of all hospitals report having fitness centers, and many other clinical facilities report offering extensive health promotion services such as medically supervised programs for high-risk individuals (Grantham, Patton, York, & Winick, 1998). Clinical settings have begun to recognize the value of providing health and fitness programs. The objective of these programs is to keep subscribers of health insurance programs healthy and avoid expensive medical procedures in the future.

Examples of popular clinical programs include preventive screenings, physical therapy, cardiac rehabilitation, water exercise therapy, childbirth and parenting education, weight management, nutrition counseling, and substance abuse treatment. Many of these programs cater to specific population groups with classes such as men's and women's health education; senior fitness; diabetes self-management; and exercise for individuals with arthritis, osteoporosis, or cardiovascular disease. By definition, fitness professionals working within clinical settings will have more contact and work in partnership with both medically based professionals and clients with diagnosed medical conditions.

Current trends in the clinical setting are not unlike those in the worksite and commercial settings. At clinical settings elaborate facilities are being built, and many offer a wide range of health and fitness programs and qualified staff to deliver these services. In addition, many facilities in this setting are beginning to offer activities that expand into other dimensions of health in addition to physical fitness. As an example, Eastern Connecticut Health Network (a combination of Manchester Memorial Hospital and Rockville General Hospital) publishes a quarterly guide called "Health Source," which offers "programs for physical, emotional, occupational, social, intellectual and spiritual dimensions of wellness." This 45-page guide includes programs with titles such as Spiritual Health and Meditation, Combining Ancient Health Techniques With Cancer Treatments, Parenting Under Stress, De-Stressing Your Finances, Supermarket Tours for Those With Diabetes, and Protecting Our Daughters' Self-Esteem.

Much like worksite settings, clinical settings have begun to develop partnerships with commercial facilities or agencies that provide expertise in the management of health and fitness facilities. This combination of commercial settings (with expertise in facility management) and clinical settings (with expertise in health promotion programming) looks very promising for the future.

Community Setting

The community setting contains many different types of health and fitness facilities. One of the largest segments of the community setting is represented by local branches of nonprofit organizations such as the Young Men's Christian Association (YMCA), the Young Women's Christian Association (YWCA), the Jewish Community Center (JCC), and city parks and recreation departments. Another large segment of this setting is community health departments and voluntary health agencies such as the American Heart Association, the American Lung Association, and the American Diabetes Association. Community settings also include health and fitness programs that exist in churches, universities, hotels, and apartment complexes.

Typically, health and fitness programs in community settings seek to fill a specific community need. Most target a specific community group and attempt to reach as many individuals in that group as resources will allow. Many of these facilities receive outside funding and are classified as nonprofit organizations for tax purposes, allowing them to offer health and fitness programs at a low cost and to provide financial assistance to individuals who could not otherwise afford to participate.

The types of programs offered in community settings are as diverse as those offered in worksite, commercial, and clinical settings, and might include parks and recreation programs for seniors, community cardiac rehabilitation programs, swimming lessons for children, youth soccer leagues, and strength training for retirees. Resources are typically more limited in the community setting, however, leading to a greater reliance on volunteers to meet many staffing needs. In addition, some programs are offered on

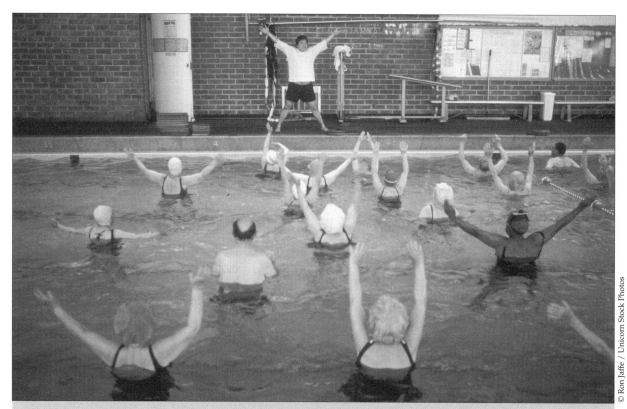

Health and fitness programs in community settings, such as this adult water exercise class at a Jewish Community Center, target a specific community group and attempt to reach as many people as possible.

a "for-profit" basis as a way of generating revenue to deliver other community service programs at little or no cost to participants. In many YMCAs, health club memberships are sold to the public as a method of generating revenue to offset the cost of nonprofit programs such as senior exercise classes or programs for individuals with special needs.

Community health and fitness projects are not limited to those offered by community-based nonprofit organizations, however. The mission to improve the health of the community has crept into the worksite, commercial, and clinical settings in recent years. Although they do not typically operate as nonprofit entities, an increasing number of organizations in these settings have expanded their missions to include contributing to the health of their surrounding communities. The motives behind these activities are varied and can include a philanthropic desire to help, improve public relations in the community, offer service opportunities to employees, reduce tax exposure, or improve long-term business health. Many examples illustrate this trend.

Many worksite, commercial, and clinical facilities also support community health and fitness programs.

The San Francisco Bay Club, a 7,000-square-meter (75,000-sq-ft) retention-based commercial health and fitness facility in the heart of downtown San Francisco, has been involved in a unique community program with the Marina Middle School. Since the beginning of the relationship, the club's staff and members have funded and staffed a variety of events and programs from after-school basketball and dance to drama classes and mentors for kids in need. The club has also been involved in school capital campaigns. The program has been so successful that in 1993 the partnership won California's state award for the best school volunteer program in the middle school category. This is an excellent example of social trustee, civic professionalism in action (see chapter 13).

In a similar fashion, many **health maintenance organizations (HMOs)** now offer an extensive menu of health and fitness programs free of charge to community members. In some cases, this is an effort to improve the overall health of potential subscribers in a geographic area. In other cases, it is a marketing strategy aimed at increasing the number of people who enroll in the HMO's health plan.

Many worksites now coordinate fund-raising events in their communities and invite employees to participate as volunteers. This is an especially interesting trend because evidence suggests that participation in volunteer work may be related to better health. One study in Tecumseh, Michigan, followed 2,700 people for close to ten years. In this study, men who did regular volunteer work had death rates two and one-half times lower than those who did not (Ornstein & Sobel, 1989).

In summary, each of the four different settings for health promotion programs has specific objectives, targets a specific population, and offers a particular menu of health and fitness programs. As a professional who may one day be seeking employment in one of these professions, it is important that you look at each organization on these merits and not place too much emphasis on the label of worksite, commercial, clinical, or community setting. As we have shown, these settings have considerable overlap, and all are rapidly expanding the scope of the health and fitness programs they offer. Many exciting professional jobs are available in each setting. Your ideal job will be the one that best matches your goals as a professional.

🔑 Because increasing overlap exists among the goals and approaches of health and fitness settings, each organization must be judged on its own merits rather than on its particular setting.

Up-Close Views of Professions in Health and Fitness

The types of jobs that are available in a health and fitness facility will depend more on the specific programs being offered than on whether it is a worksite, commercial, clinical, or community setting. The number of organizations offering high-quality health and fitness programming in each type of setting continues to grow annually. This growth has resulted in fewer differences among the settings; many different types of facilities now offer similar programs.

In this section we will describe the types of jobs that are available across the four different health and fitness settings. More important, we will explain how these jobs have evolved and continue to evolve in response to social forces and market demands. While strength and conditioning are part of an overall fitness program, and fitness and health professionals will likely deal with these issues, this is discussed in detail in chapter 15.

As you read this section, compare these job descriptions to the list you created at the beginning of the chapter. What positions can you add to your list? What job duties are different from what you imagined? We hope that you will become as enthusiastic as we are about the numerous possibilities that exist for health and fitness professionals.

Group Exercise Instructor

Once called "aerobics instructor," this job has changed greatly over the past decade. Group exercise instructors continue to lead aerobic exercise classes, but now they serve a very broad population and provide instruction on a wide variety of activities. Group exercise instructors teach outdoor activities, aquatic fitness, and exercise classes for specific populations such as pre- and postnatal women, seniors, children, and clients that need medically supervised exercise. The aerobics studio is no longer an empty room with mirrors. Group exercise instructors use a variety of equipment such as steps, slides, spinning bikes, therabands, dumbbells, and barbells. In most places, this position continues to be part-time and paid on an hourly basis.

The aging of the American population has brought an increasing number of older and higher-risk clients into the group exercise setting. We will discuss this in more depth in the next section. For now, the important thing to realize is that what was once an aerobics studio filled with young adults is now a studio filled with a diverse population of individuals. Group exercise instructors need to be dynamic, have excellent leadership skills, and enjoy working with individuals in a group setting.

Degrees in kinesiology or other health and fitness related disciplines are recommended for these positions, and certifications are usually required. Widely recognized certification programs that are appropriate for this position include the American College of Sports Medicine (ACSM) Exercise Leader program and the American Council on Exercise (ACE) Group Fitness Instructor program. Figure 14.2 provides information on how to contact these organizations.

Fitness Instructor

The fitness instructor position is an excellent entry-level position for the fitness professional with a bachelor's degree in kinesiology or another health and fitness related discipline. Fitness instructors work primarily with apparently healthy adults. Job duties typically include conducting fitness assessments and designing individualized exercise programs that incorporate strength, flexibility, and aerobic fitness components. This is an exciting job that provides an opportunity to introduce many different types of individuals to the benefits of exercise. For many sedentary adults who are joining their first health and fitness facility, fitness instructors are the initial contact person who can either encourage or discourage them in their endeavor to become more healthy and fit.

Most reputable health and fitness facilities now provide some type of health screening and/or fitness assessment for new participants. The fitness instructor is responsible for administering assessments of such things as blood pressure, body composition, aerobic capacity, muscular strength, muscular endurance, and flexibility. The results of these assessments are then used to design individualized programs that meet the client's specific health and fitness needs. Some fitness instructors stay in touch with participants as they progress with their programs. In other facilities, follow-up appointments are provided by other professionals such as personal trainers or health/fitness counselors. The fitness instructor position can be either part-time or full-time and is usually paid on an hourly basis.

Health/Fitness Counselor

The health/fitness counselor position represents a unique growth area in the health and fitness

American College of Sports Medicine (ACSM)
P.O. Box 1440
Indianapolis, IN 46206-1440
317-637-9200
http://www.acsm.org

American Council on Exercise (ACE)
5830 Oberlin Drive, Suite 102
San Diego, CA 92121-3787
619-535-8227
http://www.acefitness.org

Association for Worksite Health Promotion (AWHP)
60 Revere Drive, Suite 500
Northbrook, IL 60062
847-480-9574
http://www.awhp.org

International Health and Racquet Sportsclub
  Association
263 Summer Street
Boston, MA 02210
800-228-4772
http://www.ihrsa.org

National Strength and Conditioning Association
  (NSCA)
P.O. Box 38909
Colorado Springs, CO 80937-8909
Phone 719-632-6722
http://www.nsca-lift.org

National Wellness Association (NWA)
1300 College Court
P.O. Box 827
Stevens Point, WI 54481-0827
Phone 715-342-2969
http://www.wellnessnwi.org/nwa

Other Resources

Fitness Management Magazine
4160 Wilshire Blvd.
Los Angeles, CA 90010
Phone 323-964-4800
http://www.fitnessworld.com

Figure 14.2   List of health and fitness associations.

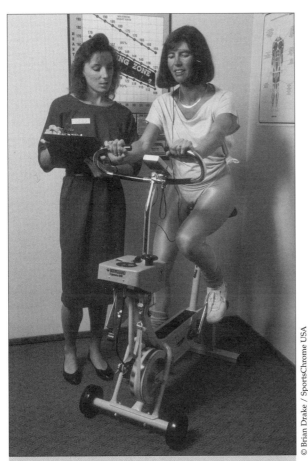

Fitness instructors conduct fitness assessments and design individualized exercise programs.

© Brian Drake / SportsChrome USA

niques are not applied universally to all clients during an initial appointment as has traditionally been the case in the fitness instructor position. Instead, health/fitness counselors assess clients' readiness for change (Prochaska & DiClemente, 1986), help them to set short- and long-term goals, and then assist them in moving at an appropriate pace toward a state of optimal health.

The Decathlon Club in Santa Clara, California, is one of the pioneers of the health/fitness counselor position. A commercial retention-based setting, the club created a new member service entitled Signature Health. Each new member meets with a Signature Health professional to have a customized Club Program designed. With an emphasis on optimal health, the customized Club Program incorporates many of the services that the club provides related to physical, emotional, intellectual, social, and spiritual health. Moreover, the Signature Health professional tracks and updates members' Club Programs through a variety of means (e.g., e-mail, interviews, phone calls) and records all information in a computerized confidential member database. Developing this database allows the Signature Health professional to filter information to identify, recommend, and market new Club Programs that are needed for specific segments of the membership. In this sense, they are very much health and fitness "promoters."

From an educational perspective, health/fitness counselors need to have a minimum of a bachelor's degree in kinesiology or another health and fitness related discipline. It is also important that they obtain certification from a nationally recognized association. Certification programs that are appropriate for this position include the ACSM Health/Fitness Instructor program and the ACE Lifestyle and Weight Management Consultant program. However, it must be noted that these certification programs do not prepare individuals completely for the health/fitness counselor position. People in this profession must make a constant effort to continue their education by reading professional journals and attending workshops, seminars, and conferences. Important organizations in this profession include ACSM, ACE, the Association for Worksite Health Promotion (AWHP), and the National Wellness Association (NWA). Figure 14.2 provides information on how to contact these organizations.

professions. In some facilities this position has replaced that of the fitness instructor. The health/fitness counselor provides guidance to a diverse population of individuals on a broad range of health and fitness topics. Many of these jobs are full-time, salaried positions and include benefits.

Health/fitness counselors have job descriptions that are consistent with O'Donnell's (1989) definition of health promotion: "the art and science of helping people change their lifestyle to move toward a state of optimal health" (p. 5). As a result, job duties are very broad and include such things as working with clients on behavior change, stress management, relaxation techniques, time management, smoking cessation, social participation, and weight management, in addition to prescribing exercise programs.

Health screening, fitness testing, and exercise program design are important skills for health/fitness counselors, but are only viewed as tools to assist them in working with clients. These tech-

While educational credentials and certifications—along with constant self-education—are essential for the health/fitness counselor, equally important is the ability to provide counseling on a broad range of health topics. Health/fitness counselors need to be organized, understand principles of behavior change, have excellent communication skills, and be effective in marketing and promoting programs and services. The health/fitness counselor position is increasingly becoming a salaried position.

Personal Trainer

The personal trainer position involves many of the same activities as that of the health/fitness counselor, but these services are typically provided on a fee-for-service basis. Some personal trainers work independently, traveling to individual clients' homes or conducting training sessions outdoors. More typically, personal trainers are employed by a facility and market their services directly to members. Most facilities pay personal trainers on an hourly fee-for-service basis, at a rate significantly higher than the hourly rates for fitness instructors or health/fitness counselors. For this reason, personal trainers have an opportunity to earn a substantial salary in comparison to other health and fitness professionals. Throughout the 1990s, personal training programs continued to grow in many health and fitness settings with many trainers earning salaries as high as $65,000 per year.

The personal trainer position provides a unique opportunity for the health and fitness professional to develop an ongoing relationship with specific clients. This relationship allows the trainer to develop a clear picture of individual clients' needs and quickly implement new strategies for behavior change. Personal trainers work with clients on a number of health issues such as weight management, stress management, physical fitness, and sport conditioning. Current trends in this position include specialization in working with specific populations such as medically based clients, older adults, and children, as well as working toward specific client goals such as injury rehabilitation, running a 10K race, or completing a triathlon.

Personal trainers need a variety of skills in order to be successful. In addition to having a strong knowledge base in fitness assessment and exer-

cise prescription, personal trainers must be excellent communicators and counselors; have strong business skills in sales, marketing, administration, and time management; and be effective in working with a diverse client population. Personal trainers are the artists of the health and fitness professions. In addition to evaluating individual client needs and designing individualized programs, personal trainers must continually present new and exciting ways to keep clients on track and excited about making changes and maintaining new health behaviors as part of their lifestyle.

Over the past decade the public has become more knowledgeable about the types of credentials and certifications that are appropriate for the personal trainer position. Simply being fit is no longer an acceptable credential. Personal trainers need to make the same effort in pursuing an interdisciplinary education as health/fitness counselors. Currently, the market dictates that educational credentials such as a bachelor's or master's degree in kinesiology or another health and fitness related discipline is very important, and certifications such as the ACSM Health/Fitness Instructor are essential to gain employment.

Personal trainers are rarely hired directly from bachelor's degree programs unless they also have extensive experience working with clients on a variety of health and fitness topics. For this reason, an aspiring personal trainer will likely begin a career as a fitness instructor or health/fitness counselor and move into a personal trainer position upon gaining considerable additional experience. Personal trainers keep skills current by attending conferences, workshops, and other continuing education programs. Important associations for the personal trainer include ACSM, ACE, and the National Strength and Conditioning Association (NSCA). Figure 14.2 provides information on how to contact these organizations.

Specialist Positions

Many health and fitness settings are now incorporating specialist positions into their programs, including health educators, clinical exercise specialists, physical therapists, and registered dietitians (see also chapter 15). Nearly all specialist positions require graduate-level studies along with a bachelor's degree in kinesiology or another health and fitness related discipline. In addition,

In Profile

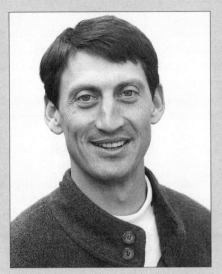

Marc Lobl
Owner of a Personal Training Studio

After graduating with a BS in exercise physiology from the University of Oregon, Mark Lobl took a position as a fitness instructor with the San Francisco Bay Club, a commercial retention-based health and fitness facility in San Francisco. Over a period of four years, he moved on to the positions of personal trainer and athletic/recreation director in this organization. During this time he also obtained his ACSM Health/Fitness Instructor certification and the NSCA Strength and Conditioning certification. Following his tenure with the San Francisco Bay Club, Mark spent three years working as a physical therapy assistant for the Asher Clinic in Larkspur, California. In 1993, while working at the Asher Clinic, Mark began working for Focus on Individual Training (FIT), a personal training studio in San Francisco. After three years of learning the business, Marc purchased FIT from the owner/founder in 1996.

Mark continues to grow a successful and highly regarded health and fitness studio with male and female clients of various fitness levels, ages, and backgrounds. Mark manages all aspects of his business including promotional activities, budgeting, accounting, payroll, facility maintenance, program planning, and business development. He provides assistance to a broad range of individual clients ranging from very well known celebrities to individuals with unique health and fitness needs. In 1996 Mark also joined the NIKE team as a fitness athlete traveling the country giving lectures and workshops on health and fitness topics, most specifically on sport training and techniques.

many of these positions require specific certifications and licensure. Specialist positions provide services that go beyond those provided by health/fitness counselors or personal trainers. These jobs can be very challenging, and also allow for greater earning potential.

What are the differences between health and fitness professionals and specialists? Let's take the example of providing nutrition information to clients in a health and fitness facility. Health/fitness counselors or personal trainers are often called on to provide basic nutritional advice to healthy adult clients. It would not be appropriate, however, for them to prescribe a specific type of diet or supplement or to make recommendations to individuals who have health risks or specific health conditions. Only registered dietitians have the appropriate qualifications to make such recommendations. This would require additional

course work than what is offered in the kinesiology department.

Injury rehabilitation provides another example of the boundaries between various professionals and specialists in a health and fitness facility. Personal trainers are required to obtain a full injury history on each client and to consider this information when designing an exercise program. An appropriately designed exercise program can help individuals prevent injuries in the future. It is not appropriate, however, for a personal trainer to design a specific program for injury rehabilitation. Physical therapists are the specialists with the appropriate knowledge and qualifications to provide injury rehabilitation services to clients. In an ideal scenario, a personal trainer would work in partnership with a physical therapist or registered dietitian. The trainer may be called on to supervise specific aspects of a program and communicate with the specialist regarding the client's progress.

As mentioned previously, most specialist positions require graduate-level education in addition to a bachelor's degree in kinesiology or another health and fitness related discipline. If you are interested in pursuing a specialist position, check with your academic advisor to find out how you can best prepare for an appropriate graduate program. For health and fitness professionals interested in working with medically based clients, ACSM offers an Exercise Specialist certification program. To contact ACSM, refer to Figure 14.2.

Health/Fitness Director

The health/fitness director is a key position in most health and fitness settings. This individual is typically responsible for managing the health and fitness services and programs that take place in a facility. In larger facilities, the health/fitness director may supervise a team of managers who handle specific responsibilities within departments. Examples of these management positions include group exercise director, personal training director, aquatics director, athletic/recreation director, and youth activities director. All of these management positions should be considered job opportunities for health and fitness professionals.

The job description for a health/fitness director position includes hiring, training, and providing support for a diverse staff of group exercise instructors, health/fitness counselors, personal trainers, specialists, and equipment maintenance personnel. In addition, health/fitness directors are responsible for business planning, managing budgets, planning facility renovations, selecting equipment, designing and marketing programs, and forecasting future trends in health and fitness programs. The health/fitness director must have a broad, interdisciplinary education that includes business planning, budgeting, marketing, and staff management in addition to a strong foundation in kinesiology.

Currently, educational requirements for the health/fitness director position emphasize academic degrees more than certifications. A degree in kinesiology is especially appropriate for students aspiring to be health/fitness directors. Many facilities require health/fitness directors to have a graduate degree in kinesiology or another health and fitness related discipline. Other requirements include experience in a position such as health/fitness counselor or personal trainer. Through experience in such positions directors gain a full understanding of individualized program design and strategies for successful behavior change. In addition, these job experiences provide valuable insight into the management responsibilities of hiring, training, and supporting staff.

Health/fitness directors need to be effective leaders. Beyond managing day-to-day operations, these individuals must be capable of articulating a vision and motivating other individuals to work toward specific goals. The health/fitness director is both a visionary who keeps current with the field of health and fitness and a mentor who supports staff members in moving toward individual goals and aspirations.

In addition to the educational recommendations listed earlier, ACSM offers a specific certification program for the health/fitness director. This certification provides verification of the knowledge and practical skills required for this position and is appropriate for professionals who have extensive experience as health/fitness directors. This certification should not be attempted prior to gaining experience in a director-level position.

Marketplace Trends and Opportunities

Across every industry, the best leaders are individuals who do extensive reading in many different fields and keep up to date on social and cultural trends. They continually ask questions about how the world around them affects their specific organization. Now that you have an understanding of the various positions available in the health and fitness professions, it is important to broaden your view by adding an understanding of the trends that affect these professions.

As a future health and fitness professional, you should be aware of the ever-changing context in which these professions are immersed. This is a very dynamic time in the health and fitness industry, with personal, social, cultural, and political issues having a powerful impact on the way we view health and fitness—and on the way we work in the profession. While it is beyond the scope of this chapter to outline all of these issues, we will deal with three major issues influencing these professions at this time: an increasing interest in a multidimensional model of wellness, health-care reform, and the aging of society.

⚷ Health and fitness professionals must understand the ways in which social and cultural forces affect their industry.

Multidimensional Model of Wellness

An important trend across all health and fitness settings is the expansion of program offerings to address other dimensions of wellness in addition to physical fitness. The multidimensional model of wellness includes five dimensions of health: physical, intellectual, emotional, social, and spiritual (Dintiman & Greenberg, 1986) (see table 14.1). Our previous description of clinical health and fitness settings provided an example of a hospital group that offers a wide variety of wellness programs and services. In addition to offering exercise programs, this hospital provides classes on topics such as meditation, parenting, and self-esteem. In our description of worksite settings, we discussed ways that worksite programs have evolved over time to provide services that not only assist employees in making changes but also support them in maintaining healthy lifestyle behaviors. In addition to offering employees state-of-the-art fitness facilities, many

worksites now offer things such as family activities, volunteer service opportunities, and programs for facilitating personal growth and improving communication skills.

As facilities expand their program offerings, they will also expand their job descriptions. If you elect to focus exclusively on the physical dimension of health, you will continue to find many exciting job opportunities. However, if you embrace the challenge of delivering services that address other dimensions of health, you are likely to find even more job opportunities.

⚷ Health and fitness programs increasingly address other dimensions of wellness in addition to physical fitness, drawing from a multidimensional model, which includes physical, intellectual, emotional, social, and spiritual well-being.

As we have shown in our description of various job categories, many health and fitness positions have already expanded to involve a broader range of responsibilities. Health/fitness counselors and personal trainers continue to design exercise programs, but are also called on to assist clients with issues such as stress management, personal growth, and involvement in social activities. The Decathlon Club's Signature Health Program (see the section on the health/fitness counselor) is an example of a program with a multidimensional wellness focus. Health/fitness directors continue to manage fitness facilities and programs, but are also responsible for managing programs that enhance intellectual, emotional,

TABLE 14.1
Dimensions of Wellness

Physical health	Biological integrity: the ability to carry out daily tasks with vigor.
Intellectual health	The ability to learn, to grow from experience, and utilize intellectual capabilities.
Emotional health	The ability to control emotions and express them appropriately and comfortably.
Social health	The ability to have satisfying interpersonal relationships and interactions with others.
Spiritual health	A guiding sense of meaning or value in life. May involve belief in some unifying force or god-like entity.

social, and spiritual health. These new responsibilities require unique skills. In short, industry leaders in all settings are looking increasingly for bright people who can deliver a broad range of services and integrate concepts of exercise and fitness into a broader definition of health.

🔑 Health and fitness professionals are increasingly being called on to integrate exercise and physical fitness into a broader definition of health.

Health-Care Reform

Another trend that has led to an increase in health and fitness programs is a national shift in health-care coverage. The old model of health care was a fee-per-service system, where people did not pay an up-front fee but instead paid for each service performed. A large percentage of health-care services are now provided on a "capitated" basis. Under the new capitation model, all subscribers pay a designated monthly fee to a health-care provider. That provider must then take care of the medical needs of all subscribers within the budget available. As an example, imagine that there is a particular health-care provider called Purple Cross with 100,000 subscribers each paying $100 per month for medical coverage. This monthly fee is paid directly by the subscriber or by his or her employer. Purple Cross receives $10 million per month in subscription revenue. All expenses related to the medical care of the subscribers, including physician fees, emergency services, and facility charges, must be paid for out of this $10 million. As a way of controlling these expenses, groups such as Purple Cross will typically enter into partnerships with physicians and hospital facilities and agree in advance on set prices for these services. After paying management operating expenses, advertising, public relations, and other administrative costs, Purple Cross gets to keep the remainder of the $10 million as profits or as a reserve for the future.

If you were the manager of Purple Cross, would you want your subscribers to have lengthy hospital stays or frequent visits to doctors' offices and emergency rooms? Obviously not. In fact, it would be ideal if all of your subscribers stayed healthy and never needed to visit the doctor at all. Of course, it is not realistic to expect that all subscribers are going to remain healthy. There will always be medical problems that need attention and accidents that require emergency services. The bottom line, however, is that some medical problems can be avoided or prevented with programs and services that target prevention.

Under this new model, exciting possibilities exist for increased funding of preventive services. The old model provided fees to practitioners for services as they were rendered. Since the majority of services rendered were for treatment after an individual became sick or injured, it was only possible for practitioners to make money when they were treating sick people. Under the new "capitation" model, many service providers are now paid a monthly fee in advance to provide for all of their patients' basic medical needs. As a result, treating sick people is not as profitable as it used to be, and many practitioners are looking for ways to deliver preventive services, such as exercise classes and fitness counseling, that are cost effective and keep their patients healthy.

Knowing that preventive services are much less costly than treatment services, some health-care providers are now using a percentage of the subscription dollars they receive to provide preventive health-care services to their subscribers. Screening programs such as prostate exams, mammographies, and blood pressure screenings can identify problems early in the disease process, which can help avoid expensive medical procedures and improve patient outcomes. Programs to reduce risk factors, such as nutritional counseling, weight loss programs, and educational classes, can prevent expensive medical procedures such as coronary bypass surgery or treatment and rehabilitation following a heart attack or stroke.

The 1996 U.S. *Surgeon General's Report on Physical Activity and Health* (USDHHS, 1996) provided a tremendous amount of evidence that regular physical activity can reduce the risk of developing heart disease. As a result of this report and other research on the benefits of exercise, many hospitals are now offering fitness facilities and programs to subscribers. Going back to our earlier example, if you were a manager in charge of preventive services at Purple Cross, who would you hire to deliver programs that assist your subscribers in becoming more physically active?

Hopefully, you have identified some of the positions described previously in this chapter. Group exercise instructors, health/fitness counselors, and personal trainers would be ideal professionals to deliver these services.

This new health-care model has already resulted in some providers building health and fitness facilities and offering more extensive health promotion programs. Blue Shield of California was one of the first health maintenance organizations (HMOs) to actively promote "lifestyle as prevention" as part of their business model. Their Lifepath program offers a health plan that not only covers subscribers' costs for doctor visits and hospital stays but also provides them with increased access and discounted fees for alternative health and wellness services, such as acupuncture, chiropractic, massage therapy, stress management techniques, and personal training. Blue Shield provides these services in partnership with a number of local health and fitness facilities in various worksite, commercial, and community settings.

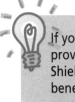

If you were shopping for a health-care provider, would you choose one like Blue Shield that offered health and fitness benefits in addition to regular medical coverage? In addition to keeping subscribers healthy, how else might Blue Shield's business benefit by offering these health and fitness services to potential subscribers?

We are at a place in the health and fitness professions with many opportunities. For the first time, physical activity is not being viewed simply as part of a recreation and leisure industry; it is increasingly seen as an integral component of the nation's health-care delivery system. Quite possibly the doctor's office of the future will have on-site fitness facilities and a staff of health/fitness counselors and personal trainers in addition to traditional medical personnel.

Physical activity is being viewed increasingly as an integral component of the nation's health-care delivery system.

Given this scenario, you may be asking yourself why more health-care providers have not expanded the number of preventive services they offer. The answer to this question is very complicated and, as a result, those in the health and fitness professions will have to be patient with the slow pace at which this change is likely to occur.

Both the rising cost of medical care and the manner in which health care is paid for in the United States are slowing the progress toward offering more preventive services. Health-care organizations are so busy developing cost-effective ways to treat people who are sick that they have taken the focus away from the development of better strategies for prevention. In addition, when employees leave their jobs, they also tend to change health insurance providers. Health insurance providers will only be motivated to invest money in preventive services when they feel confident they will reap the benefits in future cost savings.

It may take some time, but it is likely that more insurance companies will invest in prevention when the number of providers becomes reduced in particular geographic regions. For example, if

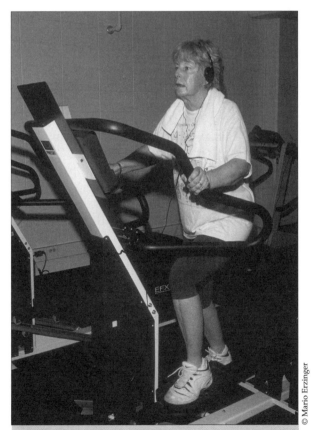

© Mario Erzinger

Physical fitness is now recognized as an important factor in the prevention of illnesses.

there are only four major health insurance providers in a specific area, these companies might all agree to provide similar prevention programs to subscribers. In this manner, each provider would know that even with the switching around that will occur as people change jobs, most subscribers will have had access to the same preventive programs throughout their lifetime. With this type of approach, health insurance companies could feel confident that their investment in prevention would result in lower overall health-care costs for their businesses.

Lastly, we need to say that while prevention programs sponsored by health insurance companies do look very promising for the future, these programs are unlikely to solve all of our nation's health-care problems. We mentioned earlier that in the United States many companies pay the cost of insurance coverage for their employees. But we also know that in the new American economy, many people get displaced from their work, subcontract, or get moved into part-time or temporary work. An estimated 42% of these workers have no health insurance coverage (Lowe, 1995). Indeed, in 1994, 40+ million American citizens were without some type of health insurance. Health and fitness professionals must recognize that the addition of insurance-sponsored prevention programs will not result in lower health-care costs for all individuals. Creative solutions to the problem of providing uninsured individuals with access to preventive programs and services will still be needed.

What are some ideas that you have for addressing the preventive needs of uninsured members of your community? Check with student health services on your campus to find out the percentage of students that are currently uninsured. What types of preventive programs are currently available to students (insured and uninsured) enrolled in your school?

Demographics

Demographic trends are radically redefining the meaning of healthy lifestyles and healthy aging within our society. According to the U.S. Census Bureau's latest population projections, the median age of the total population grew from 23 in 1900 to 30 in 1950 to 34.3 in 1995. It is expected to continue to increase steadily to 35.7 in 2000 and to peak at 38.7 in 2035. Driving this increase is the aging of the baby boom generation, the 77 million people born in the United States between 1946 and 1964 (see **http://www.census.gov/**). For the past quarter century, this generation has had a huge impact on the marketplace because of its sheer numbers. Baby boomers now account for 40% of the population over the age of 18. They are also the population segment currently in their peak earning and spending years with the highest household income of any age group.

This "age wave" (Dychtwald, 1990) raises some interesting questions. By 2011 the first baby boomers will reach the age of 65. Indeed, while there were 33 million persons over 65 in 1993, projections for 2050 show that the number will grow to an astounding 80 million, representing 20% of the population. What does this aging of America mean for the health and fitness industries? What does it mean when people say that baby boomers will not just grow older chronologically but will age youthfully? Will "middle age" be totally reinvented? What will happen when our future customers, clients, and patients retire at 65 years of age and then have another 25 years of living to do? Consider the fact that the number of senior citizens over age 85 is expected to more than triple from 3 million in 1993 to 9 million in 2030 to 19 million between 2030 and 2050. These demographic shifts will surely challenge our definition of physical activity as it relates to sport, competition, adventure, movement, pleasure, and health.

Already, industry reports for the period from 1987 to 1995 show that health club memberships rose 118% for the 55+ age group and 63% for the 35–54 age group while only 26% for the 18–34 age group. Currently, 50 million Americans have hypertension, 40 million suffer from arthritis, 20 million have lower-back pain, 18 million have diabetes, 18 million suffer from anxiety and depression, 59 million have heart disease, 95 million have cholesterol levels over 200, and 100 million carry unhealthy weight (International Health, Racquet and Sportsclub Association, 1998). Many of these health concerns can be related to age issues.

In Profile

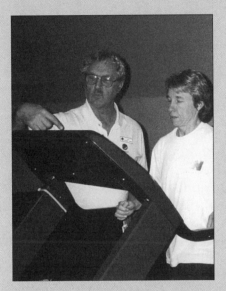

Jack Galatolo

Personal Trainer

Jack Galatolo is one of the new breed of health and fitness professionals designing programs that encompass the physical, intellectual, emotional, social, and spiritual dimensions of wellness. As a full-time personal trainer at the Pacific Athletic Club in Redwood City, California, Jack has developed a number of new and innovative programs based on some of the demographic issues we have been discussing. Indeed, his classes for seniors, such as the inspirational Lifting for Life, have been very successful. This has led the Fifty-Plus Fitness Association, a national nonprofit organization devoted to supporting community-based exercise programs, to ask Jack to design their national Challenge Camp group exercise program specially designed for older adults.

Jack is one of an increasing number of creative people who have shifted careers into the new health and fitness industries and are using their educational and life experiences to develop new and innovative relationships with particular demographic groups. Although Jack has a BA in marketing and an MA in business administration, as well as being ACSM Health/Fitness Instructor certified, NSCA Strength and Conditioning Specialist certified, USA Weightlifting Association accredited, and Arthritis Association Pace Instructor certified, it is his specific understanding of the older adult that makes him unique. This is hardly surprising. You see, Jack is the perfect role model for many of his clients because he has already retired once! In fact, he did not even enter the health and fitness profession until age 60. Prior to that, Jack owned and operated two very successful Shell Autocare service stations in San Mateo, California. It was only at age 57 that he decided he wanted to make a change. Spending the next two and a half years deciding what his new passion in life would be, he eventually enrolled in Cal State Hayward's Personal Trainer Certification program. Little did he realize he was on his way to a completely new career!

Look again at your list of job titles in the health and fitness professions. How do you think the changing demographics of society, especially the aging population, will impact the skills needed for each profession? Which of these skills do you need to improve or seek education for?

These trends are having an enormous impact on the way many American health and fitness businesses are developing their strategic plans for the next decade. Many settings are already taking advantage of this demographic shift in their hiring and programming practices.

In recognizing the baby boomers' youthfulness, prosperity, and renewed interest in outdoor activities such as camping, hiking, biking, fishing, and adventure travel, Pacific Athletic Club, a retention-based commercial facility in Redwood City, California, has also created a new twist on personal training. They have taken some of their most qualified personal trainers and turned them into "experience makers." Working in partnership with an outdoor adventure company, these trainers are given the task of creating customized, personalized, and unique active experiences for small groups of paying clients.

As an example, one trainer is currently creating a 15-day adventure trip to Patagonia where participants will hike in some of the world's most magnificent mountain regions. Prior to the trip, the trainer will lead participants in a two-month training regime (preparation). After accompanying the group on the adventure (immersion), the trainer will then return home to the club setting to relive the memorable adventure with the participants and develop a new personal program for each (retention). Unlike the traditional personal trainer, the "experience maker" includes a variety of things in the preparation phase. In preparation for the Patagonia hiking adventure, the trainer will conduct counseling sessions to determine specific goals for each individual. In addition, the trainer will organize things such as Spanish lessons, historical lectures on the Patagonia wilderness, and practical sessions on the selection of trekking clothing and equipment. Many of these services will be provided in partnership with community groups, universities,

and local businesses. All of these services are in addition to health and fitness assessments and specially designed physical activity programs to ensure that each person is "fit" enough for the adventure.

The trainer will then travel with the group of clients, using the knowledge that she has gained throughout the training period to ensure that each individual realizes the experience outcomes that he or she desires. A contracted outdoor adventure company will make all of the day-to-day arrangements and will be responsible for the logistics of the trip.

After returning to the club setting, the trainer and the participants will revisit these memorable experiences as a way of confirming accomplishments, establishing new goals, and developing new plans. It is therefore especially important that the trainer come to know the specific desires, dreams, and expectations of each individual client. Describing and reliving each person's outcome is very important and the key to the clients' full enjoyment of the experience. Trainers in dynamic positions such as these need to have an integrated understanding of the physical, intellectual, emotional, social, and spiritual components of health.

As baby boomers continue to age, acquire wealth, and gain more leisure time upon retirement, opportunities for health and fitness professionals to provide premium services, such as the two-week adventure trip to Patagonia, will increase. Given the demographics we have mentioned, what outcomes do you think clients may be looking for from such experiences? We mentioned that the Pacific Athletic Club allows only its most qualified personal trainers to deliver such programs. What qualifications do you think an "experience maker" needs? What skills might be helpful in addition to knowledge about physical training? Which of these skills do you have? Which ones could you develop?

Some health and fitness professionals are being called on to lead adventure vacations for older people.

© Marshall Smith

Many job opportunities are likely to arise as a result of the demographic patterns shaping our country. We will all witness a far more diverse nation in the coming years. By 2050 less than 53% of the population will be non-Hispanic white; 16% will be black; 23% will be of Hispanic origin; 10% will be Asian and Pacific Islander; and about 1% will be American Indian, Eskimo, and Aleut. By 2000 the Hispanic-origin population is expected to increase to 31 million. By 2015 and 2050 it will double and quadruple its 1990 size, respectively (see **http://www.census.gov/**).

How will a more diverse population impact the skills and competencies you will need to be a successful practitioner? Did you mention any of these skills and competencies in the initial list that you made at the beginning of the chapter? What are some of your ideas for health and fitness business opportunities in the future?

Inside Advice for Health and Fitness Students

An incredible transformation is currently under way as we move toward a broader understanding of health/fitness services. We are beginning to view physical activity as a key component in the health-care delivery system. We are also experiencing a considerable demographic shift in our population that challenges us to work with increasingly diverse groups of individuals.

Take one final look at the list of jobs titles, job duties, and required skills and competencies that you created at the beginning of this chapter. Now compare your list to the list provided in Table 14.2. How did your list of knowledge and skills compare to the one in Table 14.2? While our list is by no means complete, it should illustrate that a broad range of skills and competencies are now required of health and fitness professionals.

As experts in the health and fitness professions, we offer you the following advice. Today's health and fitness professional needs to obtain a broad education across several different scientific, behavioral, and humanity-based disciplines. To develop the skills and competencies listed in table 14.2, we encourage you to seek a combined degree in kinesiology and health with courses in teaching; behavior change psychology; communication; gerontology; marketing; and the sociology of race, gender, and ethnicity. Course work in theoretical kinesiology (section 2 of this text) will be extremely valuable, and other health- and fitness-related specialized courses will round out your professional practice knowledge. It is also essential that you have practical experience counseling clients on a variety of health and fitness topics, and that you can relate to a diverse population of clients from different age groups and ethnic backgrounds. Involve yourself in a health and fitness job setting through an internship or work-study to keep up to date on what is happening in this field.

When you graduate from college you will find yourself competing for jobs with individuals who have extensive practical and insightful life experiences (see profile: Jack Galatolo). For this reason you should be sure to obtain practical skills as part of your education. An increasing number of nondegree educational programs cater specifically to individuals seeking practical experience. Several universities offer two-year health and fitness educational programs. In addition, organizations such as the National Strength and Conditioning Association (NSCA), the American College of Sports Medicine (ACSM), and the American Council on Exercise (ACE) offer workshop and certification programs for health and fitness professionals. These organizations also publish extensive educational materials to help individuals with self-study programs.

In addition, be sure to read the relevant health and fitness journals and industry publications. Most of these publications are available through the associations listed in figure 14.2. Many of these publications are available to students at substantially reduced rates, and some are even provided free of charge to health and fitness professionals.

Given the competitive nature of the job market, it is essential that you maximize your

TABLE 14.2 Job Descriptions			
Job title	**Evolution**	**Job duties**	**Skills and competencies**
Group exercise instructor	This position has transitioned away from exclusively teaching aerobic dance classes. This position now involves teaching a broad range of classes to a diverse population.	Lead group exercise classes for various population groups including seniors, children, pre- and postnatal women, and medically based clients.	Bachelor's degree in kinesiology or another health and fitness related discipline preferred. Certification by a nationally recognized organization required. Additional certifications in a specialized area may also be required in order to teach specific types of classes. Strong teaching skills are a must.
Health/fitness counselor	This position has evolved from the more traditional fitness instructor position. The health/fitness counselor provides counseling on a broad range of health topics in addition to conducting fitness assessments and designing exercise programs.	Provide guidance to a diverse population in areas such as behavior change, stress management, smoking cessation, social participation, weight management, and exercise programming.	Bachelor's or graduate-level degree in kinesiology or another health and fitness related discipline required. Certification by a nationally recognized organization required. Additional skills in counseling, behavior change, cultural diversity, and teaching are a must. Marketing and promotional skills are also essential.
Personal trainer	This position has transitioned from exclusively providing individualized exercise programs to providing individualized services on a broad range of health topics.	Provide ongoing support and guidance to a diverse population of clients on topics such as physical fitness, weight management, stress management, and sport conditioning.	Bachelor's or graduate-level degree in kinesiology or another health and fitness related discipline preferred. Certification by a nationally recognized organization required. Background in exercise programming is a must. Counseling and teaching skills are a must. Business, marketing, sales, and promotion training are also essential.
Specialist positions	Examples include physical therapists, registered dietitians, clinical exercise specialists, and health educators.	Provide specialized health and fitness services to clients with special needs.	Graduate-level degree required. Additional certifications and licensure may be required in order to practice in specific states. Other specific experiences and skills will be required for each type of specialist position.
Health/fitness director	Programming all health and fitness programs that are delivered in a facility. Responsibilities include delivery of programs to address all dimensions of health.	Manage all aspects of a health and fitness department. Responsibilities include departmental leadership, staff management, programming, and all aspects of business administration.	Bachelor's or graduate-level degree in kinesiology or another health and fitness related discipline required. Additional skills in business administration, management, marketing, and promotion are required. Previous experience in an entry-level health and fitness position required.

educational experience while in college. Work with your advisor to create a degree plan that will prepare you for the current and future job market. In addition to the courses provided in your major, select elective courses that will best prepare you for the type of job that you want (see table 14.2). Take advantage of as many internship and community service learning experiences as possible. In many cases, a degree in a health and fitness discipline alone will not be sufficient to get you the job you want. In addition to having the credentials on paper, you must also be able to demonstrate that you can apply the skills that you have learned.

The authors of this chapter have spent a considerable number of years in the health and fitness industry as directors, managers, consultants, and practitioners. During this time, we have conducted literally hundreds of formal and informal job interviews of potential employees. We have often seen newly graduated students show up at interviews, excited, with degrees in hand, who were completely unprepared for the types of jobs available. In some cases, students who were interviewing for health/fitness counselor positions told us that they did not have any teaching experience because they had chosen an area of emphasis that dealt strictly with the biophysical sphere of physical activity. Because teaching courses fell within another area of emphasis (i.e., the behavioral sphere of physical activity), these students didn't believe they needed them. Don't find yourself in this situation by limiting yourself to one particular area of emphasis at the expense of gaining important skills that will help you to be successful in the job you want.

> It is essential that you maximize your educational experience while in college, being sure to select a broad spectrum of elective courses in your degree program.

Be sure to take special care choosing elective courses in your degree program. If your department does not offer a course in teaching or counseling skills, then inquire what departments on campus might. Perhaps you can speak to your advisor and have a faculty member with teaching or coaching expertise supervise you in an independent study. We can make a similar argument for classes based on business and marketing. Clearly, in our media-saturated culture, marketing skills are very important for health and fitness professionals. After all, a big part of your job as a health and fitness professional will be to motivate people to take part in the programs that you offer, and to "promote" the idea of making healthy lifestyle changes. Again, if your department does not offer a specific class in health and fitness marketing, another course on campus may provide general marketing information that you can apply to your discipline. Remember, what will matter most when you interview for a job is that you have knowledge and skills to do the job successfully. Do your homework early, and make sure that you obtain the appropriate skills along the way.

Wrap-Up

In this chapter we have described the health and fitness industry and summarized the types of settings and jobs that are currently available for health and fitness professionals. In addition, we have provided some insight into current and future trends in health and fitness and described ways in which these trends impact the industry.

The world of health and fitness is ever changing, which is partly what makes this profession so dynamic and exciting. If you are considering a career in the health and fitness professions, learn as much as you can about them. It is never too early to begin to tailor your education to your personal passions. Remember also to consider industry trends as you complete this phase of what should be an ongoing educational process. This discussion about the health and fitness professions should serve as nothing more than a point from which to begin your own process of discovery. Enjoy the journey.

Study Questions

1. Identify program objectives, target markets, and types of programs offered for each of the following health and fitness settings: (a) worksite; (b) commercial; (c) community; and (d) clinical.

2. Compare and contrast sales-based and retention-based commercial health and fitness business models.

3. Describe typical job duties for the following health and fitness positions: (a) group exercise instructor; (b) fitness instructor; (c) health/fitness counselor; (d) personal trainer; and (e) health/fitness director.

4. How will health-care reform potentially affect job opportunities in the health and fitness professions?

5. How will demographic trends in the U.S. population (e.g., aging baby-boomers) affect the health and fitness professions?

6. List the knowledge, skills, and abilities that you need to obtain in order to be competitive in the health and fitness job market.

15

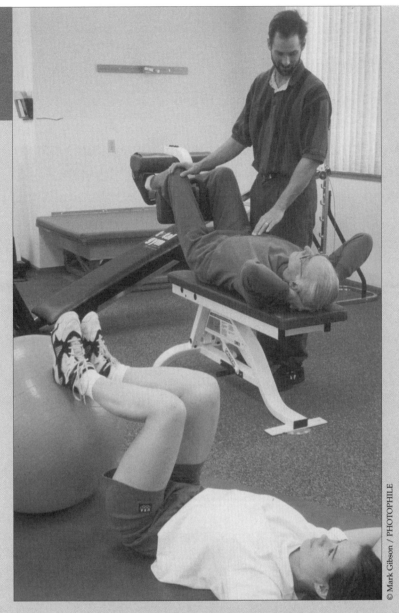

© Mark Gibson / PHOTOPHILE

Therapeutic Exercise Professions

Chad Starkey

In this chapter . . .

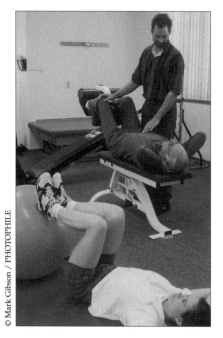

© Mark Gibson / PHOTOPHILE

A high school football player fails to get up following a play. The athletic trainer arrives on the scene and finds the athlete's left tibia fractured.

Following a stroke, a 54-year-old chief financial officer is recovering from surgery. Along her road to recovery she will meet physical therapists, occupational therapists, and cardiovascular rehabilitation specialists. Each of these professionals will contribute to her return to a successful career.

Surgeons successfully repair an infant's clubbed feet, but the child is showing a delay in walking upright. The physician refers the child to a physical therapist for the rehabilitation necessary to achieve normal development.

A 60-year-old widow suffers a brain tumor. She is unable to perform the cognitive or motor functions required for independent living (ADLs), but she is hopeful of being discharged from an assisted living facility. An occupational therapist works with her to help restore her mental abilities and help her gain the motor skills needed for independent living.

Each of these scenarios depicts real-life situations that therapeutic exercise professionals are presented with daily in work settings such as hospitals, laboratories, clinics, and sport facilities. Although their patients and clients may differ, athletic trainers, cardiac rehabilitation specialists, occupational therapists, physical therapists, and strength and conditioning coaches all apply exercise and movement experiences to improve a person's physical functioning.

Figure 15.1 illustrates the spheres of professional practice, including the sphere of therapeutic exercise. Physical activity professionals in this sphere help people restore lost function (rehabili-

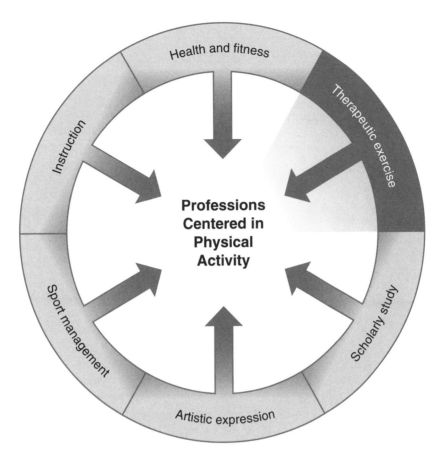

Figure 15.1 Therapeutic exercise is one of the spheres of professional practice.

tative therapeutic exercise) or acquire skills and functions considered normal or expected (habilitative therapeutic exercise).

 CHAPTER OBJECTIVES

In this chapter we will:

▌ Acquaint you with the wide range of professional opportunities in the sphere of therapeutic exercise

▌ Familiarize you with the purpose and types of work done by professionals in therapeutic exercise

▌ Inform you about the educational requirements and experiences necessary to become an active, competent professional in the area

▌ Help you identify whether one of these professions fits your skills, aptitudes, and professional desires

The World of Therapeutic Exercise

Exercise therapists are physical activity professionals who design and implement movement experiences for the purpose of restoring or improving motor function to a level that enables people to reach personal or career goals unencumbered by physical limitations. Therapeutic exercise professionals apply knowledge of human anatomy and physiology, exercise physiology, and biomechanics in structured activity programs. To develop therapeutic goals, clinicians must call upon their knowledge of the effects of exercise on the muscular, nervous, and cardiovascular systems and relate these effects to the patient's needs. Depending on the patient, workplace, and condition(s) being treated, the therapeutic goals may include restoring muscular function and strength, joint range of motion, cardiovascular and/or pulmonary function, and metabolic function.

Therapeutic Exercise, Rehabilitation, and Habilitation Defined

What is therapeutic exercise? In technical terms, **therapeutic exercise** is the systematic and scientific application of exercise and movement experiences in order to *develop* or *restore* muscular strength, endurance, or flexibility; neuromuscular coordination; cardiovascular efficiency; and other health and performance factors. In practice, therapeutic exercise is often programmed physical activity aimed at improving or restoring the quality of life. Therapeutic exercise can be classified as being rehabilitative or habilitative. In this chapter we draw a distinction between these two in order to help you understand the different types of professional work associated with this area.

> Therapeutic exercise can be classified as being rehabilitational (restoring lost function) or habilitational (helping to acquire normal function).

Broadly speaking, the term **rehabilitation** is used to describe processes and treatments that restore skills or functions previously acquired, but which have been lost due to injury, disease, or behavioral patterns. If you have ever strained a muscle or broken a bone, then you know the value of rehabilitation in helping you regain lost functions. Although rehabilitation can be in the form of ice, heat, electricity, ultrasound, or psychological counseling, we will focus in this chapter on treatments that involve physical activity.

Rehabilitation specialists require a thorough knowledge of the pathological aspects of injury and disease, the limitations they impose on human performance, and the types of treatments required to restore normal function. Because people are more than just muscles and bones, the psychological impact of the injury and the subsequent rehabilitation program must be taken into account as well. The regime used by an athletic trainer working to restore a running back's knee so he can return to competition is an example of a rehabilitative therapeutic exercise.

Habilitation, often confused with rehabilition, has a slightly different emphasis. It involves processes and treatments leading to the acquisition of skills and functions that are considered normal and expected for an individual of a certain age and status (Dudgenon, 1996). The standards or expectations that signal a need for habilitation may be vastly different for individuals of the same age. For example, different physical performance standards may be expected of a young lawyer than of a young athlete. The lawyer who is physically fit according to the definition in chapter 3 is probably not in need of habilitation—his state of physical fitness is considered normal for his age, and he does not need special physical abilities for his occupation. On the other hand, an athlete who is merely fit, but who lacks the cardiovascular endurance or strength to perform the tasks expected of her in field hockey, is a candidate for habilitation involving intensive conditioning, training, and other therapeutic exercise.

In both rehabilitative and habilitative therapeutic exercise, the status of the individual regarding any permanent disabilities or impairments, such as blindness, amputation, or paralysis, must be considered. For example, a paraplegic's functional loss of use of the lower extremities would not be a cause for rehabilitation, but a lack of upper body strength relative to that considered normal for a paraplegic may well be. Moreover, a physical therapist that is attempting to correct congenital postural problems is practicing habilitational therapeutic exercise since it involves *bringing the client to a level of functioning not previously attained.*

Obviously, health and fitness programs targeted at unfit populations may well involve habilitative therapeutic exercise since the populations served are usually performing at levels below that considered normal, and they may not have previously attained the level of health or fitness desired. Since professional opportunities in fitness and health promotion were addressed in chapter 14, they will not be considered here. We will, however, consider other types of professional services that include habilitative and rehabilitative therapeutic exercise.

Each of the professions described in this chapter is increasingly emphasizing the importance of preventing injury and disease. An athletic trainer, for example, helps to identify musculoskeletal problems such as loose joints, weak muscles, and family medical conditions that could predispose an athlete to injury or even death. Likewise, a physical therapist may assess a person's posture or evaluate a worker's biomechanics when lifting heavy objects to prevent job-related injuries. A cardiac rehabilitation specialist who performs electrocardiograms and exercise stress tests is also practicing the art of preventive medicine by identifying people who are at risk of experiencing a heart attack. By developing appropriate exercise programs to remedy these problems, these specialists help to reduce the likelihood of specific injuries and diseases.

It is not always easy to draw a clear line between habilitational and rehabilitational exercise programs. Many times they go hand in hand. For example, a therapist might not only design exercises to strengthen the muscles of the back to restore strength in a patient recovering from surgery (**rehabilitational therapeutic exercise**), but the therapist might also include exercises to prevent or reduce the possibility of reinjuring the back (**habilitational therapeutic exercise**).

> "An ounce of prevention is worth a pound of cure." Both rehabilitational and habilitational therapeutic exercise focus on developing the body's systems so they are less likely to become injured or diseased.

All of the therapeutic exercise professions discussed in this chapter involve working closely with people. These professionals work with a number of clients or patients daily, routinely discussing protocols and treatment plans with colleagues or other physical activity professionals. Do you enjoy people contact? Do you have good communication skills? If you are considering a career in therapeutic exercise, in what areas might you need to seek out further instruction and education?

Rehabilitative Therapeutic Exercise

Physical dysfunction is characterized by the inability to use one or more limbs or the torso. If you have ever broken an ankle or sprained your wrist, you have experienced physical dysfunction. Or perhaps you were born with a congenital malformation or suffered a major injury as the result of a car accident. Physical rehabilitation specialists help individuals who are suffering from physical dysfunction stemming from traumatic injury, minor congenital defects, or disease to regain the use of the affected body part or compensate for its disability. Physical therapists, occupational therapists, and athletic trainers specialize in rehabilitating these conditions. They work closely with other health-care professionals such as physicians, nurses, and dietitians.

Exercise Therapy for the Rehabilitation of Neuromuscular Injuries

Strokes, spinal cord injuries, back problems, and other injuries from automobile, industrial, sport, and home accidents can all lead to neuromuscular conditions in which the body's nervous system and/or muscles no longer function properly. In addition, physical activity carries with it the inherent risk of trauma, such as when repetitive motions at work lead to neuromuscular trauma

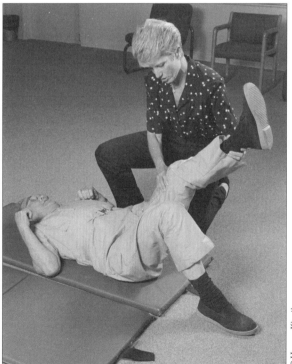

© Human Kinetics

Rehabilitative therapeutic exercise progams are used to restore the patient's functions to the preinjury level.

(see chapter 2). Not only does injury to muscles, joints, and bones directly affect the traumatized tissues, but the accompanying immobilization and associated decreased physical activity can produce much more widespread problems. Following a significant injury in which the limb's ability to function is inhibited, the resulting disuse may affect not only the entire limb, but also the activity of the entire body. Consequently, over time the efficiency of the heart and lungs may be degraded. Maybe you experienced this after injuring a bone or joint—after regaining full motion, you may have noticed that running up a flight of stairs or playing basketball left you more winded than such activities would have before your injury.

The goal of orthopedic rehabilitation programs is to restore symptom-free movement to the limb and to ensure that the body's cardiopulmonary system is restored to a level that can again accommodate the demands of activity. Restoring a limb's function consists of increasing joint range of motion, increasing muscular strength and endurance, and building cardiovascular endurance.

Although **neuromuscular injuries** directly affect the extremities, the resulting loss of function and inactivity decrease the body's cardiovascular function. Most neuromuscular rehabilitation programs also emphasize restoring the function of the heart and lungs.

Clinicians involved in this type of rehabilitation will use passive and active exercise to restore the limb to function. This is followed by strength and muscular endurance training, which serves to protect the limb. These exercises are augmented through various forms of heat and cold, electrical stimulation, therapeutic ultrasound, and manual therapy techniques. Throughout this process the therapists attempt to maintain the patient's level of cardiovascular endurance.

Most types of neuromuscular rehabilitation occur in outpatient physical therapy clinics, hospitals, and athletic training rooms.

Exercise Therapy for the Rehabilitation of Athletic Injuries. Rehabilitation of athletic injuries deserves specific attention here since the discipline of kinesiology usually offers the training for this area. You have probably witnessed an ath-

letic injury at one time or another—whether you broke a finger playing youth sports or anxiously waited during an injury time-out to find out how seriously your favorite football player was injured. Almost immediately following a sport injury, the athlete's rehabilitation begins. Restoring the body part back to its prior level of function is only one part of the rehabilitation process. Once the limb begins to regain strength, range of motion, and neuromuscular coordination, the athlete must be reintegrated into athletic activity. A unique aspect of athletic rehabilitation is the sport-specific functional progression. Here, traditional rehabilitation protocol is merged with the skills and tasks needed to compete in a particular sport.

Sports medicine is an aspect of therapeutic exercise that is exclusively dedicated to the prevention, treatment, and rehabilitation of injuries suffered by athletes. However, sports medicine is also distinct from other aspects of therapeutic exercise in that the rehabilitation protocol used is more aggressive than that used for the general population. The spectrum of sports medicine is quite broad and encompasses a range of activities that are beyond the scope of this text. Students who are interested in more information regarding sports medicine should investigate sections on the athletic trainer, the physical therapist, and the strength and conditioning specialist that appear later in this chapter.

Sports medicine involves the practice of medicine, the art of rehabilitation, and the science of research as they relate to athletic participation (Clark, 1994). The sports medicine umbrella encompasses preinjury issues including prevention, education, and counseling; injury recognition and management; and short- and long-term rehabilitation.

Exercise Therapy for the Rehabilitation of Post-surgical Trauma. Although surgery is performed to restore a person's health, the process of surgery itself is often detrimental to the body. Not only does the incision affect the involved muscles and nerves, but also the bed rest associated with the recovery process leads to decreased muscle mass and function and decreased cardiovascular efficiency. Although this effect is most easily seen when it involves the limbs, the heart and lungs are also adversely affected. Just as skeletal muscle wastes away when it is not used, cardiac muscle responds similarly. In most cases, patients recovering from long-term disability must undergo neuromuscular rehabilitation to restore normal cardiopulmonary function.

Physical Activity in Cardiopulmonary Rehabilitation

Diseases of the cardiopulmonary system include coronary artery disease, arrhythmia, hypertension, heart attacks, and emphysema. Collectively these diseases are the leading causes of death and long-term disability among adults in the United States. Undiagnosed heart disease is also the leading cause of death among young athletes (O'Connor, Kugler, & Oriscello, 1998). Early identification of people at risk for these conditions, and subsequent intervention, will reduce the likelihood of their occurrence and increase the chance of survival following an episode. Working closely with a physician, the exercise therapist may be responsible for planning, implementing, and supervising physical activity programs designed to help restore individuals to normal function.

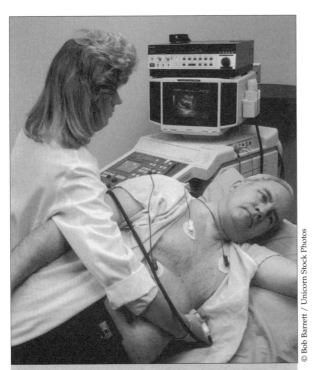

Cardiopulmonary care can begin before the onset of a patient's symptoms to identify those who are at risk of disease.

© Bob Barrett / Unicorn Stock Photos

Therapeutic exercise specialists must be aware of certain conditions that can make rehabilitative exercise a potentially deadly activity. Asthma, for example, can be especially dangerous because the lungs cannot exchange oxygen and carbon dioxide at the rate needed to support the body's metabolism during exercise. Since the risk is greatest when exercise occurs in a hot, dry environment, skilled therapeutic exercise specialists treating asthmatic clients will prescribe regimes that are much more easily tolerated by the client, such as aquatic exercise routines.

Cardiopulmonary rehabilitation includes cardiovascular exercises to improve the efficiency of the heart and lungs such as breathing exercises, walking, running, swimming, and resistance exercises such as weight training. These are prescribed at progressive levels of intensity and duration. Diagnostic tests such as stress testing, $\dot{V}O_2$max testing, electrocardiograms, and echocardiograms are used to monitor the patient's progress and adapt the level of activity accordingly.

Stress tests and other diagnostic tests are usually conducted in hospitals or other medical environments. Cardiovascular exercise programs are normally conducted in clinics, health clubs, or wellness centers with the patient also being prescribed independent programs for home use. All diagnostic tests and exercise prescribed to high-risk patients must be supervised by a licensed physician. Respiratory therapists, respiratory physical therapists, and other specialists also assist patients who are paralyzed, recovering from a heart condition, or postsurgical.

Because of the nature of the diseases being treated, most cardiopulmonary rehabilitation programs are supervised by a physician.

Exercise Therapy for the Rehabilitation of Older Populations

Humans are living longer and the percentage of the population aged 65 and over continues to grow. The natural decrease in strength and flexibility and the increase in age-related skeletal diseases such as arthritis hinder the quality of many older people's lives. As we saw in chapter 2, loss of ability to perform activities of daily living

(ADLs) and instrumental activities of daily living (IADLs) can have a profound physical and emotional effect on elderly people's lives. Also, as a person enters the latter years, the body's aerobic ability decreases, and the percentage of body fat increases, decreasing one's capacity to do physical work.

Although these conditions are somewhat inevitable, their onset can be delayed and the effects minimized through various forms of therapeutic exercise designed to increase strength, slow the loss of flexibility, and improve cardiovascular condition, thereby helping seniors to regain or maintain independent, active living. Programs that involve physical activity can decrease blood pressure, control cholesterol, reduce the risks of suffering a stroke or heart attack, and they may also lower the risk of certain types of cancer.

However, exercise in the older population is often a double-edged sword. While physical activity is required to maintain an appropriate level of fitness, the body is less capable of withstanding the forces of exercise. Clinicians working with clients with arthritis, for example, whose joints cannot tolerate the physical stresses associated with extensive walking, jogging, or running, must modify the exercise program to minimize the amount of force exerted on the joints. In this case, water aerobics could be used to maintain cardiovascular fitness without further injuring the joints.

Exercise Therapy for the Rehabilitation of Psychological Disorders

The physical benefits of exercise should now be apparent to you. But one more area is often overlooked: the psychological and emotional benefits of physical activity. Exercise is a wonderful way to reduce stress and unwind from the toils of life. People who are involved in regular physical activity tend to sleep better and suffer fewer emotional disorders.

Twenty to thirty minutes of aerobic exercise has been found to produce changes that are on a par with standard forms of psychotherapy (Raglin, 1990). In the healthy population aerobic exercise can serve to prevent the onset of some

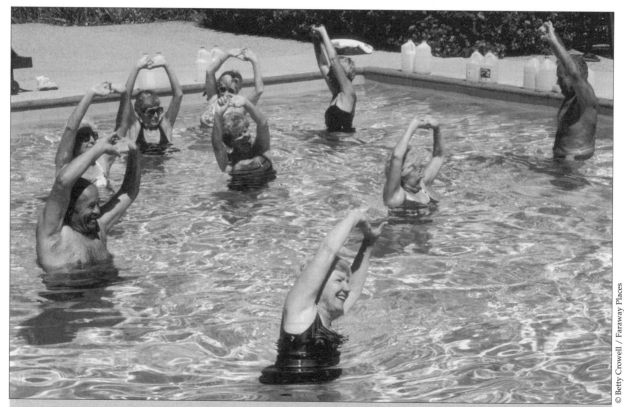

Therapeutic exercise can be prescribed to people of all ages and is especially useful in improving the lives of older citizens.

© Betty Crowell / Faraway Places

types of psychological maladies; for those suffering these types of conditions, exercise can often be considered a form of treatment. In fact, some psychotherapists prescribe exercise regimens as part of their patients' therapy programs. The older population described in the previous section can also gain psychological benefits from exercise. Elderly individuals who engage in physical activity have decreased signs of depression, increased self-image, and improved morale, all leading to a better quality of life (Singh, Clements, & Fiatarone, 1997). As an aside, smoking and alcohol cessation programs often include exercise, although scientific data has yet to show that this is effective.

Habilitative Therapeutic Exercise

Habilitative exercises help bring people in line with established physical standards such as those presented in chapter 3. The goal of this type of therapeutic exercise is to help people reach the expected level of physical fitness for their demographic classification. Throughout this text we have spoken about the relationship of physical activity to health and the physical activity professional's role of improving health through physical activity. Many of the professions described in chapter 14 also engage in habilitative therapeutic exercise. The following sections describe some of the areas in which therapeutic exercise is used for habilitative purposes.

Exercise Therapy for Specialized Habilitation

Although not recognized as such, this classification is probably the single largest role of habilitative therapeutic exercise. Specialized habilitation involves bringing specific groups of people in line with standards that exceed rather than merely meet those of the general population. These may include running a five-minute mile, having body fat within a certain range, or being able to lift a certain amount of weight.

Sports training camps, military boot camps, police and firefighter academies, and even astronaut training programs are examples of settings in which specialized habilitative therapeutic exercise takes place. Exercise specialists in this area must have a full understanding of the muscular and cardiovascular capabilities needed by people in these special groups. Often, the exercise spe-

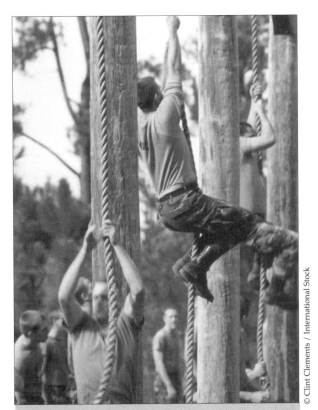

Perhaps the most common form of habilitative therapeutic exercise is that used for specialized training.

© Clint Clements / International Stock

cialist has a professional background in the specialty area. For example, a former professional baseball player with a degree in kinesiology may specialize in organizing habilitative exercise regimens for spring training camps. Such experience can help keep the exercise program in line with actual physical expectations of the baseball players involved.

Exercise Therapy for the Habilitation of Obese Populations

Physical fitness, exercising, and losing weight are a controversial American obsession. Many people overemphasize weight loss, and others ignore all aspects of healthy eating or exercise habits. Ironically, each approach is as hazardous, and potentially deadly, as the other.

Fad dieting, exercise addiction, and distorted body image have almost reached epidemic proportions among high-school and college-aged females. Medical conditions associated with such obsessions, especially anorexia and bulimia, are rising at alarming rates. At the other end of the spectrum is the overweight, sedentary portion of our population who, because of their lifestyles, are predisposed to cardiovascular disease.

Because of its role in bringing people in line with established standards, therapeutic exercise used to control weight and body mass is considered habilitational. Proper nutritional and exercise counseling are essential to promote a healthy lifestyle and to decrease the incidence of disease. Specialists such as exercise physiologists, strength and conditioning specialists, and personal trainers work in cooperation with physicians, nutritionists, counselors, and other professionals to develop and implement programs that assist people in returning to normal, functional, healthy lifestyles.

Exercise Therapy for the Habilitation of Children With Developmental Problems

In the not too distant past, children born with physical abnormalities faced living life with a functional handicap. Early identification of specific conditions followed by appropriate intervention has provided the opportunity of a fruitful life to countless people.

The goal of this type of habilitative exercise is to help the child adapt to, or compensate for, functional anatomical and physiological deficits. In certain cases the underlying condition may have been surgically corrected. Other cases may involve teaching the child how to use a prosthetic device or how to perform basic skills such as rolling over, walking, or eating in a modified manner. Exercise therapy may also be used to strengthen the muscles in children with cerebral palsy, thereby improving their walking performance.

While working with children has its own unique set of rewards, it likewise presents its own set of challenges to therapists. Issues such as communication between the therapist and child, home care problems, and schooling are unique to this population. Regardless of the challenges facing the therapist, the ultimate goal of habilitative regimens for this population is to promote physical, social, and cognitive development at a rate near the norm for the child's age group.

Exercise Therapy for Habilitation Toward General Fitness

With all of the benefits of exercise described in this text, the logical question is, Why doesn't everyone participate in exercise? The truth is that while more people are involved in exercise than at any other time, the majority of our population live sedentary lives. Although no one factor is singularly to blame for this lack of exercise, the long-time popularity of television and the recent growth in computer fixation both contribute to our "couch potato" society.

Research has shown that exercise can help prevent disease and enable people to reach their maximum life expectancy. Therapeutic exercise professionals play an important role in helping the general population achieve healthy standards of physical fitness by introducing them to exercise, through hospital-based fitness centers, commercial gymnasiums and fitness centers, employer-based wellness centers, and community-based, nonprofit agencies. Many of the professions in this areas were discussed in chapter 14.

> Societal changes have affected negatively the health of a significant portion of the population. During the industrial age a larger proportion of the population was engaged in strenuous physical activity on a daily basis. The "information age" has created a relatively sedentary group of people. Therapeutic exercise—even in the form of casual recreation—can offer a more balanced lifestyle.

> The President's Council on Physical Fitness Program is an example of habilitational therapeutic exercise for schoolchildren. The goal of this program is to increase the physical fitness of schoolchildren to a set level based on age and gender.

Therapeutic Exercise Settings

Therapeutic exercise professionals work in a variety of settings, including inpatient facilities (such as hospitals), outpatient clinics, athletic training rooms, and even clients' homes. Some are employed by others, and some are in their own private practice. While the decision to pursue a given profession in the sphere of therapeutic exercise may dictate the setting in which you work, this does not mean that you won't have opportunities to work with professionals from a wide range of work settings. Most health-care facilities employ the team approach in which representatives from several different professions collaborate in the planning and delivery of patient care.

In what type of setting would you like to work? If you are considering a career in therapeutic exercise, would you like to work in a hospital or nursing home; an outpatient clinic; for a high school, university, or professional sport team, perhaps in an athletic training room; or in your own private practice? Read on to learn more about these settings.

Inpatient Facilities

Rehabilitation hospitals provide specialized care that strives to return patients to their maximum level of function. Patients with severe conditions such as brain or spinal cord trauma, or those recuperating from severe disease, may require a long-term stay in a rehabilitation facility. Custodial care facilities such as nursing homes provide services to assist patients in the activities of daily living, as well as to meet patients' specific medical needs. In both types of inpatient facilities, the level of patient disability usually dictates the degree of coordinated effort that must be arranged among physicians, rehabilitation specialists, and social services personnel.

In addition to the skills described in this chapter, therapeutic exercise professionals who work at inpatient facilities often must also have knowledge of ambulation and patient transfer techniques, prevention of bedsores, and other skills unique to long-term care.

Outpatient Facilities

Outpatient facilities are characterized by relatively short-term patient visits (patients do not stay overnight). These types of facilities comprise the most diverse setting for therapeutic exercise

professionals and include physical therapy clinics, sports medicine facilities, and cardiac rehabilitation facilities. Outpatient facilities can have a wide range of specialized equipment to meet the needs of their clientele. The more diverse the range of patients being treated, the broader the range of equipment. Most outpatient clinics consist of examination areas, specialized treatment and rehabilitation areas, hydrotherapy pools, and open-space exercise areas. Some outpatient clinics are very specialized and accept only patients suffering from cardiovascular disease, hand injuries, or spinal conditions.

Social, economic, or other factors can often prohibit patients from traveling regularly to an outpatient facility for treatment. As a result, many outpatient clinics send therapists to patients' homes to provide both rehabilitative and habilitative home care.

Sport Team Settings

Athletic training rooms represent a very specific type of outpatient facility. Located exclusively in high schools, colleges, and professional team facilities, the first athletic training facilities were simply a table located in the corner of the men's locker room (which may help to explain the profession's male-dominated history). Although the size and complexity may vary, athletic training facilities at major colleges and universities tend to be state-of-the-art athletic health-care clinics. Facilities typically include treatment and rehabilitation areas, examination rooms, whirlpool areas, and space dedicated to pre-event preparation such as taping, wrapping, and bracing. Most professional sport training facilities, and many of those in colleges and universities, even have X-ray rooms and space where minor surgical procedures can be performed.

Many sport team settings also offer weight rooms, cardiovascular fitness centers, swimming pools, and exercise physiology laboratories. These types of facilities expand the scope and breadth of therapeutic exercise programs that can be offered to habilitate and rehabilitate athletes.

Private Practice

The thought of being one's own boss is intriguing to many people. Private practice is an entrepreneurial venture in which the professional

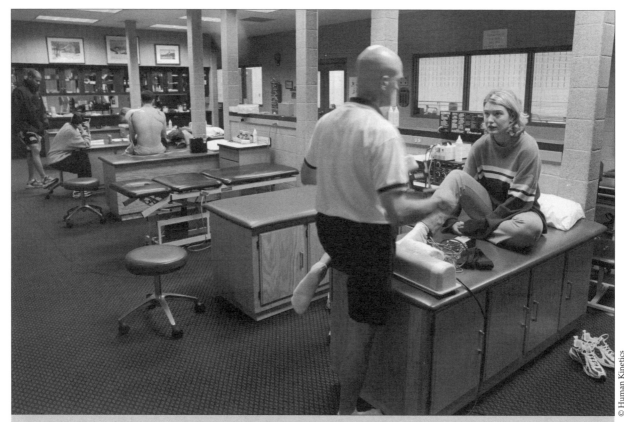

© Human Kinetics

Evolving from caged-in corners of a locker room, contemporary athletic training rooms are often state-of-the-art athletic health-care facilities.

establishes his or her own place of work. Physical and occupational therapy are capital-intensive professions requiring expensive equipment, so a business loan, personal wealth, or investors are required for start-up costs. Other expenses such as rent, utilities, and support staff must also be considered prior to venturing into private practice.

Most professionals do not begin their careers in their own practice; the transition into private practice is usually made following employment in an established clinical practice. By working first in an established practice, beginning professionals can learn about the nuances of the business world and also build up a patient base and reputation.

Before venturing into private practice, beginning therapeutic exercise professionals should first gain work experience, amass capital, and establish a strong patient base.

Up-Close Views of Professions in Therapeutic Exercise

Because of their background in the anatomical and physical principles of human movement, kinesiology students are well positioned to enter many health-care professions that use therapeutic exercise as a part of their habilitational or rehabilitational treatment regimes, including athletic training, cardiac rehabilitation, occupational therapy, physical therapy, and strength and conditioning. This section describes these professions, the settings in which they take place, and the educational requirements and credentials needed to practice in them.

You will notice that the competencies of the professions discussed here often overlap. Indeed, many people pursue multiple credentials such as athletic training and physical therapy certification, or physical therapy and strength and con-

Identify the Population You Like to Work With

People exploring a career in therapeutic exercise often first identify the population with whom they wish to work. Take a moment to think about the population you would prefer to work with. Put a check mark by the groups in the following list that seem appealing to you.

___ Infants   ___ Injured   ___ Healthy
___ Children   ___ Disabled   ___ Recovering
___ Adults   ___ Athletes   ___ Requiring long-term care
___ Senior citizens ___ Nonathletes   ___ Other: _____

ditioning certification. As the competition for the health-care dollar increases, and with the health-care job market tightening, the need for multiskilled and multicredentialed individuals will increase in the future.

The educational requirements of these professions vary depending on their focus, but most still have the common traits of a strong science base and an active clinical education component. Course work in theoretical kinesiology (section 2 of this text) will be extremely valuable, and other specialized courses and clinical practicums will round out your professional knowledge. To combat the trend toward overspecialization, the Pew Health Professions Commission (1995) has recommended that all health-care professions, including those involved in therapeutic exercise, possess a common set of competencies by 2005 (table 15.1). As this table indicates, your background in kinesiology will provide you with a well-rounded education including many of the skills that will be expected of tomorrow's health-care professional.

Differing levels of preparation and regulation are found among therapeutic exercise professions. Health-care professionals must pay close attention to state licensure requirements, especially when changing location. Table 15.2 lists the professions discussed in this chapter and the professional organizations and journals that serve them. These additional resources will allow you to explore the professions in greater detail.

Athletic Trainer

High school, college, and professional athletes are injured at staggering rates, with as many as one-

TABLE 15.1
Pew Commission Competencies for Health-Care Providers

Care for the community's health
Expand access to effective care
Provide clinically competent care
Emphasize primary care
Participate in coordinated care
Ensure cost effective and appropriate care
Practice prevention
Involve patients and families in the decision making process
Promote healthy lifestyles
Assess and use technology appropriately
Improve the health-care system
Manage information
Understand the role of the physical environment
Provide counseling on ethical issues
Accommodate expanded accountability
Participate in a racially and culturally diverse society
Continue to learn

third of the one million high school football players suffering an injury each year (DeLee & Farney, 1992; McCarthy, Hiller, & Yates-McCarthy, 1991). Combining the excitement of athletics with the demands of health care, athletic training falls entirely within the realm of sports medicine. The title *athletic trainer* can be misleading. These professionals are not coaches, personal trainers, or other performance-improving personnel. Athletic training is an allied health-care profession that addresses the prevention, evaluation, management, treatment, and rehabilitation of injuries and other

TABLE 15.2
Professional Organizations

Profession	Professional organization	Professional journals
Athletic training	National Athletic Trainers' Association, Inc. 2952 Stemmons Freeway Dallas, TX 75247-6196 214-637-6282 214-637-2206 fax www.nata.org	*Journal of Athletic Training* *Athletic Therapy Today*
Cardiac rehabilitation specialist	American College of Sports Medicine 401 W. Michigan St. P.O. Box 1440 Indianapolis, IN 46206-1440 317-637-9200 317-634-7817 fax www.acsm.org or American Association of Cardiovascular and Pulmonary Rehabilitation 7611 Elmwood Ave., Suite 201 Middleton, WI 53562 608-831-6989 608-831-5122 fax www.aacvpr.org	*Journal of Cardiopulmonary Rehabilitation* *Journal of Clinical Exercise Physiology*
Occupational therapy	American Occupational Therapy Association, Inc. 4720 Montgomery Ln. Bethesda, MD 20814-3425 301-652-2682 301-652-7711 www.aota.org	*American Journal of Occupational Therapy*
Physical therapy	American Physical Therapy Association, Inc. 1111 N. Fairfax St. Alexandria, VA 22314 703-684-3782 703-684-7343 fax www.apta.org	*Physical Therapy* *Journal of Orthopedic and Sports Physical Therapy*
Strength and conditioning specialist	National Strength and Conditioning Association 1955 Union Blvd. P.O. Box 38909 Colorado Springs, CO 80937 719-632-6722 719-632-6367 fax www.nsca-lift.org	*Strength and Conditioning* *Journal of Strength and Conditioning Research*

conditions suffered by athletes and other physically active individuals. Athletic trainers (ATs) work under the direction of a licensed medical or osteopathic physician. In addition to the direct health care of the athlete, the athletic trainer also coordinates referrals to appropriate specialists.

Employment Settings

Athletic trainers traditionally have been employed by high schools, colleges/universities, and professional sport teams. New roles are emerging for athletic trainers in hospitals, sports

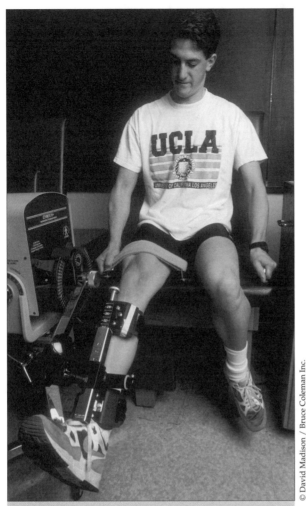

Athletic trainers use therapeutic exercise to return athletes to competition in the shortest amount of time deemed possible.

medicine clinics, industrial rehabilitation clinics, and other allied medical environments. The AT's roles and responsibilities vary depending on the work setting.

Athletic Setting. Athletic trainers are uniquely positioned to implement procedures to prevent or decrease the occurrence of sport injuries. They have the opportunity to work with the same athletes prior to an injury, immediately following the injury, and during the rehabilitation process.

States are gradually beginning to mandate athletic training coverage of high-risk, high school sports (McCarthy, Hiller, & Yates-McCarthy, 1991). Historically, athletic trainers who worked in public high schools were dual credentialed as teachers and athletic trainers. The trend toward hiring full-time athletic trainers is growing, al-

though the majority of high schools that receive the services of athletic trainers do so through contracting services from local physical therapy and sports medicine clinics and hospitals. Colleges and professional teams hire their own full-time athletic trainers.

Clinical Setting. Community recreation leagues, road races, and personal workout regimens have exposed millions of Americans to the possibility of suffering athletic-related injuries. Combine this with the fact that the majority of high school athletes do not receive the direct services of an athletic trainer, and you can understand the increase in the number of sports medicine and physical therapy clinics. The emergence of athletic trainers in these settings has spurred growth in other rehabilitation settings including corporate/industrial clinics, hospitals, and private practice. Athletic trainers' roles in these emerging, nontraditional settings may vary from those of athletic trainers in more traditional settings. These roles may also vary among states (Cormier, York, Domholdt, & Keggeris, 1993).

Athletic training practices entirely within the realm of sports medicine. Athletic trainers are responsible for the prevention, evaluation, management, treatment, and rehabilitation of athletic injuries.

Education and Credentials

Table 15.3 presents a sample of course work that would be expected in a program accredited by the Commission on the Accreditation of Allied Health Education Programs (CAAHEP). This course work is supplemented by clinical education that permits students to have affiliations with high school, college, and professional sport team athletic training rooms as well as the opportunity to learn in clinics and hospitals. The National Athletic Trainers' Association Board of Certification, Inc., (NATABOC) conducts national certification testing of athletic trainers. NATABOC certification is required to work as an athletic trainer in major colleges and universities, professional sport teams, and the U.S. Olympic Committee. Additionally, most states require NATABOC certification as a prerequisite for licensure.

In Profile

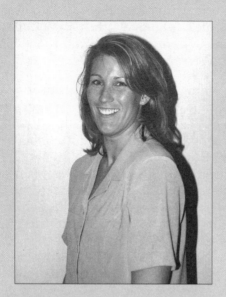

Jodie Humphrey, PT, ATC, CSCS

Sports Medicine Specialist

Jodie Humphrey, PT, ATC, CSCS, is a sports medicine professional. Truth be told, she's several sports medicine professionals. Growing up as an athlete, Jodie became interested in the plight of injured athletes. While she was still in high school, a friend who was also an athlete introduced her to the physical therapy profession. "When I enrolled in college, I learned about athletic training and had the unique opportunity to double major in athletic training and physical therapy," Jodie explains.

Jodie's purpose of majoring in both physical therapy and athletic training was to increase her expertise in the care of injured athletes, further develop her interest in orthopedic physical therapy, and open up employment opportunities. To increase her credentials further, Jodie became a certified strength and conditioning specialist to bolster her knowledge in sports-specific cardiovascular conditioning, weight programs, and even home treatment programs.

Her demanding preparation to enter the fields of physical therapy and athletic training were well rewarded. Jodie is employed at a sports medicine clinic in Massachusetts. During the mornings and early afternoons she works with older athletes and other individuals rehabilitating from orthopedic injuries. In the afternoons and on some weekends and evenings, Jodie provides athletic training services to local high schools and other athletic leagues. She also uses her wealth of knowledge and experience to sponsor workshops for people wanting to learn more about athletic injuries.

"While my classroom and clinical learning gave me the knowledge required to be a competent professional, I found myself not as prepared for other areas," Jodie explains. "Patience and a sense of perspective are needed when dealing with the health-care system, especially the insurance and legal aspects. Treatments must be carefully planned to make the best use of the allotted number of patient visits and to minimize the patient's expenses. Keen communication skills are needed to foster communication between other therapists, athletic trainers, physicians, coaches, and the athlete's family," she says. "You really need excellent time management skills to help keep on track and focused on the tasks at hand."

This sounds like a lot of work and a lot to go through, but, as Jodie says, "the rewards make it all worthwhile." To put all of this effort into perspective, Jodie notes, "The sense of accomplishment that comes across a patient's face, the gratification of someone who is able to live a functional life and be rid of the pain that has nagged them for years are rewards that cannot be measured in terms of professional success or dollars and cents."

Cardiac Rehabilitation Specialist

When supervised by cardiac rehabilitation specialists, exercise is an effective treatment for patients suffering from chronic cardiovascular, pulmonary, and metabolic diseases. Cardiac rehabilitation specialists also implement and deliver cardiovascular conditioning programs for individuals who are apparently disease free.

The American College of Sports Medicine (ACSM) offers two clinical tracks for certified cardiac rehabilitation specialists—that of exercise specialist and that of program director. Exercise testing, such as graded exercise tests, and exer-

| TABLE 15.3 |
| Sample Course Work for Athletic Training |

Acute care	Human physiology
Administration	Injury prevention
Assessment and evaluation of injuries and illnesses	Biomechanics*
	Nutrition
	Pathology
Chemistry	Pharmacology
Counseling	Physics
Exercise physiology	Statistics
Gross anatomy	Therapeutic exercise
Human anatomy	Therapeutic modalities

*Still called kinesiology at some universities.

cise prescription are the responsibility of the exercise specialist, who also provides patient education and counseling. Depending on the specialist's educational background and place of employment, job responsibilities may range from taking vital signs (blood pressure, pulse, temperature, etc.) to performing echocardiograms and electrocardiograms before, during, and after exercise.

The program director is responsible for developing and directing clinical exercise programs and, working in conjunction with a physician, has overall control of the patient's rehabilitation program. In addition to the skills described for the exercise specialist, the program director is responsible for the administration of the rehabilitation center and the education of the cardiac rehabilitation staff, and is often engaged in research.

A hospital might offer an exercise program for patients recovering from heart surgery. The program director and physician, working as a team, will collect the client's medical history and perform an evaluation of cardiopulmonary function. From these data the two will develop a structured exercise program. The exercise specialist will then work with the client in progressing through the exercise program. At regular intervals the program director, physician, and exercise specialist will reevaluate the patient's progress.

Certifications similar to the ACSM's exercise specialist and program director certifications are available to people who want to work in the fitness setting.

Employment Settings

Cardiac rehabilitation specialists are employed in hospitals, specialty clinics, health and fitness centers, and urgent care centers.

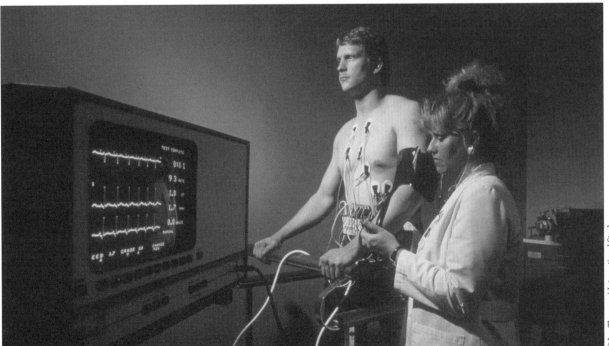

Working under a physician's direction, cardiac rehabilitation specialists design and implement cardiopulmonary programs for a wide range of patients.

© Jay Thomas / International Stock

In Profile

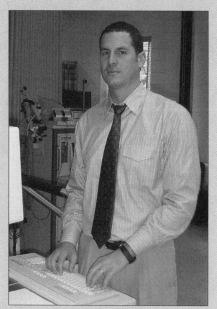

Joe Libonati, PhD

Director, Cardiovascular Center

Treadmills, people, and wires. Take a look around Dr. Joe Libonati's Cardiovascular Institute and these are the first things that you'll notice. Joe describes his laboratory as "an odd mixture of some good, old-fashioned exercise and some of the most state-of-the-art medical equipment." As the facility director, Joe is responsible for the overall administration of the institute's day-to-day operations and serves as the expert in residence to a host of physicians and a staff of cardiovascular rehabilitation specialists. Perhaps most important, Joe is responsible for exercise testing, test interpretation, and developing specific exercise programs for patients suffering from a wide range of diseases. Holding a PhD in exercise physiology, Joe is also a college professor, a researcher, and an active member of the American College of Sports Medicine.

The sequence of events leading up to Joe's entry into cardiac rehabilitation demonstrates that career choices can arise in unusual ways. "As a struggling college basketball player, I began thinking about ways to improve my athletic performance," he explains. "As I explored various exercise programs, I began to develop an interest in the body's cardiovascular system and how cells function to use energy."

After beginning his academic career as an athletic training major, Joe switched his major to exercise physiology. Following his graduation he earned a master's degree in cardiac rehabilitation and a doctorate in exercise physiology, and then he completed a postdoctoral fellowship at Boston University's Whitaker Cardiovascular Institute.

Like many people who enter the health-care professions, Joe's greatest reward is helping others. Still, despite his years of experience and wealth of academic preparation, one aspect of his job still frustrates him. "We work one on one with some patients who are very sick," he says. "Because of the nature of their illnesses, sometimes they don't make it. Losing a patient is like losing a friend, and I still have difficulty handling it." But, thanks to the efforts of Joe Libonati and others like him, many patients have gone on to live healthy, fruitful lives.

Education and Credentials

Table 15.4 presents typical course work required of individuals pursuing a career in cardiac rehabilitation. In addition to courses in these areas, students should also pursue clinical rotations and fieldwork to supplement their learning experiences.

As mentioned, the American College of Sports Medicine offers certification for exercise specialists and program directors. A bachelor's degree is required for certification as an exercise specialist, although a master's degree is preferred. Certification as a program director requires a master's or doctoral degree and several years of experience as a director of a cardiac or pulmonary rehabilitation program.

The American College of Sports Medicine offers certifications for exercise specialists who work in medical settings, such as cardiac rehabilitation specialists, and for similar professions in fitness settings, such as health/fitness instructors.

TABLE 15.4
Sample Course Work for a Cardiac Rehabilitation Specialist

Advanced cardiac life support	Echocardiography
Cardiopulmonary assessment	Electrocardiography
Cardiopulmonary disease	Exercise physiology
Cardiopulmonary physiology	Exercise prescription
Cardiovascular technology	Imaging devices
Clinical biomechanics*	Nutrition
	Pathophysiology
	Pharmacology
	Physics
	Respiratory care

*Still called kinesiology at some universities.

Occupational Therapist

Occupational therapists (OTs) assist people with physical, emotional, or mental disabilities to restore or maintain as much independence in daily living and work throughout their lives (note that the term *occupational* has roots in the word *activity*). Some of the physical care rendered by occupational therapists closely mirrors some of the rehabilitative exercises used by physical therapists. Indeed, in many rehabilitation centers a physical therapist and an occupational therapist work together on a single patient's case.

As with many allied health professions, the roots of occupational therapy can be traced to postwar veteran rehabilitation; pioneers in the profession taught craft skills to soldiers with disabilities (Ambrosi & Barker-Schwartz, 1995). Today, occupational therapists specialize in functional bracing and the modification of everyday items for the special needs of their patients. Functional bracing is the use of a supportive or assistive device that allows a joint to function despite anatomical or biomechanical limitations. Examples include derotational knee braces and wrist and hand splints that allow people to eat with a fork. Occupational specialists also work with patients on improving their concentration, motor skills, and problem-solving ability.

Contemporary occupational therapists may also specialize in task-specific, work-related rehabilitation, helping clients reacquire the motor and cognitive skill required to return to work. This type of activity may range from teaching basic skills such as coordinated movement to very specific skills such as hammering, typing, or driving a car.

To assist people suffering from disabilities, occupational therapists may be called on to evaluate the layout of schools, homes, and workplaces to suggest methods of eliminating functional barriers. Occupational therapists often employ clinical technicians called certified occupational therapy assistants (COTAs) to carry out rehabilitation plans.

Employment Settings

Occupational therapists and occupational therapy assistants work in hospitals, rehabilitation centers, nursing homes, and orthopedic clinics, and provide outpatient occupational therapy service in public and private secondary schools and colleges.

Education and Credentials

Occupational therapists are educated through professional four-year undergraduate programs or in entry-level master's degree programs. Successful completion of a two-year technical program is required for certification and/or licensure as an occupational therapy assistant (see table 15.5). Many states require that occupational therapists and occupational therapy assistants be

TABLE 15.5
Sample Course Work for Occupational Therapy

Occupational therapist	Occupational therapy assistant
Abnormal psychology	Human anatomy
Assistive technology	Human development
Biology	Human physiology
Gross anatomy	Biomechanics*
Human anatomy	Neurology
Human performance abilities	Occupational therapy procedures
Human physiology	Organization and administration
Biomechanics*	Psychology
Neuroanatomy	Psychosocial dysfunction
Occupational analysis	
Physical dysfunction	
Psychology	
Statistics	

*Still called kinesiology at some universities.

licensed. The basic requirement for licensure is completion of an accredited program and passing the American Occupational Therapy Certification Board examination.

🔑 Occupational therapists help injured or ill individuals reach their maximum level of independence by emphasizing the acquisition and retention of daily living skills.

Physical Therapist

Physical therapists (PTs) are educated to provide rehabilitative care to a diverse patient population with a wide range of injuries, illnesses, and diseases. A physical therapist may be called on to treat patients ranging from infants to seniors with conditions such as joint injury, burns, cardiorespiratory disease, neurological deficits, or other diseases.

Physical therapists combine diagnostic tests with therapeutic exercise; therapeutic modalities

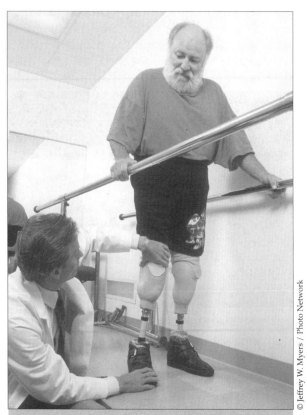

Physical therapists may practice rehabilitational or habilitational therapeutic exercise.

© Jeffrey W. Myers / Photo Network

such as ice, heat, and electrical stimulation; and manual techniques such as joint mobilization to rehabilitate or habilitate their clients. The therapy used depends on the condition being treated. Therapy for orthopedic injuries relies heavily on resistance training and proprioception activities (activities that improve knowledge of position, weight, and resistance of objects in relation to the body), while therapy designed to treat patients with disease states and neurological conditions tends to emphasize cardiovascular aspects and neuromuscular control. Entry-level education prepares students to enter the workforce as generalists, but once a person begins to practice professionally, the tendency is to begin to specialize in one of the seven areas outlined in table 15.6.

Changes in the health-care system, such as managed care and the limitation of reimbursement, have influenced the practice of physical therapy. More and more of the responsibility for patient treatment (the use of therapeutic modalities and therapeutic exercise) is being transitioned to the physical therapist assistant (PTA), while the PT performs patient evaluations and assumes a broader administrative role.

🔑 Physical therapists administer the patient's program and perform the required functional evaluations. Physical therapist assistants assume much of the hands-on patient care, functioning under physical therapists' supervision.

Education and Credentials

The wide range of potential patients and the broad scope of conditions that physical therapists treat require a vigorous and demanding academic program. For many years entry-level preparation occurred at the undergraduate level, but the physical therapy profession is increasingly emphasizing professional preparation at the master's degree level. The academic program also includes clinical affiliations that expose the student to several work settings and patient types (see table 15.7). Physical therapy programs are accredited by the Commission on Accreditation in Physical Therapy Education (CAPTE).

The American Physical Therapy Association (APTA) is the national professional organization for physical therapists. Although not specifically

TABLE 15.6
Physical Therapy Specialty Certifications

Specialty	Description
Cardiopulmonary	Treatment of patients having acute or chronic diseases of the cardiovascular and/or respiratory systems.
Clinical electrophysiology	Measurement of normal and abnormal electrical activity within the human body.
Geriatrics	Conditions related to aging or other problems associated with older members of the population.
Neurology	Treatment of patients suffering from injuries or diseases of the brain and nervous system.
Orthopedics	Treatment of patients suffering from injuries or diseases of the muscles, bones, and joints.
Pediatrics	Treatment of children in health and disease during development from birth through adolescence.
Sports physical therapy	Treatment of an athletic population, normally suffering from injuries as the result of competition.

TABLE 15.7
Sample Course Work for Physical Therapy

Physical therapist (entry-level master's degree)

Undergraduate (recommended prerequisite courses)	*Master's degree (two-year program)*
Biology	Cardiopulmonary evaluation and treatment
Chemistry	Clinical medicine
Exercise physiology	Gross anatomy
Human anatomy	Musculoskeletal evaluation and treatment
Human physiology	Neuroanatomy
Biomechanics*	Neurological evaluation and treatment
Medical ethics	Pediatric evaluation and treatment
Pathology/pathophysiology	Pediatric neurology
Physics	Pharmacology
Psychology	Psychological/social aspects of disability
Statistics/research design	Therapeutic modalities

Physical therapist assistant (two-year associate's degree)

Clinical practice	Physical therapy procedures
Human growth and development	Therapeutic exercise
Biomechanics*	Therapeutic modalities
Physical disabilities	

*Still called kinesiology at some universities.

required, the APTA does offer certification for each specialty area. Licensed professionals may also seek advanced education in physical therapy at the master's and doctoral degree level. Physical therapists who specialize in sports medicine have a strong orthopedic interest and may choose to pursue specialty certification in orthopedic and/or sport physical therapy.

Becoming a physical therapist assistant involves successful completion of a two-year associate's degree program accredited by CAPTE, the same organization that accredits physical therapy programs. Many, but not all, states require licensure for the PTA to practice. Regardless of whether they are licensed, physical therapy assistants work under the supervision of a PT to carry out the prescribed protocol. The physical therapist must perform regular reevaluations of patients under the care of a physical therapist assistant.

Licensure of physical therapists and PTAs is contingent on the successful completion of the appropriate program (i.e., PT or PTA) and passing the state examination. Historically, the physical therapist's patients were required to have a referral from a physician and physician oversight. Many states now permit direct physical therapy access, thus eliminating the need for a referral. However, a referral or physician consultation is often required for insurance reimbursement.

Physical therapists are educated as generalists, but tend to develop specialties while in the workforce.

Strength and Conditioning Specialists

Proper strength and conditioning is needed to obtain maximum physical performance, reduce the frequency of injury, and decrease the possibility of cardiovascular disease. Strength coaches design weight training programs and cardiovascular conditioning programs based on the demands inherent to specific sports and the specific needs of individual athletes. Strength and conditioning specialists may develop individualized programs in conjunction with athletic trainers, physical therapists, or physicians for athletes who have been identified as having a specific deficit or who have completed their rehabilitation program.

Certification as a strength and conditioning specialist is often combined with other professional credentials such as athletic training, exercise physiology, physical therapy, and general medicine.

Employment Settings

Strength and conditioning specialists are employed by university athletic departments, professional sport teams, health clubs, and corporate fitness centers. Likewise, a growing number of high schools are recognizing the value of having strength and conditioning specialists on staff. Individuals who have other certifications, licenses, or other areas of specialization can often implement strength and conditioning principles into their current workplaces.

Education and Credentials

Credentialing of strength and conditioning specialists is not associated with a degree program, but a bachelor's degree—and current CPR certification—is required to take the examination sponsored by the National Strength and Conditioning Association (NSCA). A degree in kinesiology is preferred. To receive certification, candidates must successfully complete a two-part examination. Passing both sections designates the person as a certified strength and conditioning specialist (CSCS).

Credentialed professionals who become certified as strength and conditioning specialists can compete more strongly in the job market and increase their salaries. Most National Strength and Conditioning Association members hold a degree beyond the level of a bachelor's degree.

Individuals interested in becoming a strength coach for a collegiate or professional team should also possess a bachelor's degree in a related field such as exercise physiology or kinesiology. Certification as a teacher would enhance the possibility of being hired as a high school strength coach. A graduate assistant position or internship position as a strength and conditioning coach also improves a person's marketability.

Do you prefer to figure out solutions on your own or would you rather be given a structured sequence of steps to follow? Clinicians devise and develop therapeutic exercise plans and are therefore called on to solve problems and make decisions. Technicians, on the other hand, are experts at performing specific sets of skills. Clinical professions include athletic training, physical therapy, occupational therapy, and higher levels of cardiac rehabilitation. Technical professions include physical therapist assistants and occupational therapist assistants.

A teaching degree is useful in gaining employment as a high school strength coach; college athletic departments often look for candidates who have a degree in kinesiology or a related field.

Inside Advice for Therapeutic Exercise Students

You should understand by now the importance of having keen knowledge of human anatomy, human physiology, and biomechanics, and of knowing the effects of exercise on healthy and unhealthy individuals, when working in the sphere of therapeutic exercise. These areas, however, represent only a partial list of the skills and knowledge required to practice in this area.

Exercise is only therapeutic when it is performed in a safe and appropriate manner. Developing and delivering appropriate therapeutic exercise routines necessitates the ability to problem-solve, to collect information regarding the patient's or client's condition, to identify the therapeutic goals, and to determine the appropriate course of action. In order to solve problems effectively, therapeutic exercise professionals must be able to access, manage, and interpret various forms of information and apply them to the current case. This often requires the use of computers and an understanding of how to access Internet sites and perform literature searches.

Although it is often taken for granted, healthcare professionals also must possess effective communication skills in order to communicate effectively across demographic, sociocultural, and professional boundaries.

Certain settings or roles will require additional areas of knowledge. For instance, professionals who work in fee-for-service environments will need to become familiar with record-keeping and insurance billing systems. A business background would be useful for practitioners in private practice, and in any type of leadership position it would be helpful to have course work dealing with management and administration.

So how does one choose an area in which to work? While reading about these occupations can

If you are interested in entering a therapeutic exercise profession, you will want to work toward a degree in kinesiology as well as become certified in a particular area. What other skills do you need to learn? Do you have good problem-solving and communication skills? Will you enjoy the business sides to these professions—billing, record-keeping, and so on? In what ways can you test the waters of these professions to see if they are for you?

provide you with an overview of this group of professions, the only way to discover what a profession is really like is to see professionals at work. Many professionals allow students to "shadow" them throughout the course of a day. Perhaps a professor or other acquaintance can help you make this connection. You may also have an opportunity to do an internship or an apprenticeship, or find a part-time or summer job in one of these areas.

Earlier in this text we discussed ethical professional conduct; its importance must be reiterated here. Therapeutic exercise professionals must adhere to basic ethical and professional principles that are often reinforced through state laws and certification guidelines. Although the particulars will vary from profession to profession and from state to state, some themes are common across the professions. First and foremost, practitioners must protect patients from harm and maintain the confidentiality of medical records. Likewise, practitioners must adhere to the profession's scope of practice—the legal parameters that define the profession. Although your instructors and supervisors will identify these issues for you, ultimately it is your responsibility to seek out this information and assure that you remain in compliance. Failure to do so could result in criminal liability.

Wrap-Up

Professions arise to fulfill a societal void. The therapeutic exercise professions fill a void by either assisting people in obtaining their desired level of physical fitness (habilitation) or helping injured individuals regain lost function (rehabilitation). Part of the attractiveness of this sphere of professional practice is the wide range of the population that is served. Highly honed athletes, newborn infants, and the geriatric population may all rely on therapeutic exercise specialists.

Almost as diverse as the population being treated are the settings in which therapeutic exercise professionals are employed. From the structured environments of hospitals and laboratories to the hectic pace of an athletic training room, the therapeutic exercise professions offer work settings that appeal to a wide range of interests. This chapter covered some of the more prominent therapeutic exercise professions such as athletic training, cardiac rehabilitation, occupational therapy, and physical therapy. If you are interested in any of these professions, we encourage you to seek more information from your professors and to explore this area in greater depth.

Study Questions

1. Describe how therapeutic exercise is used to promote healthy lifestyles.

2. Discuss the similarities and differences between habilitation and rehabilitation.

3. Identify the common overlaps among the therapeutic exercise professions described in this chapter. Does any profession make unique use of these common skills?

4. What skills and/or attributes are unique to the professions presented in this chapter?

5. Identify courses that are common among the professions presented in this chapter.

6. People obtain multiple credentials and/or specializations to make themselves more marketable. Describe some possibilities for dual credentials and preparation for more than one occupation based on the descriptions of professions in this chapter. What benefit would dual credentials and preparing for more than one occupation provide? Are there other professions that are not described in this chapter that would also lend themselves to dual credentials?

16

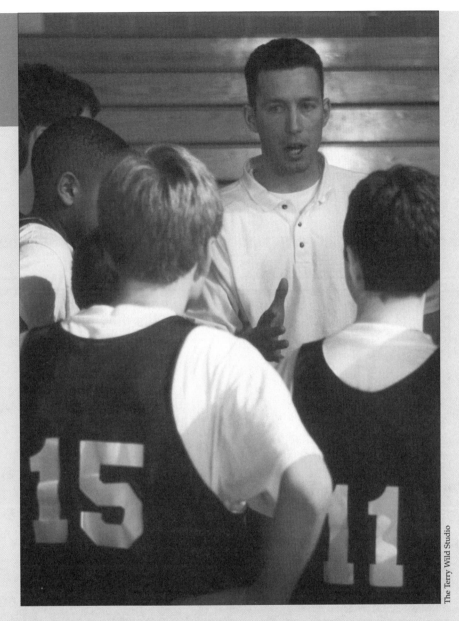

The Terry Wild Studio

Teaching and Coaching Professions

James Kallusky and Lavon Williams

In this chapter . . .

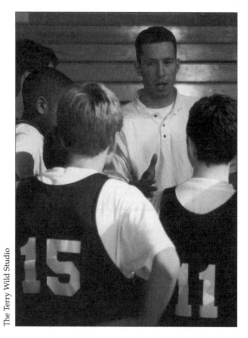

The Terry Wild Studio

A high school physical education teacher calls a meeting of all the physical education teachers in her department to discuss their budget. She will attempt to get approval to purchase some new equipment so that she can teach floor hockey.

A university volleyball coach recently had 21 talented players try out for the volleyball team. Nine of those players will have to be cut before the official roster is finalized.

The director of a Boys and Girls Club, Mr. Torres, is currently seeking assistants to help him develop an after-school physical activity program for kids at his local Boys and Girls Club. He is hoping to teach beginning swimming to 30 kids from the neighborhood.

A third-grade student displays signs of being both physically and mentally abused. Her physical education teacher is faced with reporting the girl's case to Child Protective Services.

A professional coach is afraid she may be fired because her team has not performed well recently. She knows that her team can gain the winning edge if she explains certain tactics for cheating to the players.

The preceding scenarios represent situations that challenge teachers and coaches on a regular basis. In some cases, such as that of the third-grade girl, the decision a teacher or coach makes can affect another's life deeply. Most teaching and coaching decisions, however, have far less momentous repercussions. Nevertheless, both of these professions are essentially about people,

which may be one reason many people are drawn to them.

This chapter will focus on the professions of public school teachers and coaches, community teachers and coaches, college instructors, university professors, university coaches, teaching professionals, and professional sport coaches. These professions are included in the instruction sphere of the physical activity professions shown in figure 16.1.

All the professions in the instruction sphere are concerned with developing and maintaining a certain level of fitness and motor skill performance for participants in activity settings. The participants served by those in the teaching and coaching professions vary tremendously, ranging from young children to university students and athletes to professional sport figures. Likewise, these professions take place in many different settings. Whereas a director for corporate health fitness may be confined primarily to the corporation's fitness facility, teachers and coaches may choose from a multitude of settings in which to carry out their work, including public and alternative schools, community agencies and organizations, colleges and universities, and professional sport teams.

CHAPTER OBJECTIVES

In this chapter we will:

▮ Acquaint you with the wide range of professional opportunities in the sphere of instruction

▮ Familiarize you with the purpose and types of work done by professionals in teaching and coaching

▮ Inform you about the educational requirements and experiences necessary to become an active, competent professional in teaching or coaching

▮ Help you identify whether one of these professions fits your skills, aptitudes, and professional desires

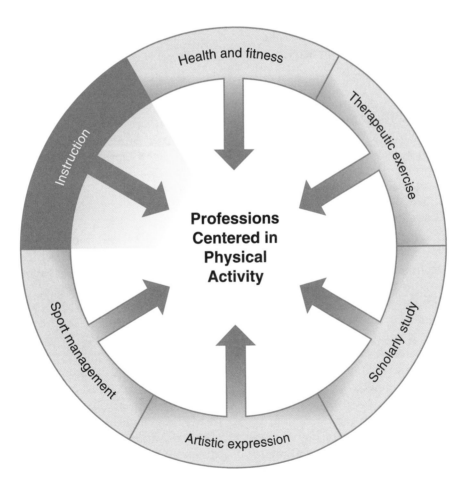

Figure 16.1   Instruction is one of the spheres of professional practice centered in physical activity.

The World of Teaching and Coaching

Teaching and coaching may be the two professions with the longest traditions in the field of physical activity. The earliest physical education teachers were specialists in training, or physical culture, as it was called. They focused on improving the health and vitality of students and other clients through various types of exercise. About the same time that teaching became established in physical education, the profession of coaching took root in colleges and in the professional ranks. Today, more than a century after their appearance, the professions of teaching and coaching continue to be two of the most popular careers sought by students entering the physical activity field.

If someone were to ask you, "Is teaching the same as coaching? Are all teachers coaches? Are all coaches teachers?" how would you respond? Teaching and coaching are similar in many ways. Both are performed by professionals who have mastered knowledge about a specific activity and the skills and techniques required for efficiently transmitting that knowledge to other people. Both require expertise in designing practice experiences to bring about learning, and conditioning experiences to enhance performance. These two types of physical activity experiences were addressed in chapter 3.

But teaching and coaching also differ in some significant ways. Teachers' efforts are usually directed toward those lacking a high level of proficiency, such as high school or college students enrolled in a beginning badminton course, middle-aged women enrolled in a beginning swimming class at the local community pool, or individuals of all ages who want to improve their golf swing by consulting a teaching professional at the local driving range. Coaches, on the other hand, typically direct their professional services toward a relatively elite population. School sport teams are commonly populated by students with above average proficiency for their age; college teams tend to be populated by an even more select group culled from the best of high school teams. And of course, professional teams are an even more highly skilled group. Still, both coaches and teachers are heavily involved in teaching, and sometimes the two terms are used interchangeably, for example, when we say someone is coaching a student to take the SAT or when we describe a coach as an excellent teacher.

So how *do* we answer the question of what distinguishes teaching and coaching? A good way to address the question is to distinguish between the *acts* of teaching and coaching and the *professions* of teaching and coaching. The acts of teaching and coaching both may be defined as attempts to alter the thinking, feelings, or behavior of a particular clientele by systematically exposing them to practice and conditioning experiences (covered in chapter 3), along with appropriate verbal and visual experiences, to bring about predetermined outcomes.

Teaching and coaching both involve instruction; in fact, the dictionary definition for coaching is very close to that of teaching. Both the gymnastics teacher and the gymnastics coach try to impart knowledge of certain routines to students/athletes, to instill in them a love of the activity, and to bring about improvements in their performances. This comes through practice and conditioning, as well as through explanations, instructions, and verbal feedback, as well as visual feedback in video replays and demonstrations.

Obviously, teaching and coaching may occur in a variety of informal contexts such as when parents attempt to teach their children how to catch a ball, or an experienced bowler teaches a friend how to approach and release the ball. As discussed in chapter 13, informal efforts by nonexperts are not examples of professional work, and for this reason they are not described in this chapter.

Figure 16.2 shows the considerable overlap in the acts of teaching and coaching. The areas not overlapping represent the clientele served. Teaching tends to be directed toward populations who lack the knowledge, attitudes, or skills required, or have forgotten or misapplied them. Although performers at all levels may be learning constantly, teaching is most often directed toward naive or inexperienced populations.

Coaching, on the other hand, is usually directed toward select or elite populations who already have acquired some degree of skill, knowledge, and attitudes essential for performance but do not display them consistently at the required level. Because of this, coaches tend to direct much of their efforts toward enhancing performance (chapter 8) rather than learning basic skills.

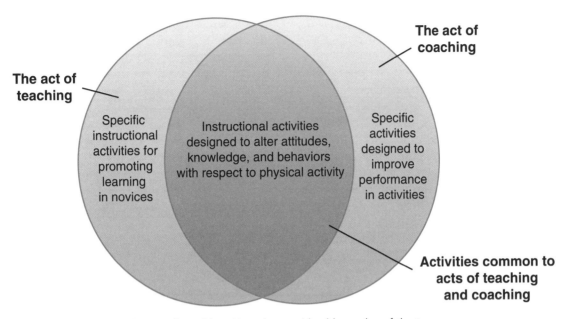

The act of
teaching

The act of
coaching

Specific
instructional
activities for
promoting
learning
in novices

Instructional activities
designed to alter attitudes,
knowledge, and behaviors
with respect to physical activity

Specific
activities
designed to
improve
performance
in activities

Activities common to
acts of teaching
and coaching

Figure 16.2   The acts of teaching and coaching. Note the considerable overlap of the two.

Thus, whereas the activities of coaching may involve a disproportionate amount of time motivating and conditioning athletes and refining and retaining acquired skills, the activities of teaching are likely to focus on the acquisition of new skills and learning how to apply them in real-life settings. The more young and inexperienced the students/athletes, the more the act of coaching becomes like teaching. And the more experienced or elite the performers, the more coaching takes on its own characteristics.

The acts of teaching and coaching are more similar than distinct, but the professions of teaching and coaching are more distinct than similar.

While considerable overlap exists between the *acts* of teaching and coaching, the same is not true between the *professions* of teaching and coaching. Teachers and coaches carry out their professional responsibilities in different occupational subcultures. These subcultures differ in many respects, but one important way is in the range and multitude of nonteaching and noncoaching duties.

Figure 16.3 shows the differences and similarities in the teaching and coaching professions. As you can see, the degree of overlap of the professions is considerably less than that of the acts of

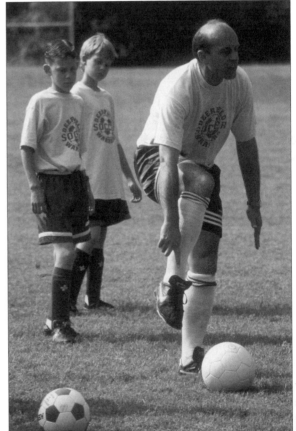

© Kim Karpeles

The more young and inexperienced the athletes, the more the act of coaching becomes like teaching.

teaching and coaching shown in figure 16.2. Whereas teachers devote the majority of their time to disseminating knowledge and molding attitudes and behaviors (teaching), coaches spend *proportionately* less time on these tasks.

Because coaches are key figures in sports, and because their success is measured in terms of the competitive outcomes of games, their attention is divided across many different tasks; teaching is only one of many. You could say that the coaching profession often does not permit much time for "coaching" (that is, teaching). Many coaches recruit, plan budgets, evaluate prospective talent, scout, schedule games, prepare for team travel, develop relationships with the media, purchase equipment, prepare facilities, and so on. Because the term *coaching* incorporates all of these "noncoaching" duties, the profession presumes a much broader array of responsibilities than simply teaching.

The answer to the question posed earlier, then, is yes, the act of teaching is essentially the same as the act of coaching. In this very narrow sense, all teachers are coaches and all coaches are teachers. But when we consider the professional responsibilities of the two roles, we see that they are really quite different. Even in cases in which people hold both roles in the same job, such as

when school physical education teachers also coach, the demands of the two roles are sufficiently distinct. So, while we recognize similarities in many of the professional responsibilities of coaches and teachers, we also need to keep in mind that each operates in distinctly different occupational subcultures, and each requires a relatively unique set of professional knowledge and skills.

Teaching and Coaching Settings

Teaching and coaching are well-established professions focusing on teaching motor skills and fitness training. Just as there are both similarities and differences in the professions of teaching and coaching, so there are similarities and differences in the worksites of these professions. Both teachers and coaches can be found in four primary work sites: community settings, K–12 schools, colleges and universities, and elite sport settings (see table 16.1). In this section we will describe briefly these worksites for both teachers and coaches, highlighting the diversity between settings and within each setting.

Teaching profession

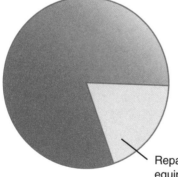

Facility preparation, scheduling and planning trips, recruiting players, scouting, reviewing game films, developing team strategy, budgeting, administration, media relations, hiring, evaluating officials and prospective talent, motivating and counseling players

Coaching profession

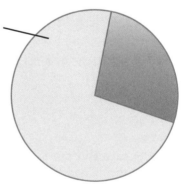

Repairing and maintaining equipment, miscellaneous institutional demands, instructional organization, assigning grades, keeping class records, advertising classes

Shaded area represents proportion of time devoted to planning, implementing, and evaluating instructional strategies for altering knowledge, attitudes, and behavior of clientele = Teaching

Figure 16.3   Differences and similarities in the teaching and coaching professions.

As previously mentioned, worksites for teachers and coaches vary tremendously. Take a few minutes to think of all of the places where you think the professions of teaching and coaching can occur.

Community Settings

Community organizations offer a variety of settings for the teacher or coach. Most of these positions are filled by volunteers, though some youth sport leagues often hire part-time coaches. Parks and recreation departments organize activities such as physical activity classes, athletic leagues, and social groups for both youth and adult leagues. Other organizations such as the YMCA, the YWCA, and the American Youth Soccer Association provide these types of opportunities primarily to children and adolescents.

Community organizations look to improve the social, physical, and moral development of the local community through physical activity including sport, exercise, and fitness activities. They rely on membership dues and private and public contributions in the form of business sponsorships of athletic teams in order to hire instructors and administrative staff to coordinate their programs. Instructors can be found in pool areas teaching swimming classes, in gymnasiums or weight rooms facilitating adult group exercise programs, in testing rooms conducting stress tests and fitness evaluations, and in conference rooms engaging in health/nutrition consulting.

Typical worksites for coaches of sport teams are on-site gymnasiums (for basketball or volley-

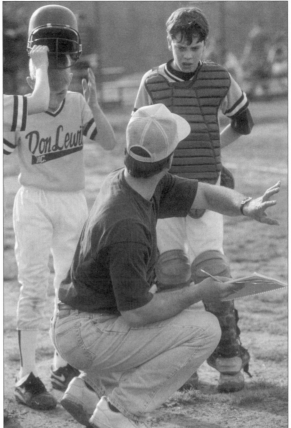

The majority of educational leaders involved in community organizations work with children and adolescents.

The Terry Wild Studio

ball); skating rinks (for ice hockey); soccer, football, softball, or baseball fields; and tracks. Generally, games are played on the organization's property, whereas it is the responsibility of the coach to find a gymnasium or field in which to practice.

TABLE 16.1			
Sites for Teaching Physical Activity and Coaching Sport			
Community	K–12 schools	Colleges and universities	Elite sport setting
• YMCA/YWCA • Boys and Girls Clubs • National Youth Sports Program • Numerous nonprofits	• Elementary schools • Junior high/middle schools • Senior high schools • Alternative schools	• Community colleges • Colleges/universities	• National/Olympic facilities • Private/public sport clubs • Professional sport arenas

K–12 School Settings

Traditionally, schools are divided into elementary, junior high, and high school. Elementary schools usually consist of kindergarten (K) and first through sixth grade, junior high usually consists of seventh through ninth grade, and high school is usually composed of tenth through twelfth grade. Instead of using the junior high school, some school districts are structured with a middle school. Under this structure, elementary schools are composed of kindergarten through fifth grade, middle schools consist of sixth through eighth grade, and high schools are composed of ninth through twelfth grade. Because of their similar structure, the term *secondary schools* are given to middle/junior high and high schools. In this section we will discuss the worksites of elementary and secondary schools.

Elementary school teachers are relatively autonomous in their work. Although teachers spend some of their day keeping the principal informed of important developments, talking with parents, and coordinating activities with other school faculty, they spend most of their time with their students. Elementary school teachers are the only K–12 teachers who spend the entire teaching day with one group of students teaching a variety of subject matters ranging from language arts to math to physical education.

Physical education at the elementary level may be the most important physical education experience students have in the public schools. A poor experience at this level can deter children's motor development or fitness and make it more difficult for them at middle and high school levels. In the early grades (K–3) the emphasis tends to be on developing fundamental motor skills and concepts such as body and spatial awareness. In the later elementary grades sports are introduced and more specialized physical activity forms are taught. Although some schools rely entirely on the classroom teacher to provide instruction in physical education, most hire elementary physical education specialists who provide instruction at least once per week. In addition, the elementary physical education teacher may serve as a resource person for the classroom teacher in physical education lessons. Teaching at the elementary level is often more rewarding than teaching at higher levels because students at this level tend to have a genuine love of physical activity and are interested in learning. The motivational problems that often plague teachers at the middle and high school levels are not normally experienced at the elementary level.

Building on the motor skills foundation students acquired at the elementary school level is one of the primary goals of the middle/junior high school physical education teacher. A primary goal of the high school physical education teacher is to build on the foundation established at the middle/junior high school level. In both cases these goals are accomplished through classroom education and school sports. The halls of secondary schools are much busier than elementary schools as students move from classroom to classroom and teacher to teacher learning a variety of subjects, one of which is physical education. Secondary physical education teachers can be found in the school gymnasium or outside on the playing field teaching individual/dual sports (e.g., tennis, gymnastics, archery), team sports (e.g., basketball, volleyball, soccer), and fitness activities (e.g., running, jogging, aerobics, weight training).

Sport teams are available at secondary schools for students interested in learning more about a specific sport and playing at a more competitive level. Traditionally, coaches also teach in the school; however, more and more states are hiring part-time coaches who are not state-certified teachers. Like physical education teachers, coaches can be found in the gymnasium or on the playing fields. Some high schools have their own stadiums.

Generally, high schools have more and higher-quality equipment for teaching and coaching than middle and junior high schools. Larger schools typically have more resources and more complex organizational structures. Although the organizational structure of physical education and sports varies from school to school, teachers generally report to a department chairperson who reports directly to the principal. With regard to their coaching duties, the same teachers, and, of course coaches, may report to an athletic director who coordinates all of the sports within a school. The athletic director reports to both the principal of the school and the athletic director of the entire school district.

One of the primary differences between the elementary and secondary school worksites involves the role of sports. Secondary schools usually have coaches; elementary schools do not.

College and University Settings

Colleges and universities are much less structured than secondary schools. As you will see in the next section, "Up-Close Views of Professions in Teaching and Coaching," less structure does not necessarily mean less work. It simply means that college teachers and coaches have greater flexibility in their schedules than do K–12 teachers and coaches.

Different types of work settings are associated with teaching and coaching at the college level. In general, colleges include two-year community or junior colleges, four-year colleges, and universities. Community colleges are more distinct from four-year colleges than four-year colleges are from universities. We will therefore examine the work setting of community colleges and then discuss colleges and universities.

Physical education teachers and sport coaches at community colleges usually coach one sport and also teach. Teaching and coaching takes place in the same facility, which generally consists of a complex of offices, gymnasiums, weight rooms, swimming pools, and an athletic training room. As with all colleges and universities, these facilities are built to accommodate spectators. Not surprisingly, the larger the school and the more emphasis the school places on sport, the larger and more well equipped the facility will be.

The worksite of some small four-year colleges is similar to that of community colleges. For the most part, however, four-year colleges are more similar to universities. Most four-year colleges and universities offer general physical activity classes and almost all sponsor sports programs. Over 600 offer degrees in physical education, kinesiology, or exercise and sport science. Because of the variety of their offerings, four-year colleges and universities hire a broader spectrum of physical activity professionals, including physical activity instructors, professors of physical education, and coaches. Unlike community colleges, four-year colleges and universities usually have separate physical education and athletic departments.

Physical activity instructors and physical education professors are housed in an academic building. This teaching facility consists of classrooms, gymnasiums, swimming pools, and office space. Playing fields are usually nearby. Kinesiology theory classes such as sport and exercise psychology, exercise physiology, biomechanics, and sport management are taught in the classroom, while the gymnasiums and fields are used for classes in physical activities and teaching methods. The administrative structure of physical education departments is similar to, but more complex than, that of secondary schools. Faculty members work within a department that is housed in a college or school that is part of a larger university. The chain of command is as follows: faculty member, department chair, college dean, university provost or vice president, and university president.

Coaches in four-year colleges and universities work in an athletic facility consisting of office space, gymnasiums and weight rooms, swimming pools, and an athletic training room. Schools offering football commonly have a separate stadium. Coaches and athletic administrators (e.g., athletic directors and their assistants) are not the only ones who have offices in the athletic facility. Compliance officers, sport marketers and promotion personnel, public relations officers, facility directors, and event directors typically have offices there as well. Although the structure of university athletic departments varies, all athletic faculty report to an athletic director, who often reports directly to the president of the university.

🔑 At community colleges and some smaller four-year colleges, physical activity personnel teach as well as coach. The roles of teacher and coach are separate at larger four-year colleges and universities, resulting in two separate worksites.

The Elite Sport Setting

Coaches and teaching professionals who work with elite athletes probably have the most diverse worksites of all teaching and coaching professionals. Some teachers and coaches work at one stable worksite, while others may teach and coach at a variety of facilities. Still others, such as itinerant golf or tennis teachers, may work out of their homes or the backs of their cars. Of those working in this setting, the worksites of coaches of professional sport teams in football, baseball, softball, hockey, and basketball are the most stable. Generally, these individuals work at a permanent facility very similar to those in colleges and universities; it contains office space, practice/game areas, weight rooms, and athletic training rooms. In this type of organization coaches often report to a general manager and team owner.

Many teachers and coaches of elite athletes, particularly those involved in individual sports, are self-employed. Such coaches are often on the road, traveling to their clients' hometowns. One example is figure skating coaches who coach high-caliber competitive figure skaters at the skaters' home rinks. Many tennis and golf coaches also travel to their clients—unless they work regularly with a nationally or internationally known athlete.

In the elite sport setting, some teachers and coaches have a stable worksite facility, while others teach and coach at a variety of facilities. Still others are self-employed and may work out of their homes.

A few individual sport coaches have the luxury of a stable worksite. For example, families of gymnasts interested in being Olympic athletes often move, or arrange for their child to move, to Houston, Texas, to learn from Bela Karolyi at his nationally known gymnastics facility. Aspiring tennis players sometimes move to Boca Raton, Florida, to take advantage of Nick Bollettieri's tennis facility.

When we think of coaching settings, we usually think of the sports we see every day on television. Coaches today, however, work in a variety of settings. Rowing, kayaking, and canoeing coaches work on rivers. With competitive rock climbing becoming more popular, we find coaches at indoor climbing walls, in the great outdoors scaling mountains, and even in towns and cities climbing stone or brick buildings.

Which teaching and coaching work settings appeal to you? Would you enjoy working in a public school setting, or does working for a nonprofit organization, perhaps at a park or all-purpose facility, appeal to you? Would you enjoy working in gymnasiums, weight rooms, and stadiums? Do you want to work with beginners or with elite athletes? Do you want to work within a school or organization, or do you want to work on your own, in a self-employed situation?

Up-Close Views of Professions in Teaching and Coaching

Do coaches require certification? What opportunities exist for teachers of physical activity in community settings? What do college and university kinesiology professors really do? This section is designed to answer questions such as these by offering brief overviews of some of the professions in the sphere of instruction. While we cannot provide all of the "ins and outs" of every profession, this section should help you decide whether these professions are for you.

Teaching

A teacher's life is filled with wonderment and reward, and thinking about teaching summons past memories in all of our lives. A teacher has the ability to impact another life immeasurably. When we think about teaching, we often think of such acts as sharing, compassion, and mentoring. These are the components that make teaching one of the noblest professions in the world. Teaching offers enormous possibilities for changing the lives of others for the betterment of society. Within the educational setting there are many different teaching positions to choose from, depending on the type of student one wishes to instruct. Someone once said, "You are a teacher first and a physical activity teacher second; never the reverse." If you agree, the world of teachers welcomes you with open arms.

🔑 Teaching is more than simply imparting subject matter to students. It is a complex and labor-intensive profession that puts the greater needs of society before the content to be taught.

K–12 Teachers

Elementary school teachers have the great responsibility of providing basic motor skills instruction to young children so that they can become skillful and efficient movers as teenagers and adults. Teachers at this level also have the privilege of working with children who are still innocent and full of wonder.

Elementary school physical education teachers usually teach 6 to 10 classes a day, each lasting thirty minutes to an hour. These teachers often instruct each class two or three times a week, thus teaching the same group of students two to three hours per week. In some states, elementary school physical educators travel from site to site, teaching in two or more schools.

Unlike elementary physical education teachers, who teach about twenty sets of students per week, or however many classes the school has, middle school and junior high school teachers usually provide instruction to a set number of students on a daily basis. Depending on the number of periods allocated to the school day, a teacher in this setting usually teaches six or seven classes daily. Therefore, physical education contact hours with students at this level are about double those with students in elementary school.

Middle school students are dealing with the powerful hormone changes that accompany puberty. Rather than viewing this challenging group of youngsters as difficult, teachers would do well to think of them as standing at a crucial crossroad in their lives as they begin to explore how they will fit into the world as adults. Middle school teachers can play a major role in their students' important processes of discovery and development.

At this stage in students' lives physical education teachers can focus on the development of more complicated movement skills, beginning sport strategies, and in-depth concepts of fitness. The idea is to prepare them not only to be successful in movement, but also to begin to understand the importance of physical activity.

Students at this level of schooling tread on the frontier of adolescence, and teachers can be instrumental in helping them explore the differences between childhood and adulthood.

High school physical education teachers, on the other hand, guard the last border before students enter adulthood. Because many students make life decisions at this point, they should be given many opportunities in classrooms and gymnasiums that will help them succeed in life. This is not an easy task. Teachers must create a learning environment that challenges students of different interests and abilities to master movement skills and perform a variety of sport, dance, and fitness activities with adeptness and efficiency. High school, for many students, is the place where they will receive their last formal academic education. This is a critical time for physical education teachers to impress on students the importance of a healthy lifestyle that includes physical activity, thus encouraging them to pursue lifelong activity with enjoyment and a sense of fulfillment.

A high school teacher's schedule is relatively similar to that of a middle or junior high school teacher, although many high school physical education teachers also coach.

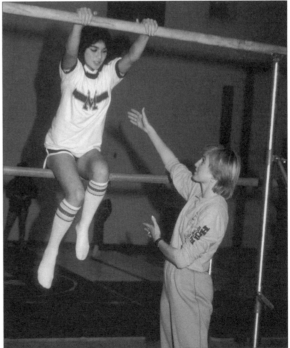

Teachers at all grade levels can have a positive impact on the lives of their students.

© Mary E. Messenger

Teachers in K–12 settings must perform other duties in addition to teaching, including grading, supervising, attending staff meetings and professional development workshops, conducting parent meetings, and being responsible for equipment purchase and maintenance. If becoming a teaching professional in the K–12 setting appeals to you, you will be happy to know that employment opportunities are plentiful. As a result of teacher retirements and reductions in class size, school districts will be looking to hire many new physical education teachers in the near future.

A physical education teacher at the K–12 grade levels is required to possess state certification. In some states, prospective teachers must complete a variety of education courses beyond the bachelor's degree to obtain this certification. These courses serve to integrate educational theory and kinesiology theory with applied professional practice. Beyond the course work, prospective teachers are typically required to pass certain state exams to secure the teaching certification. University students often spend one academic year in a certification program.

According to Ayers (1993), teachers are "asked hundreds, perhaps thousands of times why they chose teaching" (p. 5). The question can prompt many different answers. Some teach for all the "right reasons" (i.e., to help and serve society), while others have reasons that are somewhat questionable (i.e., having summers off). If one of your career goals is to have a positive impact on the lives of others, then perhaps teaching is for you.

Community College Instructors

Many high school graduates decide to continue their education at a local community college. Physical education at this level is often more focused than it is in high school. Teachers at community colleges may offer a class in one activity, say, tennis or volleyball, to a group of students for an entire semester. A physical activity instructor teaches six or more of these courses per semester. These courses are usually not required, and students take them because they want to improve their knowledge and skills in the activ-

ity. Instructors also teach courses in related areas such as health, first aid, and CPR.

Most community colleges require their physical education instructors to earn a master's degree. After completing a bachelor's degree, it takes between one and two years of full-time enrollment at a college or university to complete a master's degree program.

Like high school teachers, physical activity instructors in the community college setting often coach in addition to teaching. Being willing to coach, as well as having the qualifications to do so, will increase your chances of being hired at a community college. The outlook for employment as community college instructors is not as positive as it is for K–12 teachers, yet job opportunities are increasing as the average age of the community college instructor increases. These instructors, mainly from the baby boom era, are beginning to retire.

A career at this level offers the reward of involvement with a diverse group of students. Community colleges do not set stringent admission requirements and are reasonably affordable, thus opening their doors to a great diversity of people. Some students attend community college full time with hopes of transferring to a university. Other students attend simply because they enjoy learning about a specific field of study and may only take one or two courses each year.

A career at a community college involves working with a wide variety of students and, most likely, coaching a competitive sport team.

University Professors

Teaching at the university level usually requires a doctoral degree. This usually takes about three or four years of education beyond the master's degree. Of all the possible teaching positions in physical activity, this one requires the most knowledge about physical activity and the teaching/learning process. University professors generally teach two to four courses per semester, but their responsibilities go beyond teaching. They also engage in grant writing and research to find out more about physical activity and professional practice centered in physical activity. This is typically referred to as scholarship, which

Perry Saravalli

Assistant Professor in Physical Education Teacher Education

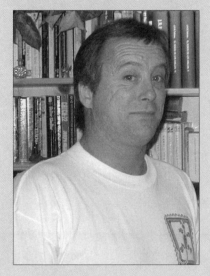

Perry Saravalli is a professor at a major university in Los Angeles. He has dedicated most of his career to serving underserved youth through developing physical activity programs in the inner city. Perry views the university as the vehicle to help strengthen his community.

For the past eight years I have served young people considered by many as detriments to our society through the use of physical activity. These youth have been under 19 years of age, and most have resided in the inner cities of Denver and Los Angeles. Several of them are now enrolled in college; several others never graduated high school. A few have since died and a few have been killed, but all of them thirsted for success.

There is no doubt that many kids' lives have been shattered like the broken windows they walk past every day. Some adults ignore the conditions altogether, while others merely suggest putting duct tape over the cracked windows in order to stop the flow of cold air. My sense is that the view through duct tape is a grim one. Rachel Carson once said, "If I had influence with the good fairy who is supposed to preside over . . . all children, I should ask that her gift to each child in the world be a sense of wonder" (Carswell & Roubinek, 1974). If I could summon that same good fairy, I would ask that all of the cracked windows be removed entirely and be replaced with new panes, preferably stained glass. Admittedly, my goals are lofty, but all these young people deserve no less. Each life, each story, is unique.

While completing my college general education requirements, I decided that I wanted to become a teacher. Since I still enjoyed participating in sports, it seemed logical that I prepare myself to teach traditional high school physical education. While enrolled in graduate school, I inadvertently met a professor who offered me another path, and, in the words of Robert Frost, "that has made all the difference." He presented to me an experience that literally changed my career and my life. In many ways, my career was transformed into a calling. The experience took place at an alternative high school which served kids who were failing in the public school system. I observed him teaching students to become more responsible for their lives, in and out of school, through physical activity.

I continued to work at the alternative school and, after completing my master's degree in physical education, I decided to pursue my doctorate at another university. By this time I had decided to become a teacher educator in physical education. It also had become apparent to me that I did not fit into the mainstream of traditional physical education methodologies. Due to continual and extraordinary support from certain professors on campus and from the local school district, I was able to immerse myself in the design and implementation of physical activity programs for underserved youth. During all of this, I was completing doctoral course work while at the same time teaching physical education at an alternative secondary school and at the university.

I've come to the conclusion that we try to teach too much of the wrong stuff in K–12 schooling. I've witnessed students receiving a barrage of outdated notions about civics when what they most needed was to learn about themselves and how to care for each other for the common good of society. For some kids, school may be the only place where these lessons can be taught and learned. Schools produce winners, but schools also produce losers, and schools aren't ready to recognize that.

→

Specific to physical education, I've seen (1) kids forced to wear uniforms for conformity's sake, (2) kids endure painstaking embarrassment for their inability to perform a skill in a particular way, (3) gender inequity, (4) meaningless grading policies based solely on attendance, and (5) a host of other absurd practices too numerous to mention here. High-quality physical education in our nation's schools is necessary for the complete development of each student. Regrettably, surfeits of physical education programs teach students simply to show up, dress out, and be competent bystanders.

Now, as a fifth-year assistant professor in physical education teacher education, I see myself reflected in the many undergraduates who are skeptical of their preparation program. Some are seeking something real to teach, while far too many are simply going through the motions and are resigned to (and, unfortunately, a few are relieved about) simply jumping through hoops until the state deems them qualified to teach physical education. If you are choosing to teach, please do not resign yourself to this mindset. It is easy to find oneself dispirited and frustrated with a system that seems short on compassion and appears powerfully resistant to change. As an antidote, therefore, you should remind yourself that small changes can make a difference and that the effort is often well worth the frustration. Recently, one of my inner-city students named her child after me. This alone should show you the power and possibilities of teaching physical activity.

also includes presenting the results at conferences and publishing the material in scholarly journals. Finally, university professors also perform service to the university (committee work) and to the surrounding region. For example, a professor might develop an in-service program for high school teachers, or involve university students in after-school physical activity programs for local elementary school children.

🔑 University professors have a wide range of responsibilities, including teaching, scholarship, and service.

Adapted Physical Activity Teachers

Within all of the educational settings, adapted physical educators are needed to provide professional services for individuals with disabilities. These disabilities can be mental, emotional, and/or physical. Adapted physical activity teachers primarily are responsible for creating a learning environment that facilitates quality instruction and considers students' varied abilities. Those who teach in this area typically have 8 to 15 students in a class, which enables them to provide specialized attention to students.

Legal mandates surrounding the civil rights of individuals with disabilities have helped to bring about a transformation "from a medical model approach [to teaching] to an educational approach" (DePauw, 1996, p. 107). As a result,

more students with disabilities are being enrolled in "regular" physical education classes. This is why all future physical activity teachers should take course work in adapted physical education. As DePauw (1996) states, "Increasingly, physical education teachers can no longer rely on highly trained adapted physical education specialists to teach students with disabilities in a segregated setting" (p. 119).

Because professionals in all spheres of physical activity will meet individuals with disabilities, adapted physical activity is not relegated only to school settings. For those who desire to specialize in adapted physical education, many job opportunities exist. These highly specialized teachers can work in a variety of settings, including schools, hospitals, and rehabilitation centers.

🔑 Adapted physical activity teachers are responsible for teaching those individuals who have disabilities, and they may work in a variety of settings.

Community Physical Activity Teachers

The community organizations that offer the majority of physical activity classes are departments of recreation and nonprofit agencies. Experts estimate that more than 50,000 professionals are needed annually to fill a variety of open positions in the nonprofit sector alone (College Preview, 1997); some of these openings are for instructional staff. Nonprofit community organizations are playing an important role in serving underserved neighborhoods. Physical activity teachers can be part of this challenge (Hellison et al., in press).

Community teachers often provide instruction to youngsters in after-school, evening, and summer programs, and many of these youth programs are physical activity based. These teachers also commonly educate older people in physical activity. Although most of the teaching positions in community agencies do not require credentials, as do public schools, most do require a bachelor's degree.

Because of the varied needs of communities, physical activity professionals at this level typically perform a variety of tasks beyond teaching. Teachers may direct physical activity programs, which may require marketing the program, budgeting the program, and overseeing a staff. In addition, physical activity specialists in community organizations may also be involved with tutoring, mentoring, literacy programs, and a host of other community services.

Traditional educational settings are not the only place an individual can teach physical activity. Many community organizations and nonprofit agencies are in need of physical activity teachers to provide quality instruction.

Teaching Professionals

We have all heard of the golf pro and the tennis pro, but who are these people? Are they teachers or are they coaches? Of course, all teachers are professionals, but in this chapter *teaching professional* refers to what is commonly called a *teaching pro*—that is, someone who offers services (private or group lessons) solely in an activity of his or her expertise. More than any other teacher, the teaching professional is very similar to a coach. In fact, many university swim, golf, and tennis coaches are teaching professionals. Outside of the university the teaching professional can be found at private, semi-private, or public teaching facilities instructing beginning, intermediate, advanced, or elite players. For example, as a certified water safety instructor you may be employed by a private club to teach swimming lessons and coach the swim or synchronized swim teams. Or, as a golf professional, you may be hired by a lo-

cal golf course to give lessons to the public and conduct golf camps or manage the pro shop or the clubhouse. And, of course, you could coach a player on the professional circuit.

Professional teachers often instruct performers of all ability levels. They may offer lessons for beginners but also coach highly skilled individuals who are competing in leagues and tournaments. Within this profession there are people who teach and people who coach, and some who do both.

The teaching professional is one who offers services (private or group lessons) solely in an activity of his or her expertise. More than any other teacher, the teaching professional is very similar to a coach.

Certification is needed to be a teaching professional in some sports. For example, individuals who teach golf are only "golf professionals" after becoming certified by either the men's Professional Golf Association (PGA) or the Ladies Professional Golf Association (LPGA); until that time they are technically called golf instructors. A similar certification system exists in other sports such as tennis and swimming. Additional activities requiring professional certification are listed in table 16.2.

Teaching professionals are typically self-employed and are commonly hired as independent contractors. Employment security for the certified professional coach depends on the satisfaction of the client and the owner or manager of the teaching facility. In this way, certified professionals have as much control over retaining their employment as any other professionals. Employment opportunities at the beginner/intermediate

TABLE 16.2 Activities Professional Teachers Teach	
Golf	Rock climbing
Tennis	Martial arts
Archery	Scuba
Boxing	Equestrian
Swimming	White-water rafting
Diving	Skiing
Skydiving	Gymnastics

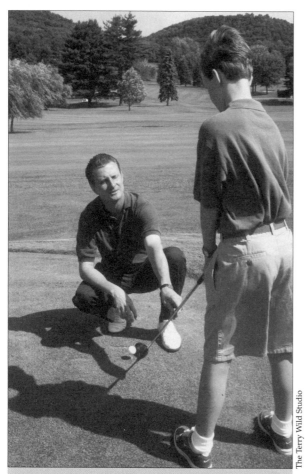

Teaching professionals instruct beginning, intermediate, advanced, and/or elite players.

The Terry Wild Studio

levels are more available than at the elite/professional levels. While many people want to learn to swim, golf, rock climb, and skydive, only a few (in relative terms) will want to work hard to become proficient enough to play at a competitive or elite level. Employment opportunities for the teaching professional are more limited than those for other teaching professions.

Coaching

We all have known people who have touched our lives as no other could. Often the emotions associated with our memories of these people—the feelings of respect, awe, deference, and admiration—feel as vibrant and real as they were when first experienced. The relationships we have developed with these people have made all the difference in our lives. For many current and former athletes, their coach is in the forefront of their

minds and hearts. Joe Paterno, head football coach at Penn State, had this to say about one of his high school coaches:

> . . . what may be his most important accomplishment, is in the relationships he has had with his athletes. He [was] more than just a coach who want[ed] to win matches. Howard Ferguson provide[d] his student-athletes at St. Edward with the unique opportunity to become the best person they can possibly be—in sport and in life. He [was] a friend who puts the time and effort into helping each one of them take advantage of every opportunity. (Ferguson, 1990, Foreword)

As with becoming a teacher, becoming a coach means building relationships that can change the life of another for the better.

Many opportunities exist for those who want to coach. Individuals can be found coaching a variety of people in many different settings—young children to adults and recreational to elite athletes. Some coaches are paid hundreds of thousands of dollars, while others do it simply for the joy it brings. Coaches can be found in sport programs in communities, secondary schools, colleges and universities, and professional sports. These different programs have different coaching requirements and philosophies, and the coaches in these programs often differ in their educational background and coaching experience.

Community Coaches

Although not technically a profession, community coaches are the most common, and sometimes are as passionate about coaching as the professional coach. These coaches usually work on a voluntary basis for local nonprofit organizations such as the YMCA, park district, community center, or Dad's Club. It is common for these volunteers to dedicate two to three evenings and weekends to their coaching duties, which may include one or two coaching meetings, practice held once or twice a week, and weekly games. The primary duties of these coaches is teaching basic skills and the rules of the game, and keeping game statistics.

Organizations dependent on volunteers are faced with the difficult task of finding qualified, certified coaches. Since many states do not have specific standards or certification requirements for the volunteer coach, anyone interested in coaching is often deemed qualified. Generally, community organizations are short of volunteers and anyone wanting to coach at this level can often find a coaching position. Often a parent of one of the team members assumes the role of coach.

Community sport organizations offer programs to a variety of age groups including adults. Coaching at the adult level tends to be very informal and unstructured and therefore will not be discussed further. The focus of this section is on the community sport organizations offering programs for young children (3 to 5 years old) through middle school (13 to 14 years old). These programs tend to de-emphasize winning and attempt to provide fair competition. Often, there is a "no cut and everyone plays" policy. These types of programs often do not keep standings or play tiebreakers, and the organizers attempt to keep the playing ability of the teams equal.

Community organizations cannot always meet the needs of the athletes, and private clubs fill this gap. Many of these private clubs have a philosophy similar to that of the community programs and play local, intraleague contests, but others are more competitive. In many private club sport programs children travel around a state or county to experience competitive interleague play. Some of these programs hire professional coaches. Pop Warner Football is a national program for children and is a good example of the type of private organization that is more competitive than community-based programs. In general, coaches at this competitive level spend more time performing the nonteaching duties associated with coaches such as scouting and recruiting new talent, viewing game films, and organizing team travel.

Community coaches volunteer in community-based sport programs that range from relatively noncompetitive to very competitive.

Professional Coaches

Professional coaches are often associated with educational institutions such as secondary schools (middle, junior high, or high schools), colleges, or universities. Some coaches, however, work with professional teams or individual athletes. Regardless of the differences among different types of coaching, they all share similar qualities and duties. All professional coaches strive to evoke each athlete's potential and guide him or her in overcoming personal challenges and achieving personal success. Coaching duties include teaching physical skills; keeping individual and team statistics; scheduling practices, games, and tournaments; and managing and maintaining equipment.

Secondary Public School Coaches. Middle, junior high, and high school coaches are often certified public school teachers who teach a full or reduced schedule and receive a stipend for taking on the extracurricular activity of coaching. They might also be nonteaching certified coaches, hired only to coach specific teams. Although the qualifications for coaches in the public schools vary by state, a teaching or coaching certification is typically required.

Secondary-level school coaches typically spend their days teaching and receive an additional stipend for coaching.

The National Association for Sport and Physical Education (NASPE) and the American Sport Education Program (ASEP)/National Federation of State High School Associations (NFSHSA) have developed curricular guidelines to help institutions of higher education, organizations, and agencies design appropriate certification programs for coaches. For example, colleges and universities that offer a coaching minor may use the National Standards for Athletic Coaches, developed by NASPE, to create an appropriate course of study for their students. Additionally, the guidelines are available for use by nationally based coaching education programs such as the ASEP/NFSHSA Coaching Principles Course (Martens, 1990). Currently, ASEP/NFSHSA is a popular certification program for interscholastic and club coaches in many states.

The ASEP/NFSHSA highlights several areas of knowledge that encompass NASPE's national standards, including (1) sport psychology, (2) sport physiology, (3) sport pedagogy, (4) developing a coaching philosophy, (5) sport management, (6) sport first aid, and (7) drug education. The first three knowledge areas were discussed in detail in chapters 9, 12, and 10, respectively.

The ASEP/NFSHSA is a popular general coaching certification program particularly among some community and secondary-level coaches. Certification requires knowledge of sport psychology, sport physiology, coaching philosophy, sport pedagogy, sport management, sport first aid, and drug education.

Successful coaches develop a sound coaching philosophy that addresses their personal coaching style and articulates what they want from the coaching experience and what they want their athletes to get out of the athletic experience. The art and science of coaching involves using correct processes to teach skills (sport pedagogy). Specifically, coaches need to teach the techniques, tactics, and strategies of a given sport; use motor learning principles in teaching skills; and plan wisely for maximum learning. Managing a team and understanding the legal and liability issues associated with sport are also critical to effective coaching. Managing any sport enterprise entails team planning, organization, appropriate staffing, leading others to team goals, and monitoring the progress toward team goals.

In the last two decades first aid and drug education have become greater concerns for coaches. As the sports medicine and athletic training fields have become more established, the coach's role has expanded to include injury prevention and emergency care facilitation. For the sake of athlete safety, coaches must, both ethically and legally, create a safe and proper playing environment. When injuries do occur, the coach should be knowledgeable enough to help trained medical personnel.

The number of contact hours coaches can have with their athletes varies depending on the governing body regulating public secondary school athletics. Typically, secondary school coaches spend approximately eight to ten hours a week in after-school practices. When competitive play begins, the number of practice hours may be reduced to eight and game hours increased to between four and six. Some coaches have early morning practice schedules; others have late afternoon or early evening schedules.

In addition to the actual time spent in practices and games, coaches have many "behind the scenes" responsibilities. To varying degrees all coaches are involved in organizing and scheduling team meetings and practices, ordering

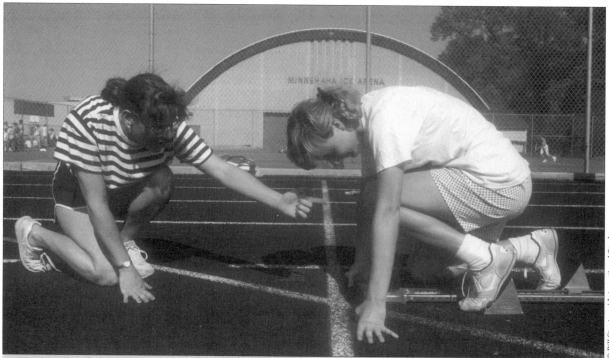

Teaching athletes important, complex skills and basic competitive strategies are primary tasks for coaches.

© Bill Stanton / International Stock

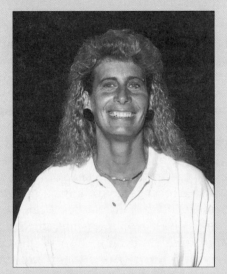

Cindy Diamond

Teacher and Coach

Cindy Diamond has 21 years of professional teaching and coaching experience. Her interest in and dedication to physical activity has a long history stemming from her high school and college experience as an athlete in softball, field hockey, basketball, and volleyball. In addition, she spent a year playing professional softball. Cindy has achieved much success in her career. She has earned the coach of the year title six times, has achieved 300 career wins in softball, has led her team to their ninth straight title as district champions, and has won the 1999 state championship title. The following is Cindy's story.

I was always successful in sport and as a result became very involved in several sport organizations, particularly the Girls' Athletic Association (GAA). My athletic experience and involvement in GAA were the foundation for my interest in teaching and coaching.

I had very positive experiences with my former teachers and coaches, and their encouragement and my own desire to work with young people influenced me to teach and coach. I wanted the chance to help girls appreciate the opportunities they have in life, particularly as they relate to involvement in physical activity. Coaching and teaching provided me with that chance.

I graduated from college with a bachelor of science degree in physical education and a teaching certificate (K–12), which also qualified me to coach at the high school level. In my career I have taught high school physical education, health, CPR, and first aid, and coached basketball, volleyball, and softball. Of all the knowledge I have gained over the last 21 years of teaching and coaching, I think that people skills and knowledge of teaching strategies are the most useful.

I think the true rewards of teaching and coaching are working with students and athletes. I take great pride in working with students and athletes to create successful teaching and coaching programs. Making a difference in students' lives, watching students and athletes learn and become skillful movers, and having them come back after they graduate to say thank you are the most valuable rewards of my career.

As with any career choice, there are challenges and difficulties. For me, the most difficult has been witnessing the decline of students' and athletes' motivation to excel, respect of authority figures, and disciplined behavior. Another challenging aspect of my job is finding time for a life outside of teaching and coaching.

Throughout my career I have learned three very valuable lessons from my students and athletes. First, physical education teachers and coaches should lead by example in promoting fitness. We should practice what we preach. Second, teachers and coaches should establish clear rules early and stick by them. Third, time management is critical. I encourage teachers and coaches to plan their work and work their plan.

For those of you considering a profession in teaching and coaching, I encourage you to take pride in preparing our children to be good leaders of tomorrow, help your students and athletes to dream big and to follow their dreams, and remember, respect is earned. If you want students to respect you, you need to respect them.

equipment, maintaining and overseeing inventory, checking athletes' eligibility, arranging transportation to and from events, talking to the media, preparing for home events, fund-raising, and organizing end-of-season banquets. The extent of coach involvement in these activities depends in part on the size of the coaching team and the number of support personnel. For example, some schools have a full-time athletic director (AD) who is responsible for organizing home contests. Other schools may have a part-time AD, who must delegate that responsibility to another coach. Likewise, some sports (especially football) require many assistant coaches to whom head coaches can delegate specific duties.

The differences in coaching at the various educational levels are a function of the athletes' developmental differences. Some middle school athletes are "diamonds in the rough" with the potential to be very good athletes, but are physically undeveloped (i.e., prepubescent and small) compared to others on the team. Others may have just gone through a growth spurt and are having to relearn a given skill in their new-sized body.

The middle school coach's primary tasks are (1) to help students interested in athletics develop a positive view of themselves as athletes and (2) to teach them important complex physical skills and the basic strategies needed to become good competitive student-athletes. Middle or junior high school coaches have the unique responsibility of introducing young athletes to the world of interscholastic sport in which athletes must balance the attention they give to their academics and their sport. These coaches also must introduce their athletes to the concept of competition in which winning takes on greater importance than it often does at the community level.

The high school coach primarily is involved with students who are interested in athletics and want to invest the time needed to become good athletes. The high school coach is granted the opportunity to build on the foundation set by the middle or junior high school coach by teaching more complex tasks and game strategies. Competition and the importance of winning take on new meaning at the high school level. The increased emphasis on winning necessitates that coaches choose their teams wisely.

With this increased emphasis on winning, high school coaches take on more duties in comparison to middle/junior high school coaches. Specifically, high school coaches spend more time reviewing game films, developing strategies specific to a given opponent, and scouting and recruiting potential team members.

College/University Coaches. Winning is clearly very important to all intercollegiate coaches; the pressure to win at this level is greater than that at the high school level. The quest of college coaches is to maximize the athletic potential of already skilled athletes, build on the foundation established in high school, and fine tune each athlete's ability in order to move them toward becoming members of the elite. Like secondary-level coaches, college coaches have many "behind the scenes" responsibilities. To varying degrees all coaches are involved in team, facility, and equipment management, and budgeting. At the college/university level, talent scouting, recruiting, fund-raising, public relations, and athletic eligibility take on greater significance. The degree of significance often depends on the type of college in which the coach is employed.

> College coaches aim to maximize the athletic potential of already skilled athletes, but they also have many other responsibilities, including team and facility management, budgeting, and recruiting.

The distribution of coaches' workloads differs between Division I and Division III schools. While coaches at Division I institutions generally hold one position, Division III coaches often have multiple job assignments such as coaching two different sports, teaching several academic or activity classes, or holding an administrative position such as assistant athletic director while also coaching. Clearly, the Division I coach has more time than the Division III coach to scout actively for new talent, recruit new athletes, and engage in more public relations functions and fund-raising events. Remember, though, that the scouting and recruiting duties are less for a Division III coach partly because these programs do not offer financial scholarships based on athletic ability.

Employment opportunities at the college/university level are not as plentiful as they are at the secondary level. Coaching at the college/university level is a goal of many high school coaches.

As there are no national or state qualifications and requirements for coaching at the college or university level, most colleges and universities searching for a prospective coach look at applicants with an established name in the sport. Typically, establishing a name requires college playing experience, coaching experience, a history of successful seasons, and being known by many other coaches and administrators. Many Division I coaches began their careers at the secondary level and moved through the lower divisions of college athletics.

In Profile

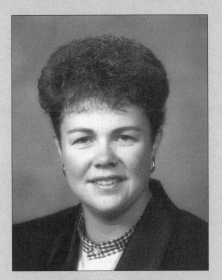

Pam Tyska

Women's Golf Coach

Pam Tyska has 13 years of experience coaching golf at a Division I university. She has played for 28 years and has risen through the ranks of amateur, collegiate, and professional golf. As a golf pro for the last 16 years, she has taught children, youth, and adults. The following is Pam's story.

As a young golfer, I was exposed to coaches I admired and who were good role models. I decided to become a university golf coach while I was an assistant golf professional at a very exclusive private country club. At the time, female head golf professionals were rare, and there was no chance of me becoming a head golf professional at such a club. I turned to collegiate coaching because the job consisted of everything I liked: traveling, teaching, being with people, and organizing events. Although I enjoy my current job, I still perceive the gender gap in golf as an obstacle to women's success in the sport.

My professional preparation consists of a bachelor of science degree in physical education with an emphasis in coaching. I also gained experience working as assistant tournament director and rules official for a women's mini tour and played on that tour for two seasons. I was an assistant golf professional for four years, and I am currently a member of both the LPGA and the PGA as well as the National Golf Coaches Association.

Of all the information I have acquired through my education and golf experience, I find that my coaching philosophy and knowing how to manage group instruction are most useful. Additionally, aspects of kinesiology, anatomy, biomechanics, and first aid have been especially helpful. Today, computer skills are a necessity.

I consider my major career accomplishment as helping some young people into careers in golf as tour professionals, teaching professionals, golf salespeople and marketers, and merchandisers. For me, however, the greatest rewards in coaching are associated with watching young people grow and mature academically, athletically, and socially.

As we all know, growing and maturing often entails some rough spots, and watching athletes go through these rough spots can be a challenge. Other challenges associated with coaching are related to budget issues. With the gender equity issues facing universities, the number of women on a team is increasing faster than the funding needed for additional staffing. Recruiting athletes is sometimes difficult, too. I coach at a small Division I university and have to compete against other universities with bigger budgets and more marketing and public relations networks.

I think the most valuable lesson I have learned is that of all the things that you can give people, the most valuable gifts are your time and attention. My experiences as a coach have consistently reinforced my belief that people, not things, are important.

Professional Sport Coaches. Earlier in this chapter we discussed the teaching professional. When thinking of teaching pros, names such as Tim Gullikson (tennis), Jim Suttie (golf), and Jim Counsilman (swimming) may come to mind. Who comes to mind when you think of professional coaches? Such a question may evoke images of Tommy Lasorda (baseball), Phil Jackson (basketball), and Mike Ditka (football). Although the number of professional sport coaches is small compared to the number of secondary school and college coaches, they typically have national prominence.

As with other professional coaching positions, facilitating athletes' performances is central to the job of the professional sport coach. The position also includes elements of administration, athlete recruitment, and public relations events and media appearances. Generally, the professional sport coach has more nonteaching duties than the teaching professional discussed earlier. For example, some sports, such as football and hockey, require coaches to spend a significant amount of time reviewing game films, and employment retention depends heavily on the performance of their team. The win/loss record in such sports is more important than those in sports such as golf and tennis. Additionally, the professional sport coach deals solely with elite athletes, whereas the teaching pro is often involved with beginning and intermediate athletes.

Employment opportunities for the professional sport coach are few and far between. The number of professional sport teams is limited, and many individuals are qualified to coach at the professional level. As in the college and university setting, no national or state qualifications are needed for coaching at the professional level. Prospective professional sport coaches need an established name in the sport; most acquire theirs by becoming known as winning coaches at the college/university level.

> Generally, the professional sport coach has many nonteaching and noncoaching duties, including administration, recruitment, and media appearances. Employment retention depends heavily on producing a winning team.

Job security for the professional sport coach is not very predictable. When you decide to coach a team sport at the professional level, you are deciding to enter an industry where success relies in large part on public support. In professional sports, public support waxes and wanes relative to a team's win/loss record. Just as the organization's success depends on producing a winning team, so does retaining your job. Many professional sport coaches thrive on this aspect of the job. They bask in the challenges of creating or maintaining a winning tradition, and there are great rewards and personal satisfaction associated with accomplishing this goal.

Sport Psychologists. Although every coach is interested in enhancing athletes' physical performance, many focus primarily on the physical side of the game. This makes sense, as athletes do become better by learning proper techniques and strategies. With a focus on the enhancement of physical skills, often the teaching of the mental skills needed for improving physical performance is neglected. You may hear a coach say to an athlete, "Concentrate!" or "Just relax," but how many times have you seen a coach teach athletes concentration or relaxation skills? Telling people who do not know how to focus their attention to concentrate is like telling individuals who don't know how to dive to perform a back somersault off the high diving board. Both the ability to concentrate and the ability to perform a back somersault are best learned with help from knowledgeable, qualified instructors.

With the increased knowledge we have gained from the study of sport and exercise psychology, more and more coaches are beginning to embrace the importance of mental skills in sport. However, few coaches feel comfortable enough to teach mental skills. As a result, some coaches opt to get a master's degree in physical education with a specialization in sport and exercise psychology and then apply what they learn in their profession. Others seek out a qualified sport psychologist.

Although there are no national certification requirements for the position of sport psychologist, the Association for the Advancement of Applied Sport Psychology (AAASP) developed a certified consulting program that requires training in both exercise and sport science and psychology. This program is designed to protect athletes from unqualified consultants.

There are two primary types of sport psychologists: clinical and educational. Clinical sport psychologists are licensed psychologists who have the skills and knowledge to treat athletes with emotional problems such as clinical depression, substance abuse, and eating disorders. Educational sport psychologists have extensive training in kinesiology and work with athletes for the sole purpose of achieving optimal performance via the development of psychological skills. Regardless of the title (clinical or educational), sport psychologists teach athletes a variety of techniques including mental imagery, relaxation, goal setting, self-talk, and concentration for the purpose of performance enhancement.

Both clinical and educational sport psychologists teach athletes a variety of techniques, including mental imagery, relaxation, goal setting, self-talk, and concentration for the purpose of performance enhancement.

In the 1980s sport psychology seemed to be only for the elite or professional athlete. Today, however, we are beginning to see sport psychologists involved in college and high school sports. As the demand for sport psychologists increases among athletes and athletic teams, so does the employment outlook for these professions. Still, the demand for sport psychologists is less than the supply, making it a difficult profession in which to find employment. Most sport psychologists work in colleges and universities teaching, conducting research, and consulting with athletes. Relatively few make a living solely as consultants.

The amount of time a sport psychologist spends with a given team or athlete and what is taught depends on the psychologist's expertise, how much time he or she is willing to give, how much time the team coach wants to spend on mental skills, and the athletes' interest in learning these skills. Sometimes a consultant will meet one to three times per week for 20 minutes to one hour with a team teaching a given skill to the entire team and then hold individual meetings with athletes who are interested in knowing more. Other times a consultant will meet with a team or group of athletes once a month or every couple of months for a half-day, full-day, or weeklong seminar and may or may not hold individual meetings with athletes. This type of structure often allows the coach and the sport psychologist to work relatively independently and within a cooperative environment.

Which teaching and coaching professions appeal to you? Are you interested in working with children or youth who are just learning physical activity skills, or would you be better suited to working with highly skilled players? If you are considering a coaching profession, what sports or activities do you want to coach? Perhaps you see yourself lecturing and doing research, working in adapted physical education programs, or exploring the psychology of sport. Whatever your leanings, do your interests match your career goals?

Summary of Teaching and Coaching Professions

As you can see, much variety exists in the sphere of instruction. Regardless of the skill, age, experience, and competitive level of the participants one works with, careers in this sphere can be extremely rewarding. By providing a variety of services, from promoting a physically active lifestyle, to helping people improve in movement skills, to developing athletic excellence, teaching and coaching professionals play an important role in the lives of the people with whom they work. Just as rewarding, if not more so, are the moments in which teachers and coaches enable individuals and teams to learn important life lessons through activity. For most teachers and coaches the biggest reward is in the lasting relationships they build with their participants, some of which grow into deep, lifelong friendships. For many, this is what brings them back year after year. Table 16.3 offers a list of teaching and coaching resources.

Inside Advice for Teaching and Coaching Students

Teachers and coaches can be very knowledgeable about the principles of communication, but not

TABLE 16.3
Teaching and Coaching Resources

Teaching Resources

American Federation of Teachers
ASHA National Office
7263 State Rt. 43
P.O. Box 708
Kent, OH 44240-0708

Association for the Advancement of Health,
Physical Education, Recreation and Dance
1900 Association Drive
Reston, VA 22091

Boys and Girls Clubs of America
1230 W. Peachtree St., NW
Atlanta, GA 30309
Phone: 800-854-CLUB
Phone: 404-815-5700
www.bgca.org
E-mail: imclemore@bgca.org

National Association for the Education of Young
Children
1834 Connecticut Ave., NW
Washington, DC 20009

National Association for Sport and Physical
Activity
An association of the American Alliance for Health,
Physical Education, Recreation and Dance
1900 Association Dr.
Reston, VA 20191-1598
Phone: 703-476-3410
www.aahperd.org/naspe/naspe-main.html

National Board for Professional Teaching Standards
26555 Evergreen Road, Suite 400
Southfield, MI 48076
www.nbpts.org

National Education Association
1201 16th St., NW
Washington, DC 20036

YMCA of the USA
101 North Wacker Drive
Chicago, IL 60606
Phone: 312-977-0031
Phone: 800-872-9622
www.ymca.net

YWCA of the USA
Empire State Building, Suite 301
350 Fifth Avenue
New York, NY 10118
Phone: (212) 273-7800
www.ywca.org

Coaching Resources

Amateur Athletic Union
Walt Disney World Resort
P.O. Box 10000
Lake Buena Vista, FL 32830-1000
Phone: 800-AAU-4USA
Phone: 407-934-7200
www.aausports.org/

Association for the Advancement of Applied
Sport Psychology
www.aaasponline.org

National Association of Intercollegiate Athletics
6120 S. Yale, Suite 1450
Tulsa, OK 74136
Phone: 918-494-8828
www.naia.org

National Collegiate Athletic Association
P.O. Box 6222
Indianapolis, IN 46206-6222
Phone: 317-917-6222
www.ncaa.org

National Federation of State High School Associations
11724 NW Plaza Cr.
P.O. Box 20626
Kansas City, MO 64195-0626
Phone: 816-464-5400
www.nfhs.org/home.html
Publications: NFHS News, NFHS Coaches' Quarterly

National Junior College Athletic Association
1825 Austin Bluffs Pkwy, Suite 100
P.O. Box 7305
Colorado Springs, CO 80933-7305
Phone: 719-590-9788
www.njcaa.org
Official publication: JUCO Review

United States Olympic Committee
One Olympic Plaza
Colorado Springs, CO 80909
Phone: 719-632-5551
www.usoc.org

Women's Sports Foundation
Eisenhower Park
East Meadows, NY 11554
Phone: 800-227-3988
Phone: 516-542-4700
www.lifetimetv.com/WoSport/

be effective communicators. Or they may know the principles of leadership, but not be effective leaders. Being a successful teacher or coach requires that one have not only knowledge, but also the skill to share the knowledge in such a way that people listen and act accordingly.

Effective teaching and coaching often entail building rapport with athletes and students and taking on many roles, some of which may appear unrelated to these professions. Teachers and coaches often serve as role models for their communities and the participants in their programs. Being ethical and trustworthy is part of that job. In addition, teachers or coaches who are social trustee, civic professionals must sometimes turn their attention from providing proper movement techniques and attend to teaching life skills.

Because assisting in participants' personal lives is part of this profession, coaches and teachers must develop a sound approach to dealing with challenging circumstances. Examining your own style of leadership will enhance your ability to address learners' personal lives appropriately, if needed, leading you to become more effective at transmitting physical activity knowledge to those learners. Real teaching and coaching goes well beyond appropriate physical activity lessons. It reaches to areas bound by uncertainty, personal reflection, and binding relationships. McDonald (1992) illustrates this:

> As soon as I finished teaching the first class I ever taught, I asked my supervisor what he thought. He told me he thought I had taught as if speaking from the next room through a tube. He was a good coach. With a single sentence, he oriented me toward the real thing. Whatever you do as you struggle to teach [or coach], he seemed to suggest, do it in person . . . and keep all relations live. (p. 1)

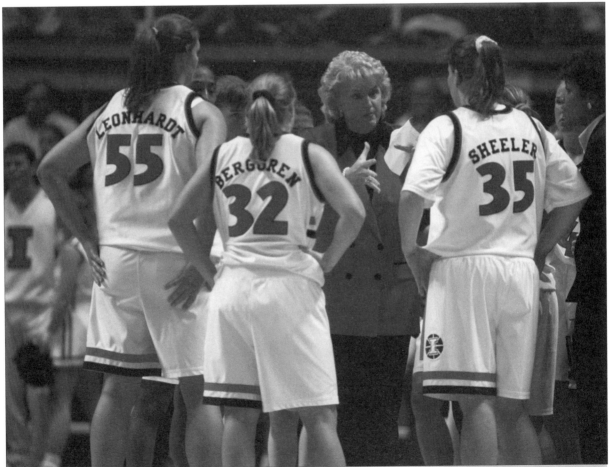

Teachers and coaches play an important role in the physical, social, and emotional development of their students and athletes.

© Human Kinetics

Successful teaching and coaching requires skills beyond scientific knowledge. Most successful teachers and coaches have "people skills" that enable them to develop rapport with their participants and foster an environment that leads to a sense of community among participants.

Are you considering a career in teaching and coaching? If so, consider whether you like dealing with people as much as you like playing your favorite sports. What other skills do you need to learn? What courses might help you gain those skills?

Successful teachers and coaches keep two critical elements at the forefront of their minds. The first is that teaching and coaching are complex skills. The second is that one only gets better at teaching and coaching by doing it. If you are interested in teaching and coaching as a career, we recommend that you seek out early practical experiences. As discussed in chapter 13, internships, practicums, field experience and courses, are opportunities to do this. Community work settings also offer practical experiences for those hoping to enter a teaching or coaching career. In addition, you can gain valuable practical experi-

ences in these professions through college courses, jobs, or volunteer opportunities.

Simply put, the more you do, the more you learn. Taking advantage of these opportunities will enhance your knowledge and skills, thus making you a more competent and effective teacher or coach when you enter the profession.

Wrap-Up

In this chapter you learned some basic information about the teaching and coaching professions. You also received an overview of possible careers within teaching and coaching and the work settings in which these careers take place. Both of these professions include instruction and offer opportunities to serve a wide range of people across many ages and ability levels. In fact, few professions offer such a wide array of populations from which to choose.

You have also met a few professionals in teaching and coaching and been privy to an inside view of their impressions of their career choices. As you can see from the stories provided by Perry, Pam, and Cindy, there are great opportunities for those who decide to enter a teaching or coaching career not only to capitalize on personal interest, but also to promote physical activity programs and serve society. As Perry noted, "Each life, each story, is unique." Through teaching or coaching you too can create a portrait of your life that is peerless.

Study Questions

1. What distinguishes teaching from coaching?

2. Describe the differences and similarities between the *acts* of teaching and the *acts* of coaching.

3. Contrast the professions and subcultures in teaching and coaching.

4. Outline the variety of work settings for teachers and coaches. Provide a description of each setting, including the possible participants, students, or clientele.

5. List the three professions in teaching and coaching that are most appealing to you. Examine and discuss the educational requirements and qualifications for these careers.

6. Consider two professions from this chapter—one teaching profession and one coaching profession—and describe the duties and responsibilities for each, including their primary purposes.

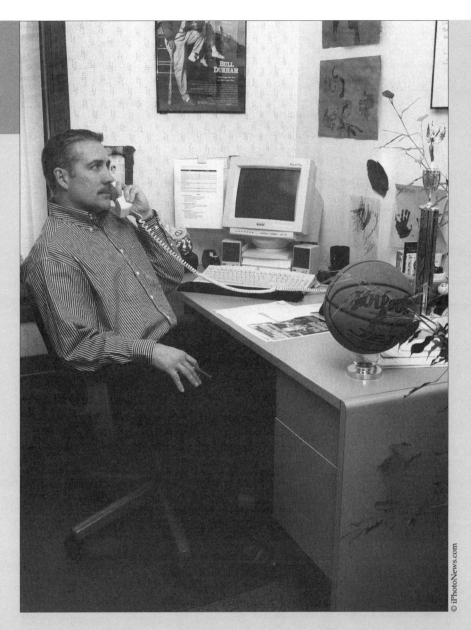

© iPhotoNews.com

17

Sport Management Professions

Lori K. Miller, G. Clayton Stoldt,
and Greg Comfort

In this chapter . . .

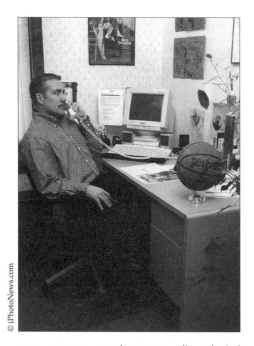

© iPhotoNews.com

A sales representative for a professional baseball team meets with a potential corporate sponsor. The topic of conversation: a proposal that the business sponsor a promotional event that will benefit the sponsor's business and help draw fans to the ballpark.

A collegiate athletic director asks several staff members to compile a report regarding gender equity within the program. The report will present data in a variety of categories relating to compliance with Title IX of the Educational Amendments of 1972.

The sports information director for a collegiate athletic program prepares a media guide after compiling statistics, selling advertisements, and writing player histories. The media guide will be distributed to surrounding colleges, coaches, the media, and fans.

The program director for a YMCA branch surveys current members regarding their level of interest in adult soccer leagues. If interest levels are high enough, the program director will make plans to add adult soccer leagues to the array of services available to its members.

The research and development department of a sporting goods manufacturer prepares a presentation on a new golf club design that may help high-handicap players improve their scores. If top management agrees that the costs are feasible, the new product could be available for distribution within a year.

All of the preceding scenarios represent decisions sport managers are confronted with on a routine basis. In each case, sport managers and employees of sport organizations make decisions that serve the consumer while enabling the sport organization to break even and/or generate a desired level of profitability.

While competition for jobs in the sport management industry is often fierce, a wide array of career options is available, and the field is growing rapidly. A recent *Sports Business Journal* profile of NBA Entertainment (NBAE), a production and programming company, illustrates the exponential growth happening in the sport industry (Miller, 1998). When formed in 1982, NBAE had a staff of 16 and provided only a game-footage library for constituents. In 1998 NBAE had over 200 employees. NBAE is currently equipped with its own studio and production facilities that produce an array of weekly television series; promotional spots; NBA and WNBA features, specials, and public service announcements; the league's Web site; corporate sales tapes; and home videos (in partnership with CBS/Fox Video) (Miller, 1998, p. 5). As a result of the incredible growth and many job opportunities in sport management, sport management comprises one of the six spheres of professional

practice centered in physical activity (see figure 17.1).

The sport management industry is thriving and offers numerous viable options for students looking for careers in sport.

The purpose of this chapter is to examine professions within the sport management industry. The career opportunities within this industry are many and varied, and rapidly expanding. Professional opportunities exist in professional sports, amateur sports, sport participation, sporting goods, and support services. And graduates with a well-rounded degree can choose from a variety of roles—from event management to human resource management to marketing management.

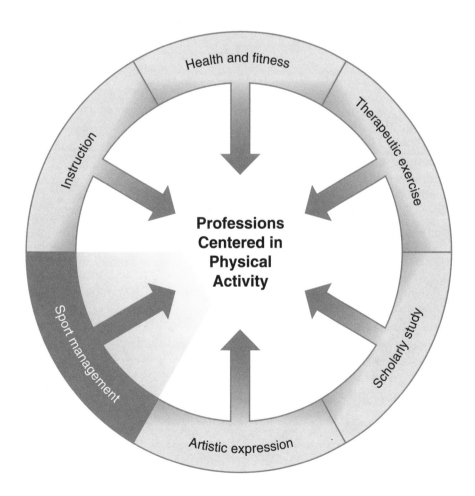

Figure 17.1   Sport management is one of the spheres of professional practice centered in physical activity.

We hope this chapter helps you decide if a career in sport management is right for you.

 CHAPTER OBJECTIVES

In this chapter we will:

■ Acquaint you with the wide range of professional opportunities in the sphere of sport management

■ Familiarize you with the purpose and types of work done by professionals in sport management

■ Inform you about the educational requirements and experiences necessary to become an active, competent professional in the area

■ Help you identify whether one of these professions fits your skills, aptitudes, and professional desires

The World of Sport Management

The sport industry, comprised of a variety of different sectors, represents the 11th largest industry in the United States (Meek, 1997). The term *sport industry* has been defined in a number of ways by various sport management scholars (Meek, 1997; Parks & Zanger, 1990; Pitts, Fielding, & Miller, 1994; Pitts & Stotlar, 1996). In this chapter we will use the following definition: "The market in which the products offered to its buyers are fitness, sport, recreation, and leisure related. These products include goods (e.g., baseball bats), services (e.g., sport marketing, health clubs), people (e.g., professional players), places (e.g., golf courses), and ideas" (Pitts, Fielding & Miller, 1994, p. 18). Based on this definition, the sport management sphere of professional practice centered in physical activity can involve career opportunities in three of the other spheres (health and fitness, instruction, and therapeutic exercise).

As defined in chapter 3, physical activity professionals are expert manipulators of physical activity experiences. In other words, their expertise lies in the manipulation of physical activity experiences to bring about improvement in performance, health, and enjoyment. They may serve as personal trainers, teachers, athletic trainers, or coaches. While many sport management professions do relate indirectly to the manipulation of physical activity itself (e.g., park and recreation directors), others focus instead on the manipulation of the elements supporting spectatorship (e.g., promotions, half-time entertainment, marketing, sports information services) in order to maximize customer enjoyment. Generally, they provide support services, facilities, and other amenities to make physical activity and spectatorship possible. For example, a sport manager may be employed as the

• marketing coordinator for a local speedway (see the following section entitled "Professional Sport Entertainment"),

• program coordinator for a YMCA (see the section entitled "Sport Participation, Nonprofit"),

• general manager for a golf course (see "Sport Participation, For-Profit"),

• athletic director in a high school (see "Amateur Sport Entertainment"),

• athletic director for a college or university (see "Amateur Sport Entertainment"),

• event manager for a triathlon (see "Sport Services"), or

• manager of a sport medicine retail store (see "Sporting Goods").

The diagrams in figures 17.2 and 17.3 represent our perception of the sport industry, based primarily on the work of Meek (1997).

Although the academic study of sport management is relatively new, management of the sport industry has a long history. In the early 1800s individuals strategized on how to promote boxing and billiards, while by the mid-1800s individuals responsible for the promotion of baseball games scrutinized the placement of baseball fields outside of urban areas. The 1880s and subsequent years brought about distribution issues that required the input of sport managers. And during the 1890s it was not uncommon for sporting goods manufacturers to hire professional advertising agencies (Fielding & Miller, 1996). By 1920 the structure (e.g., management, marketing, legal issues and related regulations, financial structure, distribution) of organizations in the sport industry was well established.

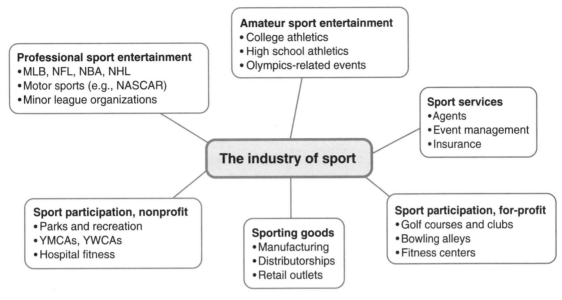

Figure 17.2 Sport industry segments.

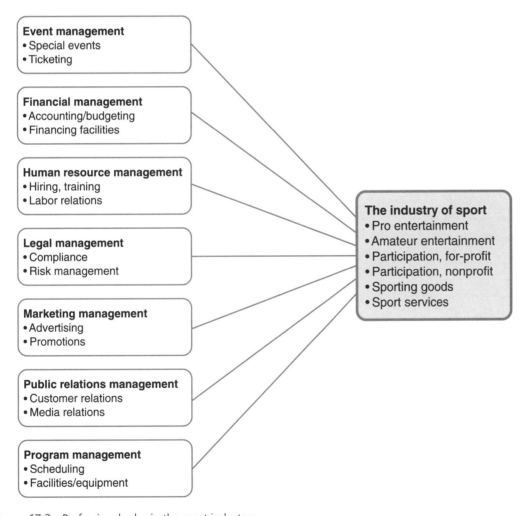

Figure 17.3 Professional roles in the sport industry.

The sport industry has grown significantly in both variety and complexity since the 1800s. Improved technology, enhanced discretionary monies and time, flexible work assignments, changing demographics and psychographics, consumer needs and desires, and other societal influences have caused the sport industry to blossom.

To consider the prevalence and popularity of sport, you need only examine your own interactions with sport and leisure during a typical day. Sport is an integral part of many people's lives, and that is good news for sport managers. "It has been estimated that the industrialized world spends more time and money amusing itself than it does actually making things," noted one *Sports Business Journal* columnist (Schoenfield, 1998, p. 1).

Think about your average week. How much time do you spend watching sport programming on television? How much time do you spend engaging in sport-related activities such as working out, golfing, or cycling? How much money do you spend on apparel featuring sport teams' logos or brand marks of sporting goods manufacturers? How much time do you spend in sport-related conversation?

The consumer's interest in, and demand for, sport and leisure alternatives has greatly influenced the job opportunities available for students of sport management.

Sport Management Settings

As indicated in figure 17.2, the sport industry can be divided into six industry segments. While a wide variety of sport organizations represent the sport industry segments, figure 17.2 offers a sampling of some of the more common organizations within each segment. Also, as indicated in figure 17.3, the professional roles in the industry are shared by all the industry segments. For instance, professional sport franchises and nonprofit sport organizations both require people working in management, marketing, and so on. Likewise, both nonprofit organizations such as the YMCA and for-profit organizations such as ice skating arenas need people with expertise in financial and legal services. The tasks listed under the different function areas (e.g., event management, financial management) are not exhaustive. Human resource management, for example, could also include motivating, compensating, retaining, evaluating, and so on. Nevertheless, figure 17.3 does provide a sense of the specific task areas within each function.

The number of tasks performed in house versus the number that are outsourced varies within the industry and within the individual sport organizations. Similarly, industry segments differ as to how each function is allocated among existing employees. Larger sport organizations often assign specialized responsibilities to individuals based on areas of expertise. On the other hand, individuals in smaller organizations are likely to be responsible for performing a variety of the different job functions indicated in figure 17.3.

Sport managers are more involved in the activities and job responsibilities surrounding the actual event than they are in the sport or activity itself.

Professional Sport Entertainment

A proliferation of **professional sport entertainment** opportunities has created an abundance of related jobs. Sport fans can be entertained by the multitude of professional major- and minor-league teams, the race car industry, boxing, golf, tennis, and so on. Expansion teams, new professional leagues, and the professional status awarded to alternative sports (e.g., beach volleyball) continue to fuel professional sport entertainment options and related career opportunities.

Each entertainment production (i.e., the game or event) represents a tremendous undertaking combining the skills, competencies, and knowledge of many individuals working in separate functional areas. As indicated in figure 17.3, each professional sport entertainment event provides career opportunities in the following areas: event management, media relations, promotions, sponsorship, advertising, risk management/insurance, accounting and budgeting, human resources, customer service, and compliance.

Amateur Sport Entertainment

The **amateur sport entertainment** industry mirrors the professional sport entertainment industry in many ways. Olympic and intercollegiate sports, for example, can be as competitive and intense as professional sports, and their sporting events often require a great deal of behind-the-scenes work. As with the professional sport entertainment industry, the entertainment alternatives are vast and the career opportunities abundant in amateur sport entertainment. Career opportunities in this industry segment include development, fund-raising, marketing, operations, ticket sales, merchandising, compliance, and student services.

Think about the last time you attended or watched on television a professional or amateur sport event. Identify as many of the periphery items or activities (e.g., concessions) associated with the main event (i.e., the game) as you can.

Sport Participation: For-Profit

For-profit sport participation organizations include fitness/health clubs, bowling alleys, roller skating rinks, miniature golf courses, country clubs, golf courses, ice skating rinks, sport parks, and more. As evidenced by earlier chapters, the health and fitness industry has many facets. An individual pursuing a career as a personal trainer, for example, would have different professional roles and educational training than a person employed in a sport management capacity.

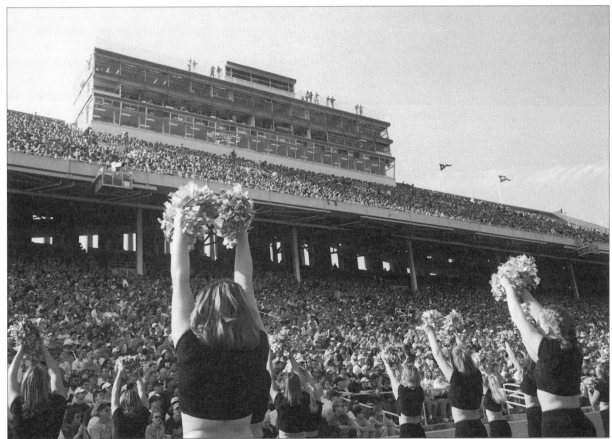

What aspects of sport management can you identify in this photo?

© iPhotoNews.com

A recent survey by the International Health, Racquet and Sportsclub Association found health and fitness clubs enjoying a 9% increase in revenue from 1996 to 1997 ("IHRSA Survey," 1998, p. 6). (From what we saw in chapter 2, this may not be reflecting an increase in active participation.) The healthy economy has created new career opportunities and allowed for growth in a multitude of other for-profit sport participation organizations as well. Such growth translates into more job opportunities for sport management practitioners.

Of particular interest to potential sport managers is the breadth of interest in sport participation (see chapter 3). The sport industry has witnessed the expansion of traditional for-profit sport participation organizations such as golf courses and ice skating centers in addition to the renewed popularity of other organizations such as martial arts academies and bowling centers.

Identify five for-profit sport participation organizations within your own local community. Does working at such an organization appeal to you? If so, what positions within the organizations do you find most attractive?

The for-profit sport participation segment has also recognized growth within existing product lines and product mixes. For example, fitness centers offer consumers traditional programs such as resistance training and aerobics as well as newer programs such as spin classes, slide aerobics, kick boxing aerobics, pump aerobics, massages, and yoga. Furthermore, as the average age of the American population continues to rise, wellness managers are designing more programs specifically for senior adults.

Employment opportunities vary, typically according to the size of the sport organization itself. Large sport participation organizations may provide job opportunities in a variety of function areas including management, marketing, promotions, program planning, human resources, risk management, and so on. Smaller for-profit sport organizations, in comparison, tend to combine a number of business functions into one person's job description.

The for-profit sport organizations are in an enviable position as their target markets and product lines expand.

Sport Participation: Nonprofit

The **nonprofit sport participation** segment also is replete with jobs for qualified sport management professionals. Nonprofit organizations providing participation opportunities in sport include YMCAs; YWCAs; Boys and Girls Clubs; and national, city, and state park and recreation departments. As in other industry segments, individual jobs in these organizations may be specialized according to one of the function areas identified in figure 17.3. On the other hand, one position may include a variety of different job responsibilities. For example, a YMCA located in a major metropolitan area may offer job opportunities in specialized function areas, whereas a Boys and Girls Club may employ one person to be responsible for all recreational-related areas.

Like many other areas in sport, significant growth has occurred in the nonprofit sport participation sector. For example, between 1978 and 1988 "there was a 114% increase in Park and Rec budgets throughout the United States" ("Park and Rec Problem," 1996, p. 2). Growth continued throughout the 1990s as park and recreation departments pursued alternative funding opportunities that combined public and private investments. YMCAs also provide expanded career opportunities. As indicated by the International Health, Racquet and Sportsclub Association, "the YMCA's across the country have put up $1 billion worth of new buildings" in the last decade ("Nonprofit Expansion and Impact," 1996).

Identify five nonprofit sport participation organizations within your own local community. Does working at such an organization appeal to you? If so, what appeals to you the most?

Sporting Goods

The **sporting goods** industry represents a significant portion of the overall sport industry. One estimate indicates that in excess of $71 billion is spent by people in the United States for sport equipment, apparel, and footwear. Another estimate indicates that 51% of all U.S. males purchased clothing with a team logo on it in 1997 (Genzale, 1998). Sport managers play a vital role in ascertaining what sport products society needs and desires. Employment opportunities in the sporting goods industry include consumer behavior research analysts, sporting goods retail store managers, manufacturing sales representatives, and many others.

Do you have a special interest in sports equipment and apparel? Perhaps you like to explore the newest merchandise on the market, or imagine designing your own. If so, a career in sporting goods may interest you.

Sport Services

As a result of the enormous growth in the sport industry, certain services have become more specialized. Today, sport managers can specialize in sport insurance, sporting event management, or providing scouting reports to coaches. This segment of the industry is known as **sport services**. The following are examples of organizations that offer sport services:

Sports & Fitness Insurance Corporation: Provides insurance for health clubs, fitness centers, martial arts studios, personal trainers, and dance schools.

DigitalScout: Provides scouting reports for football and basketball coaches.

ProServ: Provides event management services, sport marketing services, and more.

Team Marketing Report: Provides a multitude of publications dealing with professional sport ownership and financial information,

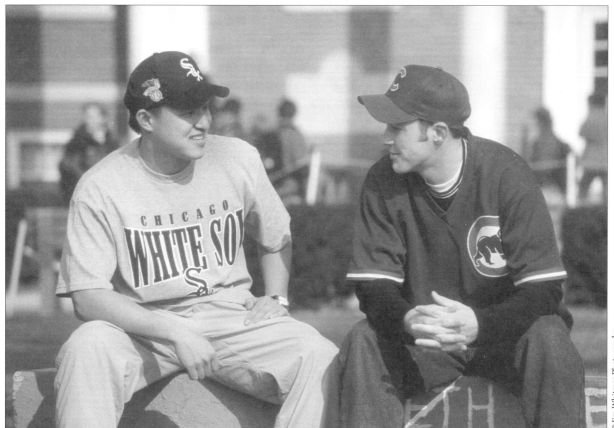

Do you have clothing with a team logo on it? The sporting goods industry is a significant portion of the overall sport industry and offers many career opportunities.

© Jim Whitmer Photography

ways to increase ticket and sponsorship revenues, sport professional leases, stadium revenue agreements, individuals making sponsorship decisions, and more.

Collegiate Licensing Association: Monitors the athletic licensing efforts of universities and colleges.

The sport service segment is likely to realize continued growth as organizations outsource job functions to reduce personnel costs while at the same time receiving specialized services for seasonal sport product offerings.

Up-Close Views of Professions in Sport Management

Many similar professional roles are performed by individuals regardless of the sport industry segment in which they are employed. For example, many of the roles and related tasks discussed in the following sections are performed in other spheres of physical activity professions and also within the different industry segments identified in this chapter. For example, event management is a responsibility of sport managers, teachers, and coaches. Similarly, risk management is a responsibility within many sport management professions, yet it is also a responsibility within the spheres of (1) physical fitness and health promotion, (2) therapeutic exercise and sports medicine, and (3) teaching and coaching. Rather than listing separate professions in the sphere of sport management, as was done in previous chapters, we chose to detail sport industry professional roles and related tasks, which are often a responsibility of one or more employees within each industry segment.

Event Management

In all physical activity professions, the staging of an event is a tremendous undertaking. Many organizations hire individuals with specific expertise in the area of **event management**. These employees are responsible for the many facets associated with hosting an event including risk management, crowd control, securement of appropriate lighting and surfaces, concessions, scheduling, sales, sponsorships, advertising, budgeting, inventory management, customer service, and more. Depending on the size and sophistication of the organization, one person may be responsible for several of the professional roles, or the roles may be assumed by individuals with specializations in given areas. A recent profile of the Coca-Cola 600 for the year 1997 illustrates the complexities of managing a sport-related event (Sluder, 1998):

- More than 400,000 people driving 53,000 vehicles attended various race-related events.

- More than 100 state troopers worked to coordinate traffic in roughly 1,200 acres of parking.

- The crowd consumed more than 5.3 million liters (1.4 million gallons) of water.

- A full-time staff of 6,000 people worked the event, 3,000 of whom handled concessions.

Clearly, event management involves considering a multitude of factors including traffic control, crowd control, resource availability, management and coordination of paid personnel and volunteers, and more. Opportunities in this area are widespread and vary from the Super Bowl to an evening of Little League baseball at a local park.

Sports commissions—local entities that attempt to attract sporting events to their cities in order to boost the local economy—have seen an enormous increase in the United States in recent years. The National Association of Sports Commissions (NASC) reports that the number of U.S. sports commissions increased 423% between 1992 and 1998 (Cawley, 1998). This increase has resulted in substantial growth in the number of events employing sport managers. Once an event is scheduled, sports commission personnel collaborate and cooperate with other sport personnel (e.g., team owners and employees, volunteers) employed in the sport industry to ensure that the event is a success. A sports commission that secures a bid to bring a bowling championship to its city, for example, would work closely with the practitioners in the local bowling community to ensure that adequate facilities are provided, customer service is exemplary, scheduling is orga-

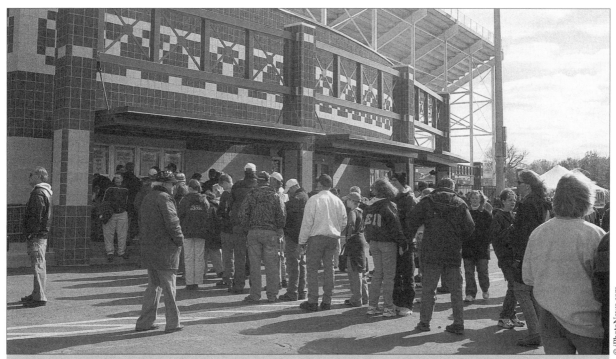

The smooth running of a sport event, including ticket sales, concessions, and crowd control, depends largely upon sport managers specializing in event management.

nized, volunteers are gathered and committed, and so on.

It is also important to note that a great deal of interdependence exists among the various sport industry segments discussed in this chapter. For instance, a city sports commission may play a key role in attracting an NCAA baseball regional to a particular municipality. However, that commission is likely working closely with a host NCAA institution, a local facility, a ticket distribution agency, and a variety of corporate sponsors. Teamwork among sport organizations is critical to secure a bid. Similarly, the hosting of a national gymnastics meet may require cooperation among parks and recreation departments, for-profit gymnastics clubs, nonprofit health clubs, universities, and high schools equipped with facilities that can be used for competition or practice.

Financial Management

Financial managers are critical to the operation of most sport-related organizations. These individuals may administer budgets, oversee income allocation, pursue development opportunities, and handle investments. Managing financial situations for sport organizations requires both a knowledge and understanding of financial basics (e.g., financial statements, investment strategies) and an understanding of the sport product. Without an understanding of the sport product, a person is not equipped to capitalize on potential revenue opportunities. For example, when budgeting for a minor-league sport, the financial manager needs to understand the cyclical nature of the sport and to know when to approach prospects for the purpose of selling inventory (e.g., fence signs, program advertising, season tickets).

Two areas of sport **financial management** that provide a significant number of opportunities are accounting/budgeting and facility finance. All sport organizations, and almost all employees in the sport industry, are involved in some manner of accounting and budgeting. Sport marketers, for example, who are responsible for promotions, advertising, and sponsorships must ensure that expenses don't exceed revenues. Similarly, sport event managers must balance expenses associated with facility rental, ushers, concession-related purchases, parking attendants, and so on, with anticipated revenues generated from tickets, sponsorships, and so forth.

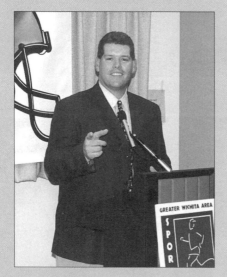

Derik Dukes

Assistant Executive Director, Greater Wichita Area Sports Commission

Derik Dukes is currently employed as the assistant executive director for the Greater Wichita Area Sports Commission, a small organization. Derik is responsible for creating bids for various events, publishing a newsletter, organizing and training event volunteers, handling all event correspondences, securing required facilities, supervising events, securing sponsorships, and more.

Derik has always been a fan of sport. Derik's father owned Dukes Diamonds, a ballpark that provided fields for youth and adult leagues. By the time Derik was 10 years old, he was helping his dad by working in concessions, umpiring, and maintaining the fields. A three-sport athlete in high school and a lifelong resident of Wichita, Derik played varsity baseball at Pratt Community College and Kansas Newman College. Derik has two undergraduate majors, one in communications and one in health and physical education. Derik also has a master's degree in sport administration from Wichita State University. Derik said his parents emphasized the importance of education throughout his childhood. Today, Derik continues to value education. He routinely reads trade magazines, newspapers, and other industry-related information. Derik also pursues opportunities to improve his computer skills by attending various workshops and computer classes. As Derik states, "Computer knowledge is part of any successful career." Derik's advice for students beginning careers in sport management follows.

- Understand that entry-level jobs are not all glamour and excitement and the pay is ridiculously low. There are so many people who love sports and want to work in sports who will do it for little to nothing just for the opportunity. Future sport administrators must be willing to work, work, and then work some more.

- The internship can be a critical stepping stone that, in part, determines the ability of the student to get a full-time job.

- Network as much as possible. Building an extensive network is always helpful because we live in a "who you know" society.

- Remain mobile. Family commitments and/or inflexibility regarding where you would like to live certainly limit the scope of career opportunities.

The Greater Wichita Area Sports Commission was formally organized in 1998. Derik says he enjoys the challenges that a young organization presents. "Being a pioneer is very difficult without vision, planning, and leadership," he says. Derik estimates that salaries for sports commission jobs range between $22,000 and $30,000 for an assistant director and between $30,000 and $70,000 for an executive director. By the year 2005, Derik would like to run his own sport business or work in a collegiate athletic department.

Financing facilities has become an important issue in the entire sport industry. Speaking of the professional sport entertainment industry segment, Bud Selig (1998), commissioner of Major League Baseball, said, "Over the last few years, we've seen the greatest stadium construction boom in (baseball's) history." Genzale (1998) reports that $2.5 billion will be spent on sports construction in the next three years. Similarly, many sport participation organizations and sporting goods establishments are looking to relocate to larger quarters or expand the distribution of their products.

⚷ The healthy economy and continued demand for sport-related products creates a positive environment for the financing of a variety of sport facilities including health clubs, swimming pools, arenas, and stadiums.

Sport organizations and their public constituents have used a variety of mechanisms to fund their projects including owner contributions, commercial loans, corporate sponsorship, government loans, taxes, and bond referendums (Miller, 1997). The growth in facility construction has provided interested individuals with a number of finance-related jobs in the sport industry. For example, Fleet Financial Group provides clients in the sport industry with guidance about investment services, private placements, asset security, and loan syndications. Similarly, some banks employ individuals specifically to assist with the financial management of particular sport events and/or organizations.

Human Resource Management

Human resource management, also known as personnel management, is possibly one of the most important of all job functions in the sport industry (Miller, 1997). Employees of sport organizations represent the organization's greatest asset. Happy and content employees are more loyal to the organization, resulting in more experienced employees and reduced costs associated with turnover. Employees are responsible for the entire sport product delivery process including customer service, sport promotions, and other crucial decisions. A gap in any job function area

dilutes the quality of the sport product. Low-quality products eventually fall below break-even financial levels, causing unprofitable sport organizations to go out of business.

Human resource managers work to combine employees' talents and desires with the needs of the sport organization to create a pleasant and legally defensible work environment. They have traditionally dealt with the hiring, training, maintenance, and dismissal of employees. Recent trends, however, reveal a far broader scope associated with human resource management. Today, human resource managers organize and manage such benefits as day care for employees' kids, employee stock ownership plans, professional development opportunities, fitness facilities, and counseling services, all designed to attract and keep high-quality employees.

⚷ Employees represent the greatest asset of any sport organization.

Human resource managers in sport organizations with unions have added responsibilities. Unions negotiate agreements with management regarding compensation, working conditions, and other issues. As evident from prior professional sport work stoppages, union and management relations are critical to the sport organization's profitability. Sport managers employed outside the professional sport domain also encounter union issues when dealing with concession and merchandising vendors, security personnel, and officials and umpires.

Think of an organization where you work or have worked in the past. Did that organization create a friendly work environment conducive to productivity and efficiency? What did they do well? What could the organization have done to improve the work environment? Does tackling such issues interest you? If so, human resource management might be the profession for you.

Darryl "Doc" Rodgers

Assistant General Manager for the Cincinnati Reds

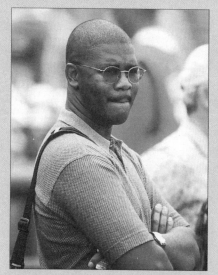

Darryl "Doc" Rodgers currently serves as the assistant general manager for the Cincinnati Reds baseball team. Doc assists the general manager in all aspects of major-league operations, including day-to-day operations, player trades, contract negotiations, and free-agent acquisitions. He also works closely with the directors of scouting and player development and has been instrumental in the development of the team's international scouting program.

Doc was a minor-league player in the Reds' organization between 1988 and 1990. In 1991 he became a pitching coach at the Reds' extended spring training camp. He served as the Cincinnati Reds' assistant for baseball operations between 1992 and 1995.

In 1995 Doc assumed the role of director of baseball administration with the Detroit Tigers. He served in this capacity until 1997 when he began his current employment with the Cincinnati Reds as assistant general manager.

Doc earned his bachelor's degree in journalism/mass communication from the University of Oklahoma in 1985. He secured his master's degree in sport management, also from the University of Oklahoma, in 1994. Doc advocates being a lifelong learner. On a daily basis, he peruses the Internet, reading the local newspaper and visiting newspaper sites from all over the country. According to Doc, "Knowledge is a necessity that sport managers cannot take lightly. Those possessing relevant knowledge will certainly do more and go farther than those without it."

Doc has three tenets of advice to students interested in careers in sport management. *First*, understand that careers will likely begin at an entry-level position. In other words, students should not plan on graduating and immediately becoming the assistant general manager for a major-league team. *Second*, Doc suggests that students know their particular sport industry segment very well. "Know everything you can about a particular sport," explains Doc. "Become an expert in the area you want to get into." *Third*, be willing to take jobs simply as a means of "getting your foot in the door." As mentioned earlier, graduating students are not likely to walk into the "dream job" upon graduating. In fact, many jobs may be less than desirable and include remedial, elementary tasks. "Maybe you have to start in the minors to get to the big leagues," he says. "If you want to work in operations and the only opening is in public relations, take it and then move over when you have the chance."

When asked about what he dislikes about his job in professional sports, Doc hesitates and then mentions the long hours and travel with some reservation. As he explains,

> I'm not sure I dislike anything about it [his job]. There's a lot of travel, and some people don't like that, but I generally enjoy it. You work long hours, but if you're doing something you like, that isn't bad. It's different every day, and the variety is motivating. The financial rewards can be great. Plus, I get to be around sports every day and meet celebrities.

Doc says that the salary range for assistant general managers and front office personnel is between $60,000 and $80,000 and $12,000 and $70,000, respectively. Doc would one day like to work as a general manager for a major-league baseball team. "Running a club as a president and chief executive officer may be an option down the road," he says enthusiastically.

Risk Management

As our society has grown increasingly litigious, risk management concerns have become more pronounced for sport administrators. Many of the issues facing sport managers today are complex and warrant advice from attorneys and other legal experts; however, all sport managers should have knowledge necessary to minimize risks within their organizations.

Risk management evolved from a predominate concern about financial losses to a more encompassing concern that includes losses of all kinds (van der Smissen, 1990). Today, the sport industry views risk management as including, but not limited to, losses resulting from inadequate or improper security, food service distribution, warnings, supervision, instruction, facility design, equipment, personnel practices, and publicity. Many sport organizations have created risk management divisions to protect against and prevent losses of all kinds. Risk management groups assist sport entities in identifying potential hazards, suggesting and implementing ways to manage potential losses, evaluating existing risk management plans, and continually improving existing risk management efforts.

Risk management is especially important in the amateur and professional sport entertainment industry segments. In addition to the concerns already listed, the entertainment industry segment is held accountable for compliance with complex rules and regulations established by governing organizations. Fearing losses to their respective athletic organizations and programs, some colleges have responded by using outside legal assistance in their compliance efforts. Many others have designated particular administrators as compliance officers, some on a full-time basis. These individuals assume leadership in helping their institutions achieve three goals (Glazier & Jones, 1991):

- Educating staff members regarding rules (usually NCAA rules) and how to obtain interpretations
- Instituting a system of checks and balances to prevent rules violations
- Conducting internal audits to gauge the effectiveness of the compliance system

The consequences of compliance-related failures have been well chronicled in the mass

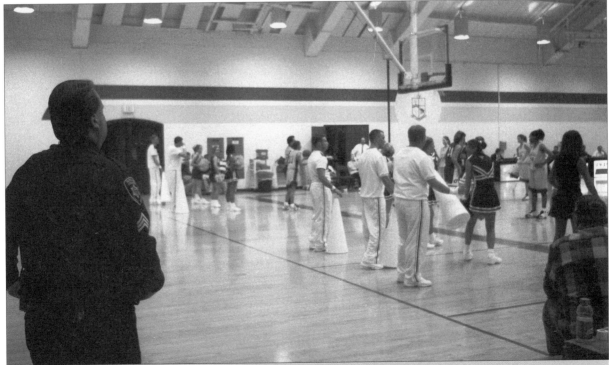

Ensuring adequate security at sporting events has become a responsibility of sport management.

© iPhotoNews.com

media. Texas Tech University and the University of Minnesota represent two institutions that made headlines in 1998 and 1999 for NCAA rule violations ("NCAA slaps Tech even harder," 1998; "These are extremely serious charges," 1999). They join a long list of programs that have faced sanctions and national embarrassment resulting in forgone revenues, loss of prestige, and competitive disadvantages. A university compliance officer strives to keep the athletic department in compliance with the rules and regulations detailed in the lengthy NCAA compliance manual; university policies and procedures; and local, state, and federal legislation and ordinances.

🔑 Risk management involves taking steps to reduce losses of all kinds. Risk management requires the support of *all* employees, from top management down to the front line.

Marketing Management

Marketing management represents a burgeoning career opportunity for qualified students. Some even suggest that the area of sport marketing and promotions is the key to success for any sport product, whether it is a new running shoe, a sport clinic, or a sporting event. A great sport product, offered at an affordable price and located in a favorable location, generates little revenue unless people are aware of it.

Sport marketers may spend time working in a variety of marketing management areas which include but are not limited to the following:

Research and Development—**Research and development** can range from sophisticated analyses of consumer opinions, economic impact studies, and so on, to focus groups or brainstorming sessions on how to better package and present products.

Sport Promotion—**Sport promotion** comprises the activities undertaken by sport marketers to promote interest in contests with the purpose of increasing attendance or television viewing of a sporting event. **Promotions** are part of what is used to "promote" and often involve special deals to consum-

ers and advertising opportunities to sponsors. Promotions come in a wide range of forms, including games, product sampling opportunities, premium giveaways, price reductions, player appearances, camps, clinics, and so on (Miller, Shaad, Burch, & Turner, 1998).

Sponsorship—**Sport sponsorship** represents an exchange between a company and a sport organization. For example, a sponsoring company may provide either cash or in-kind resources (e.g., computers, consulting expertise) in exchange for title sponsorship of an event such as the Rolex Intercollegiate Tennis Championships. Sponsorships represent powerful advertising opportunities in the form of name recognition for sponsoring companies.

Advertising—"Advertising is information placed in the media by an identified sponsor that pays for the time or space" (Cutlip, Center, & Broom, 1994, p. 10). Many sport-related organizations both purchase **advertising** to promote their events or services and sell advertising in programs, for example, as a way to generate revenues.

Merchandising—**Merchandising** efforts extend far beyond just apparel. Customers visiting sport specialty stores may choose from an array of products including computer software, toys, automobile accessories, decorations, kitchenware, and pasta shaped in the form of various team mascots. Furthermore, sport trading cards continue to be big business with some of the rare or high-demand cards commanding thousands of dollars.

Distribution—**Distribution** connects the sport product or service with the ultimate consumer. For sporting goods manufacturers, distribution concerns include building relationships with distributors and retailers, securing optimal shelf space, and maintaining low-cost product transportation systems. For sport managers in the entertainment or participation sectors, distribution concerns may include facility design, accessibility, flexibility, and attractiveness, since the sport product (e.g., game) is produced and consumed in the same location (e.g., stadium).

Students of sport management who are educated in the area of sport marketing often find they have a great deal of appeal to employers in all sport industry segments. A background in sport marketing, coupled with related job experience, provides individuals with lateral as well as vertical career opportunities.

Public Relations Management

The relationship between sport and the mass media is reciprocal, meaning each significantly influences the other (Coakley, 1998). The media needs sport to attract consumers. Sport needs the media to build fan interest. More than 8,000 sport events are televised live each year, and each week brings another new sport publication to the market (Helitzer, 1995). The NFL's recent $17.6 billion windfall in television rights fees represents the magnitude of the media's influence on the sport entertainment industry segment (Brockington, 1998). The mass media finds amateur sports attractive as well. NBC contracted to pay $715 million for the right to broadcast the 2000 Olympic games from Sydney, Australia (Helitzer, 1995). Coverage of college, high school, and other amateur sporting events represents the mainstay of various newscasts and news publications.

A number of individuals within sport organizations work in **media management**. Almost all professional and college sport organizations have at least one person assigned to media relations. These public relations practitioners, often known as sport information directors, produce media guides and programs, develop Web pages, track statistics, arrange interviews, supply story ideas, and generally service media requests. These individuals are also an integral link between the organization and its stakeholders.

Other sport managers work with the media by negotiating broadcast contracts. The importance of such work cannot be overemphasized. A report summarizing revenue sources for the Big Ten conference in 1996–97 indicated that of $63.7 million in total income, $32.9 million was a result of television royalties ("Big Ten," 1998).

While the media may be more integrally involved in sport than any other industry in the United States, **public relations** involves much more than just media relations. Sport entertainment organizations often employ individuals

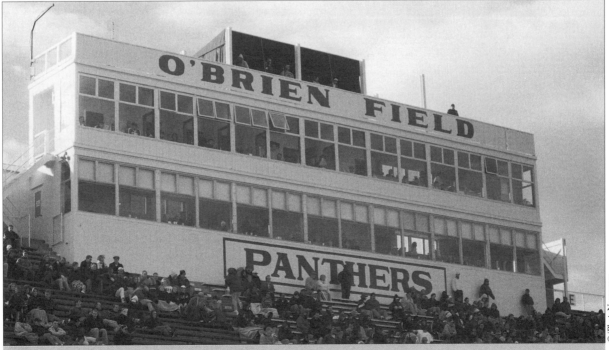

Media management is increasingly important at all levels of sport.

© iPhotoNews.com

specifically to work in fan relations, and sporting goods businesses generally realize the advantages of having customer relations employees who provide a variety of services ranging from handling complaints to giving special instructions regarding the assembly of a product.

Program Management

Program management is familiar to all sport industry segments. Health clubs, parks and recreation departments, athletic programs, and sport services all are involved with the provision and delivery of sport programs. A parks and recreation department, for example, may offer an aerobics program, an aquatics program, and a racquet sports program. Each program, in turn, is staffed with its own employees who deliver desired activities (e.g., lessons, clinics, tournaments).

Program management is discussed last because it effectively illustrates the overlap of all the other function areas. Each of the function areas discussed earlier incorporates program management considerations at some point. For example,

- *Event management*—Programs represent individual events (e.g., aerobic dance class, a single basketball game) and require that similar professional roles be performed. For example, an aerobic dance class at a health club, although only one of many program offerings, still requires planning, scheduling, equipment, monitoring, and so on.

- *Financial management*—Programs must keep expenses within budgeted amounts and generate necessary revenues.

- *Human resource management*—Programs must be staffed with qualified and competent personnel.

- *Legal management*—Programs must comply with public accommodation laws, the Americans With Disabilities Act, and other relevant legislation.

- *Marketing management*—Only programs that are demanded by the target market should be offered.

- *Public relations management*—Programs should be promoted effectively and crises handled professionally.

Think of a sport organization with which you are familiar. What programs are offered? Do you have the skills and aptitudes necessary to run such programs? If you are interested in program management, what skills would you need to develop?

Program management activities vary across function areas and sport industry segments. Two of the more common task areas include scheduling and facility/equipment maintenance.

Scheduling

Scheduling is one of the primary concerns for program managers. Many a Little League coordinator has dealt with scheduling complications stemming from too many teams with access to too few facilities. Sport entertainment administrators must also address scheduling and related considerations. For example, Texas Christian University recently canceled scheduled football games with the University of Nebraska, citing the wide disparity in the two programs' success levels ("No toughies," 1998). Scheduling travel can also be a complex procedure. Some athletic programs have administrators whose primary function is to coordinate travel.

Facility/Equipment Maintenance

Maintenance of facilities and equipment represents a crucial task for program managers. Those working in sport participation organizations must maintain and update facilities in order to meet the needs and demands of consumers. Included is the responsibility to keep present facilities and equipment clean, safe, and operative. In addition, sport managers must monitor the external environment (e.g., competitors, new product developments, and changing consumer demographics and/or psychographics) for new products and other developments that may enhance consumer offerings and satisfaction.

Employment Outlook

The sport management industry offers a wealth of job opportunities in a variety of industry segments and function areas. It is difficult to determine objectively which are the most popular industry segments, as they all appear to be hiring qualified students of sport management. A review of various trade magazines and Web sites provides insight regarding available job opportunities. Table 17.1 shows a list of job opportunities submitted to *The Insider—SportsCareers* between February 23 and August 14, 1998. In this publication alone, 2,680 jobs were advertised during a six-month time period.

The 21st century will provide many exciting employment opportunities for qualified individuals interested in sport management careers. The proliferation of amateur and professional sport teams, society's growing interest in health and fitness, progressive technology, eclectic consumers with varying needs and demands, and a healthy economy explain, in part, the promising growth.

Similarly impressive numbers of job opportunities in intercollegiate athletics were advertised in the *NCAA News*. Table 17.2 lists job opportunities in collegiate sports advertised in the *NCAA News* in a recent 12-month period.

TABLE 17.1
Job Opportunities in Sport Management

Job category	Number of jobs (approximate)
College athletics	286
Facilities	56
Health and fitness	486
Sporting goods	574
Sports media	431
Recreation administration	132
Events management	51
Professional teams	104
Professional services	508
Organizations, administration	52
Total	*2,680*

Data from *The Insider—SportsCareers* (Chandler, Arizona: Franklin Covey Publishers).

TABLE 17.2
Job Opportunities in Collegiate Sports

NCAA job market (March 1997–February 1998)	Number of jobs (approximate)
Academic coordinator	30
Academic counselor	27
Administrative assistant	17
Associate athletic director	37
Athletic director	17
Administrative business manager	20
Compliance	60
Development	48
Equipment manager	19
Executive director	15
Facilities	26
Fundraising	9
Life skills coordinator	6
Marketing/promotions	96
Public relations	17
Recreation	1
Sports information	145
Senior women's administrator	20
Ticket office	44
Recruiting	3
Operations	2
Total	*773*

As you read through the preceding descriptions of careers in sport management, did you put yourself in the picture? What positions felt the most comfortable to you? What tasks excited you? Perhaps you found yourself thinking, I'd hate to do that. Now that you have some idea of where your interests lie, what kinds of educational and practical experiences do you think will help you move toward a specific career?

Education and Qualifications

The National Association of Sport and Physical Education—North American Society for Sport Management Joint Task Force (NASPE-NASSM) developed a "competency-based minimum body of knowledge" for students of sport management (NASPE-NASSM Joint Task Force, 1993, p. 159). Competency standards exist for undergraduate, master's, and doctoral degree programs. Approximately 185 universities and colleges offer sport management degrees (Stan Brassie, personal communication, 1998). The core content (i.e., sport management knowledge) expected of students graduating with an undergraduate degree in sport management includes the following 10 competency areas.

Sociocultural dimensions in sport—Required content includes, but is not limited to, sport and gender, race, and disability; violence and deviant behavior in sport; international cultures and sport; and sport in American education.

Management and leadership in sport—Required content includes, but is not limited to, functions of management, strategic planning process, organizational structures, personal management style, theories of leadership, and human resource management.

Ethics in sport management—Required content includes, but is not limited to, professional ethics, rights, and responsibilities; theories of ethics; professional codes of ethics; and personal and management values.

Marketing in sport—Required content includes, but is not limited to, definitions of market-ing and sport marketing, marketing mix, sponsorship, preparation of the marketing proposal, merchandising, and consumer behavior.

Communication in sport—Required content includes, but is not limited to, interpersonal communication, media and sport, electronic media, print media, public speaking, mass communication and sport, and computer application.

Budget and finance in sport—Required content includes, but is not limited to, basic accounting principles; financial statements; budget development; spreadsheet utilization; and budgets as a method of control, organization, and reallocation.

Legal aspects of sport—Required content includes, but is not limited to, tort law, risk management procedures, product liability, constitutional law, contract law, administrative/strategy law, and the legal system.

Economics in sport—Required content includes, but is not limited to, delineation of micro and macro economic principles, economic impact principles, economic theory applied to stadiums and arenas, economic growth of the sport industry in the 20th century, and concepts of competitive strategy (supply and demand).

Governance in sport—Required content includes, but is not limited to, identification of governing bodies in professional and amateur sport, authority and functions of various governing bodies, requirements for membership in governing bodies, and sanctions and appeal processes used by governing bodies.

Field experience in sport management—Field experience in sport management includes practicums or internships. Students must accumulate "400 hours of hands-on field experience subsequent to the junior year . . . under the supervision of a qualified onsite professional" (NASPE-NASSM Sport Management Review Council, 1993, p. 21).

The core content (i.e., sport management knowledge) expected of students graduating with master's degrees in sport management includes the following nine competency areas:

Sociocultural context of sport—Required content includes, but is not limited to, ethnic and gender patterns causing barriers in sport, social stratification and mobility opportunities from sport, and sport as a microcosm of society.

Management and leadership in sport—Required content includes, but is not limited to, negotiation, human resource management/ development, policy development, effective management practices, leadership theory, decision making, and problem solving.

Ethics in sport management—Required content includes, but is not limited to, moral and ethical development theories, models of ethical analysis, and codes of professional ethics.

Marketing in sport—Required content includes, but is not limited to, internal and external sources of marketing information; marketing information systems; promotion methods, mix, and strategies; sport licensing; and the development of marketing, sponsorship plans, or research studies.

Public relations in sport—Required content includes employee relations, community relations, media relations, and customer relations.

Financial management in sport—Required content includes, but is not limited to, principles of budgeting, practical budgeting, sources of revenue, fund-raising methods, economic impact, and theories and methods of financial planning.

Legal aspects of sport—Required content includes, but is not limited to, tort law, risk management procedures, contract law, constitutional law, administrative/statutory law, legal research, the legal system, and labor/antitrust law.

Research in sport—Required content includes, but is not limited to, research questions and hypotheses for sport management, information retrieval, and field data collection techniques and data analysis of sport information.

Field experience in sport management—Required content includes field experiences (either practicums or internships) in sport management.

Students pursuing a doctoral degree in sport management are also expected to have a background that includes the previous content areas. Students lacking education in these areas take necessary prerequisite course work as defined by the degree-granting institution. Doctoral students receive significant training in research methodology including the "gathering, analyzing, interpreting, and reporting" of data (NASPE-NASSM Joint Task Force, 1993, p. 168). Additional academic study focuses on three areas of specialization available within the sport management doctoral degree program. Each degree-granting institution defines the specialization areas available through their particular programs, and doctoral students choose three from those the institution offers. NASPE-NASSM identifies a variety of specialization areas that doctoral institutions might offer, including, but not limited to, the following:

- Sport marketing
- Organizational theory in sport
- Sport foundations
- Sport finance
- Information management
- Managerial accounting
- Sport law
- Sport economics
- Human resource management in sport

Students earning a doctoral degree in sport management must also undertake an internship (NASPE-NASSM Joint Task Force, 1993).

Although all of the content areas listed are critical to the attainment of a quality sport management education, the internship and field experiences deserve special emphasis. Sport organizations look for people with practical, real-world sport experience. Because the sport management industry is very competitive, the references, knowledge, and work experiences that can be gained from internship/practicum site supervisors are invaluable. Consequently, the internship or field experience(s) is essential to the student's ability to secure a job.

Students may get internships working in any one of the sport industry segments discussed earlier. Responsibilities associated with each internship tend to be situation specific. For example, an internship at a Division I institution may be very specialized. In other words, the student intern may work specifically in one of the professional areas such as compliance, marketing, facilities, operations, or tickets. On the other hand, an internship at a Division III institution may combine roles. In this situation, the student intern may work in a variety of areas including marketing, facilities, operations, and tickets.

Sport management students are advised to capitalize on available internships with credible sport management organizations that provide learning opportunities.

All of the competency areas identified by the NASPE-NASSM Joint Task Force are either directly or indirectly identified in figures 17.2 and 17.3. As you can see, each function area is somewhat dependent on, and linked to, the others. Moreover, a multitude of benefits can be gained from an understanding of each area. For example, if you worked in a youth sports program, you would be better able to provide successful program offerings if you had an understanding of budgetary limitations, managerial issues, consumer behaviors, risk management principles, and societal implications. Similarly, if you worked at an Olympic event, you would have a better understanding of the intricacies involved and communication required of individuals working in different function areas of a large event. You would learn, for example, that promotions cannot be executed without the close cooperation of the people working in the area of facilities. Sound effects (e.g., music, clapping hands), lighting, fixtures, and so on, must all be coordinated so that the fans are entertained, the sponsor's promotion is flawlessly executed, and promotion participants are not injured.

When you understand how various issues and function areas influence your product, be it a sport event, clinic, or apparel item, you are better able to communicate with colleagues, employees, and customers. Your conceptual understanding makes you a valuable asset to your sport organization. In addition, by being knowledgeable in a variety of competency areas, you enhance your marketability in the profession.

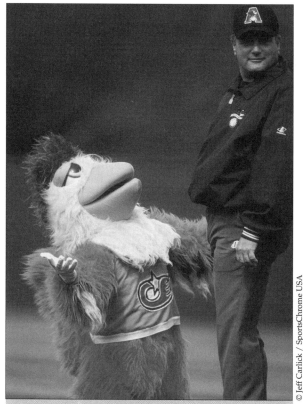

© Jeff Carlick / SportsChrome USA

The San Diego Chicken and similar mascots are used by sport managers to attract spectators and increase the entertainment value of a sport event.

Multifaceted individuals can make decisions that are in the best interest of the sport organization as a whole rather than decisions that benefit only particular business functions of the organization.

Sport management students are required to study different curriculums than students studying for careers as teachers, coaches, personal trainers, athletic trainers, and so on. As you have seen, sport management students are often not required to take courses in motor learning, exercise physiology, or anatomy and physiology. However, course work in theoretical kinesiology can significantly enhance a person's knowledge and marketability. For example, students working in the health club industry can improve their marketability by combining their sport management degree with course work in appropriate areas of theoretical kinesiology. This will enable a sport manager to make better hiring decisions and provide better supervision.

Inside Advice for Sport Management Students

As you know from reading about other physical activity professions in previous chapters, simply meeting educational requirements will not ensure your success as a sport management professional. In addition to completing the required courses and obtaining your degree, you will need practical experience in your area of interest. Such experience is invaluable in helping you improve your communication skills and enhance your problem-solving skills. Also, do not underestimate the value of a mentor, someone in the field who can give you practical insights into your new career. Finally, be sure to keep up with the profession by contacting sport management organizations and reading professional journals. Table 17.3 provides a list of resources to get you started.

Practical Experience

You should always be at work building your résumé. Practical experience is a necessity in a competitive job market such as that in the sport industry. Just about all programs have internship requirements, and the virtues of such requirements have already been described. However, the best internships often go to students with the most job experience. Try to find part-time work in the sport industry, and volunteer for special events that may arise (e.g., fun runs, triathlons, Special Olympics). Such experiences can be used to apply what you learned in the classroom to the job setting while simultaneously gaining valuable résumé material.

Mentors

Mentors are people working in a student's chosen profession who seek to provide students with learning opportunities, responsibility, knowledge, and critical contact people in the industry. Students with mentors gain insights they cannot get in the classroom, in addition to having an advocate working on their behalf when seeking future jobs. Some mentor relationships occur spontaneously when someone with education and experience takes an interest in a student. You can also arrange for a mentor directly by asking someone to be your mentor. A variety of people can serve as mentors including job supervisors, university professors, or family friends. In fact, you can have more than one mentor. Multiple mentors enhance the knowledge and opportunities to which you will be exposed.

Communication Skills

Sport managers working in virtually every function area discussed in this chapter need strong communication skills. Most undergraduate curriculums require students to take a minimum number of credit hours to facilitate development of these skills. However, because most of the jobs in the sport industry are service oriented, we encourage sport management students to take communications-related courses beyond the minimum number required. The ability to communicate effectively with others, write well, and use new communication technologies cannot be overemphasized.

Problem-Solving Skills

Sport managers making hiring decisions want qualified employees with the necessary educational and employment background to be successful on the job. Another characteristic that often distinguishes successful practitioners is their ability to analyze a problem effectively and generate creative solutions. We encourage you to enroll in courses that will assist in the development of such skills and also to seek out work experiences that require such skills. For example, by volunteering to work in a fitness center's membership drive you will gain more valuable experience than if you simply checked members in at the front desk.

Generalize

Sport-related jobs are in high demand. As previously mentioned, by working in a variety of function areas you increase your marketability. Students with broad backgrounds have more options than those who specialize at the undergraduate level. Graduate school is often a more appropriate time to seek specialization in one of the many professional roles.

TABLE 17.3
Sport Management Resources

Publications

SportsTravel
Schneider Publishing Co., Inc.
13274 Fiji Way, Fourth Floor
Marina Del Rey, CA 90292
Phone: 310-577-3700
Fax: 310-577-3715
www.sportstravelnet.com
ISSN: 1091-5354

Journal of Sport Management
Human Kinetics
P.O. Box 5076
Champaign, IL 61825-5076
www.humankinetics.com
ISSN: 0888-4773

The Sport Marketing Quarterly
Fitness Information Technology, Inc.
P.O. Box 4425
University Avenue
Morgantown, WV 26504
Phone: 304-599-3482
E-mail: fit@fitinfotech.com
www.fitinfotech.com
ISSN: 1061-6934

Fitness Management
Sales and Administrative Offices
4160 Wilshire Blvd.
Los Angeles, CA 90010
Phone: 323-964-4800
Fax: 323-964-4841
E-mail: fitmgt@earthlink.net
www.fitnessworld.com
ISSN: 0882-0481

The Sports, Parks and Recreation Law Reporter
PRC Publishing Inc.
3976 Fulton Drive, N.W.
Canton, OH 44718
Phone: 330-492-6063
ISSN: 0893-8210

Club Industry
PRIMEDIA Intertec
1300 Virginia Drive, Ste. 400
Fort Washington, PA 19034
Phone: 215-643-8000
www.clubindustry.com
ISSN: 0747-8283

Athletic Management
P.O. Box 2122
Lenox, MA 01240-9924
Phone: 607-257-6970
Fax: 413-637-4343
ISSN: 1041-5432

Journal of Legal Aspects of Sport
5840 South Ernest Street
Terre Haute, IN 47802
Phone: 812-237-2186
ISSN: 1072-0316

Street and Smith's Sports Business Journal
120 West Morehead St., Suite 310
Charlotte, NC 28202
Phone: 800-829-9839
ISSN: 1098-5972

Seton Hall Journal of Sport Law
Publisher: Seton Hall School of Law
ISSN: 1059-4310
Managing Editor
Seton Hall Journal of Sport Law
Seton Hall School of Law
One Newark Center
Newark, NJ 07102
Phone: 201-642-8239

Marquette Sports Law Journal
Publisher: Marquette Univ. Law School
Marquette University Law School
P.O. Box 1881
Milwaukee, Wisconsin 53201-1881
Phone: 414-288-5815
ISSN: 1057-6029

Entertainment & Sports Law Review
Publisher: University of Miami Entertainment &
Sports Law Review
P.O. Box 248087
Coral Gables, Florida 33124-8087
Phone: 305-284-6887

Journal of Legal Aspects of Sport
Publisher: Society for the Study of Legal Aspects of
Sport
Tom Sawyer, Executive Director
5840 S. Ernest St.
Terre Haute, IN 47802
Phone: 812-237-2186
Contact: Tom Sawyer, 812-533-0200

International Journal of Sport Management
American Press Publishers
520 Commonwealth Ave.
Boston, MA 02215-2605
Phone: 617-247-0022

Mark's SportsLaw News
members.aol.com/sportslaw/LSN.html
Mark Conrad
Fordham University
113 West 60th Street, 6th Floor
New York, N.Y. 10002
Phone: 212-636-7975
Fax: 212-744-4345
E-mail: sportslaw@aol.com

Organizations

College Sports Information Directors of America
Maxey Parrish, President
Baylor University
150 Bear Run
Waco, TX 76711
Contact: Maxey Parrish, 254-445-3063

National Association of Collegiate Directors of Athletics
P.O. Box 16428
Cleveland, OH 44116
Phone: 440-892-4000
Fax: 440-892-4407
www.nacda.com

North American Society for Sport Management (NASSM)
106 Main Street, Suite 344
Houlton, ME 04730-0991
Phone: 506-453-5010
Fax: 506-453-3511
E-mail: nassm@unb.ca
www.unb.ca/web/sportmanagement/nassm.htm

Society for the Study of Legal Aspects in Sport & Physical Activity (SSLASPA)
Tom Sawyer, Executive Director
5840 S. Ernest St.
Terre Haute, IN 47802
Phone: 812-237-2186
Contact: Tom Sawyer, 812-533-0200
http://www.ithaca.edu/sslaspa/

European Association for Sport Management (EASM)
EASM Bureau, ISEF Firenze
Viuzzo di Gattaia 9
50125 FIRENZE - ITALIA
Fax : + 39 55 241799
E-mail : easm@cesitl.unifi.it

Sport Management Association of Australia and New Zealand (SMAANZ)
Secretary SMAANZ, C/- Sport Management Program
Deakin University
221 Burwood Highway
Burwood, Australia, 3125
Contact Hans Westerbeek,
E-mail: westerbk@deakin.edu.au

Job and sport management related Internet sites

www.onlinesports.com

www.sportscareers.com

www.sports-forum.com

If you want to pursue a career in sport management, do you have the skills and aptitudes mentioned in the text? Do you communicate clearly and confidently with people? Are you adept at problem solving? What types of experiences would be useful to pursue during your undergraduate years? Would you like to have a mentor? Have you considered seeking out volunteer opportunities or part-time work within sport organizations to gain practical experience?

Ashley Jones

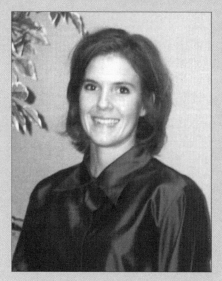

Administrative Assistant, Northern Texas Professional Golf Association Sectional Office

A 1998 sport administration graduate, Ashley Jones is beginning a career in sport management. As an administrative assistant for the Northern Texas PGA sectional office, Ashley attends to a variety of duties, including customer service and the creation of marketing proposals and board of director correspondence. She also serves as a liaison with sponsors, vendors, and new clients. The Northern Texas PGA sectional office, located at Woodbridge Golf Club in Wylie, Texas, has 11 employees. It is one of 41 sections that comprise the PGA of America and has a professional membership of 675. Its mission is to promote the enjoyment of and involvement in the game of golf and to provide services to the golf professional and the golf industry.

Like many sport administration students, Ashley faced a highly competitive job market upon graduation. However, her previous experience in the golf industry helped to distinguish her in the field. Specifically, Ashley had attended Wichita State University on a golf scholarship and had considerable experience in the industry during her playing career. More important, she spent two summers serving as an intern for the Kansas Women's Golf Association. As a result of her internship experience, Ashley developed skills in tournament direction and event management. Those skills serve her well in her current job.

Ashley readily admits that she is working as a generalist and says she sees that as a great advantage at this early stage in her career. She notes that by working in a variety of professional roles, she will both gain additional competencies and enjoy the opportunity to sample several areas of responsibility. Ashley indicates that she is especially interested in marketing and public relations activities but could discover new interests as a result of her job experience.

Ashley offers four pieces of advice to students working toward careers in sport management:

- Explore all aspects of the sport industry. It is such a broad field that you can do all sorts of things of interest. Don't shortchange yourself. Make sure you know what your options are.

- Depending on the industry sector and professional role you choose, you may need to pursue additional educational opportunities even after gaining your bachelor's degree. Some students may go on to get master's degrees in sport management. Others seek other master's degrees or even law degrees.

- Appreciate the opportunity you have to gain a degree in sport management. Despite the growth of sport, many people outside the profession still do not know that sport management degrees exist. When they learn of such degrees, many are envious of those who have them.

- You must have experience to get a job in the field. Sport managers making hiring decisions want to know how candidates have supplemented the classes they have taken with summer jobs, internships, and volunteer opportunities. Those without such experiences will not fare well in this highly competitive field.

Wrap-Up

The sport management professions offer a broad range of exciting career opportunities for qualified individuals. From sporting goods retail to commercial bowling alleys, sport managers in managerial and administrative positions are looking for individuals with a sport management education. Education, work experience, professionalism, volunteerism, networking, a good work ethic, and a positive attitude are all characteristics welcomed by sport management employers.

Individuals moving into sport management careers often find themselves holding jobs that are interesting because of the variety they offer, exciting because of the activities they involve, and challenging because of the ever-changing nature of the field. Not surprisingly, many sport administrators report high levels of job satisfaction. If you are looking for a fulfilling job and have a keen interest in sport, the sport management professions may be for you.

Study Questions

1. Discuss the breadth of the sport industry and the related career opportunities it provides with specific reference to the industry segments discussed throughout this chapter.

2. Explain how the following would help an individual succeed in the sport industry: (a) good communication skills, (b) problem-solving skills, (c) practical experience, and (d) a mentor.

3. What type of course work and related academic content does a quality sport management program provide?

4. Identify three of the functional areas within the sport industry and elaborate on the types of jobs that might be specific to these professional roles.

5. Identify two existing sport organizations for each segment of the sport industry.

6. Elaborate on the type of sport management–related job you would be most attracted to and why.

Glossary

abilities—Genetically endowed perceptual, cognitive, motor, metabolic, and personality traits that are susceptible to little or no modification by practice or training.

academic learning time—Time in which students are appropriately and successfully engaged in lesson activities.

acclimatization—Physiological adaptations to changes in natural environmental conditions (e.g., temperature, altitude).

accountability—Encouraging students to be responsible and answerable for their own actions.

active learning time—Time in which students are engaged in lesson activities.

activities of daily living (ADLs)—Self-sufficient physical activities involving personal grooming, dressing, eating, walking, and using the toilet.

activity experience—Training in, observation of, practice of, or participation in physical activity.

adenosine triphosphate (ATP)—High-energy phosphate compound used by cells to do work.

advertising—"Information placed in the media by an identified sponsor that pays for the time or space" (Cutlip, Center & Broom, 1994, p.10).

aerobic—In the presence of oxygen.

aesthetic experience—A subjective experience in which sensations appeal to our senses of beauty, grace, and artistic appreciation.

aesthetic values—Conceptions about beauty, taste, artistic production, and artistic judgment.

aggression—Behavior intended to inflict harm or injury on another person.

alveoli—Small hollow air sacs in the lungs where gas exchange between the air and blood occurs.

amateur sport entertainment—Sport industry sector comprised of organizations/events that attract spectators to watch amateur athletes compete (e.g., interscholastic and intercollegiate athletics).

amenorrhea—No more than three menses per year.

anaerobic—In the absence of oxygen.

analytical framework—Set of general ideas or concepts used to make sense of information.

anxiety—A negative response to a stressful situation characterized by apprehension and feelings of threat.

arousal—A state of physical and psychological activation or readiness.

ascetic experiences—Experiences of pain, discomfort, self-denial, sacrifice, and delayed gratification that are often associated with strenuous physical fitness and training programs.

athletic training room—A health-care facility, usually associated with high school, collegiate, or professional athletic teams, that specializes in the health care needs of athletes.

attitudes—Relatively stable mind-sets toward physical activity.

authenticity—Property of historical evidence; examination of evidence by a scholar determines that it is what it purports to be.

behavior modification—The use of extrinsic reinforcers such as reward and punishment to shape human behavior.

biochemistry—The chemistry of living organisms.

biomechanics—(a) Study of the structure and function of biological systems using principles and methods of mechanics (Hatze, 1974); (b) interdiscipline (Winter, 1985) that uses the basic laws which govern motion of all living beings to investigate human movement.

Borg scale—A rating system for determining how much effort an individual is experiencing while engaged in physical activity.

breadth of capacity—Achieving a low to moderate level of competence in a wide range of physical activities.

burnout—An extreme state of mental, emotional, and physical exhaustion that occurs due to chronic stress.

capitation—A concept whereby a health care provider is paid a pre-established amount per person per year regardless of the number of services provided.

cardiac output—The amount of blood pumped out of one side of the heart per minute.

cardiopulmonary rehabilitation—Exercise programs that are designed to improve the function of the heart, lungs, and/or vascular system.

carpal tunnel syndrome—A type of cumulative trauma disorder to the hand and wrist, usually suffered by carpenters, typists, packers, assembly line workers, and others who repeat the same movements for several hours each day.

change—State of becoming different.

choking—Popular term for performing poorly in very important, yet stressful situations.

clinical settings—Health and fitness facilities that operate within hospital or medical facilities.

closed loop theory—A theory developed by Adams (1971) that explained how slow positioning movements were controlled.

closed skill—A motor skill in which performers must coordinate their movements with a predictable, usually stationary, environment.

code of ethical principles and standards—Usually published and disseminated by professional associations to their members in order to ensure that clients' welfare is always given top priority by practitioners.

cognitive psychology—Theory based on the idea that humans process information from the environment and behave based on their appraisal and interpretation of the situation.

cognitive skills—Human acts that require complex modes of thought, including rational analysis and problem solving, in order to achieve a predetermined goal. Most professionals rely on highly developed cognitive skills.

cohesion—The tendency for groups to stick together and remain united in pursuing goals.

community settings—Health and fitness facilities that operate within community centers, churches, or other nonprofit organizations such as YMCAs or Jewish Community Centers.

competent bystanders—Well-behaved students who avoid participation without being noticed.

competition—A principle or framework for organizing physical activity in which participants compare their performances to each other's or to a standard for the purpose of increasing enjoyment.

compressive loading—When forces applied to an object push towards each other.

conditioning—The temporary end state of training reflected in the performer's possessing an adequate level of strength, endurance, and flexibility in order to carry out desired tasks.

context variables—Conditions of the learning environment.

convection—The exchange of heat between the body and a moving fluid (water or air).

credibility—Property of historical evidence; examination of evidence by a scholar determines that it is believable (i.e., consistent, accurate, valid).

critical and poetic reasoning—Skeptical criticism of traditional philosophical thinking, combined with tentative, suggestive, nontraditional analyses.

critical component—The aspect of an activity deemed most important for successfully performing that activity.

cumulative trauma disorder—Injuries to muscle, tendons, nerves, and ligaments brought about through repetitive motion of a body part.

custodial care facility—Long-term care facility that caters to the medical, rehabilitational, and specialized needs of a patient, including assistance with the activities of daily living.

deductive reasoning—Form of logic that starts with a broad, general principle and moves toward specific cases that follow from it.

degrees of freedom—The number of dimensions in which a joint can move: for example, the elbow has one degree of freedom (flexion-extension) while the hip has three (flexion-extension, lateral, rotational); often used to explain movement complexity by summing all the degrees of freedom of the joints involved in a movement.

delayed onset muscle soreness—Muscle soreness that occurs 24 to 48 hours after physical activity.

deprofessionalization—Erosion of a profession's status in society when it no longer maintains a monopoly on the provision of specific services to the community.

depth of capacity—Achieving a high level of competence in a narrow range of physical activities.

descriptive and speculative reasoning—Form of logic in which the essential qualities of one example of an object or event are described.

discipline—Organized body of knowledge considered worthy of study, usually studied in a college or university curriculum.

disinterested spectatorship—A form of watching sport contests in which the observer is nonpartisan in his or her feelings about the outcome.

dispositions—Short-term, highly variable psychological states that may affect our enjoyment of physical activity.

distribution—The process of connecting the sport product or service with the ultimate consumer.

dualism—Belief in the separateness of mind and body.

dynamical systems—A view of movement in which there is a more direct link between perception (e.g., vision) and action such that movements are organized by this direct link as opposed to the need for a motor program to control the movement

ego orientation—Defining competence in an activity on the basis of how one's performance compares with that of others; participants with this orientation tend to approach competition from an extrinsic perspective.

electromyography (EMG)—A system for monitoring and recording the electrical activity in muscles.

emblems—Body movements such as hand signals that can be translated easily into explicit messages.

emotional expression—The tendency to reveal something about our internal emotional states through physical activity.

emotions—Subjective reactions to changes in internal or external states.

Employee Assistance Programs (EAP)—Programs supported by business and industries to help employees with personal problems that may affect their work performance.

endurance—The ability to sustain physical activity for prolonged time periods.

engaged time—Time that students spend engaged in activity.

ergogenic aids—Any substance or technique (other than training) that improves athletic performance either by delaying fatigue or increasing work capacity (Anshel et al. 1991).

ergonomic work station—A safe and effective work environment where individual worker characteristics have been considered in the design and placement of equipment. Computer keyboards, chair adjustments, desk heights, and lighting are examples of equipment considerations in the creation of an ergonomic work station.

ergonomics, or occupational biomechanics—The use of a biomechanical approach to design the workplace by designing tasks, facilities and equipment to function effectively with the worker (Chaffin & Andersson, 1991).

ergonomists—Engineers who seek to improve the safety and efficiency of work through analysis of workers' movements and the conditions in the workplace.

ethical values—Conceptions about right and wrong actions of individuals.

ethnic group—Group of people who share important and distinct cultural traditions.

ethnography—Research technique that typically involves multiple research processes and includes recording notes while observing in a social setting over a relatively long period of time.

event management—The planning, organizing, execution, and evaluation of sport-related events (e.g., Super Bowl, Little League baseball tournaments).

exercise—Physical activity intended to improve one's health and/or alter the appearance of one's body.

experiential knowledge—Self-knowledge and knowledge about physical activity that is derived from performing and/or watching physical activity.

expressive movements—Movements employed in a physical activity as a way of expressing something of one's own emotion or personality; differentiated from instrumental movements.

extrinsic approaches to physical activity—Valuing physical activity because of the benefits that come from participating.

extrinsic motivation—Motivation that is derived from pursuing and obtaining rewards outside of the activity itself, such as money and status.

face-to-face contact activities—Contests such as football, wrestling, basketball, and soccer in which individuals interact with opponents' attempts to achieve the goal by physically manipulating their movements.

face-to-face noncontact activities—Contests such as volleyball, tennis, and baseball in which individuals interact with opponents in order to maximize their own chances of winning, but do not physically manipulate their opponents.

fans—Spectators who identify with a particular athlete or team and have a vested interest in the outcome of a contest.

feedback (intrinsic and extrinsic)—Information about the movement provided to the learner during and after a movement; this information may come from external (e.g., instructor, videotape) or internal sources (muscles, joints, via the nervous system).

financial management—Tasks involving financial-related activities such as the prudent investment and use of assets, monetary development opportunities, and short-term and long-term budgeting.

flow—Total immersion in an experience of peak functioning or "being in the zone."

for-profit sport participation—Sport industry sector comprised of organizations that operate for-profit and offer participation opportunities to patrons (e.g., bowling centers, fitness centers, miniature golf courses).

force—A push or a pull on a body. Forces can act from outside of the body (*external*) or from inside of a body (*internal*).

free time—Personal time that has not been encumbered with obligations; also called discretionary time.

functional learning time—Time in which students are appropriately and successfully engaged in lesson activities.

game—Activity in which rules specify a goal to be achieved and also limit the means used to reach the goal; the rules exist solely to create the activity.

game spectator knowledge—Knowledge about the game one is watching including the players, strategies, and competitive tactics.

gender—Set of norms or expectations about how we should behave that are linked to societal understandings of sexuality and procreation.

gerontology—The study of aging.

gestures—Movements used to communicate our intentions to others; they may be illustrators, emblems, or regulators.

goal setting—Establishment of objectives for motor performance (either short- or long-term)

ground reaction force (GRF)—An external force from the ground acting on a body. Based on the Law of

Action-Reaction, a GRF is created in the opposite direction but of equal magnitude as a response to a force created by the body acting against the ground. Hence, when a person pushes against the ground, the ground will create a GRF acting on the person. There are typically three different directions that GRF can act on a body—sideways, forward/backward, and vertical (upward).

growth and maturation—Growth means change in size; maturation means the process by which infants and children move toward adult status.

habilitation—Processes and treatments leading to the acquisition of skills and functions that are considered normal and expected for an individual of a certain age, status, and occupation.

habilitational therapeutic exercise—Applications of exercise in order to bring clients/patients to a level of performance not previously attained by them.

health maintenance organization (HMO)—Alternate systems of health care where payment is made in advance on a fixed contract fee basis by a certain population.

health-related fitness—Developed through physical activity experience, it refers to capacities and traits that are associated with a low risk of hypokinetic diseases.

Healthy People 2000—Health objectives set for Americans for the year 2000.

helping professions—Professions primarily committed to providing services.

hemoglobin—An iron-containing protein found inside red blood cells that carries most of the oxygen in the blood.

hidden curriculum—Everything students learn that was unintended or unplanned by teachers

high-density lipoprotein (HDL) cholesterol—Cholesterol carried in the blood bound to high-density lipoproteins.

histology—The study of tissues.

historical analysis—Research technique that typically involves description and analysis of social change and stability in particular cultures or societies during specific time periods.

holism—The characteristic of humanity that underscores the interdependence and interrelatedness of the mind, emotions, body, and spirit.

home maintenance activities—Self-sufficient activities intended to improve or repair conditions of living in one's apartment or house.

human agency—Theory suggesting that people were actively involved in developing or "constructing" their own sports.

human factors engineers—See *ergonomists*.

human resource management—Task involving, for example, the recruitment, orientation, retention, and evaluation of employees as well as benefit

program planning and the design and implementation of internal grievance procedures.

hyperplasia—An increase in muscle mass due to the splitting of muscle fibers.

hypertension—Elevated blood pressure, usually defined as a systolic pressure greater than 160 mmHg or a diastolic pressure greater than 90 mmHg.

hypertrophy—An increase in muscle mass due to the enlargement of the muscle fiber.

hypohydration—Failure to adequately replace the loss of body fluids.

hypokinetic diseases—Diseases such as heart disease, obesity, and high blood pressure that are directly associated with low levels of daily physical activity.

hypothermia—A condition in which the body temperature falls below 35 °C (95 °F) causing heart rate and metabolism to slow. Can be life threatening.

illustrators—Gestures used to demonstrate or complement what is being said.

imagery—Using all the senses to create or recreate an experience in the mind.

impersonal competition—Physical activities such as mountain climbing, long-distance swimming, and so forth, in which an individual attempts to better an established record in an activity that does not involve opponents.

individual differences—Variables within the learner that influence motor skill learning (e.g., motor abilities, reaction time, force, coordination).

inductive reasoning—Form of logic that starts with specific cases and moves toward developing a broad, general principle.

inpatient facilities—Rehabilitation hospitals, nursing homes, and other institutions where patients spend extended periods of time (several days to several months or years) for purposes of receiving medical or other health-related treatment.

instrumental activities of daily living (IADLs)—Less personal self-sufficient activities such as shopping, telephoning, cooking, or doing laundry.

instrumental movements—Movements employed in a physical activity in order to accomplish the goal of the action; differentiated from expressive movements.

insulin—A hormone that stimulates the cellular uptake of glucose.

interactional approach—A psychological approach in which behavior is viewed as being codetermined by internal characteristics (traits) as well as environmental or situational factors.

internalization—The process by which an activity gradually comes to be valued for its intrinsic qualities.

internship—Culminating educational experience for kinesiology majors planning professional careers.

It involves extended work at one our two professional sites where students work under the supervision of a veteran professional.

interviewing—Research technique that typically involves asking oral questions to a relatively small sample of individuals.

intrinsic approaches to physical activity—Valuing physical activity because of the subjective experiences embedded within the activity itself.

intrinsic motivation—Motivation that is derived from the rewards inherent or within the actual activity, such as enjoyment and feelings of accomplishment.

intuitive knowledge—Knowledge gained through physical activity that doesn't depend on rational or conscious processes.

isokinetic—An exercise in which the muscle changes length at a constant rate of velocity.

isometric—An exercise in which tension is produced by the muscle without any change in length.

isotonic—An exercise in which the muscle changes length while maintaining a constant tension.

kinematics—A description of a movement, based on mechanical physics, in which movement characteristics like position, velocity, and acceleration are recorded.

kinesiology—The discipline or body of knowledge that studies physical activity through performance, scholarly analysis, and professional practice.

kinesiology theory—Theoretical knowledge about physical activity as embodied in the subdisciplines of kinesiology.

knowledge of performance (KP)—External information about the nature of the movement (e.g, hip rotation and arm action were not coordinated during the throw) usually provided by an instructor (but a videotape could be used).

knowledge of results (KR)—External information about the outcome of the movement (e.g, missing a basket) sometimes provided by an instructor but often available just by observation.

lactate—An end product of glucose metabolism formed when inadequate oxygen is available.

lactate threshold—The exercise intensity at which blood lactate concentration increases markedly.

leadership—A behavioral process of influencing individuals and groups toward set goals.

learned helplessness—A condition in which a teacher's minimal expectations of low achieving students causes them to experience feelings of helplessness. These students may exert little effort, exhibit hostility, blame others, or concede to failure.

learning—A permanent alteration in the functioning of the nervous system that enables performers to achieve a predetermined goal consistently.

leisure—A state of being in which humans find deep satisfaction and contentment; it is often accompanied by feelings of wonder, celebration, excitement, and creativity.

leisure activities—Physical activities that nourish or maintain the disposition of leisure.

leisure studies—An area of study or department in a college or university that focuses on preparing individuals for careers in the leisure industry.

liberal studies—Also known as the liberal arts and sciences, they form the core of a higher education and are foundational for later education or life experiences.

lived body—Dynamic, ongoing life of a whole person whose mind and body are considered to be inseparably blended.

low-density lipoprotein (LDL) cholesterol—Cholesterol carried in the blood bound to low-density lipoproteins.

marketing management—Tasks involving the production, pricing, promotion, and distribution of a sport-related product or service in a way that insures mutually beneficial transactions between a sport organization and its consumers.

maximal oxygen uptake—The highest rate of oxygen uptake during heavy dynamic exercise.

mechanical, market-driven professionals—Professionals for whom technique, methodology, profit, and prestige assume priority over clients' wants and needs.

media management—Those activities designed to cultivate relationships between a sport organization and members of the mass media.

memory drum theory—Developed by Franklin Henry (1960), it proposed that rapid and well-learned movements are not consciously controlled but are run off automatically (like an older computer uses a memory drum to store and retrieve data).

mentors—Professional individuals who can provide less experienced professionals or preprofessionals with learning opportunities, responsibility, knowledge, and contact people that can contribute to the attainment of a successful career and/or continued improvement within an existing career.

merchandising—The sale of goods and services related to the sport organization (e.g., various team apparel or other products with team logos such as coffee mugs and note pads). Merchandising provides sport managers opportunities to enhance brand image, brand loyalty, and customer satisfaction and to generate revenue.

mitochondria—The part of the cell where aerobic metabolism occurs and ATP is produced.

modernization theory—Theory emphasizing that the rise of modern sport occurred during the industrial revolution as American society shifted away from being agricultural and locally oriented and developed city-based industries rooted in science and technology.

moment—The twisting, spinning, or rotational effect of a force on a body.

motivation—A complex social–psychological process that influences individuals to begin an activity and pursue it with vigor and persistence.

motor control—(a) The neural, physical, and behavioral aspects of movement (Schmidt 1988, p. 17); (b) the component of the motor behavior subdiscipline that studies these issues.

motor development—(a) Changes in the acquisition of skilled movements and in the neural, physical, and behavioral aspects of movement that occur across the life span; (b) the component of the motor behavior subdiscipline that examines the effects of age and related factors on the learning and control of motor skills. Also known as developmental motor learning and control.

motor expertise—A person with a high level of skill, usually determined by some criterion (e.g., national ranking, Division I football player)

motor learning—(a) Relatively permanent changes in skill performance that come about as a result of practice; (b) the component of the motor behavior subdiscipline that studies factors related to these changes.

motor performance fitness—Developed through physical activity experience, it is the capacity that enables individuals to perform daily activities with vigor. This type of fitness often incorporates an element of skill.

motor program—A cognitive mechanism that controls movement; you could think of it as a phonograph record where the record contains the commands to the nervous system.

motor skill taxonomy—A classification system that categorizes motor skills according to their common critical components.

motor skills—Physical activities in which performers attempt to attain specific goals by executing efficient, coordinated motor responses.

movement—Any change in the position of body parts relative to each other.

muscle fiber—An individual muscle cell.

myofibril—The part of the muscle fiber that contains the contractile elements.

myoglobin—A muscle protein that binds (stores) oxygen.

mystical knowledge—Knowledge about another dimension of reality apprehended through participation in sport and exercise.

neuromuscular injuries—Trauma to the body's bones, muscles, joints, and/or nervous system.

nonprofit sport participation—Sport industry sector comprised of organizations that operate as nonprofit organizations with tax exemption and offer participation opportunities to patrons (e.g., YMCAs).

novel learning tasks—A movement task with which the subject does not have prior experience; usually a simple movement like linear positioning or tracking.

observational learning (modeling)—The opportunity to watch either yourself (e.g., videotape) or another performer (live or videotape) as a skill is performed in order to improve your performance.

occupational biomechanics—See *ergonomics*.

open skill—A motor skill in which performers must coordinate their movements to an unpredictable, usually moving, environment.

outpatient facility—A short-term care facility where patients do not stay overnight.

oxygen debt—The amount of oxygen used during recovery from exercise to replace creatine phosphate, remove lactic acid, and return the body to resting conditions.

paradigm—Research model.

peak experiences—Special types of mystical experiences frequently experienced by runners and others engaged in strenuous sports and exercises.

pedagogy—The art or science of teaching.

pedagogy of physical activity—The study of teaching and instruction of physical activity.

perceived freedom—Feeling free to participate in an activity without a nagging sense that you have to or that you should be doing something else.

perceptions—Meaningful constructs or messages based on the interpretations of sensations from past subjective experiences.

personality—The unique blend of psychological characteristics and behavioral tendencies that make individuals different from and similar to each other.

personality states—Manifestations of personality that occur from the combination of traits and specific situations; a personality characteristic measured at one point in time.

personality traits—Relatively enduring and consistent internal attributes.

physical activity—Movement that is voluntary, intentional, and directed toward achieving an identifiable goal.

physical fitness—(a) A capacity developed through exercise enabling one to perform the essential activities of daily living, engage in an active leisure lifestyle, and have sufficient energy remaining to meet the demands of unexpected emergencies. (b) The ability to perform moderate to vigorous physical activities without undue fatigue.

physical performance capacity—Aspects of physical activity such as endurance, flexibility, and strength that are developed through training. The purpose of training is to produce well-conditioned performers.

plasma volume—The volume of extracellular fluid found in the blood.

play—Activity in which aspects of ordinary life take on meanings different from those they usually have, and ordinary events can be altered in ways that would be inappropriate in other settings.

political values—Conceptions about political and economic arrangements in relation to social morality; the public interest-goal of producing common good for all.

power—Ability to do what one wants without being stopped by others. Also the rate at which work is done (work/time or force × velocity).

practice—A type of physical activity experience that involves cognitive processing and that leads to improvement in skill (learning).

practice theory—Knowledge concerning the client, the method, and the outcomes that guides practitioners in performing their duties as professionals.

practitioners—Those who use knowledge to bring about predetermined objectives. Professionals are practitioners.

preprofessional—Professionals-in-training whose orientation to undergraduate studies is to become highly competent practitioners.

presage variables—Teacher characteristics that may affect learning.

pressure—The amount of force applied to a given amount of surface area.

pretraining—Time spent as a student in the public schools.

primary source—Historical evidence produced in the society and time period being studied.

principle of quality—Experiences that engage us in the critical components of an activity are most likely to improve our capacity to perform that activity.

principle of quantity—Increasing the frequency of experiences that engage us in the critical components of a physical activity will lead to increases in our capacity to perform that activity.

private practice—An entrepreneurial venture where a professional establishes his or her own workplace with its own client pool.

process variables—All of the events and activities in the learning environment.

product variables—Variables as they relate to the teaching outcome.

professional—A worker recognized by society for performing valuable services for clients through skilled performances that are grounded in in-depth, complex knowledge.

professional practice knowledge—Knowledge about appropriate ways to deliver professional services that is derived from an integration of scholarly study and practical experience. Knowledge that teachers derive as a result of practice and experience.

professional sport entertainment—Sport industry sector comprised of an organization/event that attracts spectators to watch professional athletes compete (e.g., NBA, NASCAR, LPGA).

profiles—A set of biomechanical and other performer-related characteristics of a given group of individuals.

program management—Those activities such as scheduling and equipment maintenance necessary for various sport organizations to address to insure operational effectiveness.

promotions—Those activities such as personal selling, sales promotions, advertising, and publicity that are designed to attract consumers to sport-related products and/or services.

psychoanalytic self-knowledge—Knowledge about one's deep-seated desires, motivation, and behavior gained through participation in sport and exercise.

psychological inventory—Standardized or objective measure of a specific sample of behavior, typically in the form of a questionnaire.

public relations—Those activities designed to promote mutually beneficial relationships between a sport organization and its key constituents.

Pygmalion effect—Impact of teacher expectations on student performance.

qualitative analysis—Evaluating aspects of a movement without use of a measuring instrument (e.g., through visual observation). Used by researchers operating within the qualitative paradigm.

quantitative analysis—An evaluation of movement based on numerical measures obtained using an instrument, e.g., a stopwatch. Used by researchers operating within the quantitative paradigm.

race—Group of people who are defined by society as different from others on the basis of genetically inherited traits.

rational knowledge—Knowledge about facts, concepts, and theories that is gained through reason, logic, and analysis.

reaction time (simple and choice)—The speed of response to a light or sound; a simple reaction time would be to press a button when you see a signal; a choice reaction time means there is more than one button to press depending on which signal you see.

receptor—A specialized nerve ending found at the end of sensory neurons that detects changes in the environment.

recreation—See *leisure studies*.

regulators—Hand and body movements used to guide the flow of conversations such as in greetings or when parting company.

rehabilitation—Processes and treatments designed to restore skills or functions that were previously acquired, but have been lost to disease, injury, or behavioral traits.

rehabilitation hospitals—Hospitals that provide specialized care to return patients to their maximum level of function.

rehabilitational therapeutic exercise—Applications of exercise and other types of physical activity in an effort to restore skills or functions that were previously acquired but have been lost to disease, injury, or behavioral traits.

research and development—Those activities that strive to generate ideas for improving sport-related products and/or services or for creating new ones that effectively meet consumer wants and/ or needs.

research on teacher education—Study of teacher educators, teacher education programs, and individuals who elect to become teachers.

research on teaching—Study of teaching and learning in the schools and in other physical activity settings.

response execution—How the skill that is selected is performed, in motor behavior research.

response selection—The process of selecting and activating a response (motor program) that is required in order to attain the skill goal.

retention—How much of learning a motor skill the performer can demonstrate after a period of no practice (the interval of time with no practice may vary).

retention-based facilities—Commercial (for-profit) health and fitness facilities that make a large percentage of profits from ongoing monthly membership dues. These facilities engage in activities that are directed at helping members to meet their goals and have a positive experience in the facility so that they will continue to pay for their membership on a month by month basis.

risk management—The prevention of loss associated with, for example, inadequate financial planning, employee management, facility and equipment maintenance, customer service, or short- and long-term planning efforts.

rituals—Physical activity employed to express symbolically some experience, truth, or value held deeply by a particular group.

sales-based facilities—Commercial (for-profit) health and fitness facilities that make a large percentage of profits from membership initiation fees and prepaid dues. As a result of this business model, sales-based facilities do not have a significant incentive to satisfy current members. This emphasis on sales can result in overcrowding and lower quality programs and services.

schema theory—Schmidt's (1975) explanation for how a motor program acquires a general set of rules from practice of similar movements.

secondary source—Historical information produced after the period being studied.

self-confidence—An individual's perception that he or she has the ability to perform a certain task successfully.

self-efficacy—How confident one feels in one's ability to perform a physical activity.

self-esteem—Perception of personal worthiness.

self-fulfilling prophecy—Influence of teacher expectations on student performance.

self-reflection—A process whereby one experiences the subjective experiences of an activity performed in the past.

sensation-seeking activities—Physical activities that involve high speed, danger, or disorientation of the body in space.

sensations—Raw, uninterpreted information collected through sensory organs.

service—Human acts intended to improve the quality of life for others.

shear loading—Two forces acting in opposite directions that create internal sliding of one part of a body across another part of a body.

side-by-side competitive activities—Contests such as golf, swim racing, and so forth, in which individuals do not directly interact in striving to accomplish the goal.

skill—The ability to execute efficiently a series of accurate, well-timed movements in order to achieve a predetermined goal. Improvements in skill brought about through practice are called learning.

social facilitation—The effects of the presence of an audience on human performance.

social life—Broad collection of relationships and ongoing activities among people, and the ways in which these relationships are understood by those involved. Synonym: social processes.

social loafing—A decrease in individual performance within groups.

social practices—Relatively specific sets of relationships and ongoing activities among people, and the ways in which these are understood by them.

social processes—See *social life*.

social sciences—Collective term for several disciplines focused on the study of contemporary social life, including sociology, anthropology, communication studies, and political science.

social trustee, civic professionals—Professionals who adhere to the creed "Healthy people and a good society first. Myself and my profession second in service of this greater good" (Lawson, 1998a).

socialization—The process by which someone learns about social life. Preprofessionals are judged to have been socialized into the profession when they understand the roles and responsibilities associated with the specific subculture of that profession.

societal analysis—Research technique that typically involves examining the sweep of social life, usually from the perspective of a broad social theory.

socioeconomic status—Social position based on wealth, education, and occupational prestige.

Socratic self-knowledge—Knowledge about our capacities and limitations that enables us to perform physical activity safely within the range of our abilities.

specificity of practice—The finding that only practice conditions that are very similar to actual game performance will benefit future game performance.

spheres of physical activity experience—Various dimensions of everyday life in which physical activity plays an important and distinctive role.

spheres of professional practice in physical activity—Categories of physical activity professions that are similar with respect to general objectives, methods, educational requirements, working environments, and other factors.

spheres of scholarly study of physical activity—A way of categorizing the subdisciplines of kinesiology according to general theories, concepts, and methods employed by scholars and researchers in the subdisciplines.

sport—Physical activity performed in order to achieve a specific goal in a manner specified by established rules.

sport industry—The sport industry is "the market in which the products offered to its buyers are fitness, sport, recreation, and leisure related. These products include goods (e.g., baseball bats), services (e.g., sport marketing, health clubs), people (e.g., professional players), places (e.g., golf courses), and ideas" (Pitts, Fielding, Miller, 1994, p. 18).

sport promotion—The activities undertaken by sport marketers to promote interest in contests with the purpose of increasing attendance or television viewing of a sporting event.

sport services—Sport industry sector often comprised of independent businesses providing needed services to existing sport organizations (e.g., monitoring of trademarks, athletic training services, marketing services).

sport spectacles—Staged competitions designed and promoted for audiences and intended to evoke an entire range of human emotions by virtue of their grandeur, scale, and drama.

sport sponsorship—The mutually beneficial exchange between a sport organization and another company or individual seeking to promote itself through sport.

sporting goods—Sport industry sector comprised of sport organizations that offer consumers the vast range of sporting equipment and apparel needed for participation in sport and physical activity.

sports commissions—Organizations typically operated by a city that serve to assist local sport organizations while also bringing new sport organizations and other sport-related events to the city for the purposes of enhanced economic activity and quality of life improvement.

sports medicine—A field of medicine and/or therapeutic exercise that specializes in the treatment, prevention, and rehabilitation of athletes and others who are involved in sports and other forms of strenuous exercise. Sports medicine also involves the investigation of training methods and practices.

stability—State of remaining the same.

stages of development (for motor skills; also might be labeled fundamental motor patterns)—Specific movement stages for basic or fundamental skills that all infants/children pass through as skills develop (e.g., throwing, locomotion, hopping).

stress—A process in which individuals perceive an imbalance between their response capabilities and the demands of the situation.

stroke volume—The amount of blood pumped out of one side of the heart per beat.

subdisciplines—A way of dividing the scholarly study of physical activity in order to facilitate teaching and research. The divisions represent extensions of established disciplines such as psychology, physiology, and history.

subjective experience—Individual reactions, feelings, and thoughts about events.

survey research—Research technique that typically involves administering a questionnaire to a relatively large sample of people.

task analysis—The systematic examination of a particular physical activity for purposes of disclosing its critical components.

task orientation—Defining competence in an activity on the basis of self-improvement; participants with this orientation often approach competitive activity from an intrinsic perspective.

technical definitions—Specialized meanings of terms used to convey information to others within a technical field. The technical definition of physical activity, for example, differs from how the phenomenon is defined and used in everyday language.

tensile loading—A type of loading where an object is being pulled apart by forces acting in opposite directions.

thematic analysis—Research technique that typically involves examining qualitative data (e.g., newspaper articles, television shows, interview data) and categorizing the content in various ways.

theoretical knowledge—Knowledge of concepts and principles and the research strategies used to discover them. Theoretical knowledge in kinesiology is knowledge about physical activity, embedded in the subdisciplines, acquired by formal study of the subdisciplines.

therapeutic exercise—The systematic and scientific application of exercise and movement to develop or restore muscular strength, endurance, and flexibility; neuromuscular coordination; cardiovascular efficiency; and other health performance factors.

thermogenesis—The generation of body heat by increasing the metabolic rate.

thermoneutral environment—A comfortable ambient temperature.

tidal volume—The amount of air inhaled or exhaled per breath.

torque—See *moment*.

training—Physical activity carried out for the express purpose of conditioning one for performance in an athletic or other type of event.

transducer—A device that converts a form of energy to a from of energy that can be measured.

transfer—After practicing a skill, the learner can perform similar skills or the same skill in a slightly different situation.

underwater weighing—The procedure in which a person's body weight is measured while completely submerged for the purpose of determining the person's body volume.

value—Conception about the importance of something.

ventilation—The process in which gases are exchanged between the atmosphere and the alveoli of the lungs.

ventilatory threshold—During a graded exercise test the point at which ventilation begins increasing at a faster rate than $\dot{V}O_2$.

vertigo—The sensation that comes from disorientation of the body in space, often experienced in conjunction with dangerous activities.

vicarious participation—Feeling as though one is engaged in a sport contest one is watching.

with-it-ness—Teacher awareness of all events transpiring in a learning environment.

work—Purposeful, utilitarian activity to make or do something.

workplace knowledge—Practical, mundane knowledge not grounded in theory that is used to perform everyday tasks in the workplace. Knowing where items are stored or how to clean, repair, or calibrate equipment are examples of workplace knowledge.

References

Abernethy, B., & Sparrow, W.A. (1992). The rise and fall of dominant paradigms in motor behavior research. In J.J. Summers (Ed.), *Approaches to the study of motor control and learning*. Amsterdam: Elsevier.

Abernethy, B., Thomas, K.T., & Thomas, J.R. (1993). Strategies for improving understanding of motor expertise (or mistakes we have made and things we have learned!!). In J.L. Starkes & F. Allard (Eds.), *Cognitive issues in motor learning* (pp. 317–356). Amsterdam: Elsevier.

Acosta, R.V., & Carpenter, L.J. (1994). The status of women in intercollegiate athletics. In S. Birrell & C.L. Cole (Eds.), *Women, sport, and culture* (pp. 111–118). Champaign, IL: Human Kinetics.

Adams, J.A. (1971). A closed-loop theory of motor learning. *Journal of Motor Behavior, 3*, 111–149.

Adams, J.A. (1987). Historical review and appraisal of research on the learning, retention, and transfer of human motor skills. *Psychological Bulletin, 101*, 41–74.

Adelman, M.L. (1986). *A sporting time: New York City and the rise of modern athletics, 1820-70*. Urbana, IL: University of Illinois Press.

Adler, P.A., & Adler, P. (1991). *Backboards & blackboards: College athletes and role engulfment*. New York: Columbia University Press.

Amar, J. (1920). *The human motor*. New York: Dutton.

Ambrosi, E., & Barker-Schwartz, K. (1995). The profession's image, 1917–1925, Part I: Occupational therapy as represented in the media. *American Journal of Occupational Therapy, 49*(7), 715–719.

American College of Sports Medicine. (1990). The recommended quantity and quality of exercise for developing and maintaining cardiorespiratory and muscular fitness in healthy adults. *Medicine and Science in Sports and Exercise, 22*, 265–274.

American College of Sports Medicine. (1993). Physical activity, physical fitness, and hypertension. *Medicine and Science in Sports and Exercise, 25*(10), i–x.

Anastasi, A. (1988). *Psychological testing*. New York: Macmillan.

Anderson, W.G. (Ed.). (1994). Building and maintaining outstanding physical education programs [Special feature]. *Journal of Physical Education, Recreation, and Dance, 65*(7), 22–49.

Anderson, W.G., & Barrette, G.T. (1978). *What's going on in gym—Descriptive studies of physical education classes* [Monograph No. 1]. Newtown, CT: Motor Skills.

Andrews, D. (Ed.). (1996). Deconstructing Michael Jordan: Reconstructing postindustrial America [Special issue]. *Sociology of Sport Journal, 13* (4).

Anshel, M.H., Freedson, P., Hamill, J., Haywood, K. Horvat, M., and Plowman, S.A. (1991). *Dictionary of the sport and exercise sciences*. Champaign, IL: Human Kinetics.

Argyle, M. (1988). *Bodily communication* (2nd ed.). London: Methuen.

Armstrong, L.E., Costill, D.L., & Fink, W.J. (1985). Influence of diuretic-induced dehydration on competitive running performance. *Medicine and Science in Sports and Exercise, 17*, 456–461.

Åstrand, P.-O. (1991). Influence of Scandinavian scientists in exercise physiology. *Scandinavian Journal of Medicine and Science in Sports, 1*, 3–9.

Atwater, A.E. (1980). Kinesiology/biomechanics: Perspectives and trends. *Research Quarterly for Exercise and Sport, 51*, 193–218.

Ayers, W. (1993). *To teach: The journey of a teacher*. New York: Teachers College Press.

Bain, L.L. (1997). Sport pedagogy. In J.D. Massengale & R.A. Swanson (Eds.), *History of exercise and sport science* (pp. 15–37). Champaign, IL: Human Kinetics.

Bain, L.L., Wilson, T., & Chaikind, E. (1989). Participant perceptions of exercise programs for overweight women. *Research Quarterly for Exercise and Sport, 60*, 134–143.

Baker, W.J. (1988). *Sports in the western world*. Urbana, IL: University of Illinois Press.

Baltzell, E.D. (1958). *Philadelphia gentlemen: The making of a national upper class*. Glencoe, IL: Free Press.

Bandura, A. (1986). *Social foundations of thought and action: A social cognitive theory*. Englewood Cliffs: Prentice Hall.

Bannister, R. (1955). *The four minute mile*. New York: Dodd-Mead.

Bar-Or, O. (1983). *Pediatric sports medicine for the practitioner.* New York: Springer-Verlag.

Barr, R.A. (1991). Recent changes in driving among older adults. *Human Factors, 33*(5), 597–600.

Barrow, J. (1977). The variables of leadership: A review and conceptual framework. *Academy of Management Review, 2,* 231–251.

Bateson, G. (1955). A theory of play and fantasy. *Psychiatric Research Reports 2: Approaches to the study of human personality,* 39–51.

Bayley, N. (1935). The development of motor abilities during the first three years. *Monographs of the Society for the Research in Child Development* (Whole No. 1, pp. 1–26).

Beevor, C.E., & Horsely, V. (1887). A minute analysis (experimental) of the various movements produced by stimulating in the monkey different regions of the cortical centre for the upper limb as defined by Professor Ferrier. *Philosophical Transactions, 178,* 153.

Beevor, C.E., & Horsely, V. (1890). A record of the results obtained by electrical excitation of the so-called motor cortex and internal capsule in the orangutan. *Philosophical Transactions, 181,* 129.

Berg, W.P., & Greer, N.L. (1995). A kinematic profile of the approach run of novice long jumpers. *Journal of Applied Biomechanics, 11,* 142–162.

Berkowitz, L. (1969). *Roots of aggression: A reexamination of the frustration-aggression hypothesis.* New York: Atherton Press.

Bernstein, N. (1967). *The coordination and regulation of movements.* London: Pergamon.

Berryman, J.W. (1973). Sport history as social history? *Quest, 20,* 65–73.

Berryman, J.W. (1975). From the cradle to the playing field: America's emphasis on highly organized competitive sports for preadolescent boys. *Journal of Sport History, 2*(2), 112–131.

Berryman, J.W. (1989). The tradition of the "six things non-natural": Exercise and medicine from Hippocrates through ante-bellum America. In K.B. Pandolf (Ed.), *Exercise and Sport Sciences Reviews, 17,* 515–559.

Berryman, J.W. (1995). *Out of many, one: A history of the American College of Sports Medicine.* Champaign, IL: Human Kinetics.

Betts, J.R. (1952). Organized sport in industrial America. *Dissertation Abstracts, 12*(1), 41. (University Microfilms #3322)

Biddle, S. (1995). Exercise and psychosocial health. *Research Quarterly for Exercise and Sport, 66,* 292–297.

Big Ten, big bucks: Major revenue sources for the Big Ten conference. (1998, August 17–23). *Street & Smith's Sports Business Journal, 1*(17), 48.

Birdwhistell, R.L. (1971). *Kinesics and context: Essays on body motion and communication.* London: Allen Lane.

Birrell, S.J. (1988). Discourses on the gender-sport relationship: From women in sport to gender relations. In K.B. Pandolf (Ed.), *Exercise and Sport Sciences Reviews, 16* (pp. 459–502). New York: Macmillan.

Black, S.J., & Weiss, M.R. (1992). The relationship among perceived coaching behaviors, perceptions of ability and motivation in competitive age-group swimmers. *Journal of Sport and Exercise Psychology, 14* (3), 309-325.

Blair, S.N., Kohl, H.W., Paffenbarger, R.S., Clark, D.G., Cooper, K.H., & Gibbons, L.W. (1989). Physical fitness and all-cause mortality: A prospective study of healthy men and women. *Journal of the American Medical Association, 262*(17), 2395–2401.

Blair, S.N., Mulder, R.T., & Kohl, H.W. (1987). Reaction to "Secular Trends in Adult Physical Activity: Exercise Boom or Bust?" *Research Quarterly for Exercise and Sport, 58*(2), 106–110.

Blix, M. (1892–1895). Die lange und spannung des muskels. *Skandinavische Archiv Physiologie, 3,* 295–318; *4,* 399–409; *5,* 150–206.

Boeck, S., & Staimer, M. (1996, December 6). NFL drug suspensions. *USA Today,* p. 1C.

Booth, F.W. (1989). Application of molecular biology in exercise physiology. In K.B. Pandolf (Ed.), *Exercise and Sport Sciences Reviews* (Vol. 17, pp. 1–27). Baltimore: Williams & Wilkins.

Bordo, S. (1993). *Unbearable weight: Feminism, western culture, and the body.* Berkeley, CA: University of California Press.

Borg, G. (1998). *Borg's perceived exertion and pain scales.* Champaign, IL: Human Kinetics.

Borg, G.A.V. (1973). Perceived exertion: A note on "history" and methods. *Medicine and Science in Sports, 5,* 90–93.

Bouchard, C., Lesage, R., Lortie, G., Simoneau, J.A., Hamel, P., Boulay, M.R., Perusse, L., Theriault, G., & Leblanc, C. (1986). Aerobic performance in brothers, dizygotic and monzygotic twins. *Medicine and Science in Sports and Exercise, 18,* 639–646.

Bowditch, H.P., & Southard, W.F. (1882). A comparison of sight and touch. *Journal of Physiology, 3,* 232–254.

Boyle, R.H. (1963). *Sport—Mirror of American life.* Boston: Little, Brown.

Bradley, B. (1977). *Life on the run.* New York: Bantam Books.

Bredemeier, B.J., Weiss, M.R., Shields, D.L., & Cooper, B.A.B. (1986). The relationship of sport involvement with children's moral reasoning and aggression tendencies. *Journal of Sport Psychology, 8,* 304–318.

Brewington, P. (1998, March 3). League adds ethnic spice. *USA Today,* p. 3C.

Brill, P.A., Burkhaulter, H.E., Kohl, H.W., Blair, S.N., & Goodyear, N.N. (1989). The impact of previous athleticism on exercise habits, physical fitness, and coronary heart disease risk factors in middle-aged men. *Research Quarterly for Exercise and Sport, 60,* 209–215.

Brockington, L. (1998, May 4–10). What NFL TV deal really cost the media. *Street & Smith's Sports Business Journal,* p. 1.

Brooks, G.A. (1994). 40 years of progress: Basic exercise physiology. In *40th anniversary lectures.* Indianapolis: American College of Sports Medicine.

Brophy, J.E., & Good, T.L. (1986). Teacher behavior and student achievement. In M.C. Wittrock (Ed.), *Handbook of research on teaching* (3rd ed., pp. 328–375). New York: Macmillan.

Brown, D.R. (1990). Exercise, fitness, and mental health. In C. Bouchard, R.J. Shephard, & T. Stephens (Eds.), *Exercise, fitness and health: A consensus of current knowledge* (pp. 607-26). Champaign, IL: Human Kinetics

Brown, W.M. (1980). Ethics, drugs, and sport. *Journal of the Philosophy of Sport, 7,* 15–23.

Brown, W.M. (1984). Paternalism, drugs, and the nature of sports. *Journal of the Philosophy of Sport, 11,* 14–22.

Bryan, W.L., & Harter, N. (1897). Studies in the physiology and psychology of the telegraphic language. *Psychological Reviews, 4,* 27–53.

Bryan, W.L., & Harter, N. (1899). Studies on the telegraphic language: The acquisition of a hierarchy of habits. *Psychological Reviews, 6,* 345–375.

Bryant, J.E., & McElroy, M. (1997). *Sociological dynamics of sport and exercise.* Englewood, CO: Morton.

Bureau of Labor Statistics. (1961). *Occupational outlook handbook* (Bulletin No. 1300). Washington, DC: U.S. Government Printing Office.

Bureau of Labor Statistics. (1982). *Occupational outlook handbook* (Bulletin No. 2200). Washington, DC: U.S. Government Printing Office.

Bureau of Labor Statistics. (1996). *Occupational outlook handbook* (Bulletin No. 2470). Washington, DC: U.S. Government Printing Office.

Buskirk, E.R., & Tipton, C.M. (1997). Exercise physiology. In J.D. Massengale & R.A. Swanson (Eds.), *History of exercise and sport science* (pp. 367–438). Champaign, IL: Human Kinetics.

Caillois, R. (1961). *Man, play, and games.* (M. Barash, Trans.). New York: Free Press. (Original work published 1958)

Carey, A.R., & Mullins, M.E. (1997, June 16). Toning up. *USA Today,* p. 1C.

Carlston, D.E. (1983). An environmental explanation for race differences in basketball performance. *Journal of Sport and Social Issues, 7*(2), 30–51.

Carr, J.H., & Shepherd, R.B. (1987). *A motor relearning programme for stroke* (p. 103, figure 4). Rockville, MD: Aspen.

Carron, A.V. (1982). Cohesiveness in sport groups: Interpretations and 'iterations. *Journal of Sport Psychology, 4,* 123–138.

Carswell, E., & Roubinek, D. (1974). *Open sesame: A primer in open education.* Pacific Palisades, CA: Goodyear.

Cauley, J.A., Donfield, S.M., LaPorte, R.E., & Warhaftig, N.E. (1991). Physical activity by socioeconomic status in two population based cohorts. *Medicine and Science in Sports and Exercise, 23,* 343–352.

Cavanagh, P.R., Simoneau, G.G., & Ulbrecht, J.S. (1993). Ulceration, unsteadiness, and uncertainty: The biomechanical consequences of diabetes mellitus. *Journal of Biomechanics, 26* (Suppl. 1), 23–40.

Cavanagh, P.R., & Williams, K.R. (1987). Relationship between distance running mechanics, running economy, and performance. *Journal of Applied Physiology, 63*(3), 1236–1245.

Cawley, R. (1998). Dream comes true for national union. *Street and Smith's Sports Business Journal, 1* (15), 25.

Celsing, F., Blomstrand, E., Werner, B., Pihlstedt, P., & Ekblom, B. (1986). Effects of iron deficiency on endurance and muscle enzyme activity in man. *Medicine and Science in Sports and Exercise, 18,* 156–161.

Chadbourne, R.D. (1990). A hard loook at running shoes. *Physician and Sportsmedicine, 18*(7), 103–104.

Chaffin, D.B., & Andersson, G.B. (1991). *Occupational biomechanics* (2nd ed.). New York: Wiley.

Chamberlin, C., & Lee, T. (1993). Arranging practice conditions and designing instruction. In R.N. Singer, M. Murphey, & L.K. Tennant (Eds.), *Handbook of research on sport psychology* (pp. 213–241). New York: Macmillan.

Charles, J. (1994). *Contemporary kinesiology: An introduction to the study of human movement in higher education.* Englewood: CO: Morton Publishing.

Children's Defense Fund. (1997). *The state of America's children.* Washington, DC: Author.

Christina, R.W. (1989). Whatever happened to applied research in motor learning? In J. Skinner et al. (Eds.),

Future directions for exercise science and sport research (pp. 411–422). Champaign, IL: Human Kinetics.

Christina, R.W. (1992). The 1991 C.H. McCloy Research Lecture: Unraveling the mystery of the response complexity effect in skilled movements. *Research Quarterly for Exercise and Sport, 63,* 218–230.

Christina, R.W., & Bjork, R.A. (1991). Optimizing long-term retention and transfer. In D. Druckman & R. Bjork (Eds.), *In the mind's eye: Enhancing human performance* (pp. 23–56). Washington, DC: National Academy Press.

Cicuttini, F.M., Baker, J.R., & Spector, T.D. (1996). The association of obesity with osteoarthritis of the hand and knee in women—A twin study. *Journal of Rheumatology, 23*(7), 1221–1226.

Clark, J.E., & Phillips, S.J. (1991). The development of intralimb coordination in the first six months of walking. In J. Fagard & P.H. Wolff (Eds.), *The development of timing control and temporal organization in coordinated action* (pp. 245–257). New York: Elsevier Science.

Clark, J.E., & Whitall, J. (1989). What is motor development? The lessons of history. *Quest, 41,* 183–202.

Clark, K.L. (1994). Working with college athletes, coaches, and [athletic] trainers at a major university. *International Journal of Sports Nutrition, 4*(2), 135–141.

Clarkson, P.M., & Haymes, E.M. (1995). Exercise and mineral status of athletes, calcium, magnesium, phosphorus, and iron. *Medicine and Science in Sports and Exercise, 27,* 831–843.

Claxton, D.B., & Lacy, A.C. (1991). Pedagogy: The missing link in aerobic dance. *Journal of Physical Education, Recreation and Dance, 62*(6), 49–52.

Clough, P., Shepherd, J., & Maughan, R. (1989). Motives for participating in recreational running. *Journal of Leisure Research, 21*(4), 297–309.

Coakley, J. (1992). Burnout among adolescent athletes: A personal failure or social problem? *Sociology of Sport Journal, 9,* 271–285.

Coakley, J.J. (1978). *Sport in society: Issues and controversies.* St. Louis: Mosby.

Coakley, J.J. (1994). *Sport in society: Issues and controversies.* St. Louis: Mosby.

Coakley, J.J. (1998). *Sport in society: Issues and controversies* (6th ed.). New York: McGraw-Hill.

Coen, S.P., & Ogles, B.M. (1993). Psychological characteristics of the obligatory runner: A critical examination of the anorexia analogue hypothesis. *Journal of Sport and Exercise Psychology, 15,* 338–354.

Coggan, A., & Coyle, E. (1991). Carbohydrate ingestion during prolonged exercise: Effects on metabolism and performance. In J.O. Holloszy (Ed.), *Exercise and Sport Science Reviews* (Vol. 19, pp. 1–40). Baltimore: Williams & Wilkins.

Coleman, J. (1961) *The adolescent society: The social life of the teenager and its impact on education.* New York: Free Press of Glencoe.

College Preview. (1997). American humanics: Training for feel-good careers, 10–13. Vol. XII, No. 4.

Connolly, K.J. (Ed.). (1970). *Mechanisms of motor skill development.* New York: Academic Press.

Contini, R., & Drillis, R. (1954). Biomechanics. *Applied Mechanics Reviews, 7*(2), 49–52.

Contini, R., & Drillis, R. (1966). Biomechanics. In H.N. Abramson, H. Liebowitz, J.M. Crowley, & S. Juhasz (Eds.), *Applied mechanics surveys.* Washington, DC: Spartan Books.

Cooper, J.M. (1977). The historical development of kinesiology with emphasis on concepts and people. In C.J. Dillon & R.G. Sears (Eds.), *Proceedings of kinesiology: A national conference on teaching.* Urbana-Champaign, IL: University of Illinois.

Cooper, J.M., & Glassow, R.B. (1963). *Kinesiology.* St. Louis: C.V. Mosby.

Cormier, J., York, A., Domholdt, E., & Keggeris, S. (1993). Athletic trainer utilization in sports medicine clinics. *Journal of Orthopedic and Sports Physical Therapy, 17*(1), 36–43.

Cottrell, N.B. (1968). Performance in the presence of other human beings: Mere presence, audience, and affiliation effects. In E.C. Simmel, R.A. Hoppe, & G.A. Milton (Eds.), *Social facilitation and imitative behavior* (pp. 91–110). Needham Heights, MA: Allyn & Bacon.

Craik, R.L., & Dutterer, L. (1995). Spatial and temporal characteristics of foot fall patterns. In R.L. Craik & C.A. Oatis (Eds.), *Gait analysis: Theory and application* (1st ed., pp. 148–158). St. Louis: Mosby.

Cratty, B.J. (1989). *Psychology in contemporary sport* (3rd ed.). Englewood Cliffs, NJ: Prentice Hall.

Crawford, S., & Eklund, R.C. (1994). Social physique anxiety, reasons for exercise, and attitudes toward exercise settings. *Journal of Sport and Exercise Psychology, 16,* 70–82.

Crews, D.J., & Landers, D.M. (1987). A meta-analytic review of aerobic fitness and reactivity to psychosocial stressors. *Medicine and Science in Sports and Exercise, 19,* S114–120.

Crosset, T.W. (1995). *Outsiders in the clubhouse: The world of women's professional golf.* Albany, NY: State University of New York Press.

Csikszentmihalyi, M. (1990a, January). *What good are sports?* Paper presented at the Commonwealth and International Conference of Physical Education,

Sport, Health, Dance, Recreation, and Leisure, Auckland, New Zealand.

Csikszentmihalyi, M. (1990b). *Flow: The psychology of optimal experience.* New York: Harper & Row.

Cureton, T.K. (1930). Mechanics and physiology of swimming (the crawl flutter kick). *Research Quarterly, 1,* 87–121.

Cureton, T.K. (1932). Physics applied to physical education. *Journal of Health and Physical Education, 1,* 23–25.

Curry, T.J. (1991). Fraternal bonding in the locker room: A profeminist analysis of talk about competition and women. *Sociology of Sport Journal, 8,* 119–135.

Cutler, N.E. (1994). Functional limitation and the need for personal care. In B.R. Bonder & M.B. Wagner (Eds.), *Functional performance in older adults* (pp. 210–222). Philadelphia: Davis.

Cutlip, S.M., Center, A.H., & Broom, G.M. (1994). *Effective public relations* (7th ed.). Englewood Cliffs, NJ: Prentice Hall.

Czaja, S.J. (1997). Using technologies to aid the performance of home tasks. In A.D. Fisk & W.A. Rogers (Eds.), *Human factors and the older adult* (pp. 311–334). New York: Academic Press.

Daly, W.M. (1972). Recent deaths. *American Historical Review, 77,* 613.

Davis, E.C. (1961). *The philosophic process in physical education.* Philadelphia: Lea & Febiger.

Davis, E.C. (Ed.). (1963). *Philosophies fashion physical education.* Dubuque, IA: Brown.

Davis, J.M., Burgess, W.A., Sientz, C.A., Bartoli, W.P., & Pate, R.R. (1988). Effects of ingesting 6% and 12% glucose/electrolyte beverages during prolonged intermittent cycling in the heat. *European Journal of Applied Physiology, 57,* 563–569.

Davis, L.R. (1997). *The swimsuit issue and sport: Hegemonic masculinity in Sports Illustrated.* Albany, NY: State University of New York Press.

Dawson, D., Hendershot, G., & Fulton, J. (1987). Aging in the eighties: Function limitations of individuals 65 years and older. *National Center for Health Statistics Advance Data 1987, 133,* 1–11.

De Grazia, S. (1962). *Of time, work and leisure.* Garden City, NY: Doubleday.

Delattre, E.J. (1975). Some reflections on success and failure in competitive athletics. *Journal of the Philosophy of Sport, 2,* 133–139.

DeLee, J.C., & Farney, W.C. (1992). Incidence of injury in Texas high school football. *American Journal of Sports Medicine, 20*(5), 575–580.

Denney, R. (1957). *The astonished muse.* Chicago: University of Chicago Press.

Dennis, W. (1938). Infant development under conditions of restricted practice and a minimum of social stimulation: A preliminary report. *Journal of Genetic Psychology, 53,* 149–158.

Dennis, W., & Dennis, M. (1940). The effect of cradling practices on the age of walking in Hopi children. *Journal of Genetic Psychology, 56,* 77–86.

DePauw, K.P. (1996). Students with disabilities in physical education. In S.J. Silverman & C.D. Ennis (Eds.), *Student learning in physical education: Applying research to enhance instruction.* Champaign, IL: Human Kinetics.

Dietz, W.H. (1990). Children and television. In M. Green & R.J. Hagerty (Eds.), *Ambulatory pediatrics IV* (pp. 39–41). Philadelphia: W.B. Saunders.

Dill, D.B. (1967). The Harvard Fatigue Laboratory: Its development, contributions, and demise. In C.B. Chapman (Ed.), *Physiology of muscular exercise* (pp. 161–170). New York: American Heart Association.

Dill, D.B. (1974). Historical review of exercise physiology science. In W.R. Johnson & E.R. Buskirk (Eds.), *Science and Medicine of Exercise and Sport* (2nd ed., pp. 37–41). New York: Harper & Row.

Dill, D.B. (1985). Arlie V. Bock, pioneer in sports medicine. *Medicine and Science in Sports and Exercise, 17,* 401–404.

Dill, D.B., Talbott, J.H., & Edwards, H.T. (1930). Studies in muscular activity. VI. Responses of several individuals to a fixed task. *Journal of Physiology, 69,* 267–305.

Dillman, C.J., Fleisig, G.S., & Andrews, J.R. (1993). Biomechanics of pitching with emphasis upon shoulder kinematics. *Journal of Orthopaedic & Sports Physical Therapy, 18*(2), 402–408.

Dintiman, G.B., & Greenberg, J.S. (1986). *Health through discovery.* New York: Random House.

Dishman, R.K. (1990). Determinants of participation in physical activity. In Bouchard, C., Shephard, R.J., Stephens, T., Sutton, J.R., McPherson, B.D. (Eds.). *Exercise, fitness, and health: A consensus of current knowledge* (pp. 75–102). Champaign, IL: Human Kinetics.

Dishman, R.K., & Sallis, J.F. (1994). Determinants and interventions for physical activity and exercise. In Bouchard, C., Shephard, R.J., & Stephens, T. (Eds.), *Physical activity, fitness, and health: International proceedings and concensus statement* (pp. 214-238). Champaign, IL: Human Kinetics.

Dishman, R.K., Sallis, J.F., & Orenstein, D. (1985). The determinants of physical activity and exercise. *Public Health Reports, 100,* 158–171.

Dodd, M., & Pearson, B. (1997, November 21). Big-time matchups underscore the big business of college ball. *USA Today,* pp. 1A, 2A.

Dodds, P. (1983). Consciousness raising in curriculum: A teacher's model. In A. Jewett, M. Carries, & M. Speakman (Eds.), *Proceedings of the third conference on curricula and theory in physical education* (pp. 213–234). Athens, GA: University of Georgia Press.

Donnelly, P. (1977). Vertigo in America: A social comment. *Quest, 27*, 106–113.

Drinkwater, B.L., Nilson, K., Chesnut, C.H., Bremner, W.J., Shainholtz, S., & Southworth, M.B. (1984). Bone mineral content of amenorrheic and eumenorrheic athletes. *New England Journal of Medicine, 311*, 277–281.

Duda, J.L. (1992). Motivation in sport settings: A goal perspective approach. In G.G. Roberts (Ed.), *Motivation in sport and exercise* (pp. 57–91). Champaign, IL: Human Kinetics.

Duda, J.L., Olson, L.K., & Templin, T.J. (1991). The relationship of task and ego orientation to sportsmanship attitudes and the perceived legitimacy of injurious acts. *Research Quarterly for Exercise and Sport, 62*(1), 79–87.

Dudgenon, B.J. (1996). Pediatric rehabilitation. In J. Case-Smith, A.S. Allen, & P.N. Pratts (Eds.), *Occupational therapy for children* (3rd ed., pp. 777–795). Baltimore: Mosby-Yearbook.

Dulles, F.R. (1940). *America learns to play: A history of popular recreation*. New York: Appleton-Century-Crofts.

Duncan, M.C., & Hasbrook, C.A. (1988). Denial of power in televised women's sports. *Sociology of Sport Journal, 5*, 1–21.

Duncan, M.C., Messner, M.A., Williams, L., & Jensen, K. (1994). Gender stereotyping in televised sports. In S. Birrell & C.L. Cole (Eds.), *Women, sport, and culture* (pp. 249–272). Champaign, IL: Human Kinetics. (Original work published 1990)

Dunkin, M.J., & Biddle, B.J. (1974). *The study of teaching*. New York: Holt, Rinehart & Winston.

Dunkle, R.E., Kart, C.S., & Lockery, S.A. (1994). Self-care. In B.R. Bonder & M.B. Wagner (Eds.), *Functional performance in older adults* (pp. 122–135). Philadelphia: Davis.

Dunning, E., Murphy, P., & Williams, J. (1988). *The roots of football hooliganism: An historical and sociological study*. London: Routledge.

Durstine, J.L., & Haskell, W.L. (1994). Effects of exercise training on plasma lipids and lipoproteins. In J.O. Holloszy (Ed.), *Exercise and Sport Sciences Reviews, 22*, 477–521.

Dychtwald, K. (1990). *Age wave*. New York: Bantam Books.

Ebihara, O., Ideda, M., & Myiashita, M. (1983). Birth order and children's socialization into sport. *International Review of Sport Sociology, 18*, 69–89.

Eitzen, D.S., & Sage, G.H. (1978). *Sociology of American sport*. Dubuque, IA: Brown.

Eitzen, D.S., & Sage, G.H. (1993). *Sociology of North American Sport* (5th ed.). Madison, WI: Brown & Benchmark.

Eitzen, D.S., & Sage, G.H. (1997). *Sociology of North American Sport* (6th ed.). Madison, WI: Brown & Benchmark.

Ennis, C. (1994). Urban secondary teachers' value orientations: Social goals for teaching. *Teaching and Teacher Education, 10*, 109–120.

Espenschade, A. (1960). Motor development. In W.R. Johnson (Ed.), *Science and medicine of exercise and sports* (p. 439). New York: Harper & Row.

Exley, F. (1968). *A fan's notes*. New York: Random House.

Fenn, W.O. (1929). Mechanical energy expenditure in sprint running as measured by moving pictures. *American Journal of Physiology, 90*, 343–344.

Ferguson, H. (1990). *The edge: The guide to fulfilling dreams, maximizing success and enjoyment a lifetime of achievement*. Cleveland, OH: Getting the Edge Co.

Fidler, G.S., & Fidler, J.W. (1978). Doing and becoming: Purposeful action and self-actualization. *American Journal of Occupational Therapy, 32*, 305–310.

Fielding & Miller (1996). Historical eras in sport marketing. In B.G. Pitts and D.K. Stotlar (Eds.), *Fundamentals of sport marketing*. Morgantown, WV: Fitness Information Technology, Inc.

Figure skating jumps in fan vote. (1997, April 24). *USA Today*, p. C1.

Fine, G.A. (1988). Good children and dirty play. *Play and Culture, 1*, 43–56.

Fink, J., & Siedentop, D. (1989). The development of routines, rules, and expectations at the start of the school year. *Journal of Teaching in Physical Education, 8*, 198–212.

Fiore, R.D., & Leard, J.S. (1980). A functional approach in the rehabilitation of the ankle and rearfoot. *Athletic Training, 15*, 655–659.

Fitnews. (1995, April). *Fitness Management*, p. 14.

Fitts, P.M., & Posner, M.I. (1967). *Human performance*. Pacific Grove, CA: Brooks/Cole.

Flacks, R., & Thomas, S.L. (1998, November 27). Among affluent students a culture of disengagement. *The Chronicle of Higher Education*, p. A48.

Fleishman, E.A. (1953). Testing for psychomotor abilities by means of apparatus tests. *Psychological Bulletin, 50*, 243–262.

Fleishman, E.A. (1956). Psychomotor selection tests: Research and application in the United States Air Force. *Personnel Psychology, 9,* 449–467.

Fleishman, E.A., & Hempel, W.E. (1955). The relationship between abilities and improvement with practice in a visual reaction time discrimination task. *Journal of Experimental Psychology, 49,* 301–312.

Fleishman, E.A., & Stephenson, R.W. (1970). Development of a taxonomy of human performance: A review of the third year's progress (Tech. Rep. No. 3). *American Institutes for Research, 726.*

Fleisig, G.S., Barrentine, S.W., Escamilla, R.F., & Andrews, J.R. (1996). Biomechanics of overhand throwing with implications for injuries. *Sports Medicine, 21*(6), 421–437.

Fraleigh, W.P. (1984). *Right actions in sport: Ethics for contestants.* Champaign, IL: Human Kinetics.

Friedman, M., & Rosenman, R. H. (1974). *Type A behavior and your heart.* New York: Knopf.

Fullerton, G.S., & Cattell, J. (1892). On the perception of small differences. *University of Pennsylvania Philosophical Series,* No. 2.

Fung, Y.C. (1968). Biomechanics—Its scope, history, and some problems of continuum mechanics in physiology. *Applied Mechanics Reviews, 21,* 1–20.

Furusawa, K., Hill, A.V., & Parkinson, J.L. (1927). The dynamics of sprint running. *Proceedings of the Royal Society of London, 102B,* 29–42.

Galton, F. (1876). The history of twins as a criterion of the relative power of nature. *Anthropological Institute Journal, 5,* 391–406.

Game plans. (1994, March 19). *The Economist,* p. 108.

Garcia, A.W., Broda, M.A.N., Frenn, M., Coviak, C., Pender, N.J., & Ronis, D.L. (1995). Gender and developmental differences in exercise beliefs among youth and prediction of their exercise behavior. *Journal of School Health, 65,* 213–219.

Gehlsen, G.M., & Seger, A. (1980). Selected measures of angular displacement, strength and flexibility in subjects with and without splints. *Research Quarterly for Exercise and Sport, 51*(3), 478–485.

Gentile, A.M. (1972). A working model of skill acquisition with application to teaching. *Quest,* Monograph XVII, 2–23.

Genzale, J., (1998, April 27–May 3). Dynamic U.S. sports industry finds a new voice. *Street & Smith's Sports Business Journal, 1*(1), 57.

Gerber, E.W. (1971). *Innovators and institutions in physical education.* Philadelphia: Lea & Febiger.

Gerber, E.W. (Ed.). (1972). *Sport and the body: A philosophical symposium.* Philadelphia: Lea & Febiger.

Gesell, A. (1928). *Infancy and human growth.* New York: Macmillan.

Giamatti, A.B. (1989). *Take time for paradise: Americans and their games.* New York: Summit Books.

Gill, D.L. (1992). Gender and sport behavior. In T.S. Horn (Ed.), *Advances in sport psychology* (pp. 143–160). Champaign, IL: Human Kinetics.

Gill, F.B. (1989). *Ornithology.* New York: W.H. Freeman.

Glassow, R.B. (1932). *Fundamentals of physical education.* Philadelphia: Lea & Febiger.

Glassow, R.B. & Broer, M. (1938). *Measuring achievement in physical education.* Philadelphia: W.B. Saunders.

Glazier, M., & Jones, K. (1991, May). A sea of rules. *College Athletic Management, III* (3), 14–18.

Goldstein, J.H., & Arms, R. (1971, March). Effects of observing athletic contests on hostility. *Sociometry, 34,* 83–90.

Gollnick, P.D., Timson, B.F., Moore, R.L., & Riedy, M. (1981). Muscular enlargement and number of fibers in skeletal muscles of rats. *Journal of Applied Physiology, 50,* 936–943.

Gonyea, W.J. (1980). Role of exercise in inducing increases in skeletal muscle fiber number. *Journal of Applied Physiology, 48,* 421–426.

Gorn, E.J. (1986). *The manly art: Bare-knuckle prize fighting in America.* Ithaca, NY: Cornell University Press.

Gorn, E.J. (Ed.). (1995). *Muhammad Ali: The people's champ.* Urbana, IL: University of Illinois Press.

Gorn, E.J., & Goldstein, W. (1993). *A brief history of American sports.* New York: Hill & Wang.

Gould, D., & Petlichkoff, L. (1988). Participation motivation and attrition in young athletes. In F. Smoll, R. Magill, & M. Ash (Eds.), *Children in sport* (3rd ed., pp. 161–178). Champaign, IL: Human Kinetics.

Gould, D., Udry, E., Tuffey, S., & Loehr, J. (1996). Burnout in competitive junior tennis players: I. A quantitative psychological assessment. *The Sport Psychologist, 10,* 322–340.

Graber, K.C. (in press). Research on teaching in physical education. In V. Richardson (Ed.), *Handbook of research on teaching* (4th ed.). Washington, DC: American Educational Research Association.

Graham, G. (Ed.). (1982). Profiles of excellence: Processes and teachers in children's physical education. *Journal of Physical Education, Recreation and Dance, 53*(7), 37–55.

Graham, G. (1992). *Teaching children physical education: Becoming a master teacher.* Champaign, IL: Human Kinetics.

Graham, G., & Heimerer, E. (1981). Research on teacher effectiveness: A summary with implications for teaching. *Quest, 33,* 14–25.

Grantham, W.C., Patton, R.W., York, T.D., & Winick, M.L. (1998). *Health fitness management.* Champaign, IL: Human Kinetics.

Graves, H. (1900). A philosophy of sport. *The Contemporary Review, 78,* 877–893.

Greendorfer, S.L. (1979). Childhood sport socialization influences of male and female track athletes. *Arena Review, 3,* 39–53.

Greenwood, E. (1957). Attributes of a profession. *Social Work, 2,* 45–55.

Griffin, P.S. (1984). Girls' participation patterns in a middle school team sports unit. *Journal of Teaching in Physical Education, 4,* 30–38.

Griffin, P.S. (1986). Analysis and discussion: What have we learned? *Journal of Physical Education, Recreation and Dance, 57*(4), 57–59.

Griffith, C.R. (1926). *Psychology of coaching.* New York: Scribner.

Griffith, C.R. (1928). *Psychology and athletics.* New York: Scribner.

Griffith, C.R. (1930). A laboratory for research in athletics. *Research Quarterly, 1*(3), 34–40.

Grossman, P.L. (1989). A study in contrast: Sources of pedagogical content knowledge for secondary English. *Journal of Teacher Education, 40*(5), 24–31.

Gruber, J.J. (1986). Physical activity and self-esteem development in children: A meta-analysis. *American Academy of Physical Education Papers, 19,* 30–48.

Gruneau, R. (1983). *Class, sports, and social development.* Amherst, MA: University of Massachusetts Press.

Guinness Book of Records. (1999). Guinness Publishing.

Guttmann, A. (1978). *From ritual to record: The nature of modern sports.* New York: Columbia University Press.

Guttmann, A. (1984). *The games must go on: Avery Brundage and the Olympic movement.* New York: Columbia University Press.

Guttmann, A. (1991). *Women's sports: A history.* New York: Columbia University Press.

Guttmann, A. (1994). *Games and empires: Modern sports and cultural imperialism.* New York: Columbia University Press.

Hagberg, J. (1987). Effect of training on the decline of VO_2max with aging. *Federation Proceedings, 46,* 1830–1833.

Hagberg, J.M. (1989). Effect of exercise and training on older men and women with essential hypertension. In W.W. Spirduso & H.M. Eckert (Eds.), *Physical Activity and Aging, The Academy Papers, 22,* 186–193. Champaign, IL: Human Kinetics.

Hagberg, J.M. (1994). Physical activity, fitness, health, and aging. In C. Bouchard, R.J. Shephard, & T. Stephens (Eds.), *Physical activity, fitness, and health: International proceedings and consensus statement* (pp. 993–1005). Champaign, IL: Human Kinetics.

Haken, H., Kelso, J.A.S., & Bunz, H. (1985). A theoretical model of phase transitions in human hand movements. *Biological Cybernetics, 51,* 347–356.

Halverson, L., Roberton, M.A., & Langendorfer, S. (1982). Development of the overarm throw: Movement and ball velocity changes by seventh grade. *Research Quarterly for Exercise and Sport, 53,* 198–205.

Hanin, Y.L. (1997). Emotions and athletic performance: Individual zones of optimal functioning model. In R. Seiler (Ed.), *European yearbook of sport psychology* (pp. 29–70). Sankt Augustin, Germany: Academia Verlag.

Hardy, L. (1990). A catastrophe model of performance in sport. In J.G. Jones & L. Hardy (Eds.), *Stress and performance in sport* (pp. 81–106). Chichester, UK: Wiley.

Hardy, S. (1982). *How Boston played: Sport, recreation, and community 1865-1915.* Boston: Northeastern University Press.

Harmond, R. (1971–1972). Progress and flight: An interpretation of the American cycle craze of the 1890s. *Journal of Social History, 5*(2), 235–257.

Hart, I. (1963). *The mechanical investigations of Leonardo da Vinci* (2nd ed.). Berkeley, CA: University of California Press.

Hartwell, E.M. (1899). On physical training. *Report of the Commissioner of Education for 1897-1898,* Vol. 1. Washington, DC: U.S. Government Printing Office.

Hastie, P.A. (1996). Student role environment during a unit of sport education. *Journal of Teaching in Physical Education, 16,* 88-103.

Hatfield, B.D., & Landers, D.M. (1983). Psychophysiology—A new direction for sport psychology. *Journal of Sport Psychology, 5,* 243–259.

Hatze, H. (1974). The meaning of the term "biomechanics." *Journal of Biomechanics, 7,* 189–190.

Hay, J.G. (1993a). *The biomechanics of sport techniques* (4th ed.). Englewood Cliffs: Prentice Hall.

Hay, J.G. (1993b). Citius, altius, longius (faster, higher, longer)—The biomechanics of jumping for distance. *Journal of Biomechanics, 26* (Suppl. 1), 7–21.

Haymes, E.M., & Wells, C.L. (1986). *Environment and human performance.* Champaign, IL: Human Kinetics.

Helitzer, M. (1995). *The dream job: $port$ publicity, promotion and marketing* (2nd ed.). Athens, OH: University Sports Press.

Hellison, D. (1995). *Teaching responsibility through physical activity.* Champaign, IL: Human Kinetics.

Hellison, D. (1996). Teaching personal and social responsibility in physical education. In S.J. Silverman & C.D. Ennis (Eds.), *Student learning in physical education: Applying research to enhance instruction* (pp. 269–286). Champaign, IL: Human Kinetics.

Hellison, D., Cutforth, N. Kallusky, J., Martinek, T., Parker, M., & Stiehl, J., (In press). *Serving underserved youth through physical activity: Toward a model of university community collaboration.* Champaign, IL: Human Kinetics.

Hellison, D.R., & Templin, T.J. (1991). *A reflective approach to teaching physical education.* Champaign, IL: Human Kinetics.

Heltne, P.G. (1989). Epilogue: Understanding chimpanzees and bonobos, understanding ourselves. In P. Heltne & L. Marquardt (Eds.), *Understanding chimpanzees* (pp. 380–384). Cambridge, MA: Harvard University Press.

Henry, F.M. (1964). Physical education: An academic discipline. *Journal of Health, Physical Education, and Recreation, 35*(7), 32–33, 69.

Henry, F.M., & Rogers, D.E. (1960). Increased response latency for complicated movements and a "memory drum" theory of neuromotor reaction. *Research Quarterly, 31,* 448–458.

Hill, A.V. (1926). Scientific study of athletes. *Scientific American, 134,* 224–225.

Hill, A.V., & Lupton, H. (1923). Muscular exercise, lactic acid, and the supply of oxygen. *Quarterly Journal of Medicine, 16,* 135–171.

Hoberman, J.M. (1992). *Mortal engines: The science of performance and the dehumanization of sport.* New York: Free Press.

Hoberman, J.M. (1997). *Darwin's athletes: How sport has damaged black America and preserved the myth of race.* Boston: Houghton Mifflin.

Hoch, P. (1972). *Rip off the big game.* New York: Doubleday.

Hong, S.K. (1973). Pattern of cold adaptation in women divers of Korea (ama). *Federation Proceedings, 32,* 1614–1622.

Hout, M., & Lucas, S.R. (1996, August 16). Narrowing the income gap between rich and poor. *Chronicle of Higher Education,* p. B1.

Howell, J., & Ingham, A. (2000). From social problem to personal issue: The language of lifestyle. *Cultural Studies*

Howell, W.C. (1997). Foreword, perspectives and prospectives. In A.D. Fisk & W.A. Rogers (Eds.), *Human factors and the older adult* (pp. 1–6). New York: Academic Press.

Hrycaiko, D., McCabe, A., & Moriarty, D. (n.d.). *Sport, physical activity and TV role models.* Ottawa, ON: Canadian Association for Health, Physical Education and Recreation.

Huizinga, J. (1950). *Homo ludens: A study of the play-element in culture.* Boston: Beacon. (Original work published 1944)

Hultman, E. (1967). Physiological role of muscle glycogen in man, with special reference to exercise. *Circulation Research, 21* (Suppl. 1), 99–114.

Hyland, D.A. (1990). *Philosophy of sport.* New York: Paragon House.

IHRSA survey reports health & fitness club $$ jumps 9 percent. (1998, August). *Club Industry, 14*(9), 6.

Income gap is widest since '40s, agency says. (1996, June 20). *Greensboro News and Record,* p. A6.

Industry may hinge on kids exercising. (1995, September). *Fitness Management,* p. 12.

International Health, Racquet and Sportsclub Association. (1992). *The economic benefits of regular exercise.* Boston: Author.

International Health, Racquet and Sportsclub Association. (1997). *Profiles of success.* Boston: Author.

International Health, Racquet and Sportsclub Association. (1998, September). IHRSA member letter. Boston: Author.

Ivy, J.L., Katz, A.L., & Cutler, C.L. (1989). Muscle glycogen resynthesis after exercise: Effect of time on carbohydrate ingestion. *Journal of Applied Physiology, 64,* 1480–1485.

Jackson, D.Z. (1989, January 22). Calling the plays in black and white. *Boston Globe,* pp. A30, A33.

Jackson, D.Z. (1996, March 27). Chasing spirits down the court at NCAA tourney. *Charlotte Observer,* p. 17A.

Jackson, J.A. (1970). *Professions and professionalization.* London: Cambridge University Press.

Jamieson, K. (1998). Reading Nancy Lopez: Decoding representations of race, class, and sexuality. *Sociology of Sport Journal, 15,* 343–358.

Jenni, D.A., & Jenni, M.A. (1976). Carrying behaviour in humans: Analyses of sex differences. *Science, 194,* 859–860.

Johnson, W.R. (Ed.). (1960). *Science and medicine of exercise and sports.* New York: Harper & Brothers.

Judd, C.H. (1908). The relation of special training to general intelligence. *Educational Review, 36,* 28–42.

Kane, R.L., Ouslander, J.G., & Abrass, I.B. (1994). *Essentials of clinical geriatrics* (3rd ed.). Boston: Allyn & Bacon.

Karpovich, P.V., Morehouse, L.E., Scott, M.G., & Weiss, R.A. (Eds.). (1960). The contributions of physical activity to human well-being. *Research Quarterly, 31*(2), part II [special issue].

Katz, S., Ford, A.B., Moskowitz, R.W., Jackson, B.A., and Jaffee, M.W. (1963). Studies of illness in the aged: The index of ADL: A standardized measure of biological and psychological function. *Journal of the American Medical Association, 185,* 914–919.

Keele, S.W., & Hawkins, H.L. (1982). Explorations of individual differences relevant to high level skill. *Journal of Motor Behavior, 14,* 3–23.

Keele, S.W., Pokorny, R.A., Corcos, D.M., & Ivry, R. (1985). Do perception and motor production share common timing mechanisms? A correlational analysis. *Acta Psychologica, 60,* 173–191.

Kelso, J.A.S. (1995). *Dynamic patterns: The self-organization of brain and behavior.* Cambridge, MA: MIT Press.

Kelso, J.A.S., & Clark J.E. (Eds.). (1982). *The development of movement control and co-ordination.* New York: Wiley.

Kent-Brown, J.A., Miller, R.G., & Weiner, M.W. (1995). Human skeletal muscle metabolism in health and disease: Utility of magnetic resonance spectroscopy. In J.O. Holloszy (Ed.), *Exercise and Sport Sciences Reviews, 23,* pp. 305–347. Baltimore: Williams & Wilkins.

Kenyon, G.S. (1968). A conceptual model for characterizing physical activity. *Research Quarterly, 39,* 96–104.

Kenyon, G.S., & Loy, J.W. (1965). Toward a sociology of sport. *Journal of Health, Physical Education and Recreation, 36*(5), 24–25, 68–69.

Kerr, J.H. (1985). The experience of arousal: A new basis for studying arousal effects in sport. *Journal of Sport Sciences, 3,* 169–179.

Khalil, T.M., Abdel-Moty, E.M., Rosomoff, R.S., & Rosomoff, H.L. (1993). *Ergonomics in back pain.* New York: Van Nostrand Reinhold.

King, A.C., Blair, S.N., Bild, D., Dishman, R.K., Dubbert, P.M., Marcus, B.H., Oldridge, N.M., Paffenbarger, R.S., Powell, K.E., & Yeager, K.Y. (1992). Determinants of physical activity and interventions in adults. *Medicine and Science in Sports and Exercise, 24*(6), S221–236.

Kinkema, K.M., & Harris, J.C. (1998). MediaSport studies: Key research and emerging issues. In L.A. Wenner (Ed.), *MediaSport* (pp. 27–54). London: Routledge.

Kircaldy, B.D., & Shephard, R.J. (1990). Therapeutic implications of exercise. *International Journal of Sports Psychology, 21,* 165–184.

Klein, A.M. (1997). *Baseball on the border: A tale of two laredos.* Princeton, NJ: Princeton University Press.

Kleinman, S. (1968). Toward a non-theory of sport. *Quest, 10,* 29–34.

The kid had it all, but just didn't like baseball. (1997, May 31). *International Herald Tribune,* p. 5.

Knoppers, A. (1987). Gender and the coaching profession, *Quest, 39,* 9–22.

Kobasa, S.C. (1979). Stressful life events, personality, and health: An inquiry into hardiness. *Journal of Personality and Social Psychology, 37,* 1–11.

Kobetic, R., Marsolais, E.B., Samame, P., & Borges, G. (1994). The next step: Artificial walking. In J. Rose & J.G. Gamble (Eds.), *Human walking* (2nd ed., pp. 225–252). Baltimore, MD: Williams & Wilkins.

Kochman, T. (1981). *Black and white styles in conflict.* Chicago: University of Chicago Press.

Kordtlandt, A. (1989). The use of stone tools by wild-living chimpanzees. In P. Heltne and L. Marquardt (Eds.), *Understanding chimpanzees* (pp. 146–147). Cambridge, MA: Harvard University Press.

Kranz, L. (1995). *Jobs rated almanac* (3rd ed.). New York: Wiley.

Krawthwohl, D.R., Bloom, B.S., & Masia, B.B. (1964). *Taxonomy of educational objectives: Handbook II: Affective domain.* New York: David McKay.

Kretchmar, R.S. (1985). "Distancing": An essay on abstract thinking in sport performances. In D.L. Vanderwerken & S.K. Wertz (Eds.), *Sport inside out: Readings in literature and philosophy* (pp. 87–103). Forth Worth, TX: Texas Christian University Press.

Kretchmar, R.S. (1994). *Practical philosophy of sport.* Champaign, IL: Human Kinetics.

Kretchmar, R.S. (1996). Philosophic research in physical activity. In J.R. Thomas & J.K. Nelson (Eds.), *Research methods in physical activity* (pp. 277–290). Champaign, IL: Human Kinetics.

Kretchmar, R.S. (1997). Philosophy of sport. In J.D. Massengale & R.A. Swanson (Eds.), *The history of exercise and sport science* (pp. 181–201). Champaign, IL: Human Kinetics.

Kroemer, K., Kroemer, H., & Kroemer-Elbert, K. (1994). *Ergonomics: How to design for ease and efficiency.* Englewood Cliffs, NJ: Prentice Hall.

Krogh, A., & Lindhard, J. (1920) The relative value of fat and carbohydrate as sources of muscular energy. *Biochemical Journal, 14,* 290–363.

Kroll, W.P. (1982). *Graduate study and research in physical education.* Champaign, IL: Human Kinetics.

LaBarre, W. (1963). *The human animal.* Chicago: University of Chicago Press.

Lane, N.E. (1995). Exercise—A cause of osteoarthritis. *Journal of Rheumatology, 22* (Suppl. 43), 3–6.

Lanier, J.E., & Little, J.W. (1986). Research on teacher education. In M.C. Wittrock (Ed.), *Handbook of research on teaching* (3rd ed., pp. 527–569). New York: Macmillan.

LaPlante, M. (1990). Disabilities of chronic illnesses and impairments. *Disability statistics report 2.* San Francisco: University of California Institute for Heart and Aging.

Latane, B., Williams, K., & Harkins, S.J. (1979). Many hands make light the work: The cause and consequences of social loafing. *Journal of Experimental Social Psychology, 37,* 822–832.

Lawson, H., Briar-Lawson, K., & Larson, M. (1997). Mapping changes for vulnerable children, youth and families: Implications for university-assisted community schools. *Universities and Community Schools, 51* (1-2), 80-84.

Lawson, H.A. (1984). *Invitation to physical education.* Champaign, IL: Human Kinetics.

Lawson, H.A. (1998a). Globalization and the social responsibilities of citizen-professionals. Unpublished paper. Address to AIESEP International Conference, Adelphi University, July, p. 7.

Lawson, H.A. (1998b). Here today, gone tomorrow: A framework for analyzing the invention, development, transformation and disappearance of helping fields. *Quest, 50,* 225–237.

Lee, A.M. (1996). How the field evolved. In S. Silverman & C. Ennis (Eds.), *Studying learning in physical education: Applying research to enhance instruction* (pp. 9–34). Champaign, IL: Human Kinetics.

Lee, A.M., Keh, N.C., & Magill, R.A. (1993). Instructional effects of teacher feedback in physical education. *Journal of Teaching in Physical Education, 12,* 228–243.

Lee, T.D., & Magill, R.A. (1983). The locus of contextual interference in motor skill acquisition. *Journal of Experimental Psychology: Learning, Memory, and Cognition, 9,* 730–746.

Lee, T.D., & Weeks, D.J. (1987). The beneficial influence of forgetting on short-term retention of movement information. *Human Movement Science, 6,* 233–245.

Leonard, W.M. (1998). *A sociological perspective of sport.* Needham Heights, MA: Allyn & Bacon

Leuba, J.H. (1909). The influence of the duration and of the rate of arm movements upon the judgment of their length. *American Journal of Psychology, 20,* 374–385.

Levine, P. (1992). *Ellis Island to Ebbets Field: Sport and the American Jewish experience.* New York: Oxford University Press.

Lewis, G.M. (1972). John Rickards Betts and the beginning of a new age in sports history. *Journal of Health, Physical Education and Recreation, 43* (3), 81–82.

Lewko, J.H., & Greendorfer, S.L. (1988). Sex differences and parental influences in sport socialization of children and adolescents. In F.L. Smoll, R.A. Magill, & M.J. Ash (Eds.), *Children in sport* (3rd ed., pp 287–300). Champaign, IL: Human Kinetics.

Locke, E.A., & Latham, G.P. (1985). The application of goal setting to sports. *Sport Psychology Today, 7,* 205–222.

Locke, L.F. (1975). *The ecology of the gymnasium: What the tourists never see.* Amherst, MA: University of Massachusetts. (ERIC Document Reproduction No. ED 104-823)

Locke, L.F. (1977). Research on teaching physical education: New hope for a dismal science. *Quest, 28,* 2–16.

Locke, L.F. (1990). Commentary: Conjuring kinesiology and other political parlor tricks. *Quest, 42,* 323–329.

Locke, L.F. (1992). Changing secondary school physical education. *Quest, 44,* 361–372.

Locke, L.F., & Griffin, P. (1986). Profiles of struggle. *Journal of Physical Education, Recreation and Dance, 57*(4), 32–63.

Lorber, J. (1994). *Paradoxes of gender.* New Haven, CT: Yale University Press.

Lortie, D. (1975). *Schoolteacher: A sociological study.* Chicago: University of Chicago Press.

Lortie, G., Simoneau, J.A., Hamel, P., Boulan, M.R., Landry, F., Bouchard, C. (1984). Responses of maximal aerobic power and capacity to aerobic training. *International Journal of Sports Medicine, 5,* 232–236.

Lowe, D. (1995). *The body in late-capitalist USA.* Durham, NC: Duke University Press.

Loy, J.W. (1974). Editor's forward. In J.R. Betts, *America's sporting heritage: 1850-1950* (pp. iii–iv). Reading, MA: Addison-Wesley.

Loy, J.W., & Kenyon, G.S. (1969a). The sociology of sport: An emerging field. In J.W. Loy & G.S. Kenyon (Eds.), *Sport, culture, and society: A reader on the sociology of sport* (pp. 1–8). New York: Macmillan.

Loy, J.W., & Kenyon, G.S. (1969b). *Sport, culture, and society: A reader on the sociology of sport.* New York: Macmillan.

Loy, J.W., Kenyon, G.S., & McPherson, B.D. (1980). The emergence and development of the sociology of sport as an academic specialty. *Research Quarterly, 51,* 91–109.

Loy, J.W., McPherson, B.D., & Kenyon, G. (1978). *Sport and social systems.* Reading, MA: Addison-Wesley.

Lucas, J.A., & Smith, R.A. (1978). *Saga of American sport.* Philadelphia: Lea & Febiger.

Madrigal, R. (1995). Cognitive and affective determinants of fan satisfaction with sporting event attendance. *Journal of Leisure Research, 27*(3), 205–227.

Magill, R.A. (1989). *Motor learning: Concepts and applications* (3rd ed.). Dubuque, IA: Wm. C. Brown.

Magill, R.A., & Hall, K.G. (1990). A review of the contextual interference effect in motor skill acquisition. *Human Movement Science, 9,* 241–289.

Maguire, J. (1994). Sport, identity politics, and globalization: Diminishing contrasts and increasing varieties. *Sociology of Sport Journal, 11,* 398–427.

Majors, R. (1990). Cool pose: Black masculinity and sports. In M.A. Messner & D.F. Sabo (Eds.), *Sport, men, and the gender order: Critical feminist perspectives* (pp. 109–126). Champaign, IL: Human Kinetics.

Malina, R.M. (1975). *Growth and development: The first twenty years.* Edina, MN: Burgess International.

Malina, R.M. (1984). Physical growth and maturation. In J.R. Thomas (Ed.), *Motor development during childhood and adolescence* (pp. 2–26). Edina, MN: Burgess International.

Malina, R.M., & Bouchard, C. (1991). *Growth, maturation, and physical activity.* Champaign, IL: Human Kinetics.

Mann, R., Griffin, F., & Yocom, G. (1998). *Swing like a pro.* New York: Bantam Doubleday Dell.

Marcel, G. (1952). *Metaphysical Journal.* (B. Wall, Trans.). Chicago: Henry Regnery. (Original work published 1927)

Marcus, B.H. (1995). Exercise behavior and strategies for intervention. *Research Quarterly for Exercise and Sport, 66,* 319–323.

Margaria, R., Edwards, H.T., & Dill, D.B. (1933). The possible mechanisms of contracting and paying the oxygen debt and the role of lactic acid in muscular contraction. *American Journal of Physiology, 106,* 689–715.

Markula, P. (1995). Firm but shapely, fit but sexy, strong but thin: The postmodern aerobicizing female bodies. *Sociology of Sport Journal, 12,* 424–453.

Martens, R. (1990). *Successful coaching.* Champaign, IL: Human Kinetics.

Martens, R., Vealey, R.S., & Burton, D. (1990). *Competitive anxiety in sport.* Champaign, IL: Human Kinetics.

Martin, R. (1997). The composite body: Hip-hop aerobics and the multicultural nation. *Journal of Sport and Social Issues, 21,* 120–133.

Martin, T.W., & Berry, K.J. (1974). Competitive sport in post-industrial society: The case of the motocross racer. *Journal of Popular Culture, 8,* 107–120.

Martinek, T. (1981). Physical attractiveness: Effects on teacher expectations and dyadic interactions in elementary age children. *Journal of Sport Psychology, 3,* 196–205.

Martinek, T. (1991). *Psycho-social dynamics of teaching physical education.* Dubuque, IA: Brown/Benchmark.

Martinek, T., & Griffith, J.B. (1993). Working with the learned helpless child. *Journal of Physical Education, Recreation and Dance, 64*(6), 17–20.

Martinek, T., & Griffith, J.B. (1994). Learned helplessness in physical education: A developmental study of causal attributions and task persistence. *Journal of Teaching in Physical Education, 13,* 108–122.

Martinek, T., & Johnson, S. (1979). Teacher expectations: Effects on dyadic interaction and self-concept in elementary age children. *Research Quarterly for Exercise and Sport, 50,* 60–70.

Martinek, T., & Karper, W. (1981). A teacher's expectations on handicapped and nonhandicapped children in mainstreamed physical education classes. *Perceptual and Motor Skills, 52,* 327–330.

Martinek, T., & Karper, W. (1984). Multivariate relationships of specific impression cues with teacher expectations and dyadic interactions in elementary education classes. *Research Quarterly for Exercise and Sport, 55,* 32–40.

Martinek, T., & Karper, W. (1986). Motor ability and instructional contexts: Effects on teacher expectation and dyadic interactions in elementary physical education classes. *Journal of Classroom Interaction, 21,* 16–25.

Massengale, J.D., & Swanson, R.A. (Eds.). (1997). *The history of exercise and sport science.* Champaign, IL: Human Kinetics.

McAuley, E. (1994). Physical activity and psychosocial outcomes. In C. Bouchard, R.J. Shephard, & T. Stephens (Eds.), *Physical activity, fitness, and health: International proceedings and consensus statement* (pp. 551–569). Champaign, IL: Human Kinetics.

McAuley, E., & Courneya, K.S. (1994). The subjective exercise experiences scale: Development and preliminary validation. *Journal of Sport and Exercise Psychology, 16,* 163–177.

McAuley, E., & Jacobson, L.B. (1991). Self-efficacy and exercise participation in sedentary adult females. *American Journal of Health Promotion, 5,* 185–191.

McAuley, E., Wraith, S., & Duncan, T.E. (1991). Self-efficacy perceptions of success and intrinsic motivation for exercise. *Journal of Applied Social Psychology, 16,* 139–155.

McCarthy, M.R., Hiller, W.D., & Yates-McCarthy, J.L. (1991). Sports medicine in Hawaii: Care of the high school athlete in Oahu's public schools. *Hawaii Medical Journal, 50*(11), 395–396.

McCloy, C.H. (1934). The measurement of general motor capacity and general motor ability. *Research Quarterly, 5* (Suppl. 5), 45–61.

McCloy, C.H. (1937). An analytical study of the stunt type test as a measure of motor educability. *Research Quarterly, 8,* 46–55.

McCloy, C.H. (1960). The mechanical analysis of skills. In W.R. Johnson (Ed.), *Science and medicine in exercise and sports.* New York: Harper & Brothers.

McCullagh, P. (1993). Modeling: Learning, developmental, and social psychological considerations. In R.N. Singer, M. Murphey, & L.K. Tennant (Eds.), *Handbook of research on sport psychology* (pp. 106–126). New York: Macmillan.

McDonald, P. (1992). *Teaching: Making sense of an uncertain craft.* New York: Teachers College Press.

McGill, S.M., & Norman, R.W. (1993). Low back biomechanics in industry: The prevention of injury through safer lifting. In M.D. Grabiner (Ed.), *Current issues in biomechanics* (pp. 69–120). Champaign, IL: Human Kinetics.

McGraw, M.B. (1935). *Growth: A study of Johnny and Jimmy.* New York: Appleton-Century-Crofts.

McGraw, M.B. (1939). Later development of children specially trained during infancy: Johnny and Jimmy at school age. *Child Development, 10,* 1–19.

McIntosh, P. (1963). *Sport in society.* London: C.A. Watts.

McIntyre, N. (1992). Involvement in risk recreation: A comparison of objective measures of engagement. *Journal of Leisure Research, 24,* 64–71.

Meek, A. (1997). An estimate of the size and supported economic activity of the sports industry in the United States. *Sport Marketing Quarterly, 6* (4), 15-22.

Meggyesy, D. (1971). *Out of their league.* New York: Paperback Library.

Meier, K.V. (1979). Embodiment, sport, and meaning. In E.W. Gerber & W.J. Morgan (Eds.), *Sport and the body: A philosophical symposium* (pp. 192–198). Philadelphia: Lea & Febiger.

Merleau-Ponty, M. (1962). *Phenomenology of perception.* (C. Smith, Trans.). New York: Humanities Press. (Original work published 1945)

Messner, M.A. (1988). Sports and male domination: The female athlete as contested ideological terrain. *Sociology of Sport Journal, 5,* 197–211.

Messner, M.A. (1992). *Power at play: Sports and the problem of masculinity.* Boston: Beacon.

Metcalfe, A. (1974). North American sport history: A review of North American sport historians and their works. In J.H. Wilmore (Ed.), *Exercise and Sport Sciences Reviews, 2,* 225–238.

Metheny, E. (1965). *Connotations of movement in sport and dance.* Dubuque, IA: Brown.

Metheny, E. (1968). *Movement and meaning.* New York: McGraw-Hill.

Metheny, E. (1975). *Moving and knowing in sport, dance, physical education.* Mountain View, CA: Peek.

Metzler, M. (1979). *The measurement of academic learning time in physical education.* Unpublished doctoral dissertation, Ohio State University, Columbus.

Metzler, M. (1989). A review of research on time in sport pedagogy. *Journal of Teaching in Physical Education, 8,* 87–103.

Miller, L.K. (1997). *Sport business management.* Gaithersburg, MD: Aspen.

Miller, L.K., Shaad, S., Burch, D., & Turner, R. (1998). *Sales success in sports marketing.* Wichita, KS: Events Unlimited.

Miller, S. (1998, May 25–31). NBAE: Making the plays pay. *Street & Smith's Sports Business Journal, 1*(5), 5.

Miller, S.C., Bredemeier, B.J.L., & Shields, D.L.L. (1997). Sociomoral education through physical education with at-risk children. *Quest, 49,* 114–129.

Mitchell, M. (1992). A descriptive analysis and academic genealogy of major contributors to JTPE in the 1980s. *Journal of Teaching in Physical Education, 11,* 426–432.

Morgan, W.J. (1994). *Leftist theories of sport: A critique and reconstruction.* Urbana, IL: University of Illinois Press.

Morgan, W.J., & Meier, K.V. (Eds.). (1995). *Philosophic inquiry in sport.* Champaign, IL: Human Kinetics.

Morgan, W.P. (1982). Psychological effects of exercise. *Behavioral Medicine Update, 4,* 25–30.

Morgan, W.P. (1985). Selected psychological factors limiting performance: A mental health model. In D.H. Clarke & H.M. Eckert (Eds.), *Limits of human performance* (pp. 70–80). Academy Papers, no. 18. Champaign, IL: Human Kinetics.

Morgan, W.P., & Goldston, S.E. (Eds.). (1987). *Exercise and mental health.* Washington, DC: Hemisphere.

Morris, D. (1994). *Bodytalk: The meaning of gestures.* New York: Crown Trade.

Morris, J.N, Heady, J.A., Raffle, P.A.B., Roberts, C.G., & Parks, J.W. (1953). Coronary heart disease and physical activity of work. *Lancet, 2,* 1111-1120.

Morrison, T., & Lacour, C.B. (1997). *Birth of a nation'hood: Gaze, script, and spectacle in the O.J. Simpson case.* New York: Pantheon Books.

Morrissey, M.C., Harman, E.A., & Johnson, M.J. (1995). Resistance training modes: Specificity and effectiveness. *Medicine and Science in Sports and Exercise, 27,* 648–660.

Murphy, W. (1995). *Healing the generations: A history of physical therapy and the American Physical Therapy Association.* Lyme, CT: Greenwich.

Nagel, T. (1987). *What does it all mean?: A very short introduction to philosophy.* Oxford, UK: Oxford University Press.

NASPE-NASSM Joint Task Force on Sport Management Curriculum and Accreditation. (1993). Standards for curriculum and voluntary accreditation of sport management education programs. *Journal of Sport Management, 7*(2), 159–170.

NASPE-NASSM Sport Management Review Council. (1993). Sport management program standards and review protocol. Available from the National Association for Sport and Physical Education, 1900 Association Drive, Reston, VA 22091.

National Association for Sport and Physical Education. (1995). *Moving into the future: National physical education standards.* New York: Mosby.

National Sporting Goods Association. (1996). *Research,* May, 1996.

NCAA slaps Tech even harder. (1998, August 4). *The Sporting News,* 2 pages. Available: http://www.sportingnews.com.

NCAA study shows extent of basketball's popularity. (1998, March 30). *The NCAA News, 35*(13), 1.

Nelson, R.C. (1970). Biomechanics of sport: An overview. In J.M. Cooper (Ed.), *Selected topics on biomechanics: Proceedings of the C.I.C. Symposium on Biomechanics* (pp. 31–37). Chicago: Athletic Institute.

Neuborne, E. (1996, October 18). Glass ceiling still in place. *USA Today,* p. 2B.

Neufeldt, V. (Ed.). (1988). *Webster's new world dictionary* (Third College Edition). New York: Simon & Schuster.

Neulinger, J., & Raps, C. (1972). Leisure attitude of an intellectual elite. *Journal of Leisure Research, 4,* 196–207.

Newell, K.M. (1990a). Physical activity, knowledge types, and degree programs. *Quest, 42,* 243–268.

Newell, K.M. (1990b). Kinesiology: The label for the study of physical activity in higher education. *Quest, 42,* 269–278.

Nideffer, R.M., & Sagal, M. (1998). Concentration and attention control training. In J.M. Williams (Ed.), *Applied sport psychology: Personal growth to peak performance* (3rd ed., pp. 296–315). Mountain View, CA: Mayfield.

Nigg, B.M. (1983). External force measurements with sports shoes and playing surfaces. In B.M. Nigg & B.J. Kerr (Eds.), *Biomechanical aspects of sport shoes and playing surfaces.* Calgary, AB: University Printing.

Nigg, B.M., & Bahlsen, H.A. (1988). Influence of heel flare and midsole construction on pronation, supination, and impact forces for heel-toe running. *International Journal of Sports Biomechanics, 4,* 205–219.

Nigg, B.M., Stacoff, A., & Segesser, B. (1984). Biomechanical effects of pain and sportshoe corrections. *Australian Journal of Science and Medicine in Sport, 16,* 10–16.

NIH Consensus Development Panel on Physical Activity and Cardiovascular Health. (1996). Physical activity and cardiovascular health. *Journal of the American Medical Association, 276,* 241-246.

Nixon, J.E., & Locke, L.F. (1973). Research on teaching in physical education. In M.W. Travers (Ed.), *Second handbook of research on teaching* (pp. 1210–1242). Chicago: Rand McNally.

No toughies. (1998, August 28). *USA Today,* p. 12C.

Nonprofit Expansion and Impact. (1996). International Health, Racquet and Sportsclub Association. Briefing paper. Boston, MA.

Novak, M. (1976). *The joy of sports.* New York: Basic Books.

Noyes, F.R., DeLucas, J.L., & Torvik, P.J. (1974). Biomechanics of anterior cruciate ligament failure. An analysis of strain rate sensitivity and mechanics of failure in primates. *Journal of Bone and Joint Surgery, 56A,* 236–242.

O'Connor, A.-M. (1999, April 29). Roar of soccer at coliseum. *Los Angeles Times,* pp. A1, A24–A25.

O'Connor, F.G., Kugler, J.P., & Oriscello, R.G. (1998). Sudden deaths in young athletes: Screening for the needle in a haystack. *American Family Physician, 57*(11), 2763–2774.

O'Donnell, M. (1989). Definition of health promotion. Part III: expanding the definition. *American Journal of Health Promotion, 3*(3), 5.

O'Donnell, M.P., & Harris, J.S. (1994). *Health promotion in the workplace.* Albany, NY: Delmar.

Ogilvie, B. (1973, November). The stimulus addicts. *The Physician and Sports Medicine,* 61–65.

Oriard, M. (1993). *Reading football: How the popular press created an American spectacle.* Chapel Hill, NC: University of North Carolina Press.

Orlick, T. (1986). *Psyching for sport: Mental training for athletes*. Champaign, IL: Human Kinetics.

Ornstein, R., & Sobel, D. (1989). *Healthy pleasures*. Menlo Park, CA: Addison-Wesley.

Osterhoudt, R.G. (1991). *The philosophy of sport: An overview*. Champaign, IL: Stipes.

O'Sullivan, M. (Ed.). (1994). High school physical education teachers: Their world of work [Monograph]. *Journal of Teaching in Physical Education, 13*, 323–441.

Owsley, C., Ball, K., Sloane, M.E., Roenker, D.L., & Bruni, J.R. (1991). Visual perceptual correlates of vehicle accidents in older drivers. *Psychology and Aging, 6*, 403–415.

Paffenbarger, R.S. (1994). 40 years of progress: Physical activity, health and fitness. In *40th anniversary lectures* (pp. 93-109). Indianapolis: American College of Sports Medicine.

Panzer, V.P. (1987). *Dynamic assessment of lower extremity loading characteristics during landing*. Unpublished doctoral dissertation, University of Oregon, Eugene.

Park and Rec Problem. (1996). International Health, Racquet and Sportsclub Association. Briefing paper. Boston, MA.

Park, R.J. (1980). The Research Quarterly and its antecedents. *Research Quarterly for Exercise and Sport, 51*(1), 1–22.

Park, R.J. (1981). The emergence of the academic discipline of physical education in the United States. In G.A. Brooks (Ed.), *Perspectives on the academic discipline of physical education* (pp. 20–45). Champaign, IL: Human Kinetics.

Park, R.J. (1987a). Edward M. Hartwell and physical training at The Johns Hopkins University, 1879-1890. *Journal of Sport History, 14*(1), 108–119.

Park, R.J. (1987b). Physiologists, physicians, and physical educators: Nineteenth century biology and exercise, *hygienic* and *educative*. *Journal of Sport History, 14*(1), 28–60.

Park, R.J. (1987c). Sport, gender and society in a transatlantic Victorian perspective. In J.A. Mangan & R.J. Park (Eds.), *From "fair sex" to feminism: Sport and the socialization of women in the industrial and post-industrial eras* (pp. 58–93). London: Frank Cass.

Park, R.J. (1989). The second 100 years: Or, can physical education become the renaissance field of the 21st century? *Quest, 41*(1), 2–27.

Park, R.J. (1992). Athletes and their training in Britain and America, 1800-1914. In J.W. Berryman & R.J. Park (Eds.), *Sport and exercise science: Essays in the history of sports medicine* (pp. 57–107). Urbana, IL: University of Illinois Press.

Park, R.J. (1995). History of research on physical activity and health: Selected topics, 1867 to the 1950's. *Quest, 47*, 274–287.

Parks, J.B., & Zanger, B.R.K. (1990). *Sport and fitness management: Career strategies and professional content*. Champaign, IL: Human Kinetics.

Pate, R.R. (1988). The evolving definition of fitness. *Quest, 40*, 174–179.

Pate, R.R., Pratt, M., Blair, S.N., Haskell, W.L., Macera, C.A., Bouchard, C., Buchner, D., Ettinger, W., Heath, G.W., King, A.C., Kriska, A., Leon, A.S., Marcus, B.H., Morris, J., Paffenbarger, R.S., Patrick, K., Pollock, M.L., Rippe, J.M., & Wilmore, J.H. (1995). Physical activity and public health: A recommendation from the Centers for Disease Control and the American College of Sports Medicine. *Journal of the American Medical Association, 273*, 402–407.

Paxson, F.L. (1917). The rise of sport. *Mississippi Valley Historical Review, 4*, 143–168.

Pearson, K.M. (1990). Methods of philosophic inquiry in physical activity. In J.R. Thomas & J.K. Nelson (Eds.), *Research methods in physical activity* (pp. 229–246). Champaign, IL: Human Kinetics.

Peiss, K. (1986). *Cheap amusements: Working women and leisure in turn-of-the-century New York*. Philadelphia: Temple University Press.

Perry, C. (1983). Blood doping and athletic competition. *International Journal of Applied Philosophy, 1*(3), 39–45.

Petrie, A. (1967). *Individuality in pain and suffering*. Chicago: University of Chicago Press.

Pew Health Professions Commission. (1995). *Critical challenges: Revitalizing the health professions for the twenty-first century. The third report of the Pew Health Professions Commission*. San Francisco: Pew Health Professions Commission.

Phenix, P.H. (1964). *Realms of meaning* (p. 171). New York: McGraw-Hill.

Phillips, P.C. (1908). Competitive athletics and scholarship. *Science, 27*, 547–553.

Pieper, J. (1962). *Leisure: The basis of culture*. New York: Pantheon Books.

Pitts, B.G., Fielding, L.W., & Miller, L.K. (1994). Industry segmentation theory and the sport industry: Developing a sport industry segment model. *Sport Marketing, 3*(4), 15-28.

Pitts, B.G., & Stotlar, D.K. (1996). *Fundamentals of sport marketing*. Morgantown, WV: Fitness Information Technology.

Pope, S.W. (1997). Introduction: American sport history—toward a new paradigm. In S.W. Pope (Ed.), *The new American sport history: Recent approaches and perspectives* (pp. 1–30). Urbana, IL: University of Illinois Press.

Posse, N. (1890). *The special kinesiology of educational gymnastics.* Boston: Lothrop, Lee & Shepard.

Poulton, E.C. (1957). On prediction in skilled movements. *Psychological Bulletin, 54,* 467–479.

Powers, S.K., & Howley, E.T. (1990). *Exercise physiology: Theory and application to fitness and performance.* Dubuque, IA: Wm. C. Brown.

Price, S.L. (1997, September 8). Spoiled sport. *Sports Illustrated,* p. 80.

Prochaska, J.O., & DiClemente, C.C. (1986). Toward a comprehensive model of change. In W. Miller & N. Heather (Eds.), *Treating addictive behaviors.* New York: Plenum Press.

Rader, B.G. (1990). *American Sports: From the age of folk games to the age of televised sports.* Englewood Cliffs, NJ: Prentice Hall.

Radin, E.L., Martin, R.B., Burr, D.B., Caterson, B., Boyd, R.D., & Goodwin, C. (1985). Mechanical factors influencing cartilage damage. In J.G. Peyron (Ed.), *Osteoarthritis: Current clinical and fundamental problems* (pp. 90–99). Paris, France: CIBA-Geigy.

Radin, E.L., Yang, K.H., Riegger, C., Kish, V.L., & O'Connor, J.J. (1991). Relationship between lower limb dynamics and knee joint pain. *Journal of Orthopedic Research, 9,* 398–405.

Raglin, J.S. (1990). Exercise and mental health. Beneficial and detrimental effects. *Sports Medicine, 9*(6), 323–329.

Ramlow, J., Kriska, A., & LaPorte, R. (1987). Physical activity in the population: The epidemiologic spectrum. *Research Quarterly for Exercise and Sport, 58*(2), 111–113.

Rarick, G.L. (1973). Stability and change in motor ability. In G.L. Rarick (Ed.), *Physical activity: Human growth and development* (pp. 201–224). New York: Academic Press.

Rasch, P.J. (1989). The history of kinesiology. In P.J. Rasch (Ed.), *Kinesiology and applied anatomy* (7th ed., pp. 3–17). Philadelphia: Lea & Febiger.

Ravizza, K. (1984). Qualities of the peak experience in sport. In J.M. Silva & R.S. Weinberg (Eds.), *Psychological foundations of sport* (pp. 452–462). Champaign, IL: Human Kinetics.

Regalado, S.O. (1992). Sport and community in California's Japanese American "Yamato Colony," 1930-1945. *Journal of Sport History, 19*(2), 130–143.

Reisberg, L. (1999, January 29). Survey of freshmen finds a decline in support for abortion and casual sex. *The Chronicle of Higher Education,* p. A47–A50.

Ricard, M.D., & Veatch, S. (1990). Comparison of impact forces in high and low impact aerobic dance movements. *International Journal of Sports Biomechanics, 6,* 67–77.

Rice, E.A., Hutchinson, J.L., & Lee, M. (1969). *A brief history of physical education.* New York: Ronald.

Riesman, D., & Denney, R. (1951). Football in America: A study in culture diffusion. *American Quarterly, 3,* 309–325.

Rink, J.E. (1983). The stability of teacher behavior over a unit of instruction. In T.J. Templin & J.K. Olson (Eds.), *Teaching in physical education* (pp. 318–328) Champaign, IL: Human Kinetics.

Rizzo, T.D., & Trigg, S.D. (1994). Getting a handle on wrist pain. *Physician and Sports Medicine, 22,* 41–42.

Robbins, S.E., & Waked, E.G. (1997). Hazard of deceptive advertising of athletic footwear. *British Journal of Sports Medicine, 31,* 299–303.

Roberton, M.A. (1982). Describing 'stages' within and across motor tasks. In J.A.S. Kelso & J.E. Clark (Eds.), *The development of movement control and coordination* (pp. 293–307). Chichester, UK: Wiley.

Roberton, M.A. (1984). Changing motor patterns during childhood. In J.R. Thomas (Ed.), *Motor development during childhood and adolescence* (p. 75). Edina, MN: Burgess International.

Roberts, M.R. (1976). *Fans.* Washington, DC: New Republic Book Company.

Rosaforte, T. (1997). *Tiger Woods: The making of a champion.* New York: St. Martin's Press.

Rosenbaum, D.A. (1991). *Human motor control.* San Diego: Academic Press.

Rosenshine, B., & Furst, N. (1973). The use of direct observation to study teaching. In M.W. Travers (Ed.), *Second handbook of research on teaching* (pp. 122–183). Chicago: Rand McNally.

Ross, H. (1996, March 10). Waiting for the call . . . . *Greensboro News and Record,* p. C1.

Rowland, T.W. (1989). Oxygen uptake and endurance fitness in children: A developmental perspective. *Pediatric Exercise Science, 1,* 313–328.

Rudolph, F. (1962). *The American college and university: A history.* New York: Vintage.

Sachs, M.L. (1981). Running addiction. In M.H. Sacks & M.L. Sachs (Eds.), *Psychology of running* (pp. 116–125), Champaign, IL: Human Kinetics.

Sage, G.H. (1997). Sport sociology. In J.D. Massengale & R.A. Swanson (Eds.), *History of exercise and sport science* (pp. 109–141). Champaign, IL: Human Kinetics.

Sage, G.H. (1998). *Power and ideology in American sport: A critical perspective.* Champaign, IL: Human Kinetics.

Sallis, J.F., Haskell, W.L., Fortnam, S.P., Vranizan, M.S., Taylor, C.B., & Solomon, D.S. (1986). Predictors of adoption and maintenance of physical activity in a community sample. *Preventive Medicine, 15,* 331–341.

Sallis, J.F., & Hovell, M.G. (1990). Determinants of exercise behavior. In K.B. Pandolf (Ed.), *Exercise and sport science reviews* (Vol. 18, pp. 307–330). Baltimore: Williams & Wilkins.

Salmoni, A.W., Schmidt, R.A., & Walter, C.B. (1984). Knowledge of results and motor learning: A review and critical reappraisal. *Psychological Bulletin, 95,* 355–386.

Salthouse, T.A. (1988). Cognitive aspects of motor functioning. In J.A. Joseph (Ed.), *Central determinants of age-related declines in motor function* (pp. 33–40). Annals of the New York Academy of Sciences, Vol. 515. New York: The Academy of Sciences.

Saltin, B. (1973). Metabolic fundamentals in exercise. *Medicine and Science in Sports, 5,* 137–146.

Santayana, G. (1894). Philosophy on the bleachers. *Harvard Monthly, 18,* 181–190.

Sarason, S. (1971). *The culture of the school and the problem of change.* Needham Heights, MA: Allyn & Bacon.

Sartre, J.-P. (1956). *Being and nothingness.* (H.E. Barnes, Trans.). New York: Philosophical Library. (Original work published 1943)

Satchell, M. (1997, July 23–28). Parks in peril. *U.S. News and World Report.*

Scanlan, T.K. (1986). Competitive stress in children. In M.R. Weiss & D. Gould (Eds.), *Sport for children and youth* (pp. 113–118). Champaign, IL: Human Kinetics.

Scanlan, T.K., Stein, G.L., & Ravizza, K. (1988). An in-depth study of former elite figure skaters: II. Sources of enjoyment. *Journal of Sport Psychology,* 65–83.

Schechner, R. (1988). Playing. *Play and Culture, 1,* 3–19.

Schempp, P.G. (1989). Apprenticeship-of-observation and the development of physical education teachers. In T.J. Templin & P.G. Schempp (Eds.), *Socialization into physical education: Learning to teach* (pp. 13–38). Indianapolis: Benchmark.

Schempp, P.G., & Choi, E. (1994). Research methodologies in sport pedagogy. *Sport Science Review, 3*(l), 41–55.

Schmidt, R.A. (1975). A schema theory of discrete motor skill learning. *Psychological Review, 82,* 225–260.

Schmidt, R.A. (1988). *Motor control and learning: A behavioral emphasis* (2nd ed.). Champaign, IL: Human Kinetics.

Schmidt, R.A. (1991). *Motor learning & performance: From principles to practice.* Champaign, IL: Human Kinetics.

Schoenfield, B. (1998, April 27–May 3). The stats that really matter now. *Street & Smith's Sports Business Journal, 1*(1), 1

Schon, D.A. (1995, November/December). Knowing in action: The new scholarship requires a new epistemology. *Change,* 27–34.

Schwartzman, H.B. (1978). *Transformations: The anthropology of children's play.* New York: Plenum Press.

Seefeldt, V., & Haubenstricker, J. (1982). Patterns, phases, or stages: An analytical model for the study of developmental movement. In J.A.S. Kelso & J.E. Clark (Eds.), *The development of movement control and co-ordination* (pp. 309–318). Chichester, UK: Wiley.

Selig, B. (1998, August 24). The commissioner speaks out. *The Sporting News, 222*(34), 10–13.

Shafer, R.J. (Ed.). (1980). *A guide to historical method.* Homewood, IL: Dorsey.

Sheehan, G. (1978). *Running and being: The total experience.* New York: Warner Books.

Sherrington, C.S. (1906). *The integrative action of the nervous system.* New Haven, CT: Yale University Press.

Shi, J., & Ewing, M. (1993). Definition of fun for youth soccer players. *Journal of Sport and Exercise Psychology* (NASPSPA Abstracts), *15,* S74.

Shields, D.L., & Bredemeier, B.J. (1995). *Character development in physical activity.* Champaign, IL: Human Kinetics.

Shinar, D., & Schieber, F. (1991). Visual requirements for safety and mobility of older drivers. *Human Factors, 33*(5), 507–519

Shorten, M. (1993). The energetics of running and running shoes. *Journal of Biomechanics, 26,* 41–52.

Shropshire, K.L. (1996). *In black and white: Race and sports in America.* New York: New York University Press.

Shulman, L.S. (1986). Those who understand: Knowledge growth in teaching. *Educational Researcher, 15*(2), 4–14.

Siedentop, D. (1980). *Physical education: Introductory analysis.* Dubuque, IA: W.C. Brown Co.

Siedentop, D. (1990). Commentary: The world according to Newell. *Quest, 42,* 315–322.

Siedentop, D. (1991). *Developing teaching skills in physical education* (3rd ed.). Mountain View, CA: Mayfield.

Siedentop, D. (1994). *Sport education.* Champaign, IL: Human Kinetics.

Siedentop, D. (1996). Valuing the physically active life: Contemporary and future directions. *Quest, 48,* 266–274.

Siedentop, D., Mand, C., & Taggart, A. (1986). *Physical education: Teaching and curriculum strategies for grades 5-12.* Mountain View, CA: Mayfield.

Silverman, S. (1990). Linear and curvilinear relationships between student practice and achievement in physical education. *Teaching and Teacher Education, 6,* 305–314.

Silverman, S. (1994). Communication and motor skill learning: What we learn from research in the gymnasium. *Quest, 46,* 345–355.

Silverman, S. (1996). How and why we do research. In S. Silverman & C. Ennis (Eds.), *Studying learning in physical education: Applying research to enhance instruction* (pp. 35–52). Champaign, IL: Human Kinetics.

Simon, J.A., & Martens, R. (1979). Children's anxiety in sport and non-sport evaluative activities. *Journal of Sport Psychology, 1,* 160–169.

Simon, R.L. (1991). *Fair play: Sports, values, and society.* Boulder, CO: Westview.

Simpson, K.J., & Pettit, M. (1997a). Jump distance of dance landings influencing internal joint forces: II. shear forces. *Medicine and Science in Sports and Exercise, 29,* 928–936.

Simpson, K.J., & Kanter, L. (1997b). Jump distance of dance landings influencing internal joint forces: I. axial forces. *Medicine and Science in Sports and Exercise, 29,* 916–927.

Singer, R.N. (1968). *Motor learning and human performance: An application to physical education skills.* New York: Macmillan.

Singh, N.A., Clements, K.M., & Fiatarone, M.A. (1997). A randomized controlled trial of progressive resistance training in depressed elders. *Journals of Gerontology, A: Biological Sciences and Medical Sciences, 52,* M27–M35.

Skarstrom, W. (1909). *Gymnastic kinesiology.* Springfield, MA: F.A. Bassette Co.

Sluder, M. (1998, June 8–14). Speedweek: Eight days in May. *Street & Smith's Sports Business Journal, 1*(7), 24.

Slusher, H.S. (1967). *Man, sport and existence: A critical analysis.* Philadelphia: Lea & Febiger.

Smith, J.K. (1979). *Athletic training: A developing profession.* Unpublished master's thesis, Brigham Young University, Provo, Utah.

Smith, R.A. (1972). *A social history of the bicycle: Its early life and times in America.* New York: American Heritage.

Smith, R.A. (1988). *Sports and freedom: The rise of big-time college athletics.* New York: Oxford University Press.

Smith, R.A., & Biddle, S.J.H. (1995). Psychological factors in the promotion of physical activity. In S.J.H. Biddle (Ed.), *European perspectives on exercise and sport psychology* (pp. 85–108). Champaign, IL: Human Kinetics.

Smith, R.E. (1998). A positive approach to sport performance enhancement: Principles of reinforcement and performance feedback. In J.M. Williams (Ed.), *Applied sport psychology: Personal growth to peak performance* (3rd ed., pp. 28–40). Mountain View, CA: Mayfield.

Smoll, F.L., & Schutz, R.W. (1980). Children's attitude toward physical activity: A longitudinal analysis. *Journal of Sport Psychology, 2,* 137–147.

Snel, J.G., Delleman, N.J., Heerkens, Y.F., & van Ingen Schenau, G.J. (1985). Shock-absorbing characteristics of running shoes during actual running. In D.A. Winter, R.W. Norman, R.P. Wells, K.C. Hayes, & A.E. Patla (Eds.), *Biomechanics IX-B* (pp. 133–137). Champaign, IL: Human Kinetics.

Snyder, E., & Spreitzer, E. (1976). Correlates of sport participation among adolescent girls. *Research Quarterly, 47,* 804–809.

Spino, M. (1971). Running as a spiritual experience. In J. Scott (Ed.), *The athletic revolution* (pp. 222–225). New York: The Free Press.

Spirduso, W.W., MacRae, H.H., MacRae, P.G., Prewitt, J., & Osborne, L. (1988). Exercise effects on aged motor function. In J.A. Joseph (Ed.), *Central determinants of age-related declines in motor function* (pp. 363–375). Annals of the New York Academy of Sciences, Vol. 515. New York: The Academy of Sciences.

Spirduso, W.W., & MacRae, P.G. (1990). Motor performance and aging. In J.E. Birren & K.W. Schaie (Eds.), *The handbook of psychology of aging* (3rd ed., pp. 184–197). San Diego: Academic Press.

Sports looking to change image. (1995, October). *Fitness Management,* p. 11.

Stacoff, A., Steger, J., Stussi, E., & Reinschmidt, C. (1996). Lateral stability in sideward cutting movements. *Medicine and Science in Sports and Exercise, 28*(3), 350–358.

Staley, S.C. (1937). The history of sport: A new course in the professional training curriculum. *Journal of Health, Physical Education and Recreation, 8,* 522–525, 570–572.

Starkes, J.L., & Allard, F. (Eds.). (1993). *Cognitive issues in motor expertise.* Amsterdam: Elsevier.

Stein, P.J., & Hoffman, S. (1978). Sports and male role strain. *Journal of Social Issues, 34,* 136–150.

Steinbreder, J. (1993, September 13). The owners. *Sports Illustrated*, pp. 64–72, 74, 76, 78, 80, 82, 84–86.

Steindler, A. (1935). *Mechanics of normal and pathological motion in man*. Springfield, IL: Charles C Thomas.

Steindler, A. (1942). What has biokinetics to offer to the physical educator? *Journal of Health and Physical Education, Nov.*, 507–509; 555–556.

Stelmach, G.E. (Ed.). (1976). *Motor control: Issues and trends*. New York: Academic Press.

Stelmach, G.E., & Nahom, A. (1992). Cognitive-motor abilities of the elderly driver. *Human Factors, 34*(1), 53–65.

Stephens, T. (1987). Secular trends in adult physical activity: Exercise boom or bust? *Research Quarterly for Exercise and Sport, 58*(2), 94–105.

Stephens, T., & Caspersen, C.J. (1994). The demography of physical activity. In C. Bouchard, R.J. Shephard, & T. Stephens (Eds.), *Physical activity, fitness, and health: International proceedings and consensus statement* (pp. 204–213). Champaign, IL: Human Kinetics.

Stevenson, S. (1997, September 7). Here's the painful truth: Injuries nagging juniors. *New York Times*, p. Y27.

Stone, G.P. (1969). Some meanings of American sport: An extended view. In G.S. Kenyon (Ed.), *Aspects of contemporary sport sociology: Proceedings of C.I.C. Symposium on the Sociology of Sport* (pp. 5–16). Chicago: Athletic Institute.

Strasburger, V.C. (1992). Children, adolescents, and television. *Pediatrics in Review, 13*, 144–151.

Stroot, S. (1996). Organizational socialization: Factors impacting beginning teachers. In S. Silverman & C. Ennis (Eds.), *Studying learning in physical education: Applying research to enhance instruction* (pp. 339–366). Champaign, IL: Human Kinetics.

Struna, N.L. (1996a). Historical research in physical activity. In J.R. Thomas & J.K. Nelson (Eds.), *Research methods in physical activity* (pp. 251–275). Champaign, IL: Human Kinetics.

Struna, N.L. (1996b). *People of prowess: Sport, leisure, and labor in early Anglo-America*. Urbana, IL: University of Illinois Press.

Struna, N.L. (1997). Sport history. In J.D. Massengale & R.A. Swanson (Eds.), *The history of exercise and sport science* (pp. 143–179). Champaign, IL: Human Kinetics.

Study shows another participation increase. (1998, April 27). *The NCAA News, 35*(17), 1.

Sugimoto, A. (1996, November). *The westernization of Japanese sport fans: The case of ouendan, a voluntary cheerleading group*. Paper presented at the annual conference of the North American Society for the Sociology of Sport, Birmingham, AL.

Suits, B. (1978). *The grasshopper: Games, life and utopia*. Toronto: University of Toronto Press.

Sutton-Smith, B. (1983). Play theory and cruel play of the nineteenth century. In F.E. Manning (Ed.), *The world of play: Proceedings of the 7th Annual Meeting of the Association for the Anthropological Study of Play* (pp. 103–110). West Point, NY: Leisure.

Sutton-Smith, B., & Kelly-Byrne, D. (1984). The idealization of play. In P.K. Smith (Ed.), *Play in animals and humans* (pp. 305–321). Oxford, UK: Blackwell.

Swanson, R.A., & Spears, B. (1995). *History of sport and physical education in the United States*. Madison, WI: Brown & Benchmark.

Taggart, A., & Alexander, K. (1993). Sport education in physical education. *Aussie Sport Action, 5*(l), 5–6, 8.

Taylor, W.C., Baranowski, T., & Sallis, J.F. (1994). Family determinants of childhood physical activity: A social-cognitive model. In R.K. Dishman (Ed.), *Advances in exercise adherence* (pp. 319–342). Champaign, IL: Human Kinetics.

Templin, T. (Ed.). (1983). Profiles of excellence: Fourteen outstanding secondary school physical educators. *Journal of Physical Education, Recreation and Dance, 54*(7), 15–36.

Templin, T., & Kollen, P. (1981). The aquatics learning lab. *Journal of Physical Education, Recreation and Dance, 52*, 15–16.

Terry, P. (1995). The efficacy of mood state profiling with elite performers: A review and synthesis. *The Sport Psychologist, 9*, 309–324.

Thelen, E., & Ulrich, B.D. (1991). Hidden skills: A dynamic systems analysis of treadmill stepping during the first year. *Monographs of the Society of Research in Child Development, 56* (1, Serial No. 223).

Thelen, E., Ulrich, D., & Jensen, J.L. (1990). The developmental origins of locomotion. In M.H. Woollacott & A. Shumway-Cook (Eds.), *Development of posture and gait: Across the lifespan*. Columbia, SC: University of South Carolina Press.

These are extremely serious charges. (1999, March 22). *Sports Illustrated*, 2 pages. Available: http://cnnsi.com/basketball/college/news.

Thomas, C.E. (1983). *Sport in a philosophic context*. Philadelphia: Lea & Febiger.

Thomas, J.R. (1980). Acquisition of motor skills: Information processing differences between children and adults. *Research Quarterly for Exercise and Sport, 51*, 158–173.

Thomas, J.R. (1997). History of motor behavior. In J.D. Massengale & R.A. Swanson (Eds.), *History of exercise and sport sciences*. Champaign, IL: Human Kinetics.

Thomas, J.R., & French, K.E. (1985). Gender differences across age in motor performance: A meta-analysis. *Psychological Bulletin, 98,* 260–282.

Thomas, J.R., & Thomas, K.T. (1989). What is motor development: Where does it belong? *Quest, 41,* 203–212.

Thomas, J.R., Thomas, K.T., & Gallagher, J.D. (1993). Developmental considerations in skill acquisition. In R.N. Singer, M. Murphey, & L.K. Tennant (Eds.), *Handbook of research on sport psychology* (pp. 73–105). New York: Macmillan.

Thomas, J.T. (1969). Keynote Address—The Army looks at biomechanics. In D. Bootzin & H.C. Muffley (Eds.), *Biomechanics*. New York: Plenum Press.

Thomas, K.T., & Thomas, J.R. (1994). Developing expertise in sport: The relation of knowledge to performance. *International Journal of Sport Psychology, 25,* 295–312.

Thompson, P.B. (1982). Privacy and the urinalysis testing of athletes. *Journal of the Philosophy of Sport, 9,* 60–65.

Thorndike, E.L. (1927). The law of effect. *American Journal of Psychology, 39,* 212–222.

Thorndike, E.L. (1932). *The fundamentals of learning.* New York: Teachers College Press.

Timson, B.F., Bowlin, B.K., Dudenhoeffer, G.A., & George, J.B. (1985). Fiber number, area, and composition of mouse soleus muscle following enlargement. *Journal of Applied Physiology, 58,* 619–624.

Tobin, G.A. (1974). The bicycle boom of the 1890's: The development of private transportation and the birth of the modern tourist. *Journal of Popular Culture, 7*(4), 838–849.

Todd, T. (1987). Anabolic steroids: The gremlins of sport. *Journal of Sport History, 14,* 87–107.

Tousignant, M. (1981). *A qualitative analysis of task structures in required physical education.* Unpublished doctoral dissertation, Ohio State University, Columbus.

Transportation Research Board. (1988). *Transportation in an aging society* (Vol. 1). Washington, DC: National Research Council.

Triplett, N. (1898). The dynamogenic factors in pacemaking and competition. *American Journal of Psychology, 9,* 507–553.

Tyson, L. (1996). Context of schools. In S. Silverman & C. Ennis (Eds.), *Studying learning in physical education: Applying research to enhance instruction* (pp. 55–80). Champaign, IL: Human Kinetics.

U.S. Bureau of the Census. (1961). *Statistical Abstract of the United States: 1961.* Washington, DC: U.S. Government Printing Office.

U.S. Bureau of the Census. (1966). *Statistical Abstract of the United States: 1966.* Washington, DC: U.S. Government Printing Office.

U.S. Bureau of the Census. (1996). *Statistical Abstract of the United States: 1996.* Washington, DC: U.S. Government Printing Office.

U.S. Department of Commerce. (1996a). Employment projections by occupation: 1996 to 2006. *Statistical abstract of the United States: 1996,* p. 420. Washington, DC: Government Printing Office.

U.S. Department of Commerce. (1996b). Participation in selected sports activities: 1994. *Statistical abstract of the United States 1996,* p. 259. Washington, DC: Government Printing Office.

U.S. Department of Commerce. (1996c). Participation in various arts activities: 1992. *Statistical abstract of the United States 1996,* p. 262. Washington, DC: Government Printing Office.

U.S. Department of Commerce. (1996d). Motion pictures and amusement and recreation services annual receipts: 1989 to 1984. *Statistical abstract of the United States: 1996,* p. 253. Washington, DC: Government Printing Office.

U.S. Department of Commerce. (1996e). Selected spectator sports: 1985 to 1994. *Statistical abstract of the United States 1996,* p. 257. Washington, DC: Government Printing Office.

U.S. Department of Commerce. (1996f). Anglers and hunters: 1991. *Statistical abstract of the United States 1996,* p. 256. Washington, DC: Government Printing Office.

U.S. Department of Commerce. (1996g). Household participation in lawn and garden activities: 1990-1994. *Statistical abstract of the United States 1996,* p. 255. Washington, DC: Government Printing Office.

U.S. Department of Commerce, Bureau of the Census. (1993). *Poverty in the United States: 1992.* (Series P60-185). Washington, DC: U.S. Government Printing Office.

U.S. Department of Commerce, Bureau of the Census. (1999, September 30). *Household income at record high; poverty declines in 1998* [Online], Available: http://www.census.gov/Press-Release/www/1999/cb99-188.html.

U.S. Department of Health and Human Services. (1990). *Healthy People 2000* (DHHS Publication No. [PHS] 91-50213). Hyattsville, MD: Public Health Service.

U.S. Department of Health and Human Services. (1995). *Healthy People 2000: Review 1994* (DHHS Pub No. [PHS] 95-1256-1). Hyattsville, MD: Public Health Service.

U.S. Department of Health and Human Services. (1996). *Physical activity and health: A report of the Surgeon General*. Atlanta, GA: U.S. Department of Health and Human Services, Centers for Disease Control and Prevention, National Center for Chronic Disease Prevention and Health Promotion; Pittsburgh: Superintendent of Documents.

Valiant, G. (1995). Perception of running shoe cushioning. In M. Shorten (Ed.), *Proceedings of the Second Symposium on Footwear Biomechanics, Abstract #16*.

Van Dalen, D.B., & Bennett, B.L. (1971). *A world history of physical education: Cultural, philosophical, comparative*. Englewood Cliffs, NJ: Prentice Hall.

van der Smissen, B. (1990). *Legal liability and risk management for public and private entitites*. Cincinnati, OH: Anderson Publishing Company.

Vealey, R.S. (1992). Personality and sport: A comprehensive view. In T.S. Horn (Ed.), *Advances in sport psychology* (2nd ed., pp. 25-59). Champaign, IL: Human Kinetics.

Vealey, R.S., & Greenleaf, C.A. (1998). Seeing is believing: Understanding and using imagery in sport. In J.M. Williams (Ed.), *Applied sport psychology: Personal growth to peak performance* (3rd ed., pp. 237–269). Mountain View, CA: Mayfield.

Veblen, T. (1967). *The theory of the leisure class*. New York: Viking. (Original work published 1899)

Vertinsky, P. (1990). *The eternally wounded woman: Women, doctors and exercise in the late nineteenth century*. Manchester, UK: Manchester University Press.

Viitasalo, J.T., & Kvist, M. (1983). Some biomechanical aspects of the foot and ankle in athletes with and without shin splints. *American Journal of Sports Medicine, 11*, 125–130.

Walling, M., & Martinek, T. (1995). Learned helplessness: A case study of a middle school student. *Journal of Teaching in Physical Education, 14*, 454–466.

Wankel, L.M. (1985). Personal and situational factors affecting exercise involvement: The importance of enjoyment. *Research Quarterly, 56*(3), 275–282.

Wankel, L.M. (1988). Exercise adherence and leisure activity: Patterns of involvement and interventions to facilitate regular activity. In R.K. Dishman (Ed.), *Exercise adherence: Its impact on public health* (pp. 369–396). Champaign, IL: Human Kinetics.

Wankel, L.M., & Krissel, P.S.J. (1985). Methodological considerations in youth sport motivation research: A comparison of open-ended and paired comparison approaches. *Journal of Sport Psychology, 7*, 65–74.

Weber, E. (1971). Gymnastics and sports in fin-de-siecle France: Opium of the classes? *American Historical Review, 76*(1), 70–98.

Weiss, M.R. (1991). Psychological skill development in children and adolescents. *The Sport Psychologist, 5*, 335–354.

Weiss, M.R., & Klint, K.A. (1987). "Show and tell" in the gymnasium: An investigation of developmental differences in modeling and verbal rehearsal of motor skills. *Research Quarterly for Exercise and Sport, 58*, 234–241.

Weiss, P. (1969). *Sport: A philosophic inquiry*. Carbondale, IL: Southern Illinois University Press.

Welch, P.D. (1996). *History of American physical education and sport*. Springfield, IL: Charles C Thomas.

Wells, K.F. (1950). *Kinesiology*. Philadelphia: W.B. Saunders.

Whorton, J.C. (1982). *Crusaders for fitness: The history of American health reformers*. Princeton, NJ: Princeton University Press.

Wickstrom, R. (1970). *Fundamental movement patterns*. Philadelphia: Lea & Febiger.

Widule, C.J. (1980). The contributions of Ruth B. Glassow to pedagogical kinesiology. In J.M. Cooper & B. Haven (Eds.), *Proceedings of the Biomechanics Symposium* (pp. 101–118). Bloomington, IN: Indiana State Board of Health.

Wiggins, D.K. (1980). The play of slave children in the plantation communities of the old south, 1820-1860. *Journal of Sport History, 7*(2), 21–39.

Wild, M. (1937). *The behavior pattern of throwing and some observations concerning its course of development in children*. Unpublished doctoral dissertation, University of Wisconsin-Madison.

Wild, M. (1938). The behavior pattern of throwing and some observations concerning its course of development in children. *Research Quarterly, 9*, 20–24.

Willett, W.C., Manson, J.E., Stampler, M.J., Colditz, G.A., Rosner, B., Speizer, F.E., & Hennekena, C.H. (1995). Weight, weight change, and coronary disease in women. *Journal of the American Medical Association, 273*, 461–465.

Williams, A.F., & Carsten, O.L. (1989). Driver age and crash involvement. *American Journal of Public Health, 79*, 326–327.

Williams, J.F. (1964). *The principles of physical education* (8th ed.). Philadelphia: Lea & Febiger. (Original work published 1927)

Williams, J.M., & Straub, W.F. (1998). Sport psychology: Past, present, future. In J.M. Williams (Ed.), *Applied sport psychology: Personal growth to peak performance* (3rd ed., pp. 1–12). Mountain View, CA: Mayfield.

Williams, K.R. (1993). Biomechanics of distance running. In M.D. Grabiner (Ed.), *Current issues in biomechanics* (pp. 3–32). Champaign, IL: Human Kinetics.

Willis, J.D., & Campbell, L.F. (1992) *Exercise psychology*. Champaign, IL: Human Kinetics.

Willis, P. (1982). Women in sport in ideology. In J. Hargreaves (Ed.), *Sport, culture and ideology* (pp. 117–135). London: Routledge & Kegan Paul.

Wilmore, J.H., & Costill, D.L. (1994). *Physiology of sport and exercise*. Champaign, IL: Human Kinetics.

Wilson, B., & Sparks, R. (1996). "It's gotta be the shoes": Youth, race, and sneaker commercials. *Sociology of Sport Journal, 13*, 398–427.

Wilson, W. (1977). Social discontent and the growth of wilderness sport in America: 1965-1974. *Quest, 27*, 54–60.

Winograd, C.H., Lemsky, C.M., Nevitt, M.C., Nordstrom, T.M., Stewart, A.L., Miller, C.J., & Bloch, D.A. (1994). Development of a physical performance and mobility examination. *Journal of Geriatrics Society, 42*(7), 743–749.

Winter, D.A. (1985). *Biomechanics and motor control of human gait*. Waterloo: ON: University of Waterloo Press.

Winter, D.A. (1991). *The biomechanics and motor control of human gait: Normal, elderly, and pathological* (2nd ed.). Waterloo, ON: University of Waterloo Press.

Woodworth, R.S. (1899). The accuracy of voluntary movement. *Psychological Review, 3* (Suppl. 2).

Yanker, G. (1983). *The complete book of exercise walking*. Chicago: Contemporary Books.

Young, M.C. (Ed.). (1997). *The Guinness book of world records*. New York: Guinness Media.

Zaichowsky, L.B. (1975). Attitudinal differences in two types of physical education programs. *Research Quarterly, 46*, 364–370.

Zajonc, R.B. (1965). Social facilitation. *Science, 149*, 269–274.

Zakarian, J.M., Hovell, M.F., Hofstetter, C.R., Sallis, J.F., & Keating, K.J. (1994). Correlates of vigorous exercise in a predominately low SES and minority high school population. *Preventive Medicine, 23*, 314–321.

Zeigler, E.F. (1964). *Philosophical foundations for physical, health, and recreation education*. Englewood Cliffs, NJ: Prentice Hall.

Zillman, D., Bryant, J., & Sapolsky, B.S. (1979). The enjoyment of watching sport contests. In J.H. Goldstein (Ed.), *Sports, games and play: Social and psychological viewpoints* (pp. 297–336). Hillsdale, NJ: Lawrence Erlbaum.

Zillman, D., & Cantor, J.R. (1976). A disposition theory of humor and mirth. In T. Chapman & H. Foot (Eds.), *Humor and laughter: Theory, research, and applications*. London: Wiley.

Zwiren, L.D. (1989). Anaerobic and aerobic capacities of children. *Pediatric Exercise Science, 1*, 31–44.

Index

About the Contributors

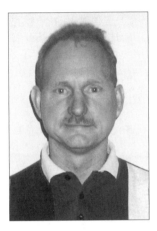

Greg Comfort, EdD, is an assistant professor and serves as coordinator of the undergraduate program in sport administration. Dr. Comfort joined the sport administration team at Wichita State University after teaching courses in sport sociology, sport history, sport law, sport psychology, sport facility and design, and serving as coordinator for field experiences, interim internships and practica for 11 years at Liberty University. Dr. Comfort's previous experience as a coach and athletic director allow him to bring a practitioner's approach to the teaching of leadership theory and organizational behavior in the classroom and in the sport administration program.

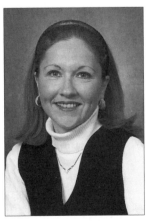

Kim C. Graber, EdD, is an assistant professor in the department of kinesiology at the University of Illinois at Champaign/Urbana. She received her BS at the University of Iowa, her MA at Teachers College Columbia University, and her EdD at the University of Massachusetts at Amherst. Her research interests include teacher socialization, teacher education, faculty micropolitics, and research methods. She has published numerous articles in a variety of peer-refereed journals, has written several book chapters, and currently is writing a textbook. She is a member of the editorial board of the *Journal of Teaching in Physical Education* and is a regular reviewer for other jour-

nals. She received recognition for Outstanding Scholarship in Teacher Education from the Association of Colleges and Schools of Education in State Universities and Land Grant Colleges and Affiliated Private Universities. She also has served as chair of the Curriculum and Instruction Academy, National Association for Sport and Physical Education.

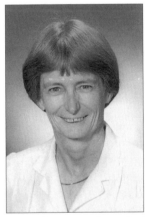

Emily M. Haymes, PhD, is a professor of the department of nutrition, food and exercise science at Florida State University. She received her BA from Drury College in 1961, her MS from Florida State University in 1962, and her PhD from Pennsylvania State University in 1973. She coauthored a book on *The Environment and Performance* with Christine Wells. Her papers have been published in several journals, and she is frequently invited to speak at conferences and has presented more than 80 papers. Dr. Haymes received a University Teaching Award in 1986 and a Teaching Incentive Award in 1995 from Florida State University, and the Citation Award from the American College of Sports Medicine in 1996. She is a member of the editorial boards of *Medicine and Science in Sports and Exercise, Sports Medicine,* and *International Journal of Sport Nutrition* and a member of the Scientific and Medical Advisory Board of Life Fitness.

Jeremy Howell, PhD, is an assistant professor of exercise and sport science at the University of San Francisco. He received his PhD from the University of Illinois at Champaign/Urbana. His research interests focus on transformations in the cultural industries associated with the production, promotion, and consumption of sports and fitness events, goods, and experiences. He has ex-

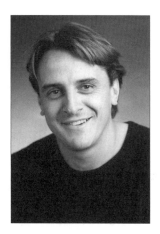

tensive health and fitness industry experience and serves on the advisory boards of a number of Bay Area health, fitness, and technology corporations. He is also on the editorial board of the *Journal of Sport & Social Issues*.

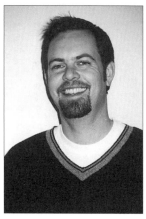

James Kallusky, EdD, is an assistant professor of teacher education for the department of kinesiology and physical education and executive director for Youth Agency Administration Studies at California State University, Los Angeles. He is cofounder of the Urban Youth Leader Project, a national partnership that focuses on physical activity programs for underserved youth. From university students and teachers to directors of national and community agencies, James' work is best described as "youth development." He received his BA degree (1989) and MA degree (1991) in physical education at California State University, Chico. His doctorate degree was completed in 1997 at the University of Northern Colorado.

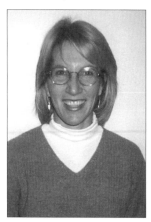

Lori K. Miller, EdD, is a professor in sport administration at Wichita State University. She also serves as Wichita State University's chair for the department of kinesiology and sport studies. MIller has written 3 textbooks, 6 book chapters, and 38 articles. She has also been involved in over 40 sport management-related presentations at international, national,

state, and local levels. She has served on the executive board for both the North American Association of Sport Management and the Society for the Study of Legal Aspects in Sport and Physical Activity. Miller has received research awards from both the University of Louisville and Wichita State University, and she received a Teacher of the Year award in 1996 from the University of Louisville School of Education. Miller has a masters in business administration from the University of Louisville and a masters in education in physical education from Texas A&M University. Lori earned her doctor of education degree from Texas A&M–Commerce.

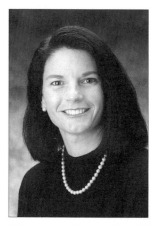

Sandra L. Minor, MS, is an assistant professor in the department of public health at Southern Connecticut State University. She was previously the director of fitness operations for Western Athletic Clubs in San Francisco. Sandy is a PhD candidate in health education at Texas Woman's University. She has her masters of science degree in exercise physiology and fitness management from the University of Oregon and is certified as a Health/Fitness Director by the American College of Sports Medicine. In addition, she has served on the certification and education subcommittee for the American College of Sports Medicine and was selected as the 1991 IHRSA/CYBEX Fitness Director of the Year.

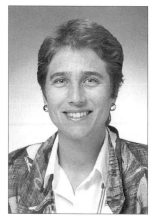

Kathy Simpson, PhD, received her doctorate in biomechanics from the University of Oregon. She is currently an associate professor in the department of exercise science at the University of Georgia. Her research focuses on factors influencing force loading on the lower extremity during high impact landings and on running mechanics of runners with lower extremity amputations. Dr. Simpson is a fellow of the Research Consortium of the Alliance of American Alliance for Health, Physical Education, Recreation and Dance (AAHPERD) and of the American College of Sports Medicine (ACSM). She has served as chair of the Biomechanics Academy of AAHPERD and is currently serving as a member of the executive board of the Biomechanics Interest Group of ACSM and as a section editor for *Research Quarterly for Exercise and Sport*.

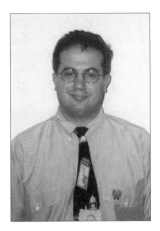

Chad Starkey, PhD, ATC, is an associate professor and athletic training program director at Northeastern University in Boston, MA and serves as the chair of the National Athletic Trainers' Association Education Council. Dr. Starkey has published several textbooks on orthopedic injury evaluation and therapeutic modalities, and he is a consultant to the National Basketball Association to study the rate of injury and illness. Dr. Starkey was recently appointed to the editorial board of the *Journal of Sport Rehabilitation*.

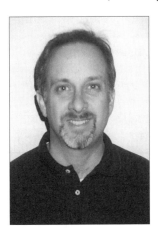

G. Clayton Stoldt, EdD, is an assistant professor and serves as coordinator of the graduate program in sport administration. Prior to joining the Wichita State University faculty, Dr. Stoldt spent 10 years working in college athletics at Oklahoma City University, serving as a sports information director, a play-by-play broadcaster, and development officer. He has also served as an adjunct instructor at the University of Oklahoma and Oklahoma City University. Dr. Stoldt's teaching background coupled with his practical sport administration experience are genuine assets as he brings expertise to his classes in sport marketing, sport public relations, and sport sociology.

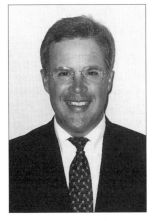

Thomas J. Templin, PhD, is a professor and head of the department of health, kinesiology, and leisure studies at Purdue University, West Lafayette, Indiana. He is a graduate of Indiana University (BS, 1972; MS, 1975) and the University of Michigan (PhD, 1978). Templin was appointed at Purdue in 1977 in sport pedagogy where he began his research on teacher socialization and the lives and careers of physical education teachers. He has written numerous articles and book chapters on these topics primarily with his pedagogy colleagues, Paul Schempp and Andrew Sparkes. He has coedited two books and coauthored, *A Reflective Approach to Teaching Physical Education* with Donald Hellison. Templin was appointed as department head in 1996 and has written and presented on administration and leadership within HKLS in various forums. He has served on various committees within AAHPERD and was coeditor of the *Journal of Teaching in Physical Education* from 1983-1988.

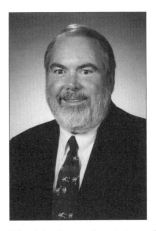

Jerry R. Thomas, EdD, has taught research methods and children's motor development for more than 30 years, most recently as a professor and chair of the department of health and human performance at Iowa State University. Previously, Dr. Thomas has taught as a professor at Florida State, Louisiana State, and Arizona State Universities. Dr. Thomas has written more than 125 published papers, including many on children's motor skills. He is past president of the American Academy of Kinesiology and Physical Education and NASPSPA. In addition, his scholarly work in physical activity has earned him the titles of C.H. McCloy Lecturer for children's control, learning, and performance of motor skills; Alliance Scholar for the American Alliance for

Health, Physical Education, Recreation and Dance (AAHPERD); and Southern District AHPERD Scholar.

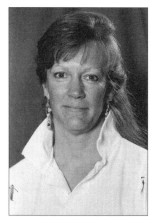

Katherine Thomas Thomas, PhD, is an associate professor of health and human performance at Iowa State University, where she teaches a variety of teacher education and motor development courses. Dr. Thomas previously has taught at Arizona State University, Southeastern Louisiana University, and Southern University, Baton Rouge. Her research focuses primarily on skill acquisition in sport and exercise and the relation of physical activity to health. She has numerous publications on physical activity and health, and skill acquisition. She has external grant funding in excess of $800,000 to study physical activity and is the physical activity consultant for the USDA's Team Nutrition. Dr. Thomas is author and coauthor of five textbooks. Dr. Thomas is a member of the American Alliance for Health, Physical Education, Recreation and Dance (AAHPERD) and the North American Society for the Psychology of Sport and Physical Activity. She received her doctorate in physical education from Louisiana State University in 1981.

Robin S. Vealey, PhD, is a professor in the department of physical education, health, and sport studies at Miami University in Ohio. She teaches courses in sport psychology, coaching effectiveness, and children in sport. She has received the Distinguished Scholar Award from the Australian Psychological Society, is listed in the U.S. Olympic Committee Sport Psychology Registry,

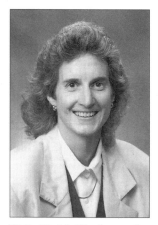

served as editor of the journal *The Sport Psychologist*, and is recognized as a Fellow, Certified Consultant, and Past President of the Association for the Advancement of Applied Sport Psychology (AAASP). Dr. Vealey has worked as a sport psychology consultant for the U.S. Ski Team, U.S. Field Hockey, elite golfers, and numerous college and high school athletes. A former collegiate basketball player and coach, she now enjoys the mental challenge of golf.

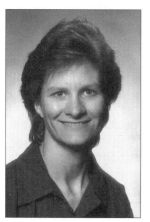

Lavon Williams, PhD, received her doctorate in exercise and sport science from the University of North Carolina at Greensboro. She is currently an assistant professor in the department of kinesiology and physical education at Northern Illinois University. Her research focuses on motivational processes in physical activity contexts. Specifically, she has examined how individuals' thoughts about ability impact their perceptions of the physical activity environment. Dr. Williams is a fellow of the research consortium of the American Alliance for Health, Physical Education, Recreation and Dance and is a member of the Association for the Advancement of Sport Psychology (AAASP) social psychology committee. She also serves on the editorial board for the *AAASP Newsletter* and for the *Research Quarterly for Exercise and Sport*.

About the Editors

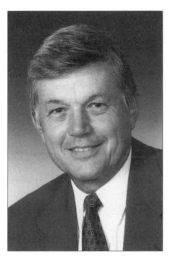

Shirl J. Hoffman, EdD, is a professor of exercise and sport science at the University of North Carolina at Greensboro where he was head of the department for ten years. He has served at all levels of higher education, from research university to liberal arts college. Hoffman has published extensively on a variety of topics, including sport philosophy and ethics, sport sociology, and motor learning and performance. He also has been a frequent commentator on problems in kinesiology and higher education. He is former editor of *Quest* and associate editor of the *Chronicle for Physical Education in Higher Education.*

Hoffman is a member of the American Academy of Kinesiology and Physical Education and the National Association for Physical Education in Higher Education. He gave the Dudley Sargent Lecture to the National Association for Physical Education in Higher Education in 1998.

Hoffman and his wife, Claude, reside in Greensboro, North Carolina. He enjoys walking, swimming, golf, and traveling.

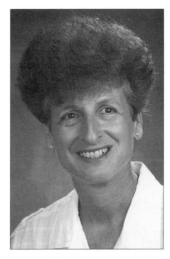

Janet C. Harris, PhD, is professor and chair of the department of kinesiology and physical education at California State University, Los Angeles. Harris was editor of *Quest* from 1989 to 1991 and served as president of the AAPHERD Research Consortium from 1992 to 1993. Two of her most noted publications include "Broadening Horizons: Interpretive Cultural Research, Hermeneutics, and Scholarly Inquiry in Physical Education" and "Using Kinesiology: A Comparison of Applied Veins in the Subdisciplines," both of which appeared in *Quest.*

Harris is a fellow of the American Academy of Kinesiology and Physical Education and a member of the National Association for Physical Education in Higher Education. She served as the Amy Morris Homens Lecturer for the National Association for Physical Education in Higher Education in 1992.

Harris received her PhD from the University of California, Berkeley. She resides in Los Angeles and enjoys urban hiking, working out, and people-watching.